Drugs in psychiatric practice

Drugs in psychiatric practice

Edited by

Peter J. Tyrer, MD, MRCP, DPM, FRCPsych

Consultant Psychiatrist, Mapperley Hospital, Nottingham

Butterworths
London · Boston · Durban · Singapore · Sydney · Toronto · Wellington

First published 1982

© **Butterworths & Co (Publishers) Ltd. 1982**

British Library Cataloguing in Publication Data

Drugs in psychiatric practice.
  1. Psychopharmacology
  I. Tyrer, Peter J.
  616.89′18   RC350.C54
ISBN 0–407–00212–X

Filmset by Northumberland Press Ltd, Gateshead, Tyne and Wear
Printed by Cambridge University Press, Cambridge

Preface

There are many books on psychotropic drugs and the authors of each new volume are often hard pressed to justify their addition to the pile. This book offers no dramatic claims for novelty or erudition; it is only intended to be a useful aid to the prescriber and the student. Drug treatment in psychiatry is now a subject in which the links between basic science and clinical practice are beginning to be unravelled, so it is now possible to explain how and why drugs act in a certain way instead of merely giving instructions on what to do. The reader is therefore kept abreast of recent advances in pharmacology in each of the chapters so that he can understand the basis for prescribing habits. The book is not a pharmacopoeia and drug dosage is only mentioned when certain clinical effects are highly dependent on dosage. When dosages are not described the recommended range given in the *British National Formulary* (1982) can be implied.

There are a bewildering number of drug names used throughout the world. To make reference easier a separate drug index gives the approved and proprietary names of the compounds used in psychiatry. An index of the clinically important drug interactions is also included.

I am very grateful to the contributors for helping to give the book a coherence it would not otherwise possess and to Butterworths for encouragement throughout its preparation. Many others have given unstinting help. I thank in particular my wife, Ann, Marlene Whitaker and Linda Humphreys for secretarial assistance, Dr Bridget Jack and Charles Marsden for giving expert advice, Dr Angus Mackay for his collaboration at the initial planning stage and Fiona Norman and Celia Timson for their willing assistance on pharmaceutical issues, for compiling the drug index and checking structural formulae. I should be grateful to know of any errors that have escaped our scrutiny so that they can be corrected.

P.J.T.
Nottingham

Reference

British National Formulary No. 3 (1982), London: British Medical Association and The Pharmaceutical Press.

Contributors

Thomas R. E. Barnes, MB, MRCPsych,
Wellcome Research Fellow, Psychiatric Research Unit, University of Cambridge Clinical School, Addenbrooke's Hospital, Trumpington Street, Cambridge.

Jean Phillipe Boulenger, MD, Charge de Recherché INSERM,
Institute of Psychiatry, De Crespigny Park, London.

Paul K. Bridges, MD, PhD, FRCPsych,
Senior Lecturer in Psychiatry, Guy's Hospital Medical School, London.

Patricia Casey, MB, MRCPsych,
Research Fellow and Honorary Senior Registrar, Mapperley Hospital, Nottingham.

S. Checkley, BA, BM, BCH, MRCP, MRCPsych,
Consultant Psychiatrist, The Maudsley Hospital, Denmark Hill, London.

Peter Jenner, MD, MRCP,
Senior Lecturer, University Department of Neurology, Institute of Psychiatry and King's College Hospital Medical School, Denmark Hill, London.

Malcolm Lader, DSc, PhD, MD, FRCPsych,
Professor of Psychopharmacology, Institute of Psychiatry, De Crespigny Park, London.

Angus V. P. Mackay, MA, BSc, PhD, MB, ChB, MRCPsych,
Physician Superintendent, Argyll and Bute Hospital, Lochgilphead, Argyll, Scotland and MacKintosh Lecturer in Psychological Medicine, University of Glasgow.

Philip C. McLean, MB, DPM, MRCPsych,
Director Regional Addiction Unit, Mapperley Hospital, Nottingham.

Charles A. Marsden, PhD,
Wellcome Senior Lecturer, Department of Physiology and Pharmacology, University of Nottingham.

C. David Marsden, MSc, FRCP, MRCPsych,
Professor of Neurology, Institute of Psychiatry, and King's College Hospital Medical School, Denmark Hill, London.

Richard H. Mindham, MD, MRCP, FRCPsych,
Professor of Psychiatry, University of Leeds, Nuffield House, Leeds.

David M. Shaw, PhD, FRCP, FRCPsych,
Member of the External Scientific Staff of the Medical Research Council, Whitchurch Hospital, Cardiff.

Anthony Philip Thorley, MB, MRCP(Lond), MRCPsych,
Director Regional North Addiction and Drug Dependency Unit, St Nicholas Hospital, Gosforth, Newcastle upon Tyne.
Carol Trotter, MB, ChB, MRCPsych,
Consultant Psychiatrist for the Elderly, St James Hospital, Portsmouth.
Peter J. Tyrer, MD, MRCP, FRCPsych,
Consultant Psychiatrist, Mapperley Hospital, Nottingham.
Stephen Tyrer, MB, BChir, MRCPsych,
Wellcome Senior Lecturer in Psychiatry, Research Unit in Psychological Medicine, University of Newcastle upon Tyne.

Contents

Introduction

All doctors in clinical practice use psychotropic drugs and psychiatrists use them almost exclusively. The science of their properties, psychopharmacology, has developed dramatically in the past 20 years and new findings with implications for clinical practice are reported many times a year. Indeed, such is the pace of change that by the time this book is published it will already be out of date. This in itself poses problems for the practitioner, for those using the drugs are not in the same position as colleagues in other medical disciplines. Drug treatment is only one of the therapeutic modes in which psychiatrists have to operate, for they are also expected to have a sound working knowledge of the psychotherapies, learning theory and social psychiatry, as well as neurology and general medicine. Small wonder that the late Henry Miller suggested that a psychiatrist should 'not only first be a physician but ideally a superlative physician' (Miller, 1967) with an inspiring breadth of knowledge that dwarfed his colleagues.

In practice few can aspire to this level of competence. Yet the general practitioner or psychiatrist is expected to use all the treatments at his disposal from the standpoint of informed knowledge rather than from following the ritual of the cookbook. Proper use of drugs must involve some knowledge of their pharmacology; this may be unpalatable for those who turn to psychiatry to escape from scientific medicine, but it is inescapable. At the same time this knowledge has to be selective, for pharmacology is a discipline that even exceeds psychiatry in its production of words, and only a fraction of this is relevant to the clinician. For this reason all standard texts on drug treatment in psychiatry devote a substantial part to the principles of pharmacology and the mode of action of drugs, and many involve pharmacologists as authors (Shepherd, Lader and Rodnight, 1968; Hollister, 1973; Simpson, 1976; Silverstone and Turner, 1978; Van Praag, 1978; Barchas et al., 1978; Lader, 1980).

This book is for the clinician, whether he be general practitioner, hospital physician or psychiatrist, and is designed so that it can be used as both a general text and an easy source of reference. The problems of classification, nomenclature and evaluation of drugs are described in the early chapters and the essential of pharmacokinetics, a rapidly expanding aspect of psychopharmacology, given by Dr Boulenger and Professor Lader. The chapters between 4 and 12 all follow a similar pattern. Each major drug group is described in terms of its chemistry, pharmacology and toxicology, pharmacokinetics, clinical use and adverse effects. Structural formulae of the drugs are also given; in each case the basic formula is given although the drug may be marketed as

1

one of its salts. The amount of space given to each of these aspects varies greatly, but throughout the aim is to give the reader a rounded view that should help to rationalize the use of these drugs in practice. Comparisons between drugs of the same or differing groups are also discussed so that the practitioner has some guidelines affecting his choice of drug. Some overlap between the chapters has naturally followed from these comparisons but is kept to a minimum. In an ideal world, a range of comparative studies assessing the value of the drug in competition with other non-pharmacological treatments would be of greatest help but very few have been carried out to date. Nevertheless, both the comparisons between drugs and other treatment and the value of them in combination are being used increasingly and, where adequate comparative data exist they are given. The last chapters of the book are concerned with the special issues of drugs in child psychiatry and psychogeriatrics, and with the use of drugs in the treatment of eating and sexual disorders.

The main clinical features of psychiatric disorder are not described separately although to some extent these become apparent in discussing the indications for drug treatment. The reader, however, is expected to understand the terminology of clinical psychiatry and, if new to the subject, may need to have available a general textbook on the subject (e.g. Klein *et al.*, 1980) to understand some of the difficulties involved in relating clinical diagnosis to drug effects.

Because so many judgements in psychiatric treatment are personal and idiosyncratic it is important to give references when discussing issues that are contentious or in a state of flux. This has necessarily led to a substantial number of references but this should help those who wish to extend their inquiries. Some bias is bound to be present in a subject that is still in its infancy but this can be reduced by giving authority to statements that would otherwise be unsupported.

The final choice of whether to use drug treatment and which individual drug to prescribe has to be a personal one. To help this decision comparisons are made between the different treatments towards the end of each chapter. Here the contributors often give their choice of drug and their justification for it. This should aid the clinician in making his own choice but is not a dictum. There is sufficient open discussion of the issues in the body of the text to enable him to come to an informed decision, one that correctly perceives the balance of advantage and risk, and which lies at the heart of good prescribing.

References

BARCHAS, J. D., BERGER, P., CIARANELLO, R. D. and ELLIOTT, G. R. *Psychopharmacology: From Theory to Practice*, Oxford University Press, New York (1978)
HOLLISTER, L. E. *Clinical Use of Psychotherapeutic Drugs*, Charles C. Thomas, Springfield, Illinois (1973)
KLEIN, D. F., GITTELMAN, R., QUITKIN, F. and RIFKIN, A. *Diagnosis and Drug Treatment of Psychiatric Disorders: Adults and Children*, 2nd edn, Williams and Wilkins, Baltimore (1980)
LADER, M. *Introduction to Psychopharmacology*, Upjohn, Michigan (1980)
MILLER, H. Depression, *British Medical Journal* 1, 257–262 (1967)
SHEPHERD, M., LADER, M. and RODNIGHT, R. *Clinical Psychopharmacology*, English Universities Press, London (1968)
SILVERSTONE, T. and TURNER, P. *Drug Treatment in Psychiatry*, 2nd edn, Routledge and Kegan Paul, London (1978)
SIMPSON, L. L. (Ed.). *Drug Treatment and Mental Disorders*, Raven Press, New York (1976)
VAN PRAAG, H. *Psychotropic Drugs: A Guide for the Practitioner*, MacMillan, London (1978)

Chapter 1

Classification of psychotropic drugs

P. J. Tyrer and C. A. Marsden

Putting things into order is one of the activities that correlates with intelligence, and classification is the science of order. An outsider looking at psychopharmacology might be excused the conclusion that it was an activity carried out by the less able, because the classification of psychotropic drugs is a classification only in name. It resembles the description of plants and animals in pre-Linnaean days, lacking any coherent theme and varying greatly from country to country. Perhaps we await a new Linnaeus to show us the key to order in psychopharmacology but there are no indications at present how this could be achieved.

What is a psychotropic drug?

Any drug that influences mental functioning can be regarded as a psychotropic drug. If this is taken literally most drugs in medicine are psychotropic ones, because so many of the unwanted or secondary effects of drugs are related to the central nervous system. There is considerable literature on the psychiatric side effects of medical drugs (Shader, 1972) and many examples are given in later chapters, but it would be very confusing to have, for example, digoxin, hypotensive drugs and atropine all classified as psychotropic agents when their main clinical use is outside psychiatry. Most classifications make a pragmatic distinction on the basis of the major clinical use of the drugs, so a psychotropic drug is one whose major effects are on mental function. These effects may be central or peripheral and a direct action on the central nervous system is not a *sine qua non* of their psychotropic activity.

Types of classification

Chemical

The chemistry of drugs is related to their pharmacological properties and the relevance of chemistry in classification is clear from the naming of drug groups such as the tricyclic antidepressants, benzodiazepines and hydrazine monoamine oxidase inhibitors. The chemist involved in the synthesis of new drugs knows that certain molecular configurations are likely to have predictable pharmacological activity and, indeed, whenever a major class of psychotropic drugs is discovered a host of new compounds is synthesized immediately afterwards, which has a similar range of pharmacological activity.

Unfortunately the chemist cannot synthesize an entirely new compound and have much idea about its pharmacological spectrum of activity. There are no rules that he can follow to ensure the effects that he wants and it is significant that only about 0.1 per cent of all compounds synthesized and screened in pharmacology ever get to testing in man. It is also ironic that the psychotropic drug with the simplest structure, the inorganic compound lithium carbonate, has the most complex clinical effects. For these reasons no serious chemical classification of psychotropic drugs has ever been made. Nevertheless, the structural formulae of the important psychotropic drugs are given in this book because they can be instructive in illustrating differences and similarities in the pharmacological actions of drugs.

Pharmacology

The important clinical actions of a drug follow from its pharmacological activity. The most logical classification of psychotropic drugs is one that concentrates on their pharmacological properties. This is sometimes possible with drugs that have their major actions on peripheral organs, such as the heart and kidney, because their activities in animals are clearly related to those in man. The psychotropic drugs are different; animal models of psychiatric disorder are difficult to construct (Chapter 3), and so much depends on clinical testing in man. The record of advances in treatment to date has not been one that supports the pharmacological classification of drugs. Most progress has been made by fortuitous clinical observations that have then been tested by the pharmacologist.

One of the original classifications of psychotropic drugs is based on their supposed pharmacological effects. Its terminology derives from the concept of psycholepsy, first described by the well-known French psychiatrist, Janet. He used psycholepsy to describe reduction in 'tension psychologique' (Janet, 1903), and in modern terminology this is closer to the neurophysiological concept of arousal than the specific feeling of tension associated with anxiety.

In 1954 Delay used the concept of psycholepsy to introduce the term 'neuroleptics' to describe the drugs he and Paul Deniker had introduced to psychiatry in the form of chlorpromazine. Delay (1961) subsequently separated psychotropic drugs into three groups; psycholeptics, psychoanaleptics and psychodysleptics. Psycholeptics are drugs that reduce arousal and therefore depress mental functions. Psychoanaleptics have the converse effect of increasing arousal, stimulating intellectual activity and mental function. Because their main clinical use is concerned with the elevation of depressed mood they are often called thymoleptics. The third group, psychodysleptics, is now rarely used in treatment. These drugs produce new and distorted arousal that is qualitatively different from normal and their influence in psychiatry is largely negative, creating psychopathology rather than alleviating it. This pathology can be considerable with the creation of what used to be called 'model psychoses'. The term psychodysleptic has a bewildering number of synonyms, including psychotomimetics, psycholytics, hallucinogens, psychedelics and phantastica, which only indicates that none of them is satisfactory.

Delay and Deniker further subdivided the psycholeptics into

(1) hypnotics, whose principal action is to induce sleep,

(2) neuroleptics, which lead to 'psychomotor inhibition', neurovegetative changes and reduction in psychotic symptoms, and
(3) tranquillizers, which reduce agitation and anxiety.

American workers, particularly Kline (1959), felt that the amphetamines and other stimulant drugs were different from the tricyclic antidepressants and monoamine oxidase inhibitors and incorporated the latter into a group called the psychic energizers.

Thus psychotropic drugs became classified into three main classes and five subgroups. Although there are many aspects of this classification that are easy to criticize in retrospect it represents a formidable achievement. Before Delay and Deniker formulated these subdivisions there was no acceptable classification in psychopharmacology and, although many modifications and additions have been made since, the same general principles are used today.

Although the basic classification was accepted readily, the idea of psycholepsy did not go down as well. It has a spurious objectivity that when examined closely does not have any real pharmacological correlates. The terms 'neurovegetative syndrome', 'psychomotor inhibition' and 'tonus', which enter frequently into the definition of the subgroups, are not immediately understandable to pharmacologists working in basic science or clinical work. It therefore became difficult to find the dividing lines between the drug groups. This uncertainty led to the development of a classification based on clinical use.

Clinical

Soon after Delay and Deniker's classification the World Health Organization (1958) issued a classification that was based primarily on the clinical uses of the drugs. It, and its later modification (WHO, 1967), was very similar to the French classification although it used different terminology (apart from retaining the terms neuroleptic and psychodysleptic) (*Table 1.1*). By basing itself on clinical use it avoided being tied to the somewhat diffuse concept of psycholepsy and was more flexible in accommodating new additions. Of course, if the clinical use of a compound changed with experience it was difficult to relocate it in the system, and if, as so often is the case, drugs had more than one clinical action, such as neuroleptics having primary sedative effects in low dosage and antipsychotic ones in higher dosage, it was impossible to accommodate these in the classification.

Most psychiatrists have adopted a clinical classification of drugs in the past 20 years. It is far from satisfactory because it is essentially a floating classification with no pharmacological or physiological base, suitable for description but not for prediction. Attempts to elaborate it by, for example discussing the effects of drugs on 'target symptoms' (Freyhan, 1960) rather than clinical syndromes, have been generally unsuccessful.

Shepherd (1972) has suggested that a universally acceptable classification might be achieved by a procedure called 'facet analysis' whereby all the factors relevant to the activity of a drug such as chemistry, pharmacology, psychology, sociology, physical and psychiatric illness are separately coded and incorporated into a multidimensional theme, from which a suitable classification could be developed. This has not been attempted on a large scale and there is a danger that classification would be split into too many subdivisions unless suitable weightings were attached to the different variables.

TABLE 1.1 Comparison of French and WHO classifications of psychotropic drugs

Pharmacological (after Delay and Deniker, 1961)		Clinical (after WHO, 1958 and 1967)	
Main class	*Subclasses*	*Main class*	*Subclasses*
Psycholeptics	Neuroleptics	Neuroleptics	Phenothiazines Butyrophenones Thioxanthenes
	Hypnotics Tranquillizers	Anxiolytic sedatives	Barbiturates Propanediols Benzodiazepines
Psychoanaleptics	Stimulants	Psychostimulants	Amphetamine group Caffeine
	Thymoleptics	Antidepressants	Monoamine oxidase inhibitors Tricyclic antidepressants
Psychodysleptics	—	Psychodysleptics	Lysergic acid diethylamide Mescaline Psilocybin Dimethyltryptophan Cannabis

Neurochemical

In recent years there have been important advances in the understanding of neurochemical transmission. This has been mainly along two lines. Firstly, there has been an increase in our understanding of the factors that regulate the synthesis, storage, release and receptor interactions of the neurotransmitters identified from 1950–1970. These include the amines—noradrenaline, dopamine, 5-hydroxytryptamine and acetylcholine, and amino acids—γ-aminobutyric acid (GABA), glutamic acid and glycine. Secondly, during the past decade there has been an explosive growth in the number of putative neurotransmitters, in particular, the possibility that up to 30 small peptides may have transmitter or neuromodulator functions in mammalian CNS. While the evidence for such a role is good for a few of the plethora of candidates, for example, methionine- and leucine-enkephalin, β-endorphin, substance P and thyrotrophin releasing hormone (TRH), for most it is scanty, particularly as almost nothing is known about the synthesis, storage, release and metabolism of these compounds (for review *see* Hökfelt *et al.*, 1980).

With this increase in information and understanding of both the pharmacological actions of drugs used in psychiatry and the possible neurotransmitter dysfunctions associated with particular psychiatric disorders, it is inevitable that attempts to classify the drugs within a neurochemical framework have been made. This approach has been helped by observations showing that the pharmacological effects of several psychotropic drugs on neurotransmission correlate roughly with their clinical effects (e.g. Seeman *et al.*, 1976; Briley, 1981). At present however, this classification is based on our understanding of the amine neurotransmitters and only very preliminary attempts have been made to incorporate the putative peptide neurotransmitters/neuro-modulators. It is apparent that during the next decade the classification may be modified substantially as more information becomes available about the role of neuropeptides in behaviour and disease.

The characteristics of the monoaminergic transmitters on which the classification is based is shown in *Figure 1.1* (for general review *see* Cooper, Bloom and Roth, 1978). In outline the transmitters are synthesized in the pre-synaptic nerve ending, using enzymes produced in the cell body, and transported down the axon. They are stored in this region within vesicles until released in a Ca^{++} dependent manner following the arrival of the action potential at the nerve ending. Following their release into the synaptic cleft the transmitter molecules interact with post-synaptic receptors initiating changes in the post-synaptic membrane. They may also interact with receptors on the pre-synaptic nerve ending membrane—so-called pre-synaptic or autoreceptors—of the nerve ending from which the transmitter was released, thereby exerting feedback control over the release of that transmitter. Alternatively the transmitter can interact with pre-synaptic receptors situated on nerve endings of nerves releasing a different transmitter subsequently modulating the release of the second transmitter by a pre-synaptic action. An example of this pre-synaptic modulation is the proposed pre-synaptic inhibition by enkephalin of substance P release from some sensory primary afferent endings within the substantia gelatinosa of the spinal cord (Jessell and Iversen, 1977). The action of the transmitter may be terminated by enzymatic breakdown

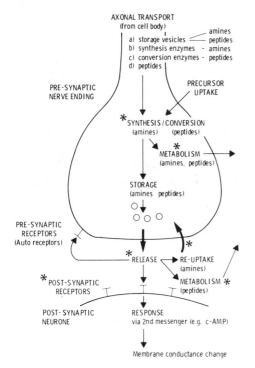

Figure 1.1 Generalized characteristics of a neurotransmitter. Note the differences outlined between the established amine transmitters and the putative peptide transmitters. (* Main sites at which psychotropic drugs act)

(acetylcholine), re-uptake into the pre-synaptic nerve ending (noradrenaline, dopamine and 5-hydroxytryptamine (5-HT)) or a combination of both (e.g. GABA). In the case of the monoamines there is also the intraneuronal mitrochondrial enzyme monoamine oxidase (MAO) which appears to regulate the concentration of intraneuronal transmitter.

While the putative peptide transmitters share many of these characteristics such as granular storage, Ca^{++} dependent release and enzymatic degradation, there are some important differences. In particular, the major site of synthesis is the cell body and then the peptide is transported to the nerve ending. Alternatively, a precursor could be formed in the cell body which is then broken down into active forms at the nerve ending. However, the importance of the latter process in the brain is not known, as the only well-documented examples relate to hormones in the pituitary, such as vasopressin.

From such information it is apparent that drugs can influence neurotransmission by either facilitating or inhibiting the mechanism involved. Transmitter function may be facilitated firstly, by increasing the amount of transmitter available for release—such as precursor administration (e.g. levodopa in parkinsonism), or inhibition of intraneuronal metabolism (e.g. MAO inhibitors). Alternatively, transmitter release can be enhanced (e.g. amphetamine increases release of dopamine and noradrenaline in the brain) or its removal from the synaptic cleft can be delayed, thereby prolonging receptor stimulation (e.g. the monoamine re-uptake inhibitors or acetylcholine esterase inhibitors). Finally drugs may act as direct receptor agonists (e.g. apomorphine and bromocriptine stimulate dopamine receptors). The identification of multiple receptor types—the two forms of β adrenoceptor are well established and there seems to be also dual α receptor forms and up to four types of dopamine receptor—will certainly complicate this area of drug classification.

The benzodiazepines facilitate GABA transmission but not via a direct effect on GABA neurons. There are specific benzodiazepine binding sites in the brain (Squires and Braestrup, 1977) and there is evidence that these sites are normally occupied by an endogenous GABA modulatory factor (Guidotti, Toffano and Costa, 1978). This has led to a search for the endogenous ligand and present findings indicate that it is a compound closely related to β-carboline-3-carboxylate (β-CCE) (Braestrup, Nielsen and Olsen, 1980). The benzodiazepines appear to antagonize the GABA inhibitory effects of the endogenous ligand. A similar situation may exist in relation to the 5-HT re-uptake system and the high affinity ^{3}H-imipramine binding sites in the brain (Briley, 1981).

Drugs that decrease synaptic transmission act in a converse fashion. Thus transmitter release can be decreased by reducing the amount of transmitter available by inhibiting synthesis (e.g. α-methyl-p-tyrosine inhibits the conversion of tyrosine to dopa—these are not important drugs clinically but are valuable experimental tools) or preventing storage (e.g. reserpine depletes catechol and indole amines by preventing vesicular storage). Other drugs may prevent transmitter release; these include the sympathetic neuron blocking drugs such as guanethidine and bretylium. Clinically however, the most important drugs of the ones that decrease transmitter action are those which block post-synaptic receptors by binding to the receptor and so preventing access to the natural agonist—the released transmitter—to the receptor. Drugs of this type include the antipsychotic drugs which block central dopamine receptors. Other examples are the use of cholinergic receptor blocking drugs in the treatment of parkinsonism or β-adrenoceptor blocking drugs to treat peripheral anxiety symptoms (*Table 1.2*).

While such a classification is particularly useful to the experimental pharmacologist, in the clinical field it needs to be used carefully as it is easy to derive the simple equation that because a drug has a certain pharmacological action and it is used to treat a certain psychiatric disorder, the action and treatment are causally related. It is important to remember that there is no such thing as a pharmacologically pure psychotropic drug. Neuroleptics for example, are antagonists of various receptors and it has only been by skilfully designed trials that a relationship between their effects on dopamine receptors (rather than one of many other receptors) and their clinical use has been established (*see* Chapter 4). A similar debate now surrounds the link between the monoamine re-uptake inhibition by tricyclics and their antidepressant activity (Maas, 1979). Such debates are inevitable in a rapidly expanding field such as neurotransmitter research.

Classification of drugs used in this book

No satisfactory classification of psychotropic drugs exists but at present a simple descriptive listing based on clinical use is the best available (*Table 1.2*). This is both understandable and flexible to change. The reader will readily see the connection

TABLE 1.2 Neurochemical classification of psychotropic drugs

Neurochemical classification	*Classification used in this book*
Dopamine-receptor blocking drugs	Antipsychotic (antischizophrenic) drugs
Dopamine precursors Dopamine agonist drugs Acetylcholine receptor blocking drugs	Antiparkinsonian drugs
Dopamine receptor blocking drugs α-Aminobutyric acid (GABA) facilitating drugs Cholinergic agonist drugs	Antidyskinetic drugs
α-Aminobutyric acid (GABA) facilitating drugs	Central antianxiety drugs
β-Adrenoceptor blocking drugs	Peripheral antianxiety drugs
Monoamine re-uptake inhibitors (MARI)	Tricyclic antidepressants Newer antidepressants (some)
Monoamine oxidase inhibitors (MAOI)	Monoamine oxidase inhibitors (delayed psychostimulants)
5-Hydroxytryptamine precursors	Amine precursors
—	Lithium carbonate
5-Hydroxytryptamine receptor agonists	Psychostimulants/hallucinogens (acute psychostimulants)
—	Drugs of addiction Antiaddictive drugs
—	Drugs modifying sexual behaviour

between this and earlier classifications although the number of drug groups has increased dramatically since the 1960s. Although the neurochemistry of these drugs does not explain all their clinical actions it is very encouraging to find that so many drugs of similar clinical profile have equivalent effects on neurotransmission. If a systematic classification is to be evolved in psychopharmacology the neurochemical path looks to be the most promising to follow.

References

BRAESTRUP, C., NIELSEN, M. and OLSEN, C. E. Urinary and brain β-carboline-3-carboxylates as potent inhibitors of brain benzodiazepine receptors, *Proceedings of the National Academy of Science* **77**, 2288 (1980)

BRILEY, M. Alteration in brain receptors in affective disorders. In *Neuroendocrine Regulation and Altered Behaviour* (Eds. P. D. HROLINA and R. L. SINGHAL). pp. 299–314. Croom Helm, London (1981)

COOPER, J. R., BLOOM, F. E. and ROTH, R. H. *The Biochemical Basis of Neuropharmacology*, 3rd edn, Oxford University Press, New York (1978)

DELAY, J. *Méthodes Chimiothérapiques en Psychiatrie*, Masson et Cie, Paris (1961)

FREYHAN, F. A. On classifying psychotropic pharmaca, *Comparative Psychiatry* **2**, 241–247 (1960)

GUIDOTTI, A., TOFFANO, G. and COSTA, E. An endogenous protein modulates the affinity of GABA and benzodiazepine receptors in rat brain, *Nature, London* **275**, 553–555 (1978)

HÖKFELT, T., JOHANSSON, O., LJUNGDAHL, Å., LUNDBERG, J. and SCHULTZBERG, M. Peptidergic neurons, *Nature, London* **284**, 515–521 (1980)

JANET, P. *Les Obsessions et la Psychaesthénie*, Alcan, Paris (1903)

JESSELL, T. M. and IVERSEN, L. L. Opiate analgesics inhibit substance P release from rat trigeminal nucleus, *Nature, London* **268**, 549–551 (1977)

KLINE, N. S. (Ed.) *Psychopharmacology Frontiers*, Little, Brown & Co., Boston (1959)

MAAS, J. W. Neurotransmitters and depression, Too much, too little or too unstable, *Trends in Neuroscience* **2**, 306–308 (1979)

SEEMAN, P., LEE, T., CHU-WONG, M. and WONG, K. Antipsychotic drugs doses and neuroleptic/dopamine receptors, *Nature* **261**, 717–719 (1976)

SHADER, R. (Ed.). *Psychiatric Complications of Medical Drugs*, Raven Press, New York (1972)

SHEPHERD, M. The classification of psychotropic drugs, *Psychological Medicine* **2**, 96–110 (1972)

SQUIRES, R. F. and BRAESTRUP, C. Benzodiazepine receptors in rat brain, *Nature, London* **266**, 732–734 (1977)

WORLD HEALTH ORGANIZATION. *WHO Technical Report Series, No. 152*, WHO, Geneva (1958)

WORLD HEALTH ORGANIZATION. *WHO Technical Report Series, No. 371*, WHO, Geneva (1967)

Chapter 2

Pharmacokinetics and drug metabolism— basic principles

J. P. Boulenger and M. Lader

'The sole aim of drug therapy should be to produce maximum benefit at minimum cost, both in terms of real and potential toxic side effects and money. These aims cannot be achieved however, without a better understanding of pharmacokinetics than most medical practitioners possess.'

(V. Marks, 1980)

Pharmacokinetics, the study of the time-course of drug absorption, distribution, biotransformation and elimination in the body, has become increasingly important in recent years. Previously, psychotropic drugs were essentially prescribed on the basis of clinical experience, the physician trying to produce the best therapeutic effect with the fewest side effects and without toxicity. However, if the patient failed to respond to the treatment, the physician did not know whether the drug had reached its sites of action in sufficient amount or whether the patient was truly 'refractory'.

The pharmacokinetic approach, already established in the treatment of infectious diseases and epilepsy, was first used in psychopharmacology with the introduction of lithium salts. Much information is now available about pharmacokinetic properties of other psychotropic drugs and a basic understanding in this field has become increasingly relevant to psychiatrists over the past few years. For example, when confronted with such different sleep disorders as initial insomnia, repeated awakenings or early morning waking, it would be difficult to prescribe rationally a hypnotic drug without knowing its half-life and the delay in its peak plasma level.

The psychiatrist cannot know all the pharmacokinetic details of every psychotropic agent, i.e. its absorption characteristics, distribution, liver metabolism, kidney excretion and drug interactions. The purpose of this chapter is to introduce some basic principles and to point out their relevance to the rational use of therapeutic agents. Where relevant, the important pharmacokinetic features are dealt with in the chapters on the individual drugs.

Definitions and basic principles in pharmacokinetics

Pharmacokinetics aims to provide a mathematical model for the description and prediction of the time-course of drugs within the body. This is achieved by measuring the drug concentrations in plasma and sometimes other body fluids, e.g. urine, saliva or

11

cerebrospinal fluid (CSF), over a period of time following administration. The pharmacokinetic variables obtained from these data are essential factors for rational therapy. For each drug they give important information about:

(1) the optimal dosage intervals,
(2) the time-lag and duration of action of a single dose,
(3) the delay of maximal effect of repeated doses,
(4) the influence of physiological (e.g. sex, pregnancy, age) as well as pathological states upon the usage of the drug,
(5) the likelihood of drug interactions.

However, these variables represent mean values for populations of normal adults and can vary widely for the same drug between individuals. Thus, if such variation is suspected the dosage regimen needs adjustment for some people according to their own pharmacokinetic properties. This may be pertinent in those who fail to respond to treatment or develop severe side effects during usual dosage regimens.

Compartments

The pharmacokinetic model describes the body as one compartment or more often a series of compartments in which the drug is homogeneously distributed and submitted to the same kinetic processes. Theoretically, on anatomical and physiological grounds, one could describe several categories of body spaces, i.e. plasma, highly perfused tissues (liver, heart, lungs, brain, kidney), poorly perfused tissues (muscles, skin), fat and other with negligible perfusion (bones, teeth, hair). However, for the pharmacokinetics of most drugs, the body can be regarded as two compartments. These compartments often lack any physiological meaning but offer an accurate model to describe the fate and the time-course of the drug in the body.

In the two-compartment model (*Figure 2.1*), it is assumed that the drug penetrates into the plasma, which is a part of the first or central compartment, then diffuses immediately and uniformly throughout the whole volume of this compartment (V1). Thus, the drug concentration in the central compartment (Cl) equals the plasma concentration. From the central compartment the drug is either eliminated, or diffuses to the peripheral, second compartment. The sum of all irreversible drug elimination from the central compartment is represented by a rate constant, kel; k 1 – 2 and k 2 – 1 are the rate constants for the drug transfer, respectively, from compartment 1 to

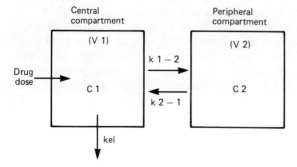

Figure 2.1 The two-compartment pharmacokinetic model. V1 and V2 (ℓ) are the volumes of the respective compartment, C1 and C2 (mg·ℓ^{-1}) the drug concentrations, kel, k 1 – 2 and k 2 – 1 (h^{-1}) the first order rate constants of drug elimination and transfer between compartments

compartment 2 and from the latter to the former. Usually, kel, k 1 − 2 and k 2 − 1 are assumed to be first-order rate constants, i.e. the rate depends upon the drug concentration in the compartment from which the drug is eliminated, absorbed or transferred. This results in an exponential relationship between drug concentrations and time. The rate constants are expressed as a fraction of the drug concentration submitted to elimination, absorption or transfer per unit of time, i.e. usually h^{-1} (/hours). This contrasts with zero-order kinetics where a constant amount of drug is eliminated per unit of time independent of its concentration in the respective compartment, e.g. phenytoin or ethanol. In this case the plot of the concentrations versus time will be a straight line. Some other drugs, like phenobarbitone, are eliminated by a first-order kinetic process at low plasma concentrations but have zero-order kinetics at high concentrations due to saturation of elimination processes.

The existence of several compartments can be inferred from plotting the plasma concentration of the drug against time on a semilogarithmic scale. The number of compartments corresponds to the number of different slopes, i.e. to the number of exponential functions composing the curve.

Intravenous injection in a single-compartment model

The single-compartment model does not correspond to the kinetics of most drugs. However, its description is simple and useful for the understanding of such important parameters as the biological half-life ($T_{\frac{1}{2}}$), the apparent volume of distribution (Vd) and the total body clearance (Cl tot). In this model, the drug injected intravenously is immediately distributed throughout the volume of the compartment. The plot of plasma concentrations versus time both in normal and semilogarithmic ordinates is illustrated in *Figure 2.2*.

The integration of the semilogarithmic curve

$$\log_e Cl = Co − kel \cdot t$$

gives

$$Cl = Co_e − kel \cdot t$$

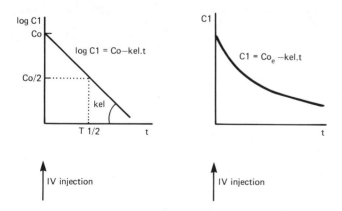

Figure 2.2 Schematic graph of plasma drug concentrations versus time in a one-compartment model after IV injection. The plasma concentrations are plotted using both normal (right graph) and semi-logarithmic (left graph) ordinates, and the equation of Cl (t) given above the curve

where Co is the drug plasma concentration immediately after the injection and kel the first-order elimination rate constant. These data can be used to obtain three important pharmacokinetic parameters:

(1) *The biological half-life ($T_{\frac{1}{2}}$)* which is the time required for the plasma drug concentration to decrease by half. This time is a constant for a given drug in a given individual if the elimination is a first-order kinetic process. Half-life can be calculated graphically as indicated in *Figure 2.2* or by the formula:

$$T_{\frac{1}{2}}(h) = \frac{0.693}{kel\,(h^{-1})}$$

where kel, the elimination constant, is the slope of the linear curve obtained from the semilogarithmic plot. $T_{\frac{1}{2}}$ will be large for drugs which are eliminated slowly and small for drugs which are eliminated rapidly. The biological half-life is an important parameter to determine the dosage interval of a drug and the delay necessary to achieve steady-state on repeated administration or complete elimination after cessation. In both cases this delay is roughly equal to five times the $T_{\frac{1}{2}}$. In some instances $T_{\frac{1}{2}}$ can help to understand the duration of action of a drug after acute administration.

(2) *The apparent volume of distribution (Vd)* is a purely theoretical ratio ($\ell \cdot k^{-1}$), without any physiological meaning, between the amount of drug present in the body ($mg \cdot kg^{-1}$) and its plasma concentration ($mg \cdot \ell^{-1}$). It is usually calculated to notional time zero immediately after an intravenous injection (IV) of a dose D:

$$Vd\,(\ell \cdot kg^{-1}) = \frac{D\,(mg \cdot kg^{-1})}{Co\,(mg \cdot \ell^{-1})}$$

For most psychotropic drugs Vd is large because of their distribution throughout the body fluids and their significant uptake by the tissues due to their lipophilic properties. A Vd of about $10\ \ell \cdot kg^{-1}$ will mean that the average drug concentration in tissues is ten times higher than in plasma, indicating important binding to tissue proteins.

(3) *The total body clearance (Cl tot)* is the fraction of the apparent volume of distribution which is completely cleared from drug per unit time. Thus, Cl tot is a general index of all the elimination mechanisms leading to a disappearance of the drug from the central compartment. These mechanisms are mainly contributed by hepatic metabolism and renal elimination.

$$Cl\,(ml \cdot min^{-1} \cdot kg^{-1}) = Vd\,(ml \cdot kg^{-1}) \cdot kel\,(min^{-1})$$

The total body clearance is directly proportional to the elimination constant and thus is commonly used to quantify the drug elimination.

Intravenous injection in a two-compartment model

Most often for psychotropic drugs the body acts as a two-compartment model, i.e. the plot of the plasma concentration logarithm versus time has two linear portions (*Figure 2.3*) instead of one in the previous model.

The first part of the curve is called the alpha (α) or distribution phase because the rapid decrease of central compartment concentrations is mainly due to the penetration of the drug into the peripheral compartment. Equilibrium is achieved when the penetration of the drug into the peripheral compartment equals the output of drug

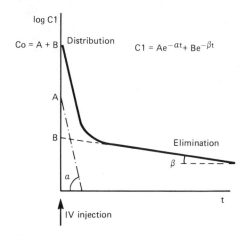

Figure 2.3 Schematic graph of plasma drug concentrations versus time in a two-compartment model after IV injection. The plasma concentrations are plotted on a logarithmic scale

from this compartment to the central one. The second part of the curve, called beta (β) or elimination phase, is mainly due to irreversible elimination from the central compartment.

The concentration curve can be broken down into two components as shown in *Figure 2.3* and the values of α, β, A and B can be obtained respectively from the slopes and the intercepts of these components. From these parameters Vd, Cl, V1 and V2, can be calculated as well as two different half-lives, one referring to the distribution phase ($T_{\frac{1}{2}}\alpha$) the other referring to the elimination phase ($T_{\frac{1}{2}}\beta$). $T_{\frac{1}{2}}\beta$ is the most commonly used and referred to simply as the 'half-life'.

Other modes of administration

ORAL AND INTRAMUSCULAR (IM) ADMINISTRATION

If the drug is administered orally or IM, the absorption process must be taken into account to describe the drug behaviour. Usually this process has a first-order kinetic and is described by an absorption constant k_a (h^{-1}). The plot of plasma drug concentrations versus time gives in both cases similar types of curves (*Figure 2.4*).

The maximum plasma concentration (Cl max) achieved, referred as the peak plasma concentration, and the delay of this peak (t max) are indicators of the rate of absorption. These parameters can be important in understanding the efficacy and delay of action of drugs given in acute doses. Furthermore, the area under the curve of drug concentrations versus time (AUC) can be calculated. The AUC is proportional to the fraction of the administered dose which is absorbed and reaches the general circulation. A comparison can be made with the AUC obtained after IV injection of the same dose to assess the extent of the drug absorption (*cf.* section on bioavailability).

INTRAVENOUS (IV) INFUSION

When an IV infusion is given at a constant rate Q ($ml \cdot min^{-1}$) the plasma drug concentration increases progressively and, if the infusion is long enough, reaches a steady-state level, i.e. remains constant (*Figure 2.5*).

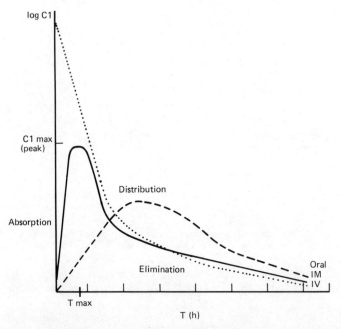

Figure 2.4 Schematic graph of plasma drug concentrations versus time after oral (---), IM (——) or IV (.....) administration in a two-compartment model. The same dose is administered to the same patient. Notice that the rate of absorption is shown as quicker after IM than oral administration (not invariable in practice). The extent of absorption, as estimated by the area under the curve, is similar in both cases

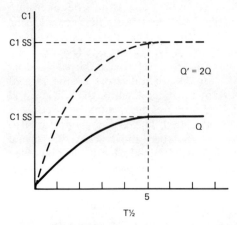

Figure 2.5 Schematic graph of plasma drug concentrations versus time during an IV infusion. The dotted line represents the curve obtained for an infusion of the same drug with a rate $Q' = 2Q$. Time is expressed as multiples of the drug half-life ($T_{\frac{1}{2}}$). Cl SS is the steady-state concentration

The delay necessary to reach the plasma steady-state concentration (Cl SS) depends only upon the half-life of the drug ($T_\frac{1}{2}$). After five times $T_\frac{1}{2}$, 97 per cent of the Cl SS is achieved. Therefore, as most drugs have a $T_\frac{1}{2}$ longer than 1 h, steady-state concentration cannot be attained during a single infusion. The magnitude of the Cl SS is directly related to the infusion rate Q and inversely proportional to the drug clearance

$$\text{Cl SS (mg} \cdot \text{ml}^{-1}) = \frac{Q \, (\text{mg} \cdot \text{min}^{-1})}{\text{Cl} \, (\text{ml} \cdot \text{min}^{-1})}$$

The increase of the rate of an infusion will therefore lead to a higher plasma drug steady-state concentration but will not shorten the time needed to reach it.

Multiple administration

If the administration of an oral dose is repeated on a regular basis at a constant interval T (h) the pharmacokinetic principles defined for a continuous IV infusion can be used. The mean steady-state concentration ($\overline{\text{Cl SS}}$) depends upon the fraction of the initial dose absorbed and reaching the general circulation (FD), the drug clearance (Cl) and the dose interval (T):

$$\overline{\text{Cl SS}} \, (\text{mg} \cdot \text{ml}^{-1}) = \frac{FD \, (\text{mg})}{\text{Cl} \, (\text{ml} \cdot \text{min}^{-1}) \cdot T \, (\text{min})}$$

As for IV infusions, the steady state is nearly reached after 5 $T_\frac{1}{2}$. This delay is clinically important because a drug cannot be expected to have its maximum effects until the steady-state plasma concentration has been reached. At that time, a modification of the dose will lead to a proportional modification of $\overline{\text{Cl SS}}$ after a new delay of 5 $T_\frac{1}{2}$.

Steady state does not mean constancy of concentrations but equilibrium between absorption and elimination processes. The plasma drug concentrations still vary after each dose between a maximum and a minimum.

Knowledge of the drug half-life ($T_\frac{1}{2}$) for a given patient provides some important facts about multiple dosing:

(1) the longer the $T_\frac{1}{2}$ the longer the delay to reach the steady state,
(2) the longer the $T_\frac{1}{2}$ the smaller the plasma concentration fluctuation between the doses. Furthermore, dosage intervals can be up to two-thirds of the half-life without fluctuations becoming too marked. Many psychotropic drugs, e.g. amitriptyline and diazepam, have half-lives sufficiently long for once-daily dosage.
(3) if the half-life increases (e.g. in hepatic or renal failure) the steady-state plasma concentration will increase if the daily dose remains the same.

Absorption

A drug enters the circulation either by being placed there directly or by absorption from depots such as the gastrointestinal tract, the muscles or subcutaneous tissue. The latter two sites represent the parenteral mode and the gut represents the enteral mode.

Some drugs such as iron, methyldopa, and several amino acids are actively absorbed by specific carrier mechanisms. Most, however, diffuse into the body. To do so the molecule must be either very small or non-ionized and lipid soluble. Most psychotropic drugs are weak bases that exist in two forms: the non-ionized form (non-dissociated) and the ionized form (dissociated). The degree of dissociation depends on the pH of the medium and the drug is half-ionized at the pH of the solution indicated by its pK_a

(negative logarithm of the dissociation constant). Due to their high liposolubility and the low proportion of their ionized form, most psychotropic drugs are generally extensively absorbed.

Intravenous injection (IV)

An obvious advantage of the intravenous method of drug administration is that the drug enters the circulation with the least delay. Moreover, intravenous administration is easy to control, especially if an infusion rather than a bolus injection is used. Abreaction is an example of controlled injection. Intravenous infusions are a useful way of building up body concentrations as has been advocated in the case of clomipramine. The disadvantages of intravenous injection are that dangerously high concentrations can occur during the bolus injection and that once injected the drug cannot be removed, whereas an emetic or stomach lavage can remove an oral overdose.

Intramuscular injection (IM)

Intramuscular injections are commonly used by psychiatrists not only to quieten the disturbed patient with tranquillizers but also as long-acting depot injections. Blood flow through resting muscles is about 0.02 to 0.07 $ml(min \cdot g)^{-1}$ tissue and may increase tenfold during emotional excitement. Thus, the agitated or frenzied, disturbed patient should rapidly absorb antipsychotic injections. However, for some drugs like diazepam or chlordiazepoxide, the extent and rate of absorption are less after IM injection than after oral administration. Highly lipid-soluble formulations of drugs such as fluphenazine decanoate in oil are absorbed very slowly from the fatty tissues of the muscle.

Oral administration

Psychotropic drugs are absorbed along the whole length of the gastrointestinal tract, mostly by a mechanism of passive diffusion depending upon the concentration gradient across the cell membranes, and the absorption surface. The site of maximum absorption depends on the chemical properties of the drug: stomach for weak acids (barbiturates, phenytoin) and neutral materials (ethanol); intestine for weak bases (antidepressants, antipsychotics).

Gastric absorption is favoured by an empty stomach, and decreased or delayed by food intake. Thus, if rapid action is required, drugs should be given on an empty stomach. For a smoother, delayed absorption, the drug should be taken after meals. In some instances however, the extent of drug absorption is increased by food intake (propranolol, phenytoin, carbamazepine). In some patients, an increase in gastrointestinal motility due to anxiety can lead to a quicker absorption of drugs like diazepam.

Drug interactions

Other substances can affect gastrointestinal absorption of psychotropic drugs. A modification of gastric pH by antacids can modify the degree of dissociation (ionization) of drugs like diazepam or chlordiazepoxide and delay their absorption. With clorazepate, antacids decrease the hydrolysis of the drug to nordiazepam which takes place in the stomach and can reduce the sedative effects of single doses. Anticholinergic drugs like tricyclic antidepressants and some antipsychotics can decrease the motility and delay the emptying of the stomach. Thus, the extent of absorption can be increased for drugs absorbed in the stomach and decreased for those absorbed in the intestine.

Bioavailability

Bioavailability strictly refers to the relative amount of an administered drug which reaches the general circulation but is sometimes used to mean the rate at which it occurs. Bioavailability is commonly referred to as a fraction of the drug dosage and is calculated by comparing the area under the curve (AUC) of the given formulation with the AUC obtained after IV administration (which guarantees complete absorption):

$$\text{Bioavailability (per cent)} = \frac{\text{AUC after oral or IM dose}}{\text{AUC after IV dose}} \cdot 100$$

The rate of absorption is estimated as the delay to the peak plasma level and its value, i.e. the quicker a drug is absorbed the higher and the sooner will be its peak plasma level (*Figure 2.6*).

All the factors influencing absorption can modify the bioavailability of a drug. Differences in the product formulation is another factor which can lead to important modifications in the rate and extent of absorption of a drug. This has been clearly documented for drugs like phenytoin, digoxin, aspirin and to a lesser extent for some psychotropic drugs like chlorpromazine, dextroamphetamine, chlordiazepoxide, methaqualone and amitriptyline. Furthermore, the amount of hepatic metabolism of

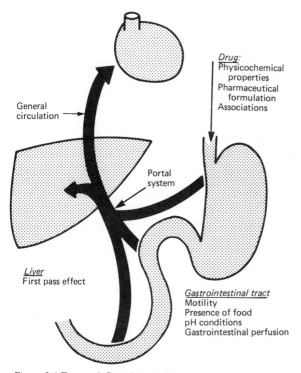

General circulation

Drug:
Physicochemical
   properties
Pharmaceutical
   formulation
Associations

Portal
system

Liver
First pass effect

Gastrointestinal tract
Motility
Presence of food
pH conditions
Gastrointestinal perfusion

Figure 2.6 Factors influencing the bioavailability of a drug administered orally

the drug during its passage from the portal system to the general circulation can influence the bioavailability of drugs. As shown later, this hepatic 'first-pass' effect is especially important for some psychotropic drugs.

Protein binding and distribution

Most drugs are distributed throughout the body fluids in the water phase of plasma. From there, they reach their sites of action at a rate depending on the blood flow through the organ and on the ease with which the drug can pass across lipoprotein membranes. Only drug which is not bound to plasma protein (i.e. the unbound or 'free' drug) is able to cross the membranes and reach the site of action. Thus, plasma protein binding is another crucial factor governing drug distribution within the body.

Plasma protein binding

Tricyclic antidepressants, phenothiazines and benzodiazepines are highly and strongly bound to plasma proteins. The amount of free drug is usually less than 10 per cent of the plasma drug concentration, and remains constant for a wide range of concentrations. However, binding varies among individuals and the free fraction varies about twofold across most subjects. The characteristics of protein binding depend strongly on the chemical structure of the drug. While acidic drugs bind mainly to serum albumin, basic drugs, like most of psychotropic drugs, can also be bound to lipoproteins, α_1-glycoproteins and globulins. In the case of imipramine and chlorpromazine the binding to lipoprotein is even as high as that to albumin.

The binding is reversible and can be modified by different factors:

(1) *The plasma drug concentration.* Usually the percentage of binding increases linearly with the plasma drug concentration until it reaches a plateau and then remains constant. Thus, the percentage of drug binding is a meaningless value unless the drug concentration is specified.
(2) *The plasma protein concentration.* While variations in plasma albumin concentrations are narrow and usually in the direction of decreasing concentrations, large fluctuations in both directions are possible for other proteins. Thus a decrease, or sometimes an increase in protein binding of psychotropic drugs can be observed in pathological conditions. These conditions are detailed in *Table 2.1*. Furthermore a decrease of serum albumin concentration can be observed in different physiological conditions, e.g. ageing or pregnancy.
(3) *The presence of other substances* which can compete with the drug for binding sites or modify their affinity by inducing structural changes in the tertiary conformation of the protein. This can be due to other drugs administered concomitantly or to changes in concentration of physiological substances e.g. bilirubin, free fatty acids or urea.

For psychotropic drugs which are highly bound, a small decrease in binding can cause a large increase in the free fraction. As the free fraction is the only part susceptible to diffusion, glomerular filtration and hepatic metabolism, its increase will lead to an increase of these processes. Thus, the increase of the free drug concentration in plasma will usually be transient due to the large volume of distribution of these drugs. After a variable period of transition the original drug concentration at its sites of action is re-established.

TABLE 2.1 Pathological conditions affecting plasma concentrations of different proteins

Modification of plasma protein concentration	Pathological conditions
Hypoalbuminaemia	Hepatic diseases, renal failure, burns, cardiac failure, nephrotic syndrome, surgery, malnutrition, cancer, inflammatory diseases
Hyper -α_1-glycoproteinaemia	Crohn's disease, rheumatoid arthritis, inflammatory diseases
Hypo -α_1-glycoproteinaemia	Hepatic diseases, nephrotic syndrome, malnutrition
Hyperlipoproteinaemia	Hyperlipoproteinaemia of different types

Important clinical consequences are unlikely to occur with psychotropic drugs as a result of modifications of their binding, given their wide apparent therapeutic concentration range. However, adverse reactions to phenytoin, diazepam and flunitrazepam have been reported to be more common in hypoalbuminaemic patients.

Ideally the free concentration of a drug should be measured when studying the relationships with therapeutic effects. However, even in physiological conditions with human proteins, binding studies are difficult, poorly reproducible and not fully predictive of the extent of binding *in vivo*. Consequently, other methods have been developed to estimate the concentration of free drug at its sites of action, e.g. measuring the drug concentration in saliva or cerebrospinal fluid (CSF) (*Figure 2.7*). These methods are based on the assumption that only the free drug diffuses into the

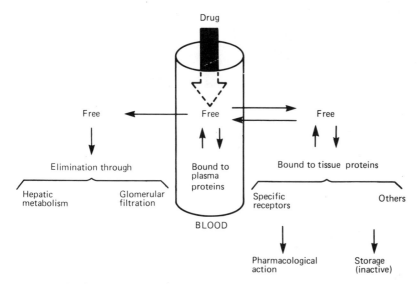

Figure 2.7 The drug protein binding and its dynamic equilibrium between blood and tissues

given fluid without intervention of any active process. Good correlations with plasma free drug have been described for CSF concentrations of diazepam, phenytoin and nortriptyline and for saliva concentrations of phenytoin, carbamazepine and diazepam.

Distribution

Psychotropic drugs are extensively distributed to brain and other body tissues. The drug may enter the brain directly from the circulation or indirectly from the cerebrospinal fluid. Areas of brain vary in vascularity, the cortex having a richer blood supply than white matter. The brain is the best supplied of all organs; it comprises only 2 per cent of the body weight but receives 15 per cent of the cardiac output. Thus, drugs should equilibrate rapidly between brain and blood. Some drugs, however, do not enter the brain easily, giving rise to the concept of the 'blood–brain barrier'. However, more recently it has become recognized that there is no such absolute barrier and that the rate of diffusion from blood to brain depends on a number of physicochemical factors.

PROTEIN BINDING

Highly bound drugs will diffuse into the brain slowly because their plasma free drug concentration is low. After equilibration, the concentration in the CSF is usually close to the free plasma water concentration because the fluid is virtually protein-free. Brain tissue proteins, by contrast, can strongly bind many psychotropic drugs, forming a central pool. This binding takes place either on inactive sites of storage, or on active sites responsible for the pharmacological effects. Such specific sites called 'receptors' have now been established for antipsychotics, opiates, benzodiazepines and tricyclic antidepressants. Drug protein binding in tissues is reversible and varies in parallel with the modifications of drug concentrations.

IONIZATION

As with absorption from the gut, the drug diffuses into the brain in its non-ionized form. Thus, at the plasma pH of 7.4, or the slightly lower pH values of extracellular fluid, knowledge of the dissociation constant (pKa) of the drug allows the non-ionized proportion to be calculated.

LIPOPHILICITY

The brain is a highly lipid tissue, and the lipid solubility of a drug gives a good indication of how rapidly the drug will enter the brain. This factor is the most important of the three. Most psychotropic drugs are highly lipophilic and enter the brain expeditiously. Dopamine and 5-HT have low lipophilicity and fail to diffuse into the brain. Finally, simple cations or anions such as lithium and bromide diffuse readily because the molecules are small.

Metabolism

Some drugs, mainly those that are relatively lipid insoluble or ionized, are excreted unchanged by the kidney; barbitone and lithium are examples. However, most highly lipophilic drugs like psychotropic drugs diffuse readily across body membranes and will be reabsorbed by diffusion from the glomerular filtrate in the kidney. Such substances have a very low renal-clearance rate and persist in the body. To be eliminated, drugs of this type must be metabolized to derivatives that are more polar, i.e. more soluble in water and less in lipids. This process is not 'detoxication' since the metabolite may be more active than its parent.

Drug metabolism takes place mainly in the liver and occurs in two phases:

(1) *Oxidation* is the most common form of drug metabolism. The reactions are carried out by enzymes located in the microsomal fraction of the liver and involve oxygen and an unusual cytochrome, P 450, which activates the oxygen. These enzymes catalyse a variety of reactions including hydroxylation, N-dealkylation, O-dealkylation and sulphoxide formation, to provide the drug with a group which can react with the conjugation agent. Some drug oxidations are not catalysed by the typical liver microsomal enzymes. Examples are the alcohol and aldehyde dehydrogenases, which oxidize ethanol to acetaldehyde and then to acetic acid. Another group, the monoamine oxidases, are widely distributed mitochondrial enzymes that oxidatively deaminate a whole range of substances.

Other types of reactions like hydrolysis and reduction are uncommon.

(2) *Conjugation* consists in the coupling of molecules such as glucuronic acid, acetyl radicals and sulphate to form less lipid-soluble and hence easily excretable metabolites. The molecular weight of the complex is increased so that active transport excretion can also take place.

Psychotropic drugs are extensively metabolized, often through several pathways. As a result of this, several metabolites may appear in the plasma, and most of the time almost no drug is excreted unchanged. The metabolites may be pharmacologically inactive, or active with the same or different properties than the parent drug.

Another aspect of the metabolism of psychotropic drugs is the wide inter-individual variability. The differences in the rate of metabolism are probably the major source of variability among individuals in the pharmacological action of a given drug.

Some other practical aspects of the drug hepatic metabolism need further discussion.

First-pass metabolism

After oral absorption a drug must pass through the liver before it reaches the general circulation. The rate of metabolism occurring in the liver is referred to as the hepatic 'first-pass' effect. This effect can be quantitatively very important. For example, more than 90 per cent of orally administered fluphenazine is oxidized in the liver after absorption before even reaching the systemic circulation and some individuals metabolize phenothiazines almost entirely. These patients in particular may benefit from a switch to depot administration of antipsychotic drugs, which obviates first-pass metabolism.

For antidepressants the inter-individual variability of the first-pass effect is wide: from 20 to 70 per cent for imipramine and nortriptyline. Consequently the bioavailability of the drug will vary in the same proportions between subjects. The clinical consequences of such differences depend on whether or not the metabolism creates active metabolites, and on the pharmacological profile of those metabolites.

Inhibition of drug metabolism

In multiple drug therapy different drugs may compete for a common enzymatic site of metabolism. This can lead to an inhibition of the biotransformation of one of the drugs and to its accumulation. For example, dicoumarol inhibits the metabolism of phenytoin and tolbutamide and consequently may induce severe adverse effects due to the high plasma concentration of these drugs. Disulfiram may have the same effect on the metabolism of phenytoin, tolbutamide, chlordiazepoxide and diazepam. Furthermore, disulfiram inhibits aldehyde dehydrogenase thus causing the accumulation of acetaldehyde after the ingestion of ethanol. Acetaldehyde accumulation is believed to produce the unpleasant flushing, throbbing, nausea, and vomiting of the 'disulfiram reaction'. Phenothiazines and haloperidol inhibit the metabolism of tricyclic anti-depressants, leading to an increase of their steady-state concentration. The clinical consequences of this concentration increase are unknown but probably limited.

The inhibition of intestinal monoamine oxidase (MAO) by MAO inhibitor (MAOI) antidepressants is another example. This inhibition is irreversible, and the effects of the drug wear off only when new enzyme has been synthesized. The MAOIs thus potentiate the action of amines that are broken down primarily by MAO. The chief example is tyramine, a constituent of fermented foods such as cheese. On ingestion, tyramine is not metabolized by the inhibited MAO, but instead reaches the circulation and releases noradrenaline from the noradrenergic nerve endings. Thus, a potentially fatal hypertensive crisis may ensue from the combination of a MAOI and a tyramine-containing food.

Hepatic diseases are another factor of drug metabolism inhibition, oxidation being usually more impaired than conjugation. The total clearance of drugs such as barbiturates, narcotic analgesics, chlordiazepoxide and diazepam can be reduced in patients with hepatic function impairment. Thus patients with liver disease are unduly sensitive to these drugs, which means that the dose should be reduced.

Stimulation of hepatic metabolism

Several drugs administered for a few days may induce an increase in concentrations of microsomal metabolizing enzymes due both to an increased synthesis and a decreased destruction. The induction leads to a stimulation of the inducing-drug metabolism and may produce an apparent condition of drug tolerance. Furthermore, due to the non-specificity of these enzymes, which can deal with a wide variety of substrates, the metabolism of other drugs can be accelerated. Consequently, enzyme induction is a major potential mechanism of drug interaction.

Barbiturates are a well-known example of inducing drugs. Patients treated chronically with barbiturates metabolize the drugs more rapidly than do non-exposed persons. The concurrent administration of phenobarbitone with chlorpromazine or nortriptyline produces liver enzyme induction, more rapid metabolism of the psychotropic drugs, and a drop in their plasma concentrations. Other barbiturates also induce enzymes and counteract other psychotropic drugs. Antiparkinsonian drugs such as orphenadrine are powerful liver inducers and should not be given routinely with antipsychotic medication. Enzyme induction by alcohol partly explains the tolerance that alcoholics have to alcohol and the cross-tolerance they have to barbiturates; cellular changes are also an important factor. Phenytoin is also a powerful enzyme inducer and can interact with other drugs. Many drugs are inducers in animals, but species differences are important and each drug must be assessed in man. For example, benzodiazepines are good inducers in rats, but induction is of no clinical importance in man. Among other psychotropic drugs known to induce their own metabolism are glutethimide, chloral hydrate, meprobamate, chlorpromazine, and the anticonvulsants, carbamazepine and primidone

Caffeine, cigarette smoking, adrenal steroids, sex hormones, dicoumarol and phenylbutazone are also capable of induction. This probably explains why the incidence of drowsiness during chlorpromazine or diazepam treatment is lower in smokers than in non-smokers.

Induction usually occurs within a few days of drug administration and wears off a week or so after the drug is discontinued. The phenomenon can be quite marked, resulting in a 50 per cent reduction in plasma concentration of the drugs. Response to enzyme inducers is partly genetically controlled. Another example of genetically determined differences in drug metabolism is acetylation. Isoniazid and probably phenelzine are metabolized mainly by acetylation: about half the population acetylate rapidly, the other half slowly. Higher concentrations of unmetabolized drug are maintained in the slow metabolizers, with greater chance of side effects, but clinical response seems less influenced.

Some physiological conditions can affect hepatic metabolism. The microsomal enzymes that metabolize drugs are not fully active until about eight weeks after birth. Hence neonates metabolize most drugs slowly. Conjugation to form glucuronides is less deficient. Furthermore, especially in the premature infant, the blood–brain barrier is immature so that centrally acting drugs penetrate the brain readily and have enhanced effects. Thus, babies in the first month or two of life, especially the newborn, are usually very sensitive to psychotropic drugs. Adults and children metabolize drugs similarly, but smaller doses must be used in children, especially prepubertal children, because of their smaller Vd. During pregnancy, the rate of hepatic metabolism of drugs like phenytoin and barbiturates can be increased and thus the clinical effects of the drug may be diminished.

Excretion

Each day 190 ℓ of plasma water are filtered through the glomeruli, all but 1.5 ℓ being reabsorbed. Only drug dissolved in free (i.e. unbound) plasma water can be filtered, and lipid-soluble non-ionized drugs, including most psychotropic drugs, are re-absorbed because they diffuse back in the tubules.

This resorption cannot occur with lipid-insoluble (water-soluble) drugs, which, along with their metabolites, are therefore cleared from the plasma. The pH of the urine is an important factor influencing the rate of drug excretion. Thus, it is the non-ionized form of the drug that tends to diffuse across the tubule cells back into the bloodstream. Weak acids tend to be excreted in alkaline urine because they form ions, whereas weak bases remain in acidic urine as they are non-ionized. For example, amphetamine, a weak base, is excreted rapidly in urine of low pH but slowly and erratically in alkaline urine. Acidification of the urine with ammonium chloride therefore hastens the excretion of amphetamine in cases of overdose. Conversely, barbiturates, being weak acids, are excreted more rapidly if the urine is made alkaline by administering bicarbonate.

Lithium is a prime example of a drug for which renal excretion is quantitatively important. A decrease in clearance due to renal impairment may cause an increase in plasma lithium concentrations and lead to severe side effects. Conversely, the increase in renal clearance observed at the end of pregnancy may induce a decrease of both in plasma concentration and the therapeutic effect of lithium salts.

Drugs can also be excreted by the liver cells into the bile. Biliary excretion is a major route of elimination of drug metabolites, especially glucuronides. In some cases the metabolite can be reabsorbed from the intestine, a process that forms the enterohepatic cycle. The existence of such a cycle may explain why some drugs have their clinical effects increased after meals when much bile is excreted into the intestine.

Other ways of excretion are the expired air, the saliva, the sweat and the intestine. Some basic drugs can be excreted into the stomach after IV administration. Furthermore the lactating mother is likely to secrete lipophilic drugs into the milk. This is known to occur with diazepam, which has been reported to have appreciable effects on the baby. Milk excretion may also occur with other benzodiazepines, lithium, meprobamate, barbiturates, imipramine, phenytoin and phenothiazines which thus should be avoided during lactation.

Pharmacokinetics and pharmacological effect

Variability in response to a given drug varies widely in psychopharmacology. On the basis of the fundamental pharmacological relationship $E = f(C \times S)$ where the clinical effect (E) is described as a function of the concentration of drug at the site of action (C) and of the sensitivity of that site of action (S), the variability of drug response can be examined as follows:

(1) *The function relating the effect to the concentration × sensitivity combination.* This function is not always linear and one example of complex relationship concerns nortriptyline. In this case there is believed to be a parabolic relationship between clinical response and plasma concentration, both low and high concentrations being associated with a lack of response. However, the function may be assumed to be the same among individuals and thus does not seem to be involved in the inter-individual variability in drug response.

(2) *The receptors' sensitivity, i.e. the responsiveness of tissues.* This factor is probably critical, but attempts to assess receptor sensitivity have until now only been indirect. Examples of such attempts are the measurement of the K_i values for MAOIs, the prolactin response to antipsychotics, or the growth hormone response to clonidine. In practice there is no way by which the sensitivity of the receptor response in man to any psychotropic drug can be estimated directly. This reflects the lack of knowledge of the precise biological mechanisms of action underlying the clinical properties of psychotropic drugs as well as the inaccessibility of human brain response systems.

(3) *The concentration of drug at its site of action.* This factor cannot be measured directly for the same reasons as indicated above. But, because the therapeutic response to drugs usually correlates better with the plasma concentration than with the drug dosage, it is assumed that the former is a better indicator of the drug concentration at its site of action than the latter. However, such estimations are only an approximation of receptor site concentrations because of complicating factors such as plasma binding, active metabolites, penetration and binding in the brain. Consequently it is not usually possible to define for a given drug an optimal concentration but only a therapeutic range wherein the majority of patients will experience maximal therapeutic effects for minimal toxicity and side effects. Two different situations have to be considered in the attempt to correlate plasma drug concentrations and clinical effects (*Figure 2.8*).

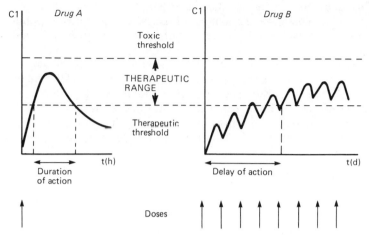

Figure 2.8 Theoretical relationships between drug plasma concentrations (Cl) and clinical effects for drugs administered in acute dosage (A) or in repeated dosages (B)

Acute dosage

In psychopharmacology, drugs administered on an acute basis are mainly hypnotics and antianxiety agents. For both types of drugs, when groups of patients are compared, no precise correlation is found between the plasma concentration and the clinical effects but the higher concentrations usually correspond to the patients having the greater effects. The correlation is not increased when drugs without active metabolites are used, e.g. lorazepam, or when these metabolites are taken into account, e.g. N-desmethyldiazepam for diazepam.

However, if the comparison is done within the same subject, there is usually a good correlation between dose, plasma peak concentration and clinical effect. Thus, when using hypnotics, one should begin to administer small doses to test the patient's sensitivity, then progressively increase the doses until the therapeutic effect is achieved.

Other pharmacokinetic properties like $T_{\frac{1}{2}}$ or the delay of the peak plasma concentration are important guides for acute administration of drugs. These two variables are not always related and oxazepam is a good example of a drug with a short $T_{\frac{1}{2}}$ but a long delay of peak plasma concentration, e.g. 3–4 h.

For patients with sleep disorders, a drug should be chosen which is rapidly eliminated, i.e. a short $T_{\frac{1}{2}}$ is desirable, in order to avoid an impairment of psychomotor functions during the following day. Furthermore, when the $T_{\frac{1}{2}}$ is long the drug will not be completely eliminated when the next dosage is given, leading to a progressive accumulation of the drug in the body. The time of the plasma peak concentration is usually correlated to the maximum effect of the drug. For example, diazepam is used for the treatment of acute anxiety and triazolam for difficulties falling asleep, both drugs having their peak plasma concentration within the first hour following oral administration.

Repeated dosage

In patients receiving medications for a long period of time it is not possible to follow blood concentrations continuously. Blood must be drawn at a given time regularly during treatment. This time is usually between 8 am and 10 am, before the patient has received the morning dosage. Therefore, the sample is taken after a delay corresponding to the maximum dosage interval and the concentration is likely to reflect the lowest of the day.

The attempt to correlate plasma drug concentrations and clinical effects will only be made when the steady state is reached because one can expect the drug will have its maximal effects at that time. The steady-state plasma concentrations (Cl SS) vary considerably between individuals: after repeated administration of the same dose the variability in Cl SS is about 10- to 20-fold for the majority of psychotropic drugs. The main factors involved in the variability of Cl SS are summarized in *Table 2.2*.

TABLE 2.2 Main factors of variability in steady-state concentration (Cl SS) of a given drug

Pharmacological	Drug dosage* Drug physicochemical properties Pharmaceutical formulation Route of administration Duration of treatment (if induction)* Co-prescription of other drugs*
Individual	Age Weight Genetic factors influencing metabolism Pathological factors* Pregnancy
Others	Compliance Diet Time of administration of the drug* Cigarettes Alcohol

*Indicate the most common reasons for an unexpected variation of Cl SS in a given subject.

The free drug concentration, which is more likely to reflect concentrations at receptor site, has been proposed to be more relevant in correlation studies with clinical effects. However, this measure is of little value in practice for several reasons:

(1) the technical difficulty of measuring binding accurately,
(2) the small inter-individual variability in binding (twofold) compared to the variability in steady-state concentrations (at least tenfold),
(3) for each individual, the percentage of drug bound is a constant.

Except for lithium, only a few positive results have emerged from attempts to correlate steady-state plasma concentrations and clinical effects of psychotropic drugs. The best documented examples of positive correlations are those related to adverse effects, e.g. the sedative and hypotensive effects of chlorpromazine, the extrapyramidal effects of haloperidol, and the cardiotoxicity of tricyclic antidepressants. In most of the cases, attempts to correlate Cl SS with therapeutic results remain controversial, e.g. for tricyclic antidepressants. Several reasons may explain this absence of correlation:

(1) Some drugs have an irreversible action which is maintained despite the disappearance of the drug from plasma. This is the case of drugs qualified as 'hit-and-run' like MAOIs and reserpine.

(2) Receptor sensitivity may be modified so drug concentrations bear no constant relation to receptor effects. With benzodiazepines such modifications may explain the tolerance developing over time for sedative effects and the increased sensitivity of elderly people to the same effects.

(3) The presence of active metabolites, with different pharmacokinetic properties and sometimes a different mode of action. This is the case with most psychotropic drugs except a few like haloperidol, lorazepam or oxazepam.

(4) The inability to confirm in man that plasma concentration reflects the concentration at receptor sites. When the drug has an active transport mechanism, the plasma concentration will clearly not reflect that at the receptor site.

(5) The selection of patients, their diagnosis and subtyping, or the choice of outcome criteria may be irrelevant. Furthermore, the measures available, e.g. the rating scales, may lack precision. The absence of data about the rate of spontaneous remissions is another factor which can make the interpretation of such studies difficult.

In practice, lithium is the only psychotropic drug whose plasma concentrations are routinely monitored because a correlation exists between plasma concentrations and clinical responses. Furthermore, there is a narrow range between therapeutic and toxic levels of the drug. For other psychotropic drugs the measurement of plasma concentrations will only be helpful in some particular situations, summarized in *Table 2.3*.

TABLE 2.3 Main reasons for the monitoring of psychotropic drugs

Therapeutic failure at usual dosages.
Exaggerated adverse drug reaction at usual dosages.
Drugs whose clinical efficacy is related to a minimum steady-state concentration.
Drugs with a narrow therapeutic range.
Diagnostic of drug intoxications.
Drugs likely to induce their own metabolism.
Evaluation of pharmacokinetic consequences of drug interactions.
Evaluation of pharmacokinetic consequences of diseases.
Necessity to maintain plasma concentrations as low as possible (children, pregnancy, coexisting disease, elderly patients).

Conclusions

In this brief review, only some of the advances in pharmacokinetics have been outlined. We have concentrated on showing that psychotropic drugs are subject to the same principles as other drugs with respect to their disposition in the body. Absorption, distribution, metabolism and excretion are all processes which can be studied and the appropriate values, e.g. for plasma half-life, assigned to each drug from a knowledge of its physiochemical and biological properties. Thus, therapy can be made more rational by ensuring that adequate drug concentrations reach the presumed site of action.

Nevertheless, psychotropic drugs act on the most complex and highly organized organ in the body, the brain. While the biochemical and physiological mechanisms associated with various forms of mental illness remain obscure, the mode of action of the majority of psychotropic drugs also remains obscure. Luckily, we have discovered, mostly by accident, a series of drugs more or less effective in many psychiatric conditions. Until rational treatments are developed, however, we can at least use our empirical therapies in as logical a way as possible. The most important consideration is that we constantly bear in mind the fact that we are using drugs, and that these drugs are capable of being studied. Both the pharmacokinetics and the pharmacodynamics of the important psychotropic drugs should be part of the clinical working knowledge of the psychiatrist.

References

BALDESSARINI, R. J. Status of psychotropic drug blood level assays and other biochemical measurements in clinical practice, *American Journal of Psychiatry* **136**, 1177–1180 (1980)

BENET, L. Z. and SHEINER, L. B. Design and optimization of dosage regimens; pharmacokinetic data. In Goodman and Gilman's, *The Pharmacological Basis of Therapeutics*, 6th edn, p. 1675–1737, MacMillan, New York (1980)

BURROWS, G. D. and NORMAN, T. R. (Eds.). *Psychotropic Drugs. Plasma Concentration and Clinical Response*, Marcel Dekker, New York (1981)

CIBA FOUNDATION SYMPOSIUM 74 (New Series). *Drug Concentrations in Neuropsychiatry*, Excerpta Medica, Amsterdam (1980)

CURRY, S. H. *Drug Disposition and Pharmacokinetics. With a Consideration of Pharmacological and Clinical Relationship*, 2nd edn, Blackwell Scientific Publications, Oxford (1977)

DANHOF, M. and BREIMER, D. D. Therapeutic drug monitoring in saliva, *Clinical Pharmacokinetics* **3**, 39–57 (1978)

GIBALDI, M. *Biopharmaceutics and Clinical Pharmacokinetics*, 2nd edn, Lea and Febiger, Philadelphia (1977)

GOTTSCHALK, L. A. and MERLIS, S. (Eds.). *Pharmacokinetics of Psychoactive Drugs: Blood Levels and Clinical Response*, Spectrum Publications, New York (1976)

GREENBLATT, D. J. and KOCH-WESER, J. Clinical pharmacokinetics (in two parts), *New England Journal of Medicine*, 702–705 and 964–970 (1975)

KOCH-WESER, J. Bioavailability of drugs (in two parts), *New England Journal of Medicine* **291**, 233–237 and 503–506 (1974)

KOCH-WESER, J. and SELLERS, E. M. Binding of drugs to serum albumin (in two parts), *New England Journal of Medicine* **294**, 311–316 and 526–530 (1976)

KRISTENSEN, M. B. Drug interactions and clinical pharmacokinetics, *Clinical pharmacokinetics* **1**, 351–372 (1976)

LADER, M. Clinical psychopharmacology. In *Recent Advances in Clinical Psychiatry* (vol. 2), p. 1–30 (Ed. K. GRANVILLE-GROSSMAN), Churchill Livingstone, London (1976)

LADER, M. Biological monitoring of psychotropic drug treatment: usefulness and limitations. In *Neuropsychopharmacology* (Eds. B. SALETU *et al.*) p. 585–590, Pergamon Press, Oxford (1979)

MARKS, V. Clinical monitoring of therapeutic drugs, *Annals of Clinical Biochemistry* **16**, 370–379 (1979)

MELANDER, A. Influence of food and the bioavailability of drugs, *Clinical Pharmacokinetics* **3**, 337–351 (1978)

MORSELLI, P. L., CUCHE, H. and ZARIFIAN, E. Pharmacokinetics of psychotropic drugs in the pediatric patient, *Advances in Biological Psychiatry* **2**, 70–86 (1978)

PIAFSKY, K. M. Disease-induced changes in the plasma binding of basic drugs, *Clinical Pharmacokinetics* **5**, 246–262 (1980)

POTTER, W. Z., BERTILSSON, L. and SJÖQVIST, F. Clinical pharmacokinetics of psychotropic drugs. Fundamental and practical aspects. In *Handbook of Biological Psychiatry* 6, 71–134 (1981)

RAWLINS, M. D. Variability in response to drugs, *British Medical Journal* **4**, 91–94 (1974)

SCHOOLAR, J. C. and CLAGHORN, J. L. (Eds.). *The Kinetics of Psychiatric Drugs*, Brunner Mazel, New York (1979)

SCHUMACHER, G. E. Use of pharmacokinetic principles in drug therapy: a suggested topic outline and reading list, *American Journal of Hospital Pharmacy* **33**, 590–595 (1976)

SHADER, R. I. and GREENBLATT, D. J. Clinical indications for plasma level monitoring of psychotropic drugs, *American Journal of Psychiatry* **136**, 1590–1591 (1979)

TILLEMENT, J. P., LHOSTE, F. and GIUDICELLI, J. F. Diseases and drug protein binding, *Clinical Pharmacokinetics* **3**, 144–154 (1978)

WILLIAMS, R. L. and MAMELOK, R. D. Hepatic disease and drug pharmacokinetics, *Clinical Pharmacokinetics* **5**, 528–547 (1980)

Chapter 3

Evaluation of psychotropic drugs

P. J. Tyrer

It is important for those who prescribe psychotropic drugs to know something about their evaluation. This is not a 'cut-and-dried' issue; all drugs reach the clinician in a stage of imperfect knowledge about their pharmacological effects. Evaluation constantly accompanies use and even when a drug has been established for many years it can still produce surprises, as, for example, in the case of tardive dyskinesia following long-term antipsychotic drug therapy. In one sense every doctor who prescribes a drug is also evaluating it. When assessing the value and risks of a new drug one has to know what stage of evaluation this has reached, otherwise fair comparisons cannot be made. These stages are

(1) animal studies,
(2) experimental studies in volunteers,
(3) experimental studies in patients,
(4) clinical trials,
(5) marketing,
(6) short-term clinical evaluation,
(7) long-term clinical evaluation.

Animal studies

When a new drug has been discovered its effects need to be evaluated in animals before it can be introduced to man. Psychotropic drugs are more difficult to test than most others, because there are no really satisfactory animal models of mental disorders. Nevertheless animal studies have proved invaluable, both in screening new drugs that might be considered to have psychotropic effects, and to provide a profile of pharmacological activity of drugs that are sufficiently promising to test further. To date, animal studies have not been particularly helpful in making major breakthroughs in psychotropic drug treatment which have almost all followed from clinical observations, but they have been essential in testing the many compounds that are considered to have psychotropic activity.

It is beyond the scope of this chapter to go into details of the types of animal studies used in initial testing of drugs but a crude subdivision is shown in *Table 3.1*. More detailed discussion of these tests and their limitations in interpreting the findings in

TABLE 3.1 Some common screening tests in animal psychopharmacology

Drug type	Screening test in animals	Significance
Antipsychotic drugs	Reduction of spontaneous activity and exploratory behaviour	Linked to extrapyramidal side effects and dopamine blockade
	Produce hypothermia	Hypothalamic effects
	Antagonism of dexamphetamine and apomorphine toxicity	independent of antipsychotic ones
Antianxiety drugs	Increase in spontaneous activity and exploratory behaviour	Spontaneous activity and exploration are suppressed, and
	Reduction in conditioned avoidance behaviour	avoidance behaviour increased by anxiety, so change indicates antianxiety effects
Antidepressants	Antagonism of tetrabenazine and reserpine sedation and hypothermia	Both measures of increased central monoamines available for neurotransmission
	Potentiation of pyrexia produced by noradrenaline	
Monoamine oxidase	Antagonism of tetrabenazine and reserpine sedation and hypothermia	As for antidepressants
	Potentiation of amines	Important in assessing food and drug interaction
Lithium carbonate	No appropriate test to evaluate prophylactic action in affective disorder	
Drugs of addiction	Increase in self-stimulation and drug-seeking behaviour	Equivalent to drug-seeking behaviour in man

human mental disorder are to be found elsewhere (Maxwell, 1968; Kumar, 1976; Spencer, 1976; Mackay, 1981).

Although many of the tests in laboratory animals mimic their use in man there are many others that bear no relation to the use of the drugs in clinical practice. The giving of drugs to produce abnormal behaviour, which is then altered by giving the drug under test, is an acceptable form of screening but not a good animal model of mental disorder. Thus the ability of antidepressants to potentiate the convulsant activity of a drug such as picrotoxin is common to almost all members of the group but has nothing to do with their antidepressant effects. It reflects the tendency of antidepressants in man to be epileptogenic and is normally correlated with antidepressant effects. But when an antidepressant is discovered which has no epileptogenic properties, such as nomifensine, the picrotoxin test is negative even though antidepressant efficacy is well established clinically.

For this reason no animal pharmacologist will be rash enough to predict the possible clinical effects of a drug from one test alone. A profile of activity is established from a battery of experiments and this enables some conclusions to be drawn about the area of clinical interest. The animal studies cannot really be more specific than that in terms of potential clinical efficacy. Where they are more accurate is in predicting and testing toxicity. In most countries there now exists strict controls on the testing of new drugs so that no new compound can be released for experiments in man until it has been cleared of toxic effects in therapeutic dosage. Both acute and chronic toxicity, teratogenicity and effect on fertility require evaluation; these are complex and expensive procedures (Greenwood and Todd, 1977). The thalidomide tragedy is the most notorious of earlier failures to take these precautions before clinical use, but there have been many others, including the failure to detect the food and drug interactions of monoamine oxidase inhibitors before they were used in clinical practice (Doll, 1969).

Animal studies are also valuable in what could be called the post-evaluation phase of psychotropic drug use. Whether or not a drug proves to be valuable in clinical use it may still be a valuable experimental tool in research work. Reserpine now has little use in medicine and none at all in psychiatry yet it is universally used in animal testing of psychotropic drugs. Animal studies may also be useful in determining the mechanism of action of drugs in producing both desired and unwanted effects and have proved to be useful models of clinical syndromes such as tardive dyskinesia (Clow *et al.*, 1979). There are also some drugs, still regrettably few to those who believe in scientific medicine, that have been introduced from pharmacological deduction rather than clinical serendipity. Levodopa was introduced to treat Parkinson's disease after it was established that there was dopamine deficiency in the nigrostriatal area of the brain in the disease. L-Tryptophan was similarly introduced into psychiatry as an antidepressant on pharmacological grounds and has proved to be of some value (*see* Chapter 9). These developments have followed from neurochemical rather than behavioural evidence and it seems likely that the clinicians of the future will look increasingly to the neurochemist for guidance on his use of psychotropic drugs. At present we still have far to go before the links between laboratory and prescription are constant and predictable. The recent exciting discovery of the opioid peptides (Hughes *et al.*, 1975) is a case in point. Although the discovery of these peptides and their important analgesic activity must be relevant to psychiatric practice their use to date has been frustrating and disappointing and there are as yet no clinical indications for their use (Verebey, Volavka and Clouet, 1978).

Experimental studies in volunteers

Before psychotropic drugs are given to patients it is common for volunteers to take them in acute dosage, and often in chronic dosage as well. This is usually considered necessary by clinical investigators (Blackwell, 1972) although there are sound arguments for missing out volunteers and using the drug with the patients who have the illness requiring treatment (Oates, 1972). There are several reasons for choosing volunteers, including much greater control of experimental design, ethical ones (patients should not be asked to take a new drug until it has been shown to be safe in man) and the assessment of unwanted effects and appropriate dosage levels for clinical response. These are matters that cannot be decided in the rat or other animals; the considerable inter-species differences in drug response make it essential for the clinical investigator to re-test in man before deciding on appropriate dosage.

There are problems with studies in volunteers that make interpretation of the findings difficult. One is that volunteers do not constitute a random sample of the population. They often become involved for curious psychopathological reasons. In one early study of 56 volunteers for a psychopharmacological study Lasagna and Felsinger (1954) found 15 to be psychiatrically ill (12 with neuroses, three with psychoses), three to have personality disorders and one to have a severe peptic ulcer. It is perhaps predictable that those who volunteer to take psychotropic drugs have some personal interest in the subject and are rarely innocents abroad. Nevertheless, there are at best only dilatory attempts to screen volunteers and exclude these who might be considered unrepresentative of the population at large. Generalizations are naturally made from volunteer studies as though the participants constituted a random sample. Whilst subjective measurements are still such an important part of assessment of psychotropic effects every attempt should be made to make the population tested as homogeneous as possible and this applies as much to volunteers as to patients.

A more serious criticism of results from volunteer studies is that they may be quite different from the same studies carried out with patients. This is self-evident when looking at the major clinical effects of the drug so that improvement in mood would not be expected in a normal subject taking an antidepressant, but it is also true of unwanted effects. It is also assumed that if unwanted effects are demonstrated in volunteers the same effects will be shown by patients. This can lead to mistaken conclusions, as for example in the study of hangover effects of hypnotics. In 1970 it was reported that single doses of nitrazepam and amylobarbitone sodium produced significant impairment on behavioural tests (and altered EEG frequency) 18 h afterwards (i.e. hangover effects persisted for most of the following day) (Malpas et al., 1970). Soon afterwards Betts and his colleagues (1972) showed significant impairment of driving skills after single doses of similar hypnotics in an ingenious experiment in which subjects carried out driving manoeuvres on a special track. Both these studies were widely reported and quoted to illustrate the dangers of hypnotics in impairing judgement and competence. In 1974, however, Malpas and her colleagues repeated their original study except that subjects took their hypnotics for seven nights instead of one only. This time there were no differences in hangover effects between nitrazepam, amylobarbitone sodium and placebo and the EEG differences were only one-fifth of those found in the earlier study. Although some of the discrepancy between the findings of the two studies could be explained by the development of tolerance following repeated dosage, the important difference was that the second study was with patients and the first was with volunteers. As it is the patients who take these drugs it is much more appropriate to rely on the findings with them than to extrapolate from studies with volunteers, particularly when in this instance, the volunteer findings aroused such alarm.

Another source of concern is over the status of so-called volunteers, as they are often induced to take part or are just 'drafted'. This can give rise to ethical problems. For example, for many years the Addiction Research Centre in Kentucky, USA, used volunteers serving prison sentences for drug offences to test the effects of hallucinogens and other potentially addictive drugs. Although it is often easy to induce people to volunteer for such experiments when they constitute a captive population, particularly when taking part may lead to concessions in prison or early parole, it does not follow the principle of informed consent. Bearing in mind that experiments with hallucinogens carry serious long-term risks (Cohen and Ditman, 1963) this use of volunteers would not pass any ethical committee nowadays. Perhaps most volunteers in drug studies are employees of the pharmaceutical companies or of the clinical institutes testing new drugs. It is difficult to know to what extent such participants are genuine volunteers, with a real wish to test out some of the products they are involved with manufacturing or marketing, or are reluctant volunteers, who only come forward because they feel it will count against them if they do not.

One way around these problems is to have a register of volunteers which is vetted by an independent agency so that inappropriate people do not take part. In the UK this has repeatedly been advocated by Professor Paul Turner of St Bartholomew's Hospital but has not received official approval. Another suggestion has been to involve local ethical committees in the assessment of all studies with human subjects, and to give particular attention to the inducements made to volunteers, medical screening and assessment of the scientific merits of the study as well as ethical ones (Smith, 1975). Because volunteer studies are not subject to the same jurisdiction as research studies with patients the legal liability is not spelt out in the same way. For this reason it is better to obtain written consent and, sometimes, a formal contract is signed to protect the volunteer.

Despite these reservations about the use of volunteers it seems likely that no alternatives will be available in the forseeable future. Provided that volunteers are recruited ethically and involved in experimental studies which are properly designed to answer strict pharmacological and pharmacokinetic questions rather than ones of clinical efficacy, their use is justified. Volunteer studies and the first experimental ones in patients together constitute Phase 1 studies.

Experimental studies in patients

The first studies in patients are tentative and seldom involve controlled clinical trials. Initially small doses are used and only given singly. If all goes well higher doses near to those predicted from animal studies will be given, often in repeated dosage. Pharmacokinetic studies with measurement of plasma levels are common and with some drugs administration of radioactively labelled compounds (with short half-lives) may enable a fuller pharmacokinetic profile of distribution, metabolism and excretion to be made. Ethical problems may also arise here and proper consent must be obtained.

If these studies establish that the new drug is safe and its clinical pharmacology can be predicted it will then be used in open clinical studies. Patients with a disorder suitable for treatment with the drug will receive the compound for the appropriate length of time for clinical response to be noted. At this stage flexibility is important and the duration of treatment and dosage may be altered with different groups of patients. There are many restrictions in these studies; children, the elderly and women of childbearing age are usually excluded. In the UK a Clinical Trial Certificate has to be obtained before a drug is released for use with patients and this is by no means automatic. The pharmacology and chemistry of the drug, and its use to date in animals and man has to be submitted together with a full protocol of the proposed clinical work. According to the International Federation of Pharmaceutical Manufacturers' Associations (1975) the UK requires more scientific information before a trial certificate is granted than any other country, but most developed countries have similar, but sometimes less stringent, requirements with the exception of Japan, which does not require formal submissions before a clinical trial of a psychotropic drug is undertaken.

Early clinical trials

The first open studies with patients are primarily needed to establish dosage, duration of treatment and safety. Once these have been completed satisfactorily more formal trials can be begun. These are at first uncontrolled and cover a range of possible uses as well as different dosage regimens. For example, a new antianxiety drug is likely to be evaluated as a hypnotic by taking it as a single dose at night, as an anxiolytic by taking it (in lower dosage) during the day, as a possible therapy for alcohol and drug withdrawal states, and in lower dosage as a sedative in psychogeriatrics. The results will be a rough pointer towards its future clinical indications, although this is sometimes decided in advance by information derived from market research rather than clinical pharmacology. A range of unwanted effects will also be detected in the studies and the dosage range may need to be revised.

This stage of the investigation of the drug moves outside the portals of the pharmaceutical companies and pharmacological institutes to the places where the consumer is usually seen. Because most patients are seen in general practice it is very common for general practitioners to be involved in these early clinical trials. Because general practitioners are quite independent of the drug industry and do their work in addition to their normal clinical practice, these studies are not under the same rigorous controls as earlier ones. There has been some criticism of the quality of this work and a few isolated instances of abuse in that fictional patients and results are manufactured to fill the practitioner's 'quota'. It would be unfair to criticize the pharmaceutical industry too harshly over these incidents. There is a bottleneck at the clinical testing stage of drug evaluation because relatively few doctors are trained clinical investigators, but a better system needs to be devised. Nevertheless, assessment by general practitioners can be a very important part of evaluation if it is done by the right people. Although it is common practice to include standard rating scales in such assessments it is often preferable to allow the practitioner to widen the scope of his evaluation to detect all forms of change, both unexpected and predicted. The good general practitioner knows his patients well and is best placed to make these judgements. As one authority, who is both a clinical investigator and a general practitioner, comments 'we are highly sensitive assessors in much the same way as a mother is a highly sensitive assessor of a child' (Salkind, 1976), and it is no coincidence that so many new drug effects are detected in the general practitioner's surgery rather than in the hospital clinic. This is particularly true of Type B (bizarre) adverse reactions that are qualitatively abnormal and pharmacologically unexpected (Rawlins, 1981).

Later in these investigations, which formally constitute Phase 2 of clinical studies, controlled trials are initiated. These compare the new drug with existing drug therapies and often with placebo in appropriate disorders. In the UK, the General Practitioner Research Group under Dr David Wheatley is one of the main bodies involved in these studies.

Controlled clinical trials

Although controlled trials are often used in Phase 2 studies of drug evaluation they are the essential part of Phase 3 studies, which place the new drug on the therapeutic map. The aim of most controlled trials in evaluation is to test the efficacy of the new drug against no treatment and against established drug therapy. Thus the aim of the trial is quite straightforward but for mainly ethical reasons such trials have aroused controversy. Joyce (1968) has compared them with the town-dweller's pig, an animal that is highly useful but whose activities always seem to lead to criticism from others. The ethical concern mainly stems from placebo-controlled trials. In scientific terms a 'no treatment' group in psychopharmacology has to be a placebo group, because the power of the placebo is considerable. If patients think they are getting an active treatment they are likely to improve, particularly if they have such disorders as anxiety, mild depression or psychosomatic conditions. Giving them a placebo tablet is considered to be necessary deceit in order to allow for this (non-pharmacological) effect in the new drug under test.

It is now taken for granted that a drug has not proved its therapeutic worth until at least one well designed controlled trial has shown it to be superior in efficacy to placebo. What is often not appreciated by those who criticize drug treatment in psychiatry is that no other branch of psychiatry has such an effective means of separating the valuable wheat of therapeutic merit from the redundant chaff of useless remedy. Behaviour therapy, psychotherapy, social skills training, other physical treatments such as ECT and milieu therapy depending primarily on setting rather than specific treatment, all have difficulties in adjusting to double-blind procedure and have some of the disadvantages of 'open' trials (*Table 3.2*). Although it is often possible to use single-blind procedure in evaluation, with one party, usually the assessing therapist, ignorant of the nature of therapy, the patient normally has to be aware of the treatment. He will often detect (i.e. break the blind) of 'dummy' treatments which superficially look like active therapy but have no systematic content. If the patient can differentiate between active and controlled therapy it is easy for the information to be passed on to the assessor, covertly or openly, and thereby involve the bias of the assessor when he makes his judgement. This bias is a very significant component of apparent outcome; in psychiatric treatment more so than most others the truism applies of the investigator finding what he expects to find. So the patient, who improves but should have failed to respond to an expected inferior treatment, is mysteriously removed from the final analyses on grounds of 'suitability' and others who seem to have got worse in the eyes of everybody else somehow get impressive ratings of improvement if the treatment is thought by the assessor to be a good one. To the outsider this appears to be fiddling the results. It may be, but it is more common for investigators to be unaware of the extent to which their therapeutic prejudices are exposed.

A properly designed double-blind trial is free from these sources of error, but proper design is often expensive and time-consuming. Above all, it involves commitment by the participants. Drug trials are growing at an alarming rate and it is difficult to believe that they all involve committed investigators who will always carry out procedures

TABLE 3.2 Main differences between controlled double-blind and open trials

Open trial (uncontrolled)	Controlled double-blind trial
Assesses safety and unwanted effects primarily	Assesses efficacy primarily
Does not allow for non-pharmacological factors responsible for improvement	By using a placebo control group non-pharmacological factors are compensated
Usually few criteria for entry	Strict criteria for entry to ensure a homogeneous sample
Improvement measured by change from initial ratings	Improvement measured by relative difference in improvement between active and control groups
Random selection preferable	Random selection essential so that groups are comparable
Bias may be present	Bias removed if neither patient nor doctor breaks the double blind

painstakingly in order to arrive at the truth. A bad double-blind trial is worse than no trial at all; it gives a spurious impression of authority that will only mislead.

There are many types of clinical trial and those interested in the range and advantages of different approaches are referred to Johnson and Johnson (1977). In principle, multicentre trials involving many participants are preferable, but they often suffer through lack of commitment (*Lancet*, 1981) and are hardly appropriate for rapid evaluation. Some designs yield more rapid results than others, such as sequential analysis, and others, such as cross-over designs, may be necessary if it is felt that all patients should be exposed to an active treatment.

Different designs, if selected and carried out appropriately, will still allow comparable results. The important results to the practising clinician are the differences in efficacy between two or more treatments. Superiority of a new drug over placebo has to be established, preferably before it is compared with other active treatments, although ethical concern may prevent a full placebo-controlled trial being carried out in conditions such as severe depressive illness because of the suicide risk. If later studies show the new drug to be equivalent in efficacy to an established drug for the disorder this may not mean what it implies, that there are no therapeutic differences between the two drugs. The absence of measurable differences could be a consequence of poor design or selection, insufficient patients, untrained assessors or incompetent statistical analysis. As there are few ethical problems in comparing one supposed effective treatment with another, such trials are more popular even though interpretation of their results is more difficult. These factors are relevant when it comes to interpreting the published trials of a newly introduced drug, particularly as so much of the information available is provided by the manufacturers of the compound.

Marketing

The pharmaceutical industry, like all private industry in a capitalist society, is governed by profit and loss. Only about 1 in 3500 drugs synthesized actually gets as far as a controlled clinical trial and less than 1 in 20 of them will be marketed. There is therefore a tremendous amount invested in the launch of each new drug, and nowadays the success or failure of one compound can make or break a company. A successful launch can only come through successful marketing; the clinician must be persuaded to use the drug in at least a few patients otherwise the compound is bound to fail. Marketing has now become a science with its origins in psychology and is highly sophisticated. It is important to realize that a drug's initial success is as much related to the quality of its marketing as its intrinsic therapeutic merits. Successful marketing involves good presentation or 'packaging' and the right blend of conviction, novelty and honesty. Pharmaceutical manufacturers do not falsely misrepresent their products but they do present them in their most favourable light, and this will have the maximum impact if it also appears to be objective. The published word has lost a great deal of its impact in marketing and the pharmaceutical representative is often the key to persuasion.

The aim of marketing, to sell the product, and the aim of therapeutics, to find the best remedy, may coincide but do so less often than we would like. In psychopharmacology there are innumerable examples of drugs littering the pages of pharmacopoeias that have no right to be there, either because they are expensive placebos with no significant pharmacological value or because they are replicas of earlier compounds that have proved to be successful. The dangerous compounds have been weeded out by the Committee on Safety of Medicines in the UK and equivalent regulatory bodies in other countries, but there are no restrictions on the introduction of 'me-too' drugs (*Drug and Therapeutics Bulletin*, 1976) that masquerade as advances and only confuse the practitioner. The drug salesman is not unduly concerned about this; as long as he can get the new drug selling well it matters little about the clinical significance of the introduction. Doctors have no reason to criticize his attitude, but it shows that they should be vigilant and well informed so that they can detect the unnecessary drugs. Once this is done the drugs need no longer be prescribed: the sales will fall and the company will withdraw the drug from the market, so once again clinical and marketing policy will coincide.

Each unnecessary drug on the market reflects inadequate medical training as much as overzealous marketing. By far the greatest proportion of psychotropic drugs are prescribed by general practitioners, and as these drugs are prescribed more than any other group (Skegg, Doll and Perry, 1977) they represent a large part of the commercial market. It is therefore natural for the marketing men to direct a great deal of promotional material towards general practitioners, who respond by prescribing energetically if not always appropriately (Tyrer, 1978). Psychiatrists and medical schools can only reverse this trend by giving more attention to psychotropic drug treatment in the medical curriculum and by keeping general practitioners up to date once they have completed their training. Exhortation to the pharmaceutical industry to take more note of their 'ethical' label and spend less on advertising and promotion will get nowhere whilst the commercial return on these activities greatly exceed their cost (Comanor and Wilson, 1967). If those in the medical profession fail to grasp the nettle governments will do it for them, in a cruder and less appropriate way.

Early and late clinical evaluation

Once a drug is accepted as having therapeutic value by clinicians it will sell itself (although continued advertising will usually increase its share of the market). Clinical experience in practice continues to be the most valuable source of information about a drug, because although it is less economical in terms of time and numbers of patients studied in the controlled clinical trial, it encompasses a broader range so that unexpected benefits and disadvantages of the drug are detected. Not all these later observations prove to be correct and many have to be put to the test of a controlled trial, but much more is discovered about a new drug after its introduction to general clinical practice than is known before.

There is a general rule that needs to be borne in mind when assessing the merits of drugs in clinical practice; a compound cannot be regarded as definitely safe or indubitably effective until it has been in use for at least ten years. The longer a drug is on the market the less popular it is likely to be as later discoveries tend to be in the field of unwanted rather than desired effects. If a drug is to satisfy the requirements of marketing the initial toxicological tests have to be satisfactory and most drugs start their clinical life with a 'good press'. Later the constant trickle of adverse reports and qualifications about their use bring them down to the level of the other drugs that preceded them, or, if the adverse effects are particularly serious, lead to the drugs being withdrawn from clinical use. Teratogenic adverse effects and those that only develop after chronic use are particularly difficult to detect in early studies, as are the type B (bizarre) effects of drugs (Rawlins, 1981). The type A (augmented) effects are predictable from initial pharmacological testing and are dose-dependent but type B effects are only detected by keen observation and deduction. In the UK doctors are advised to report all suspected adverse effects on yellow cards to the Committee on Safety of Medicines, and similar systems exist in other countries.

In choosing a drug it is therefore important to know what stage it has reached in its life history. If one reads heady reports of a major advance in treatment and finds that the drug has only just been introduced, it is fair to treat the claim with some scepticism. We live in an age in which novelty is mistaken for progress and psychopharmacology has often been a victim. There is another reason for not abandoning the well-tried and tested drugs prematurely. The proper use of each drug requires knowledge of not only its clinical effects and indications, but also its unwanted effects in acute and chronic dosage, its interactions with other drugs, its full dosage range and its duration of treatment. This information is not obtained overnight and the doctor who concentrates on using drugs that he knows well will ensure greater confidence, compliance and clinical response in his patients than his colleague who is superficially more informed and up to date, but whose prescribing practice is fickle and disorganized, responding to every breath of promotional wind that blows across his surgery.

References

BETTS, T. A., CLAYTON, A. B. and MACKAY, G. M. Effects of four commonly-used tranquillizers on low speed driving performance tests, *British Medical Journal* **4**, 580–584 (1972)

BLACKWELL, B. For the first time in man, *Clinical and Pharmaceutical Therapy* **13**, 813–823 (1972)

BLACKWELL, B. and SHEPHERD, M. Early evaluation of psychotropic drugs in man: a trial that failed, *Lancet* **2**, 819–822 (1967)

CLOW, A., JENNER, P., THEODOROU, A. and MARSDEN, C. D. Striatal dopamine receptors become super-sensitive when rats are given trifluoperazine for six months, *Nature* **278**, 59–61 (1979)

COHEN, S. and DITMAN, K. S. Prolonged adverse reactions to lysergic acid diethylamide, *Archives in General Psychiatry* **8**, 475–480 (1963)

COMANOR, W. S. and WILSON, T. A. Advertising, market structure and performance, *Review of Economics and Statistics* **49**, 423–440 (1967)

DOLL, R. Recognition of unwanted drug effects, *British Medical Journal* **2**, 69–76 (1969)

DRUG AND THERAPEUTICS BULLETIN. The Medicines Act and 'me-too' drugs **14**, 65–66 (1976)

GREENWOOD, D. T. and TODD, A. H. From laboratory to clinical use. In *Clinical Trials* (Eds. F. N. JOHNSON and S. JOHNSON), pp. 13–35, Blackwell, Oxford (1977)

HUGHES, J., SMITH, T. W., KOSTERLITZ, H. W., FOTHERGILL, L. A., MORGAN, B. A. and MORRIS, H. R. Identification of two related pentapeptides from the brain with potent opiate agonist activity, *Nature* **258**, 577–579 (1975)

INTERNATIONAL FEDERATION OF PHARMACEUTICAL MANUFACTURERS' ASSOCIATIONS. *Requirements for Drug Registration*, IFMPA, Zurich (1975)

JOHNSON, F. N. and JOHNSON, S. *Clinical Trials*, Blackwell, Oxford (1977)

JOYCE, C. R. B. Psychological factors in the controlled evaluation of therapy. In *Psychopharmacology: Dimensions and Perspectives* (Ed. C. R. B. JOYCE), pp. 215–242, Tavistock, London (1968)

KUMAR, R. Animal models for screening new agents: a behavioural view, *British Journal of Clinical Pharmacology* **3**, Suppl. 1, 13–17 (1976)

LANCET. Multicentre depression (Editorial), *Lancet* **2**, 564 (1981)

LASAGNA, L. and VON FELSINGER, J. M. The volunteer subject in research, *Science* **120**, 359–361 (1954)

MACKAY, A. V. P. Assessment of antipsychotic drugs, *British Journal of Clinical Pharmacology* **11**, 225–236 (1981)

MALPAS, A., ROWAN, A. J., JOYCE, C. R. B. and SCOTT, D. F. Persistent behavioural and electroencephalographic changes after single doses of nitrazepam and amylobarbitone sodium, *British Medical Journal* **2**, 762–765 (1970)

MALPAS, A., LEGG, N. J. and SCOTT, D. F. Effects of hypnotics on anxious patients, *British Journal of Psychiatry* **124**, 482–484 (1974)

MAXWELL, D. R. Principles of animal experimentation in psychopharmacology. In *Psychopharmacology: Dimensions and Perspectives* (Ed. C. R. B. JOYCE), 57–93, Tavistock, London (1968)

OATES, J. A. A scientific rationale for choosing patients rather than normal subjects for Phase 1 studies, *Clinical and Pharmaceutical Therapy* **13**, 809–811 (1972)

RAWLINS, M. D. Clinical pharmacology: adverse reactions to drugs, *British Medical Journal* **282**, 974–976 (1981)

SALKIND, M. R. Assessment of drugs in general practice, *British Journal of Clinical Pharmacology* **3**, Suppl. 1, 69–72 (1976)

SKEGG, D. C. G., DOLL, R. and PERRY, J. Use of medicines in general practice, *British Medical Journal* **1**, 1561–1563 (1977)

SMITH, R. N. Safeguards for healthy volunteers in drug studies, *Lancet* **2**, 449–450 (1975)

SPENCER, P. S. J. Animal models for screening new agents, *British Journal of Clinical Pharmacology* **3**, Suppl. 1, 5–12 (1976)

TYRER, P. Drug treatment of psychiatric patients in general practice, *British Medical Journal* **2**, 1008–1010 (1978)

VEREBEY, K., VOLAVKA, J. and CLOUET, D. Endorphins in psychiatry, *Archives of General Psychiatry* **35**, 877–888 (1978)

Chapter 4

Antischizophrenic drugs

A. V. P. Mackay

Introduction

Historical perspectives

The management of pyschiatric disorders has long provided an arena for arcane practices. Ancient Greece, the birthplace of so much of the cultural heritage of western medicine, appears to have fostered a lively interest in the chemical modification of mental state. Homer reports a nameless drug, given to Helen of Troy by Polydamna, which was apparently capable of inducing tranquillity without clouding of consciousness. A glimpse of things to come perhaps, but millenia were to pass before any modern correlate of Polydamna's drug emerged to transform the treatment of the major functional psychoses. Diagnosis must precede treatment and it was during the late nineteenth and early twentieth centuries that the classification of mental disorder matured to a state compatible with specific remedies. The description and delineation of the major functional psychoses illuminated clear targets for chemotherapy in the form of manic-depressive psychosis and the schizophrenias. During the first half of the twentieth century schizophrenic patients were liable to the exhibition of several bizarre physical remedies, including the barbiturates (to induce prolonged sleep), insulin (to induce coma) and leptazol (to induce epileptiform fits). Psychiatrists could not have been accused of nihilism in matters therapeutic—everything was tried; drugs, shocks, even brain surgery. Nevertheless, disturbed wards remained distressing and long-stay wards overcrowded; psychopharmacology had as yet made no impact. The impact, when it came, was clear and indisputable and its reverberations signalled the birth of contemporary psychopharmacology (Caldwell, 1970; Hollister, 1977). The drug was chlorpromazine, the time 1952 and the place the Val-de-Grace military hospital in Paris.

The French surgeon, Laborit, had decided in 1947 that in order to control the physical reaction to surgical stress the autonomic nervous system had to be inhibited. In 1949 he began to use the antihistaminic drug promethazine for this purpose. He was struck by its central actions, observing that patients became calm and relaxed without being heavily sedated, and appeared to suffer less pain. Laborit was not satisfied however, and in collaboration with the Parisian anaesthetist Huguenard, tested a whole range of drugs active on the autonomic nervous system; the majority of them belonging to the *phenothiazine* family. Vital support in this quest came from the French drug house Specia, through their Rhone–Poulenc laboratories. They initiated a

42

systematic programme of drug synthesis and in December, 1950 one of their chemists, Charpentier, produced a phenothiazine (code number RP 4560) which was weakly antihistaminic but also adrenolytic and parasympatholytic. This was chlorpromazine, and in May of the following year Laborit was delighted to find that this new drug produced tranquillity without lowering consciousness. Laborit, a man of extra-ordinary vision, saw great potential for this drug in the management of psychiatric illness. At first the Parisian psychiatric fraternity did not agree, their recent experiences with various drugs having rendered them rather pharmacophobic.

The first psychiatrists persuaded by Laborit to use the new drug were his own colleagues at the Val-de-Grace—Hamon, Paraire and Velluz. The first psychotic patient to be treated showed dramatic improvement and the word quickly spread. It was now January, 1952 and four weeks later chlorpromazine was introduced to the nearby St Anne's psychiatric hospital where Delay, Deniker and their colleagues correctly evaluated the therapuetic importance of the drug. Results were reported at the Centennial of the Société Medico-Psychologique and the occasion was dramatic and of profound international importance. During 1952 chlorpromazine raced through the mental hospitals of France and entered Italy. A symposium in Basle in 1953 was devoted entirely to the therapeutic use of chlorpromazine and between 1953 and 1954 it had crossed the channel to the UK and the Atlantic Ocean to North America.

The discovery of the antipsychotic activity of a quite unrelated plant alkaloid, reserpine, was made at about the time chlorpromazine became available. Although this drug is not now used in the treatment of schizophrenic illness, it must be acknowledged as probably the first effective antipsychotic drug to be documented in modern times (Hollister, 1977). The parent plant from which the pure alkaloid is derived is *Rauwolfia serpentina*, a climbing shrub found in India, extracts of which were described in ancient Hindu writings as a remedy for snakebites, hypertension, insomnia and insanity. In 1931 Sen and Bose published a claim that rauwolfia was useful in the management of severely disturbed patients and over the following 20 years this claim was supported by several reports. Reserpine, the active principle, was isolated in 1952 and Kline was soon thereafter to report on its antischizophrenic activity. As it was responsible for a high incidence of depressive illness, reserpine was soon to be abandoned as a treatment for schizophrenic illness in favour of chlorpromazine and its relatives. Curiously, its place in the history of psychopharmacology is assured on account of this unwanted side effect of depression (a crucial component of the biogenic amine hypothesis for depressive illness) and also in view of its usefulness as a reliable pre-clinical pharmacological tool which can be used to deplete neuronal stores of monoamines.

In the years following the discovery of chlorpromazine there was intense activity by groups of synthetic chemists exploring the pharmacological properties of structural variants of the tricyclic phenothiazine prototype. This activity produced two families of 'second generation' antipsychotic agents—the thioxanthenes and butyrophenones which, together with the phenothiazines, were to provide the main pharmacological repertoire for the treatment of schizophrenic illness for a period of well over 20 years.

The *thioxanthene* family is structurally related to the phenothiazines. In the course of systematic work, Petersen and colleagues succeeded in synthesizing a series of tricyclic compounds with preserved antipsychotic efficacy but reduced toxicity by replacing the phenothiazine nucleus with a thioxanthene nucleus. Chlorprothixene, clopenthixol, thiothixene and flupenthixol are the thioxanthene analogues of chlorpromazine, perphenazine, thioproperazine and fluphenazine respectively (*Figures 4.1* and *4.2*).

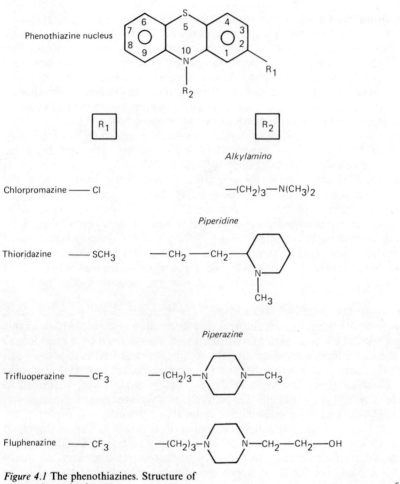

Phenothiazine nucleus
S
5
10
N
R1
R2
R1
R2
Alkylamino
Chlorpromazine —— Cl
—(CH2)3—N(CH3)2
Piperidine
Thioridazine —— SCH3
—CH2 —CH2—
N
CH3
Piperazine
Trifluoperazine —— CF3
—(CH2)3—N
N—CH3
Fluphenazine —— CF3
—(CH2)3—N
N—CH2—CH2—OH

Figure 4.1 The phenothiazines. Structure of commonly used subtypes

S
CF3
CH
CH2
CH2
N
N
CH2
CH2
OH

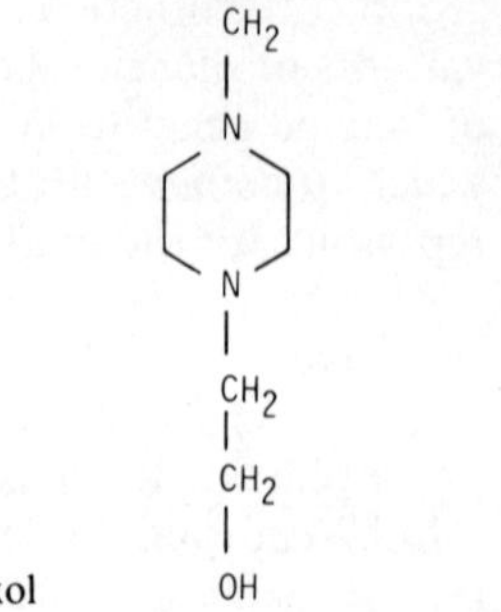

Figure 4.2 Flupenthixol

The *butyrophenones* are the most potent and among the most selective antipsychotic agents, developed almost single-handedly through the brilliant efforts of Paul Janssen at Beerse in Belgium. They were the progeny of a methodical 'production line' approach to drug development. The starting point was a bicyclic chemical (4-phenyl-4-piperidinol) from which compounds with both chlorpromazine-like and morphine-like activity evolved, and eventually emerged with relatively pure and very potent activity. Chemically quite unrelated to the phenothiazines, the haloperidol molecule (*Figure 4.3*) is structurally reminiscent of γ-aminobutyric acid (GABA).

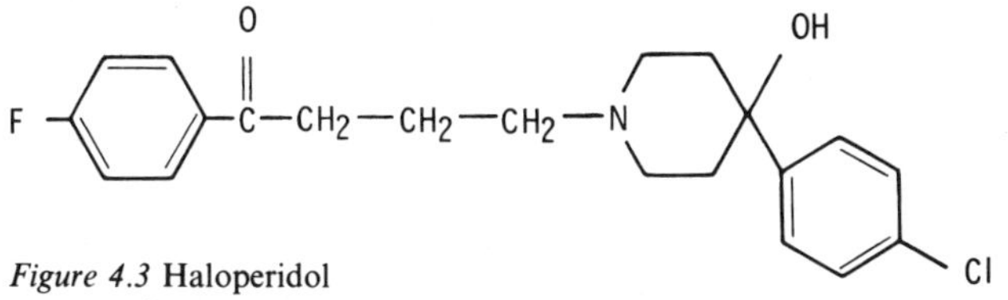

Figure 4.3 Haloperidol

Successful clinical trials of haloperidol were first reported in 1958 and by 1960 the drug was in common use in Europe.

While sporadic developments occurred in the 1960s and early 1970s, the third and most recent generation of antipsychotic drugs is still in the throes of proper clinical evaluation. Pimozide, fluspirilene and penfluridol represent a completely new class of potent and long-active drugs; derivatives of *diphenylbutylpiperidine* (*Figure 4.4*).

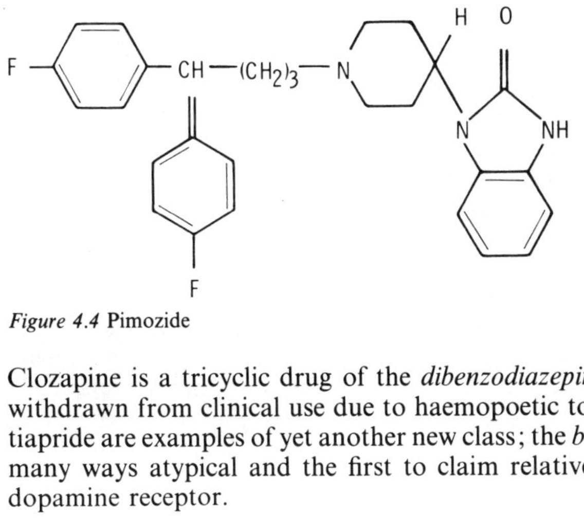

Figure 4.4 Pimozide

Clozapine is a tricyclic drug of the *dibenzodiazepine* family, but the drug has been withdrawn from clinical use due to haemopoetic toxicity. Sulpiride (*Figure 4.5*) and tiapride are examples of yet another new class; the *benzamide* derivatives, which are in many ways atypical and the first to claim relative specificity at one subspecies of dopamine receptor.

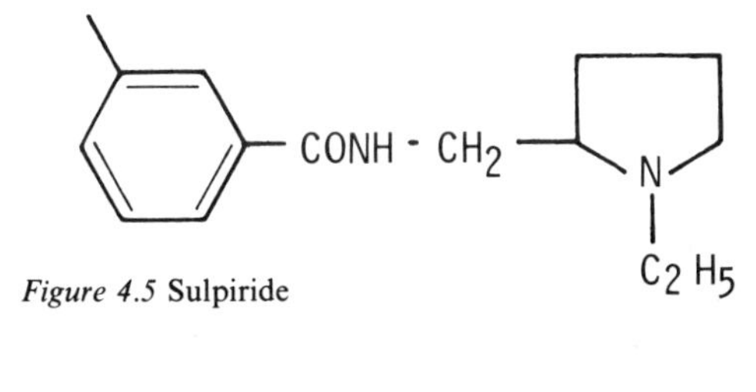

Figure 4.5 Sulpiride

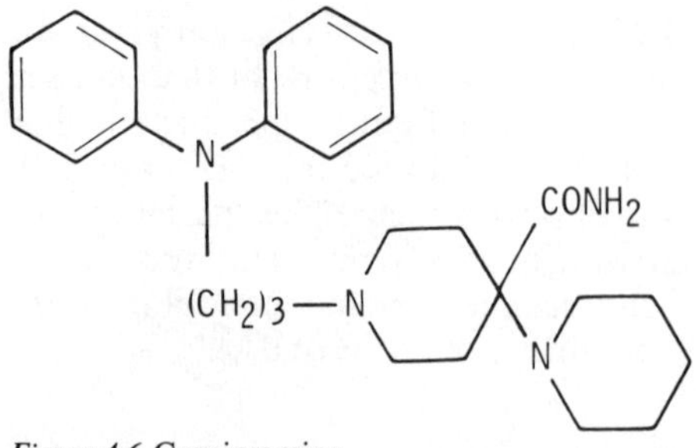

Figure 4.6 Carpipramine

It is perhaps fitting that one of the most recent developments in the general field of antischizophrenic chemotherapy brings this historical account back full circle to its starting point at the Specia drug house and to Professor Paul Deniker and his colleagues at St Anne's Hospital in Paris. Specia have produced an agent, carpipramine (*Figure 4.6*), which contains a tricyclic moiety reminiscent of imipramine but with a butyrophenone-like side-chain. The drug has a most unusual pharmacological profile and in limited preliminary studies by Deniker, carpipramine is reported to have particularly beneficial effects on certain intractable aspects of schizophrenic psychopathology (Deniker, 1978).

Nomenclature

The term 'neuroleptic' has been used to refer to the group of drugs, alternatively referred to as 'major tranquillizers' or 'ataractics', which made their debut in Europe with the introduction of chlorpromazine. Neuroleptic was the term proposed by Delay and Deniker in 1955 to the French Academy of Medicine and was derived from the term 'psycholepsis' coined by Janet for his concept of reduced psychological tension. Neuroleptic was meant to designate substances which reduced extrapyramidal function while having effects on mental state. This is a rather odd and unsatisfactory definition, depending as it does on the occurrence of neurological side effects in conjuction with psychotropic actions. In the fourth edition of Goodman and Gilman neuroleptics are described as drugs which 'cause general quiescence and a state of psychic indifference to environmental stimuli but do not produce sleep'. As Shepherd, Lader and Rodnight (1968) have pointed out, such a behavioural definition also lacks precision and scarcely covers the wide use of this group of drugs in the treatment of schizophrenia, where environmental indifference may already be a feature of the illness. The drugs were first used to reduce psychomotor excitement, then established as a symptomatic treatment for acute, and later chronic, schizophrenia. Thus terms such as 'antipsychotic' and 'antischizophrenic' agent have tended to coincide with the term 'neuroleptic', implying some specific remedial action. However, the relationship between the manifestations of schizophrenia and its pathology remains so obscure that symptomatic improvement cannot be regarded as radical treatment, and clinical evidence barely warrants the assumption of a specific antipsychotic or antischizophrenic action. While it is true that the majority of patients suffering from the acute symptoms of schizophrenic illness and paranoid psychosis will benefit from treatment with this class of drugs, so also will patients suffering from mania and from psychomotor agitation associated with affective psychoses and organic psychoses.

Thus none of the currently used terms appear to be satisfactory for the definition of agents used in the treatment of schizophrenic illness; 'neuroleptic' requires associated neurological impairment and 'antischizophrenic' perhaps misleadingly implies total specificity. In the absence of anything better, however, the terms antischizophrenic agent and antipsychotic agent will be used here interchangeably. They are preferred to the term neuroleptic since some of the drugs referred to are virtually devoid of extrapyramidal side effects. Specificity is not claimed, the terms will be used merely in a pragmatic sense in that the drugs to which they refer have been found useful in the treatment of psychotic illness in general, and schizophrenic illness in particular.

Unconventional chemotherapy

The vast majority of drugs included in this chapter can be thought of as conventional to the extent that their historical development has followed some sort of natural progression based upon the essential pharmacological ingredients of chlorpromazine. There are, however, other agents whose use in the treatment of schizophrenia could not have been predicted by accepted animal screening methods and whose pharmacology differs in fundamental respects from chlorpromazine and its many descendants. Their history is relatively short and their proper clinical evaluation is at an early stage.

β-blockers

Following an anecdotal report in 1971, interest has grown in the use of high doses of propranolol in the treatment of schizophrenic illness. Recent reports cast doubt on the efficacy of propranolol (Peet *et al.*, 1981a) and no studies to date have been carried out with other β-receptor antagonists. As a departure from conventional antischizophrenic chemotherapy this remains an area of theoretical interest, particularly in the context of arousal mechanisms, but clinical application may be premature.

Endorphin-related chemotherapy

One of the most significant developments in neurobiology of the past decade has been the demonstration that the mammalian brain, human included, contains morphine-like chemicals in the form of small proteins, or peptides, which interact with central opiate receptors. The generic name 'endorphin' has been used to describe this family of peptides and the more popular endorphins comprise met- and leu-enkephalin (5 amino-acid chain) and β-endorphin (31 amino-acid chain). The endorphins exist in discrete neuronal systems in the brain and probably perform physiological functions as neurotransmitters and neuromodulators. There is no clinical evidence for primary disturbance of central endorphin systems in the major psychoses, apart from scattered reports of diminished pain perception in chronic schizophrenic patients (Marchand, 1955; Watson, Chandarana and Merskey, 1981; Buchsbaum *et al.*, 1981). Behavioural experiments with rats have demonstrated that direct injection of endorphin material into the brain can induce motor abnormalities which have been variously interpreted as schizophrenia-like or like the extrapyramidal impairment induced by anti-schizophrenic drugs. Based upon these rather crude and diametrically opposed inferences, two broad therapeutic strategies have been assessed in schizophrenic patients. One is based upon the assumption that schizophrenic illness is associated with excessive release of endorphins, suggesting treatment with the opiate receptor antagonist naloxone. The other is based upon the assumption that schizophrenic illness is associated with reduced endorphin activity, suggesting treatment with natural endorphins or their more stable synthetic analogues (Ruther *et al.*, 1982). Neither therapeutic approach has so far proved to be of general clinical use but this remains an area of intense research activity.

The endorphin era has seen the revival of haemodialysis as a treatment for schizophrenic illness, stimulated by claims that a psychotogenic atypical endorphin (β-leu^5-endorphin) was present in excess in the blood of schizophrenic patients and that this psychotogen was dialysable (Palmour, Ervin and Wagemaker, 1977). Attempts to replicate the detection of this abnormal peptide in body fluids of schizophrenic patients have failed (Berger, 1981) and a double-blind evaluation of haemodialysis in the treatment of schizophrenia has likewise failed to reveal any therapeutic effect (Diaz-Buxo *et al.*, 1980).

Pharmacology

The dopamine hypothesis

The dopamine hypothesis states that the therapeutic actions of antischizophrenic drugs depend upon their ability to block central dopamine receptors. The formulation of this, the most coherent hypothesis for the therapeutic action of conventional antischizophrenic drugs, represents one of the most intriguing pieces of clinical pharmacological detective work in recent years. There are two lines of origin for the hypothesis. In the early 1950s the clinicians originally responsible for the therapeutic evaluation of chlorpromazine noted that parkinsonism was a common accompaniment of the antipsychotic action of the drug. This observation preceded by more than a decade the pioneering work of Hornykiewicz and his colleagues which was to demonstrate that idiopathic and post-encephalitic parkinsonism were associated with substantial degeneration of dopamine (DA)-releasing neurons in the nigrostriatal tract, leading to loss of dopaminergic transmission in the caudate-putamen. The other major source of the DA hypothesis arose out of clinical and pre-clinical observations of the effects of amphetamine psychosis. Connell (1958) was the first to suggest that a psychosis 'indistinguishable from acute or chronic paranoid schizophrenia' was a not uncommon phenomenon in habitual abusers of large doses of amphetamine. Although the facsimile may not be exact, there is general agreement that amphetamine psychosis provides the best available pharmacological model of schizophrenia (Snyder, 1973; Angrist *et al.*, 1974) and that the psychotogenic effect is due to a direct action of the drug and is not mediated through sleep deprivation or requiring a previous history of, or predisposition to, schizophrenia. Similar psychotogenic actions are observed with the DA precursor levodopa. The model psychoses induced by amphetamine and levodopa are readily reversed by antischizophrenic drugs.

AMPHETAMINE IN ANIMALS

Amphetamine has numerous behavioural actions in animals; suppressing eating, stimulating locomotor activity and, in high doses, causing striking forms of stereotyped behaviour in which the animal constantly repeats selected items from its behavioural repertoire in a meaningless fashion. Randrup and his colleagues in Denmark (for review *see* Randrup and Munkvad, 1974) first suggested that stereotyped behaviour in response to amphetamine might represent an animal model for amphetamine psychosis and schizophrenia. They also suggested that these effects of amphetamine depended critically upon an interaction of the drug with dopaminergic mechanisms in the brain.

BRAIN DA SYSTEMS AND BEHAVIOUR

DA-containing neurons are localized mainly in the midbrain. The zona compacta of the substantia nigra contains dopaminergic neurons (A-9 cell group) whose axons form the nigrostriatal tract projecting to the caudate nucleus and putamen. The globus pallidus also receives a small, but diffuse, DA innervation and the function of these various elements of the basal ganglia appear to include involuntary sensorimotor coordination and the maintenance of a balanced motor output. Medial to the substantia nigra lies another group of DA containing cells, designated A-10, which surrounds the interpeduncular nucleus and these cells (with their axonal projections) form the so-called mesolimbic and mesocortical DA systems. The former includes axonal projections to the nucleus accumbens, the olfactory area, septal nuclei and amygdala, and the latter includes projections to the frontal, cingulate and entorhinal cortex (Iversen, 1980). The functions of the mesolimbic DA system may be intimately involved in processes of behavioural arousal and motivation and the mesocortical systems appear to react to environmental stress (Iversen, 1980).

A series of careful studies, involving pharmacological and neurosurgical manipulations, has shown quite clearly that the behavioural effects of amphetamine in animals are mediated through DA. Amphetamine is known to release DA from dopaminergic neurons and the stereotyped behaviour is mediated through increased DA release in the nigrostriatal tract, whereas increased locomotor responses are mediated largely through a similar action on mesolimbic systems. These behaviours induced by amphetamines are DA-dependent and independent of any important contribution by brain noradrenaline systems (Kelly, Seviour and Iversen, 1975). The behaviours are selectively blocked by small doses of antischizophrenic drugs; indeed, the ability of a drug to block amphetamine-induced stereotypy in animals has become a standard screening test of proven predictive value in the commercial development of antischizophrenic drugs.

NEUROCHEMICAL STUDIES

More direct support for the DA hypothesis for the mode of action of antischizophrenic drugs has come from in vitro biochemical and pharmacological investigations of DA receptors. This approach was launched in 1972 by Greengard and Kebabian and their colleagues at Yale University (Kebabian, Petzold and Greengard, 1972) with the demonstration that adenylate cyclase (the enzyme which converts ATP into cyclic AMP) which is enriched in brain areas receiving DA innervation can be stimulated in vitro by the addition of DA. This proved to be a receptor-mediated stimulation and the DA-stimulated adenylate cyclase thus became the first in vitro model in which DA receptor pharmacology could be investigated directly. Results from this system showed that most conventional antischizophrenic drugs were potent DA receptor antagonists, with an order of antagonist potency roughly equal to clinical therapeutic potency. There were, however, some discrepancies; particularly with the butyrophenones, whose apparent antagonist potency in the adenylate cyclase system was far less than clinical potency would have predicted.

An even more direct assessment of DA receptor interaction with antischizophrenic drugs came from the work of Snyder and Creese and their colleagues at Johns Hopkins Medical School. With the advent of radioactively labelled DA antagonists and agonists of high specific activity it became possible to quantify precisely the affinity of antischizophrenic drugs for the DA receptor. When crude membrane preparations of

DA-innervated areas, such as the caudate nucleus, are incubated with a radioactively labelled DA receptor ligand such as ^{3}H-haloperidol, the potency with which an unlabelled antischizophrenic drug can compete with the labelled ligand for binding to the tissue is proportional to the affinity of the unlabelled drug for the DA receptor. Through the application of ligand binding studies such as these it became clear that the clinical potency of a drug as an antischizophrenic agent was very closely related to its ability to bind to DA receptors (*Figure 4.7*). There was an equally close relationship between receptor binding data and potency in the earlier animal behavioural models such as antagonism of amphetamine-induced stereotypy.

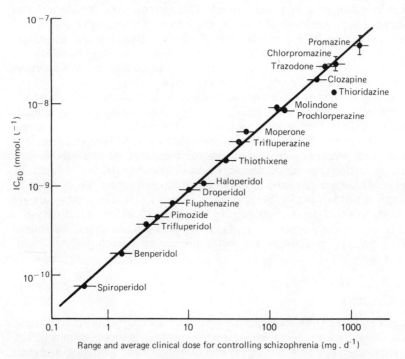

Figure 4.7 Comparison of the clinical potencies of neuroleptic drugs, measured as average daily dose in treating schizophrenia, with potencies of the same drugs in displacing ^{3}H-haloperidol from dopamine receptor binding sites *in vitro* (concentration of drug required to displace 50 per cent of specific haloperidol binding). (From Seeman *et al.*, 1976)

Although the strength of the association between DA receptor antagonism and clinical effect was persuasive support for the DA hypothesis, the compelling observation was that for no other transmitter receptor model is there a correlation at a level even approaching that seen for DA; ability to bind to receptors for noradrenaline, 5-HT and histamine has been shown to have little relationship to clinical potency (Peroutka and Snyder, 1980). The possibility of putting the DA blockade hypothesis to a stringent test in a clinical setting arose from the availability of geometrical isomers (cis: α and trans: β) of the thioxanthene flupenthixol (*see Figure 4.2*). The isomers are chemically similar and differ only in their three-dimensional configuration, a property governing receptor interaction. Only the α-isomer possesses DA receptor antagonist properties and therefore a comparison of the antischizophrenic activity of α- and

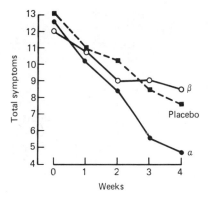

Figure 4.8 The clinical effects of α- and β-flupenthixol compared with placebo in recently admitted patients with acute schizophrenia (from Johnstone *et al.*, 1978)

β-flupenthixol provides an interesting direct test of the relationship between DA receptor blockade and antipsychotic activity. In a clinical trial of the two isomers against placebo in the treatment of acute schizophrenic illness, only the α-isomer was found to possess pharmacotherapeutic activity (Johnstone *et al.*, 1978) (*Figure 4.8*). This result rules out many alternative mechanisms of therapeutic action, including non-receptor-mediated membrane effects. While this observation on its own does not rule out an action at 5-HT receptors (the α-isomer being more active than the β-isomer as a 5-HT receptor antagonist), this mechanism seems highly unlikely in view of the complete lack of correlation between 5-HT receptor affinity and antipsychotic activity in a wide range of psychotropic drugs.

So, in summary, the ability to act as an antagonist at central DA receptors is at present the single best predictor of antischizophrenic activity of a drug.

DA receptor subtypes

It has recently become clear that DA, in keeping with the majority of its fellow neurotransmitters, interacts with more than one type of receptor in brain. Designated 'D1' and 'D2', the D1 receptor appears to be linked to adenylate cyclase activation (therefore analogous to the β-adrenergic receptor) whereas the D2 is not. Established antischizophrenic drugs (such as chlorpromazine) show little selectivity between D1 and D2 receptors and, although not completely selective, the butyrophenones show preferential affinity for the D2 receptor. A new family of antipsychotic drugs, the substituted benzamide derivatives (such as sulpiride, *see Figure 4.5*) appear to be highly selective antagonists at D2 receptors.

D1 and D2 receptors appear to co-exist in most DA-innervated areas of the brain. The only site so far shown to possess exclusively one sort is the pituitary gland, where only D2 receptors exist on mammotroph cells which react to DA released from the hypothalamus by reducing their output of prolactin. While the relative significance of D1 and D2 receptors for the antischizophrenic activity of DA antagonists can only be fully evaluated once a specific D1 antagonist is made available, it can be said at present that all of the known clinical effects of DA antagonists (including antipsychotic activity, extrapyramidal side effects and hyperprolactinaemia) can be sufficiently explained through an interaction with D2 receptors.

Non-DA-related pharmacology

With the advent of techniques to label neurotransmitter receptors in the brain by the use of radioactive ligands it has become possible to investigate directly the interaction of antischizophrenic drugs with several discrete types of receptor. In addition to a potent interaction with DA receptors, antischizophrenic drugs are also active at muscarinic acetylcholine (ACh), α-noradrenergic (NA), serotonergic and histamine H_1 receptors. In several instances these drugs are just as potent or even more potent at neurotransmitter receptor sites other than DA. While non-DA related receptor interactions do not appear to be related to general antischizophrenic activity, they undoubtedly contribute to the total clinical profile of the drug and in particular to the various side effects, both desirable and undesirable.

Anticholinergic activity

The majority of conventional antischizophrenic drugs possess the ability to block muscarinic ACh receptors in the mammalian brain, but their potency in this respect varies very widely (*Table 4.1*). Anticholinergic activity bears importantly upon two aspects of the clinical use of this group of drugs; peripheral autonomic side effects and extrapyramidal side effects.

Blockade of ACh receptors in the iris will produce blurring of vision and increased intra-ocular pressure through pupillary dilatation and similar actions in the gastro-intestinal tract and genitourinary system will produce symptoms such as dry mouth, constipation and urinary retention (*see below*).

TABLE 4.1 Relative affinities of antischizophrenic agents for muscarinic cholinergic receptor sites in brain

Drug	Affinity for muscarinic receptor	Parkinsonian side effects
Phenothiazines		
Alkylamino: chlorpromazine	10	+
Piperidine: thioridazine	119	±
Piperazine: fluphenazine	1.25	+ + + +
Thioxanthenes		
α-Flupenthixol	2.56	+ + +
Butyrophenones		
Haloperidol	1.16	+ + + +
Spiroperidol	0.6	+ + + +
Diphenylbutylpiperidines		
Pimozide	4	+ +
Dibenzodiazepines		
Clozapine	204	±
Substituted benzamides		
Sulpiride	0.06	
(Reference agent: Benztropine	4347)	

Affinity for the muscarinic receptor defined as the reciprocal $\times 10^{-5}$ of the IC-50 value, defined as the molar concentration of drug capable of inhibiting the specific binding of ^{3}H-Pr BCM to rat brain homogenates by 50 per cent. Figures calculated from the data of Fjalland, Christensen and Hythel (1977)

Transmitter interactions in the basal ganglia

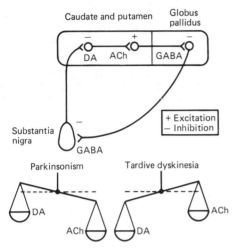

Functional consequences of changes in transmitter balance

Cholinergic interneurons in caudate and putamen are probably inhibited by nigrostriatal dopaminergic (DA) neurons. These cholinergic neurons send out short axons which ramify within caudate/putamen, releasing acetylcholine (ACh) which excites GABA-containing neurons. GABAcidic neurons provide a short-axon connection between caudate/putamen and globus pallidus from which other GABA-containing cells send long axons back to substantia nigra. Following this simple functional circuit around from substantia nigra, it will be seen that the following process occurs: increased activity in substantia nigra DA neurons *leads to* decreased activity of ACh neurons *leads to* decreased activity of short-axon GABA neurons *leads to* increased activity of long-axon GABA neurons *leads to* decreased activity of substantia nigra DA neurons

For normal extrapyramidal function the influences of DA and ACh need to be in balance. When DA transmission is substantially decreased (as in Parkinson's disease or in the face of neuroleptic drug treatment), ACh neurons are disinhibited and their activity increases. Under normal conditions the balance would be redressed through the feedback loop above, but if the imbalance is too great then pharmacological treatment may be required. Logical treatment in this case would involve either potentiating DA transmission or inhibiting ACh transmission. Conversely where DA transmission is increased (as may be the case in tardive dyskinesia) the logical pharmacological approach would be either to inhibit DA transmission or potentiate ACh transmission.

Figure 4.9 Dopamine-acetylcholine balance and extrapyramidal function (from Mackay, A. V. P., 1980)

On the other hand, anticholinergic activity in the extrapyramidal motor system may be clinically beneficial, in the short term at least. In the basal ganglia there appears to exist a reciprocal interaction between DA and ACh transmission such that a functional balance between the two is necessary for normal extrapyramidal function (*Figure 4.9*). In parkinsonism there is effectively a reduction in the relation of DA:ACh transmission due to an absolute drop in DA output. Redress of the functional balance by administration of an ACh blocker such as benztropine (Cogentin) or procyclidine (Kemadrin) will tend to restore extrapyramidal performance. All conventional antischizophrenic drugs are DA receptor blockers and at therapeutic doses will tend to induce a pharmacological facsimile of Parkinson's disease. However, with some drugs this extrapyramidal action is offset by a propensity to block ACh receptors, thus minimizing the net effect upon the ratio of DA:ACh transmission. This principle is well illustrated within the phenothiazine family in which piperidinyl compounds (such as thioridazine) rarely produce parkinsonism whereas piperizinyl compounds (such as fluphenazine and trifluoperazine) frequently produce moderate to severe extra-pyramidal impairment, with the aliphatic alkylamino compounds, such as chlor-promazine, occupying a middle position (*Table 4.1*). Therefore, as far as extra-pyramidal function is concerned, giving thioridazine is crudely equivalent to giving fluphenazine plus an anti-ACh antiparkinson drug. This intriguing pharmacological bonus explains the apparently puzzling anomaly of why, if anti-DA activity is important for treating schizophrenic illness, all antischizophrenic agents at anti-schizophrenic doses do not induce similar intensities of extrapyramidal side effects. This scheme linking anticholinergic activity and extrapyramidal side effects requires that the relative affinities of the drugs for the DA and ACh receptors do not follow each other in parallel. For example, regardless of absolute affinities, if fluphenazine had only $\frac{1}{100}$ the affinity of thioridazine for DA receptors as well as for ACh receptors, the two drugs should elicit extrapyramidal side effects to the same extent at effective

TABLE 4.2 Relative affinities of antischizophrenic agents for the α-noradrenergic (NA) and dopamine (DA) receptor sites in brain

Drug	Affinity for α receptor	Affinity for DA receptor	Ratio of affinity for α NA receptor: DA receptor	Sedation and hypotension
Phenothiazines				
Alkylamino: chlorpromazine	192	98	1.96	+ + +
Piperidine: thioridazine	185	67	2.76	+ + +
Piperazine: fluphenazine	101	1111	0.09	±
Thioxanthenes				
α-Flupenthixol	100	1000	0.1	
Butyrophenones				
Haloperidol	83	714	0.12	±
Spiroperidol	55	4000	0.01	
Droperidol	1429	1000	1.43	+ +
Diphenylbutylpiperidines				
Pimozide	55	1250	0.04	
Dibenzodiazepines				
Clozapine	58	8	7.25	+ + +
(Reference agent: Phentolamine	277	0.5	554)	

Receptor affinity defined as the reciprocal $\times 10^{-6}$ of Ki (inhibitor constant) for drug when competing with ^{3}H-WB-4101 (for α receptors) or ^{3}H-haloperidol (for DA receptors) for binding to rat brain homogenates. Figures calculated from the data of Peroutka *et al.* (1977)

antipsychotic doses. In fact, this is not the case; affinities at the two receptors show no correlation, the affinity of fluphenazine for the DA receptor being at least ten times greater than thioridazine (*Table 4.2*). This suggests that therapeutic antischizophrenic DA receptor blockade requires approximately ten times higher brain concentrations of thioridazine than of fluphenazine. At those much higher brain concentrations, thioridazine will block cholinergic receptors and hence minimize extrapyramidal impairment (Snyder, Greenberg and Yamamura, 1974).

Antinoradrenergic activity

Among the most prominent side effects of conventional antischizophrenic drugs are sympatholytic effects such as orthostatic hypotension and sedation. Both sedation and hypotension can be attributed to blockade of central and peripheral α-noradrenergic receptors. In a series of antipsychotic drugs the tendency to produce autonomic and sedative side effects is roughly related to their affinity for the α-noradrenergic (NA) receptor. The absolute affinity of some antipsychotic agents for the NA receptor is even greater than that of a classic α-antagonist such as phentolamine (*Table 4.2*). It must be remembered that the therapeutic antischizophrenic brain concentrations of these drugs will be determined by satisfactory blockade of DA receptors. The extent to which an antipsychotic agent would block α-receptors at therapeutic dose levels would then be not purely related to absolute potency as a α-blocker, but to the *ratio* of its potency as an α-blocker to potency as a DA blocker (Peroutka *et al.*, 1977; *Table 4.2*). Drugs with high ratios would be expected to exert substantial α-blockade. This prediction appears to be borne out in practice; drugs such as fluphenazine, α-flupenthixol and haloperidol have low ratios and are not usually sedative or hypotensive at therapeutic doses, whereas chlorpromazine, thioridazine, droperidol and clozapine have high ratios and show the greatest tendency to sedation and orthostatic hypotension. Therefore the ratio of α-NA to DA affinity may represent a useful predictor of sedation and the incidence of autonomic sympatholytic side effects.

Antihistamine activity

Ability to block central H_1 histamine receptors is yet another pharmacological property of most antischizophrenic drugs. Most potent H_1-antihistamines possess prominent sedative properties and drugs such as chlorpromazine, thioridazine and droperidol have antihistaminic potencies equivalent to the classic antihistamines such as chlorpheniramine (Quach et al., 1979). Antihistamine activity would be expected to enhance any sedative action arising out of the coincidental ability to block central α-NA receptors.

Antiserotonin (5-HT) activity

Many antischizophrenic drugs have high affinity for central serotonin (5-HT) receptors, but no statistically significant correlation exists between this pharmacological property and clinical therapeutic potency. The clinical effects of central 5-HT antagonism are less clear than those associated with blockade of central DA, ACh, NA or histamine receptors. The drugs fluspirilene, droperidol, benperidol, spiroperidol and pipamperone are particularly potent antagonists at 5-HT receptors (Peroutka and Snyder, 1980). Both fluspirilene and pipamperone have been reported to be particularly effective in relieving schizophrenic hallucinations. While these drugs differ by more than 100-fold in their clinical antischizophrenic potencies and in *in vitro* activity at DA receptors, they have equally high potency at 5-HT receptors. Since the 5-HT system has been implicated in hallucinogenesis it is interesting to speculate that at least some of their anti-hallucinatory action may derive from blockade of central 5-HT receptors.

Pharmacokinetics

PHENOTHIAZINES

While the characteristics of individual phenothiazines vary somewhat, certain main pharmacokinetic characteristics are common:

(1) wide tissue distribution resulting from high lipid solubility,
(2) high degree of tissue binding—for example, more than 95 per cent of chlorpromazine in plasma is bound to plasma protein leaving only a small percentage in bioavailable form,
(3) efficient and rapid elimination by hepatic metabolism,
(4) auto-induction of hepatic and intestinal muscosal enzymes,
(5) very wide individual range of plasma concentrations within any group of patients taking the same oral dose.

More than 80 per cent of an oral dose of chlorpromazine is metabolized by liver and by enzymes present in the intestinal mucosa (collectively termed 'first-pass metabolism'). Intramuscular chlorpromazine will avoid first-pass metabolism and it is important to appreciate that, on average, an intramuscular dose of chlorpromazine will be equivalent to about *five times* the oral dose. The overall plasma elimination half-life of chlorpromazine has been estimated at between 10–20 h. There exist over 150 theoretical metabolites of chlorpromazine (*Figure 4.10*), but only 7-hydroxychlor-promazine (7-OH CPZ) and chlorpromazine sulphoxide (CPZ-SO) occur in plasma at approximately the same concentrations as the parent molecule (Mackay, Healey and Baker, 1974). CPZ-SO is biologically inactive but 7-OH CPZ is of potential importance for the clinical effects of chlorpromazine since its DA receptor blocking potency is roughly equivalent to the parent molecule. The proportion of 7-OH CPZ which exists in unbound form in plasma is about ten times higher than chlorpromazine. It is therefore arguable that the therapeutic effects of chlorpromazine are mediated to an appreciable extent by its 7-OH metabolite (Snyder, 1981).

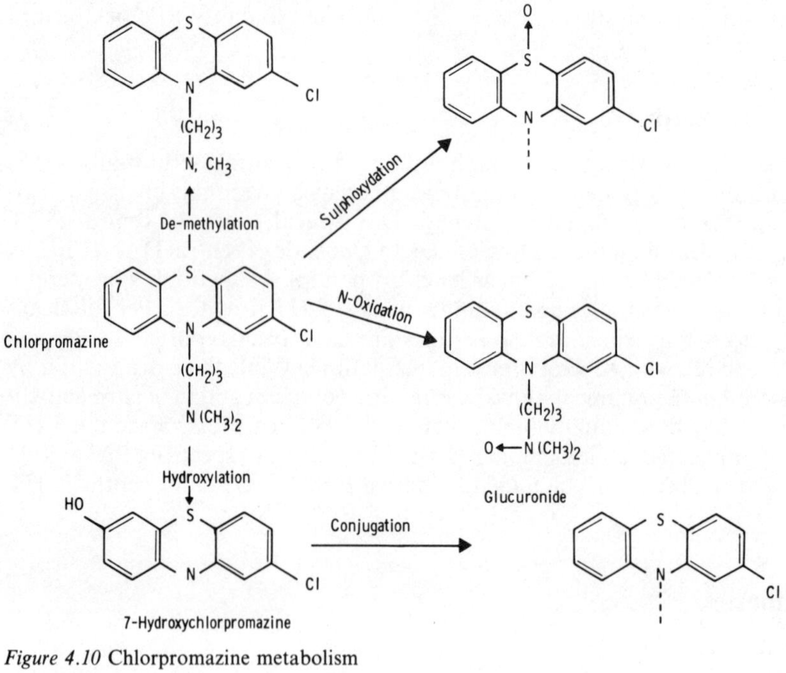

Figure 4.10 Chlorpromazine metabolism

The pharmacokinetics of thioridazine are similar to those of chlorpromazine but its strong anticholinergic actions on the gut can modify its own absorption. Major metabolites include mesoridazine, and free levels of this metabolite in plasma are 50 times higher than thioridazine. Mesoridazine is roughly equipotent with thioridazine as a DA receptor antagonist and thus most of the therapeutic activity of the parent drug may be accounted for by the metabolite (Snyder, 1981).

BUTYROPHENONES

Haloperidol is metabolized in the liver and no biologically active metabolite has so far been demonstrated. Approximately 60 per cent of the drug is bioavailable after oral administration and the plasma elimination curve is multiphasic with a plasma half-life of 12–38 h (Forsman *et al.*, 1977). There is no evidence of enzyme auto-induction and a closer relationship between oral dose and plasma level has been observed than for the phenothiazines.

THIOXANTHENES

These are absorbed and metabolized in ways essentially similar to phenothiazines, except that metabolism to ring-hydroxylated metabolites is uncommon.

Relationship of plasma drug concentration to clinical effect

While clinical pharmacological activity in this area has been sustained for well over a decade, it still remains to be established for any antischizophrenic agent that a clear and useful relationship exists between plasma levels and clinical result. For only one phenothiazine, butaperazine, has a crude relationship been established between plasma concentration and therapeutic outcome in a small number of schizophrenic patients. There appears to be an optimal plasma level or 'therapeutic window' and this relationship is much clearer for the concentration of drug in red blood cells than in plasma (Garver *et al.*, 1977). It may be that the physicochemical factors regulating drug entry into erythrocytes are similar to those governing entry into strategic sites in the brain.

Long-acting antischizophrenic agents

In order to facilitate drug administration over long periods, two ways of reducing the required frequency of administration have been developed. Firstly, by increasing the elimination time of an orally administered drug and, secondly, by dispensing the drug in a vehicle which can be injected intramuscularly to form an absorption depot.

The diphenylbutylpiperidines such as pimozide, fluspirilene and penfluridol provide examples of potent antischizophrenic drugs with remarkably long biological half-lives after oral administration. Pimozide has an elimination half-life in man of 53 h (McCreadie *et al.*, 1979) and penfluridol and fluspirilene remain biologically active for between one and two weeks following a single dose. Fluspirilene is an injectable drug and is dispensed in an aqueous solution of microcrystals from which the drug is released quite rapidly.

A widely employed mechanism for achieving sustained action is that of slow release of an ester of the active drug from an oily vehicle. Fluphenazine hydrochloride possesses an alkyl-piperazine side-chain that allows it to be esterified with long-chain fatty acids (*Figure 4.11*). Among the commonly used phenothiazines only fluphenazine and perphenazine have this property. On a molar equivalent basis, fluphenazine is about ten times more active than chlorpromazine as a DA receptor antagonist and the effective duration of oral fluphenazine is 24 h. However, when fluphenazine hydrochloride is esterified with a long-chain fatty acid (such as decanoic acid) and dissolved in sesame oil, the duration of effect following a single intramuscular injection can be from one to four weeks. The rate of liberation of the ester from the oily depot is inversely proportional to the length of the fatty acid chain—fluphenazine enanthate persists for approximately one week and fluphenazine decanoate (Modecate) for two to four weeks. Once injected the drug ester, still in the oil, is fairly rapidly redistributed about the body in 'secondary depots' in fat. The ester cannot penetrate the brain but

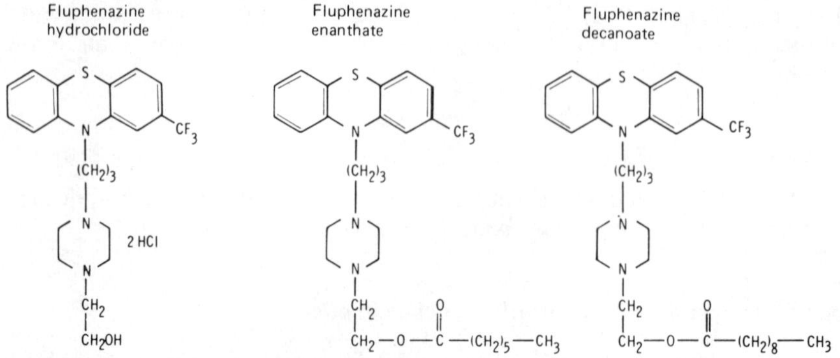

Figure 4.11

must first diffuse out of the oily vehicle into the aqueous phase of tissue fluids where hydrolysis will cleave the fatty acid from the active drug. Hydrolysis occurs in the liver, at the primary injection site and at secondary depots (Groves and Mandel, 1975). In most important respects the pharmacokinetics of α-flupenthixol decanoate (Depixol) are similar to fluphenazine decanoate. Haloperidol decanoate has also recently been marketed for depot use.

The most popular injection sites for depot drugs are the deltoid, thigh or buttock muscles but it should be appreciated that regional blood flow can vary significantly between sites and according to local muscular activity. This may affect the rate of release of the ester from the oily depot and its removal from the injection site. Blood flow is usually greatest in deltoid, followed by thigh and buttock. The volume of injection will also bear upon the speed of absorption—assuming a crudely spherical injection depot, the absorption rate will be proportionately higher for smaller injection volumes.

Work by Wiles and his colleagues in Oxford, using a sensitive radioimmunoassay for fluphenazine, has shown that after a fleeting initial peak of fluphenazine immediately following injection, plasma concentrations of drug are roughly constant over a two-week injection cycle in patients established on fluphenazine decanoate. Plasma levels of fluphenazine decline remarkably slowly after discontinuation of chronic treatment. In many patients drug is still detectable in plasma for up to *six months* after the last injection, and hyperprolactinaemia (a reflection of biological activity) persists for similar periods (Widstedt, Wiles and Kolakowska, 1981). This strikingly long elimination time should be taken into account when interpreting results from any study involving the withdrawal of patients from depot drugs.

Neuroendocrine markers

The fact that the release of certain anterior pituitary hormones is directly affected by DA transmission in the tuberoinfundibular system offers the possibility of monitoring the presence in plasma of DA antagonist drugs by monitoring circulating hormone levels. Dopaminergic cell bodies lying in the arcuate nucleus of the hypothalamus send short axons to the median eminence whence DA is released into the hypothalamo–hypophyseal portal system to reach DA receptors on endocrine cells of the anterior pituitary. DA normally inhibits the release of prolactin and stimulates the secretion of growth hormone; thus pharmacologically active concentrations of antischizophrenic drugs will produce hyperprolactinaemia and reduced circulating levels of growth hormone.

The hyperprolactinaemic response to antischizophrenic agents has been extensively studied. Administration of drug is associated with marked, prompt and sustained rises in plasma prolactin concentrations. During withdrawal from medication prolactin levels drop back to normal. While hyperprolactinaemia may offer a biological marker for DA receptor-active concentrations of drug in plasma, it may not reflect accurately the situation at DA receptors in the brain. For example, it is now clear that whereas brain DA receptors show tolerance to the effects of chronic blockade, pituitary receptors show no such tolerance. Furthermore, it appears that prolactin estimations are of limited usefulness in predicting or monitoring clinical response because the prolactin system is too sensitive. That is, maximal prolactin rises are attained at drug doses insufficient for clinical response. In practical terms, the absence of a prolactin response would indicate the unlikelihood of clinical response, but the presence of a prolactin response has no predictive value (Lader, 1980).

Non dopamine-related drugs

PROPRANOLOL

This drug was established on the basis of its peripheral neuropharmacology as an antagonist at adrenergic β-receptors. Noradrenergic β-receptors have been demonstrated in the mammalian CNS in areas such as frontal cerebral cortex, basal ganglia, hypothalamus and medulla. Evidence has accumulated that β-receptor antagonists such as propranolol have the ability to antagonize certain biochemical and behavioural actions in which 5-HT is involved (Green and Grahame-Smith, 1976; Middlemiss, Blakeborough and Leather, 1977). At the high doses of propranolol claimed to be of some benefit in the treatment of schizophrenic illness, it is impossible to say with certainty whether any effect is being mediated centrally and/or peripherally, and whether β-adrenergic or 5-HT receptor interactions are operative. Insofar as arousal may exert potent effects on the likelihood of schizophrenic breakdown it may be that an arousal-reducing action of propranolol is fundamental to any therapeutic action. Recent summaries of the role of NA in stress-induced arousal indicate an NA–DA interaction (Iversen, 1980) and it may be at that point that NA blockers such as propranolol and DA blockers such as the conventional antischizophrenic drugs converge on a final common therapeutic pathway.

The pharmacokinetic properties of propranolol in humans are complicated (Greenblatt, Shader and Koch-Weser, 1976). There is a very high rate of first-pass clearance by the liver and a variety of metabolites. The drug is widely distributed with ready access into the brain. Propranolol is removed rapidly from the body, with an elimination half-life from plasma of 2–5 h.

OXYPERTINE

This is an indole derivative with a phenylpiperazine side-chain whose main pharmacological effects are qualitatively similar to reserpine. It depletes neuronal stores of monoamines by inhibiting uptake and storage by intraneuronal vesicles. Unlike reserpine, it has an amine-selective action; depleting NA vesicles predominantly, with less potent effects on DA stores and only weak effects on 5-HT stores. It is generally less potent than reserpine, is more readily reversible and is claimed to be free of depressive side effects—perhaps by virtue of its sparing effect on 5-HT transmission. Rarely used in the west, most clinical experience with oxypertine in the treatment of schizophrenic illness has been derived in Japan.

Endorphin-related drugs

Drugs acting to inhibit or potentiate central endorphin transmission can interact with at least two species of endorphin receptor (Chang, Hazum and Cuatrecasas, 1980) (*Table 4.3*). One sort, the 'μ' or morphine receptor, has highest affinity for morphine-like compounds and is found in the dorsal horn of the spinal cord, periaqueductal grey matter, thalamus and raphë nucleus. These areas are concerned with the processing of sensory information and it is likely that morphine exerts its analgesic actions through interaction with opiate receptors in midbrain and spinal cord. The other type, the 'δ' or enkephalin receptor, has preferential affinity for the enkephalins and their stable synthetic analogues and is enriched in forebrain structures such as hippocampus, frontal cerebral cortex, amygdala and corpus striatum. While stimulation of the morphine receptor produces mainly analgesia, stimulation of enkephalin receptors produces complex behavioural responses in animals which may hold more significance for psychiatry.

TABLE 4.3 Opioid receptor subtypes

	μ (*Morphine*)	δ (*Enkephalin*)
Morphine	+ + +	+
β-Endorphin	+ + +	+ + +
met-Enkephalin	+	+ + + +
Naloxone	+ + +	+
Main responses	Analgesia	Behavioural effects

(Modified from Chang. Hazum and Cuatrecasas. 1980)

Of the agents investigated clinically, the opiate antagonist naloxone has been most widely tested. The drug is a classic opiate receptor blocker. It is very poorly absorbed after oral administration and must be given systematically. Naltrexone, a closely related opiate antagonist, can be given orally but has recently been withdrawn from clinical use due to toxicity. Naloxone has preferential affinity for the morphine receptor (*Table 4.3*).

Synthetic β-endorphin must be administered systematically, and after intravenous administration the elimination from plasma is very rapid (biphasic elimination curve with half-lives of 15 and 39 min) although CSF β-endorphin concentrations remain raised by approximately 50 per cent 6 h after intravenous injection of β-endorphin (Berger, 1981). Stable synthetic enkephalin analogues are now available for clinical experimentation but they too must be given systematically.

The endorphin fragment des-tyrosynyl-γ-endorphin (DTγE) possesses behavioural activity in rats reminiscent of chlorpromazine but lacks typical morphine-like activity (de Wied *et al.*, 1978). Like most other agents used to influence central endorphin systems, it cannot be given orally.

Clinical efficacy

Acute therapy

THE PHENOTHIAZINES

Of all the drugs used in psychiatric practice none have been evaluated as widely as the phenothiazines in the treatment of schizophrenic illness. The decade following the introduction of chlorpromazine saw the emergence of an impressive American phenomenon—the Multicentre Veterans Administration Collaborative Study. These and similar trials undertook the careful evaluation of a range of phenothiazines in huge samples of patients (numbered in the high hundreds) and employing standardized clinical rating instruments. The first large VA collaborative study of this sort was published in 1960 (Casey *et al.*, 1960a). In 37 VA Hospitals 805 male schizophrenic patients under the age of 51 were randomly allocated to receive either chlorpromazine, promazine, phenobarbitone or placebo in a double-blind cross-over design. Chlorpromazine emerged with flying colours and phenobarbitone emerged no better than placebo. Promazine (a relatively weak DA receptor blocker) occupied an intermediate position. Two additional monolithic studies were soon to follow (Casey *et al.*, 1960b; Laskey *et al.*, 1962) and with a collective patient sample of 1152 they addressed the important question of relative efficacy of various antipsychotic agents. The accumulated evidence of many such trials has been usefully reviewed (Davis, 1965; Davis and Cole, 1975; Davis and Garver, 1978) and the evidence in support of the therapeutic action of the phenothiazines in the management of schizophrenic illness is indisputable. In general, roughly two-thirds of patients are seen to improve significantly under phenothiazine treatment, only one-tenth fail to improve to some degree and virtually none get worse. On average, most of the therapeutic gain occurs within the first six weeks of treatment although individual variation is wide (Davis and Garver, 1978).

The crucial question of whether chlorpromazine and its relatives were merely a new class of sedatives or 'chemical straightjackets' was specifically explored by Goldberg and colleagues (1965). Re-analysis of the results of an earlier collaborative trial (NIMH-PSC, 1964) confirmed that the clinical effects of phenothiazine treatment went far beyond simple sedation.

It is also quite clear that, on average, there is nothing to choose between the phenothiazines of the three chemical subgroups (aliphatic, piperidine, piperazine) in terms of overall efficacy or therapeutic profile—the only distinctions lie in side effects (*see below*). The notion that certain of the piperazine phenothiazines possess 'activating' rather than sedating properties has entered clinical mythology, but this is based on the most slender evidence. The myth holds that chlorpromazine or thioridazine are treatments of choice for excited patients because of their sedative action, and that fluphenazine or trifluoperazine are best for withdrawn patients because of alerting properties. These beliefs have never been demonstrated to be true (Davis and Cole, 1975): chlorpromazine and thioridazine are sedative (*Table 4.2*) but it is not clear that fluphenazine or trifluoperazine are 'activating', unless the side effect of akathisia is interpreted in this way.

Despite the absence of any clear indication that any phenothiazine is a more effective antipsychotic agent than the prototype chlorpromazine, psychiatrists continue to observe clinically that patients who fail to respond to one drug will occasionally show a good response to another. Given an adequate trial of one agent it would seem sensible to change to another in the face of therapeutic failure. The reasons for differential individual response are probably numerous, including the straightforward one of bioavailability.

THE BUTYROPHENONES

Haloperidol, the prototype and main representative of this group of antipsychotic agents, was synthesized and clinically tested in the late 1950s. Its main therapeutic place in psychiatric disorder is undoubtedly in the management of manic illness, but efficacy against acute schizophrenic illness has also been shown. Motor hyperactivity appears particularly amenable to this drug and one of the earliest demonstrations of clinical efficacy was in the treatment of the syndrome of Gilles de la Tourette.

The quantity of published experience with haloperidol in the management of schizophrenic illness is much less than for the phenothiazines and is confined mostly to European trials (Davis, 1965). In general, properly controlled trials have consistently shown haloperidol to be superior to placebo and to be as effective as chlorpromazine. For reasons that are not altogether clear, haloperidol has never achieved the clinical popularity of the phenothiazines as the first treatment of choice in schizophrenic illness. Haloperidol is more commonly used as a second-line agent in patients who show an inadequate response to phenothiazines.

The administration of very high doses of antipsychotic drugs to abort a psychosis ('rapid neuroleptization') was first reported by Mountain in 1963. This megadose strategy was later adopted by Oldham and Bott (1971) with haloperidol. It has been reported that high dosage haloperidol (100 mg daily) might evoke improvement in the mental state of chronic drug-resistant schizophrenic patients, albeit at the expense of some deterioration in ward behaviour (McCreadie and MacDonald, 1977). Recent trials in which low and high dose regimens of haloperidol have been compared in the management of acute schizophrenic psychoses have, however, failed to show any advantage of high over routine dose levels (Donlon et al., 1980; Neborsky et al., 1981). A curious phenomenon reported with high dose haloperidol was a threshold effect of increasing doses on extrapyramidal impairment. A potent DA receptor blocker with weak anticholinergic activity like haloperidol is naturally prone to producing parkinsonian side effects. It was observed that as doses were increased, a threshold was reached above which extrapyramidal side effects not only levelled off in intensity but actually lessened (Sangiovanni et al., 1973; McCreadie and MacDonald, 1977). It has been suggested that this is due to a ceiling effect of maximal DA receptor blockade, over which increasing doses of haloperidol start to exert significant anticholinergic activity. However, the occurrence of this extrapyramidal phenomenon appears to be in some doubt (Neborsky et al., 1981). Not only does there seem to be no clear support for the efficacy of high dose regimens in the routine management of acute schizophrenic illness, but such a practice is best avoided for fear of increasing the likelihood of long-term neurotoxicity.

THE THIOXANTHENES

Chlorprothixene and thiothixene are marketed in the USA and there is ample evidence that they are effective antischizophrenic agents (Davis and Garver, 1978). Flupenthixol, the thioxanthene analogue of fluphenazine, is the one most commonly used in the UK. A recent clinical trial in the UK not only demonstrated the antischizophrenic efficacy of α-flupenthixol but also highlighted two issues of general importance; the significant early placebo component in recovery from acute schizophrenic illness in hospital (patients tend to improve somewhat merely by removal to a non-stressful hospital environment), and the fact that the pharmacological influence on recovery takes at least two to three weeks to become apparent (Johnstone *et al.*, 1978) (*see Figure 4.8*). The time-course of the pharmacotherapeutic action of α-flupenthixol suggests that although the antipsychotic effect may depend upon DA receptor blockade, such blockade may be necessary only to allow other, longer-term, restorative processes to take place. An interesting extension to this study was the observation that patients whose arousal in response to an auditory stimulus did not habituate tended to show a poorer antipsychotic response to medication than those who did habituate (Frith *et al.*, 1979).

THE DIPHENYLBUTYLPIPERIDINES

This is a relatively new class of potent and long-acting antipsychotic agents and includes pimozide, fluspirilene and penfluridol. While their clinical efficacy has been established reasonably but not rigorously, the use of pimozide continues to increase in the UK. Although pimozide was clinically available in Europe in 1970, systematic evaluation has occurred slowly. Pimozide has now been shown to be effective in acutely ill schizophrenic patients (Freeman, 1979) and to be effective in reducing the rate of relapse in schizophrenic patients discharged from hospital (Falloon, Watt and Shepherd, 1978). Penfluridol is used as a long-acting oral medication which can be taken once weekly and its efficacy as a prophylactic antischizophrenic agent has been demonstrated (Davis and Garver, 1978). Fluspirilene is given intramuscularly in aqueous solution. The drug has not yet been evaluated in a sufficient number of double-blind placebo controlled studies to allow definite conclusions but the available evidence suggests that fluspirilene may also be an effective maintenance drug when given once weekly.

THE SUBSTITUTED BENZAMIDES

This new class of compounds, which includes metoclopramide, sulpiride, sultopride and tiapride was introduced into clinical use in the 1960s by Justin Besançon and colleagues in France. Most of the relevant clinical literature is French and there is a dearth of published reports from double-blind placebo controlled studies. Open studies have shown that sulpiride has antipsychotic properties in chronic and withdrawn schizophrenic patients and that it produces parkinsonian side effects (Davies and Garver, 1978).

Evidence for the antipsychotic efficacy of metoclopramide is conflicting and requires clarification (Borenstein and Bles, 1965; Stanley and Wilks, 1979). As yet there is no conclusive information on the two clinically most important questions relating to these D2 DA receptor blockers; does their clinical profile offer advantages over the older and less specific DA receptor antagonists, and are they less prone to extrapyramidal side effects? The answer to the latter question is at present the clearer and it seems to be no.

OTHERS

Propranolol
It is always useful to have at one's disposal a drug, or group of drugs, which act in a way quite different from the therapeutic mainstays and which offer some advantages in terms of side effects or prospect of response in the drug-resistant case. Propranolol

might be considered in this category although thorough evaluation in treatment-resistant schizophrenic patients remains to be done. Claims that propranolol is effective either alone or in combination with conventional agents in both acute and chronic schizophrenic illness (Atsmon *et al.*, 1971; Yorkston *et al.*, 1977; Yorkston *et al.*, 1981) have not been substantiated by some (Peet *et al.*, 1981a; Myers *et al.*, 1981). While the question of the place, if any, of propranolol in the management of schizophrenic illness must remain open, it seems likely that the interpretation of any beneficial effect observed when the drug is used in combination with a phenothiazine is complicated by the fact that propranolol increases the bioavailability of the phenothiazine (Peet *et al.*, 1981b; Yorkston *et al.*, 1981).

It has been a matter for concern that large oral doses of propranolol have been recommended as necessary for any antipsychotic effect, although recent studies claim encouraging results and little toxicity at daily doses under 1 g. Nonetheless, caution needs to be exercised (Tyrer, 1980); hallucinations have been a reported side effect at relatively modest doses of β-blockers. Several other side effects are attributed to propranolol, the most important being fatigue, depressed affect, bradycardia, hypotension (and occasionally paradoxical hypertension), congestive cardiac failure, dizziness and sleep disturbances. Unlike conventional DA-blocking antipsychotic agents, propranolol causes neither hyperprolactinaemia nor extrapyramidal impairment.

Oxypertine

This unconventional drug may also fall into the category of an adjunct to established antischizophrenic medication. Two early controlled trials in the west were encouraging (Davis, 1965) and the drug has recently been used quite widely in Japan. It is a monoamine depletor (*see above*) and appears to avoid the depressive side effects typical of reserpine. It may therefore turn out to have useful synergistic actions with the DA receptor blockers in the treatment of refractory cases. Early reports of a selective beneficial effect on variables such as poverty of speech and motor retardation have not so far been substantiated.

Endorphin-related agents

The manipulation of central endorphin systems in the treatment of schizophrenic psychoses is at an early experimental stage and the agents available for this purpose are few. Clinical strategies have so far aimed crudely at either inhibiting or stimulating endorphin transmission.

Of the agents investigated clinically the opiate antagonist naloxone has been most widely tested. There are conflicting reports about its efficacy in the treatment of schizophrenic illness (Mackay, 1980) but the results of a World Health Organization Multicentre Collaborative Study tend to support earlier suggestions that it may be of benefit in some patients suffering from intractable auditory hallucinations (Pickar and Bunney, 1981).

The opposite strategy has most commonly involved the systemic administration of β-endorphin or one of its stable analogues. Administration of synthetic β-endorphin to schizophrenic patients has been variously reported to evoke either deterioration or improvement which is statistically significant but clinically unimportant (Gerner *et al.*, 1980; Berger *et al.*, 1980). Double-blind evaluation of a met-enkephalin analogue (FK-33-824) has failed to reveal any significant therapeutic effect in schizophrenic illness (Ruther, Gerd and Nedopil, 1982). Early clinical trials of the endorphin fragment DTγE were encouraging, but subsequent work has shown this peptide to be at best of limited efficacy in a small subgroup of schizophrenic patients (Manchanda and Hirsch, 1981).

Clinical results so far are therefore not very encouraging but it must be remembered that apart from the obvious limitations imposed by the need to give all of these agents systematically, the proper clinical evaluation of endorphin-active agents in schizophrenic illness must await the availability of a wider range of receptor-specific drugs.

Nature of improvement with antischizophrenic drugs

From the very first, it was clear to clinicians using chlorpromazine and its descendants that here was a group of drugs that were not simply sedative or tranquillizing. This led to a re-examination of the cognitive and perceptual abnormalities that are the hallmarks of schizophrenic illness. The early efficacy trials employed diagnostic criteria and indices of improvement which relied heavily upon the views of Eugen Bleuler. Bleuler's 'fundamental' symptoms (thought disorder, affective blunting, ambivalence and autistic behaviour) were all found to be responsive to the phenothiazines. In recent years, diagnostic habits and foci for therapeutic improvement have moved from Bleuler's list of fundamental phenomena to a list of symptoms which are more readily defined, and therefore more readily rated. These are embodied in the Present State Examination (PSE), a highly reliable diagnostic instrument of proven operational value (Wing, Cooper and Sartorius, 1974). It has been shown that the nuclear syndrome of the PSE (thought insertion, thought broadcast, thought commentary, thought withdrawal, auditory hallucinations of voices speaking about the patient, delusions of control and delusions of alien penetration) resolves steadily over the first few weeks of treatment of acute schizophrenic psychosis with chlorpromazine (Phillipson *et al.*, 1977). It thus appears that even when viewed through a different and more rigorous experimental instrument, there is clear evidence of general improvement in the clinical features which distinguish schizophrenic illness. This is not to say that the therapeutic extent of these drugs is confined to the symptoms of schizophrenia—it must be emphasized again that they appear to be antipsychotic in general and antischizophrenic in particular.

POSITIVE VERSUS NEGATIVE PHENOMENA

An important issue which has not been satisfactorily resolved is whether this group of drugs is effective in ameliorating the so-called negative, as opposed to the positive or productive phenomena of schizophrenic illness. It is clinical experience that negative phenomena such as flattened affect, poverty of speech, slowness, underactivity, social withdrawal and lack of motivation tend to be relatively refractory to medication. There is no doubt that positive phenomena such as delusions and hallucinations which are typical of the acute psychosis respond well to medication, but it is the negative features (or defect state) which contribute most to the crippling stigmata of chronic schizophrenic illness. The early multicentre trials of the phenothiazines seemed to show that, indeed, these negative features responded just as well as the positive. However, clinical impression does not accord with this and a recent drug trial showed preferential improvement in positive symptoms (Johnstone *et al.*, 1978). It has been suggested that this apparent discrepancy may arise out of differences in what was actually measured. The early trials made behavioural ratings of negative *features* of the disease (such as social withdrawal and lack of self-care) which are not uncommon in the acute stages of the illness, whereas negative *symptoms* are only rateable through clinical interview. When symptoms are elicited, it seems that conventional antischizophrenic medication is relatively ineffective against the defect state typical of chronic schizophrenic illness (Mackay and Crow, 1980).

Chronicity and failure of functional restoration are as much essential features of schizophrenia as are the signs and symptoms of the disease. Many patterns of individual morbidity exist, but chronic schizophrenic illness carries a poor prognosis. While there is little doubt that medication reduces the probability of relapse into florid psychosis, there is absolutely no evidence that suppression of florid psychotic episodes affects the long-term course and eventual outcome of the schizophrenias (Ciompi, 1980).

Social environment, arousal and drugs

In research on chronic schizophrenic patients there have been many indications that drug treatments and social treatments are not alternatives but must be used to complement each other. The better the environmental conditions, the less the need for medication; the poorer the social milieu, the greater the need for drugs. If the phenothiazines and their descendants work, at least in part, by reducing a high level of physiological arousal (Venables and Wing, 1962; Goldberg, Klerman and Cole, 1965) then they should be most effective in conditions of social over-stimulation. The elegant studies of the MRC Social Psychiatry Unit have shown that the emotional climate generated between the patient and the relative with whom he lives has a direct influence on the likelihood of relapse. In particular, the intensity of 'expressed emotion' (EE) and the time spent in enforced face-to-face contact with the relative are critical factors. It appears that maintenance antischizophrenic medication exerts a protective action against the damaging effects of high EE, reducing the risk of psychotic relapse to a level

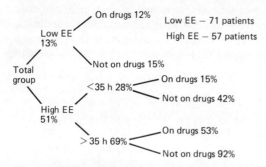

Low EE — 71 patients

High EE — 57 patients

Figure 4.12 Nine-month relapse rates in a group of 128 schizophrenic patients analysed according to expressed emotion (EE) rated in a relative and time per week in contact with that relative (from Vaughn and Leff, 1976)

similar to that for patients in an ideal non-threatening environment (*Figure 4.12*). It has further been shown that patients in a high EE environment have a particular pattern of hyper-arousal (Tarrier *et al.*, 1979) which might represent a target for therapeutic drug action (Sturgeon *et al.*, 1981).

Maintenance therapy

There is abundant evidence that once an optimal level of remission from the acute stage of schizophrenic illness has been achieved, the risk of relapse into florid psychosis is substantially reduced if patients continue to take medication (Davis, 1975). It appears that while the majority of patients derive some benefit from continued medication, there is a small group (some 15 per cent) who will remain well for long periods without medication (Hogarty and Ulrich, 1977). Two important questions arise; firstly, who to treat chronically with drugs, and secondly, for how long should drug therapy be maintained? The answer to the first is, unfortunately, quickly dealt with—the characteristics of this group are unclear. The only prediction that can be made on present evidence is that patients being discharged to low EE environments will have a relatively good prognosis even in the absence of medication.

The duration of drug administration must be guided by knowledge of the extent of any protective effect of medication in the patient who remains well, and by knowledge of the risks of long-term toxicity (*see below*). Sophisticated long-term prospective follow-up studies have shown that relapse rates in drug-maintained patients are at least twice those of patients maintained on placebo. While risk of relapse does decline the longer a patient remains well, at the two and a half year stage the risk in drug-free patients is still nearly three times higher than in drug treated patients (Hogarty and Ulrich, 1977). There is evidence from one study that even in patients who have remained well for three to five years on medication, replacement of antischizophrenic medication by a benzodiazepine results in a four-fold higher rate of relapse in the subsequent 18 months (Cheung, 1981). If a patient remains well over a prolonged period of maintenance chemotherapy clinical intuition might suggest that the risk of relapse is so reduced as to render continued medication unnecessary. Such intuition can be unsound and dangerous.

Most relapses occur within three months of stopping medication and it has been proposed that rather than being a natural expression of the underlying disease process, such a relapse is a drug-induced supersensitivity psychosis; a mesolimbic dopaminergic rebound following prolonged DA receptor blockade (Chouinard and Jones, 1980). This possibility makes the interpretation of most studies of maintenance medication rather difficult (Mackay, 1981).

Choice of drug for maintenance therapy

The choice of maintenance medication is governed by efficacy, ease of administration, toxicity and avoidance of non-compliance. For the phenothiazines, such as flu-phenazine, there is equivalent efficacy with both oral and depot intramuscular preparations. Maintenance therapy using multiple daily dosage of oral preparations is accompanied by a high rate of default. Injected depot preparations are usually preferred, for while they do not eliminate overt default (open refusal), they undoubtedly eliminate covert default since administration is always professionally supervised. It has been shown that provided patients are seen regularly at a systematic follow-up clinic, daily oral pimozide is as effective as fortnightly injections of fluphenazine decanoate (Falloon, Watt and Shepherd, 1978). Johnstone and Freeman (1973) found that 15–20 per cent of patients receiving intramuscular medication dropped out of treatment, mostly within the first six months. The reasons for default are largely attributable to unwanted side effects, in particular an awareness of extrapyramidal symptoms such as akathisia, akinesia, tremor and dystonia (Van Putten, 1974).

There is nothing to choose between the two most popular depot intramuscular preparations used in the UK, fluphenazine decanoate and α-flupenthixol decanoate. Clinical efficacy and prevalance of a variety of side effects are essentially equal at dose equivalents of 25 mg fluphenazine or 40 mg of α-flupenthixol (Knights *et al.*, 1979).

Unwanted effects

The price paid by patients for treatment with antischizophrenic drugs is quite high in the form of unwanted side effects. A good working knowledge of the full range of unwanted effects is essential if the clinician is to react quickly and appropriately to relieve unnecessary distress, to prepare the patient against emergence of these side effects, and to weigh the benefits of medication against the cost—particularly when embarking upon chronic therapy.

Antipsychotic drugs have a high therapeutic index (i.e. the ratio of fatal to therapeutic dosage is large). Most phenothiazines have a rather flat dose-response curve and can therefore be used over a wide dose range. Death from overdose is extremely rare. However, short of threat to life, this group of drugs is guilty of a long list of unwanted effects and should be treated with great respect.

Most commonly encountered side effects are *dose-related* and understandable in the light of the known pharmacological actions of this group of agents. These can be classified into effects on the extrapyramidal system, other CNS effects, autonomic effects, endocrine effects, skin and eye effects. Other, less common side effects are not clearly dose-related and probably reflect an *idiosyncratic* or allergic response by the patient and are therefore largely unpredictable.

Extrapyramidal side effects

Dysfunction of the extrapyramidal motor system is the commonest of the unwanted side effects of antischizophrenic chemotherapy. While it is now generally agreed that overt extrapyramidal side effects are not a *conditio sine qua non* for therapeutic effectiveness, any antipsychotic agent which substantially inhibits central DA transmission will carry the risk of such disorders, acute and chronic. The nature, prevalence and management of drug-induced extrapyramidal side effects have been reviewed in detail (Marsden, Mindham and Mackay, 1981).

Overall, at least 30 per cent of all patients receiving antischizophrenic medication will suffer extrapyramidal dysfunction. There is a wide inter-drug variation, the most troublesome in this respect being the newer, more selective and potent DA antagonists which are devoid of anticholinergic activity (*see above*). With them, the prevalence of extrapyramidal disorder is over 50 per cent, and in the case of the depot intramuscular preparations, can be as high as 80 per cent (Knights *et al.*, 1979). Many of these untoward reactions occur early in the course of drug treatment, particularly after systemic administration, and it is important to appreciate that this may represent the patient's earliest experience of this form of treatment.

Acute toxicity

ACUTE DYSTONIC REACTIONS (ACUTE DYSKINESIAS)

An acute dystonia is often the earliest extrapyramidal disorder to appear, the great majority occurring within 4–5 d of starting therapy, and an appreciable number of cases occur within the first few hours. This is perhaps the most dramatic of the drug-induced disorders of striopallidal function. The syndrome consists of intermittent or sustained muscular spasms and abnormal postures which are both clinically striking and profoundly distressing to the patient. The five commonest manifestations of acute dystonia are torticollis, contraction of the tongue, trismus, oculogyric crisis and opisthotonus. Oculogyric crisis is characterized by a brief prodromal fixed stare followed by upward and lateral rotation of the eyes. If the eyelids are forced open against blepharospasm the irides are typically found hidden beneath the upper canthus of the eye, leaving only the sclerae visible. Associated with these alarming ocular signs, the head is usually tilted backwards and laterally, the mouth is open and the tongue protruded. Erroneous diagnoses for acute dystonia have included tetanus, status epilepticus, meningitis and encephalitis.

Acute dystonic reactions are most likely to occur in young males under the age of 30, and are clearly dose-related. Care should be exercised over the choice of initial dose, particularly when instituting depot therapy (when a test dose is advisable), and account should be taken of the patient's age, sex and weight rather than blind adherence to the manufacturer's recommended test dose. Acute dystonias are spontaneously reversible as plasma drug concentrations fall but the urgency of the clinical situation usually demands positive therapeutic action in the form of an intramuscular injection of an anticholinergic drug such as procyclidine, to which the dystonia will respond rapidly and dramatically.

AKATHISIA

This is a state of motor restlessness of which the cardinal diagnostic feature is a *subjective* feeling of motor unease or inner tension ('impatience musculaire': Van Putten, 1975). The unfortunate patient feels unable to keep still and must constantly move in an attempt to relieve his discomfort. The subject constantly shifts his legs and taps his feet and, in severe cases, may pace up and down. Such florid agitation may be misinterpreted as an exacerbation of psychotic behaviour, leading to an inappropriate increase in drug dosage. Akathisia is probably grossly underdiagnosed. Following the administration of antischizophrenic drugs it appears more slowly than acute dystonia but more rapidly than parkinsonism. Women are almost twice as frequently affected as men. Unlike the other acute extrapyramidal syndromes it tends to respond poorly to anticholinergic medication. Reduction in dosage is the most effective method of management but if this is not possible, benzodiazepines have been found beneficial. It has been proposed that this rather odd but common extrapyramidal syndrome is caused by inhibition of DA transmission not in the nigrostriatal tract but in mesocortical DA pathways projecting from the ventral tegmentum to the frontal cortex (Marsden and Jenner, 1980).

PARKINSONISM

Antischizophrenic drugs can induce an exact facsimile of classic Parkinson's disease; the cardinal signs of rigidity, tremor, bradykinesia, with a variety of subsidiary clinical features such as changes in gait and posture, excessive salivation, difficulty in speaking and swallowing, characteristic frozen facies, and greasy skin.

Bradykinesia is especially common, occurring soon after starting treatment, and frequently the only sign of parkinsonism to occur. The face is blank and expressionless, accessory movements are lost; the arms fail to swing on walking and gesture on talking disappears. Voluntary movement becomes slow in initiation and execution, and reduced in amplitude. The voice becomes soft and handwriting small (micrographia is a sensitive and easily recorded clinical sign). Like akathisia, bradykinesia may pose problems of diagnosis and interpretation. The lack of spontaneity and general slowness may be interpreted as part of the defect state of chronic schizophrenia. 'Akinetic depression' is a term coined by Van Putten and May (1978) to capture the negative subjective accompaniment of bradykinesia. It is vital to distinguish a drug-induced parkinsonian syndrome, which may be amenable to anticholinergic drug therapy, from a natural feature of schizophrenic illness. A brief diagnostic trial with an anticholinergic antiparkinson drug probably represents the only straightforward means available by which to make such a distinction.

Drug-induced parkinsonism occurs roughly twice as commonly in women as in men of the same age. Most cases will appear within two weeks of starting treatment but this is quite variable and it is not uncommon for signs to develop after weeks or months with no change in dose level and for no apparent reason. The incidence of drug-induced parkinsonism rises steeply after middle age and there is a suggestion that a family history of Parkinson's disease raises the likelihood of the drug-induced syndrome (Marsden, Mindham and Mackay, 1981).

The ideal management of drug-induced parkinsonism is reduction in dose of the antischizophrenic agent. Where this may not be possible, for example in the early stages of treatment of the acute psychosis, exhibition of an antiparkinson drug may be required for a limited period. Anticholinergic agents are the most widely used drugs for this purpose. Surprisingly, the published evidence for their effectiveness in Parkinson's disease itself is rather sparse, and procyclidine is one of the few of this class which has been compared favourably with placebo (Mindham, 1976). While some evidence exists for the effectiveness of orphenadrine and benztropine in the treatment of drug-induced parkinsonism, the evidence in favour of procyclidine again seems the clearest.

Anticholinergic medication is not without dangers and considerable drawbacks. A toxic confusional state may occur, particularly in the elderly, as may all of the autonomic effects of atropine-like drugs. Anticholinergic drugs will usually exacerbate an existing tardive dyskinesia and may unmask latent dyskinesia (see below). They may also contribute to the development of hyperthermic episodes, which can be fatal. Hyperpyrexia may result from a combination of peripheral inhibition of sweating by the anticholinergic, and a central effect on thermoregulatory centres by concurrently administered phenothiazines (Westlake and Rastegar, 1973). A number of reports have claimed that anticholinergics attenuate the therapeutic actions of antischizophrenic drugs. Such an attenuation may be explicable on a pharmacokinetic basis, the anticholinergic drug causing a reduction in plasma concentrations of the antipsychotic drug by impairing its intestinal absorption (Rivera-Calimlim, 1976) although this effect has been disputed (see Cooper, 1978).

There is considerable evidence that chronic antiparkinsonian medication is not required by the vast majority of patients receiving antischizophrenic drugs. Where originally indicated by definite neurological signs, the need for anticholinergic medication usually disappears even if the patient continues to receive the same dose of antipsychotic medication. In about 90 per cent of patients the anticholinergic drug can be withdrawn after three months with no return of parkinsonian signs. The principles of treatment with anticholinergic drugs for drug-induced parkinsonism are outlined in Chapter 5 (p. 104).

Chronic toxicity

While some cases of drug-induced parkinsonism may appear late in the course of treatment and may persist for prolonged periods, the commonest long-term extrapyramidal complication, tardive dyskinesia, is of a very different nature.

TARDIVE DYSKINESIA

Within five years of the introduction of phenothiazine drugs for the treatment of psychoses Schonecker (1957) drew attention to an involuntary choreo-athetoid dyskinesia, apparently associated with antipsychotic medication, which was distinguishable from the acute dystonias and from parkinsonism on the basis of both phenomenology and time-course. Uhrbrand and Faurbye (1960) coined the term tardive dyskinesia to denote an involuntary hyperkinesia which was characteristically late in appearance during treatment with antischizophrenic drugs.

The disorder occurs most commonly after approximately two years of uninterrupted drug teatment but individual variability is wide. The core of the disorder is the bucco-linguo-masticatory (BLM) syndrome consisting of involuntary pursing and smacking of the lips, rolling or thrusting of the tongue, puffing of the cheeks and lateral chewing jaw movements. This cephalic dyskinesia may be associated with choreic movements of the limbs and rhythmic dystonic contraction of axial muscles giving rise to paroxysmal torticollis and pelvic thrusting. In the elderly, the BLM syndrome predominates, in children and adolescents the trunk, arms and hands are commonly affected and here the character of the movements is often more dystonic than choreic. Muscle tone is usually reduced but the BLM syndrome can co-exist with features of drug-induced parkinsonism such as cog-wheel rigidity in the limbs. It is the exception rather than the rule for patients to report distress from tardive dyskinesia, more commonly a complaint will come from relatives or nursing staff. Arousal plays a key role in determining the severity of movements; tardive dyskinesia disappears during sleep and is intensified by anxiety, although embarrassment may force the patient to suppress voluntarily the movements for limited periods.

Estimates of prevalence vary widely but well executed studies in both the UK and USA have recorded prevalence rates between 40 and 50 per cent of all patients receiving antischizophrenic medication—whether in-patients or out-patients (Marsden, Mindham and Mackay, 1981). Two differential diagnoses may cause some confusion and misunderstanding. Firstly, there may be a superficial similarity between tardive dyskinesia and the bizarre mannerisms and stereotypies of chronic schizophrenia but most authorities agree that the abnormal movements of schizophrenia are of a different character (Mackay, 1981b) and are much less common than tardive dyskinesia. Secondly, a BLM syndrome identical to tardive dyskinesia can occur in old people who have never been exposed to antischizophrenic medication and in them the syndrome is a variant of senile chorea. There is, however, no doubt that the incidence of orofacial dyskinesia in all age groups and for all diagnoses is highly significantly increased by chronic exposure to antischizophrenic drugs.

Of the many variables, in both patients and medication history, which have been investigated for a relationship with risk of tardive dyskinesia, the *age* of the patient stands out clearly as increasing the risk. There is a sharp increase in prevalence after middle age and this is not merely related to the length of time a patient has been exposed to medication—the ageing brain seems particularly susceptible to this disorder. There is no clear evidence incriminating any one sort of antischizophrenic drug—any drug which inhibits central DA transmission for long periods runs the risk of inducing tardive dyskinesia.

A particularly serious aspect of tardive dyskinesia is the fact that in between one-third and one-half of patients the dyskinesia is irreversible. Withdrawal of the offending drug usually causes a paradoxical worsening of the condition and in a considerable proportion of cases the abnormal movements will then gradually abate, although improvement may continue for up to three years. Factors which appear to militate against reversibility are the duration of drug therapy, age and the duration of obvious dyskinesia. Caution needs to be exercised in the use of periodic drug withdrawals ('drug holidays') as a strategy for avoiding irreversible long-term side effects; Jeste and colleagues (1979) have found that 'drug holidays' may actually make it more likely that dyskinesia will become irreversible.

The neurobiological basis of tardive dyskinesia is not yet clear but the most coherent hypothesis suggests that tardive dyskinesia reflects relative dopaminergic overactivity in the nigrostriatal tract. Chronic occlusion of central DA receptors by an anti-schizophrenic drug results in compensatory proliferation of the DA receptors. The hypothesis states that in tardive dyskinesia this DA receptor 'supersensitivity' may express itself as neurological disorder if there is a failure of normal homeostatic mechanisms. The result is a functional overactivity of dopaminergic transmission relative to cholinergic (and perhaps GABAcidic) transmission in the basal ganglia—the diametric opposite of Parkinson's disease (*see Figure 4.9*).

Since there is no generally accepted treatment for tardive dyskinesia *prevention* must be the most important consideration and the following guidelines are suggested:

(1) antipsychotic drugs exhibited for serious indications only,
(2) use of the minimum effective dose for the shortest time,
(3) regular (monthly) neurological examination. Early detection and drug withdrawal will maximize chances of reversibility. Earliest signs are often detected in the tongue—observed retracted in the open mouth,
(4) particular care in patients over the age of 50.

Once a tardive dyskinesia has appeared, any concomitant anticholinergic medication should be withdrawn since this will tend to intensify the abnormal movements. The antischizophrenic drug should, if possible, be withdrawn gradually. If complete withdrawal is clinically unjustifiable then dose reduction is the next best strategy. In cases where tardive dyskinesia is irreversible in the face of drug withdrawal or dose reduction (and this may take months or years to assess), a therapeutic trial of a benzodiazepine (such as clonazepam) may evoke some improvement (Sheppard, Mackay and Kitson, 1982).

In the case of a serious iatrogenic disorder such as tardive dyskinesia it seems prudent to advise all clinicians using long-term antischizophrenic drugs to make a clear statement in the case-notes of the clinical indications for such therapy. If, as will often be the case, it is judged clinically inadvisable to withdraw the offending drug in the face of emergent tardive dyskinesia, recognition of the disorder should be made in the case-notes along with a statement explaining why in that par-ticular case, the psychiatric risks of drug withdrawal outweigh the neurological benefits.

Other CNS effects

EEG EFFECTS

The EEG frequency slows, with increased theta and delta waves, a decrease in alpha waves and fast beta activity, and some increase in burst activity and spiking. The seizure threshold is lowered, particularly by the aliphatic phenothiazines such as chlorpromazine. Butyrophenones have variable and unpredictable effects. The likelihood of frank epileptic fits is more in patients with a history of epilepsy or a condition which predisposes to seizures. Therefore the aliphatic phenothiazines are to be avoided in patients prone to epileptic attacks or in withdrawal from general CNS depressants such as alcohol or the barbiturates. High potency agents (such as fluphenazine) can be used relatively safety in epileptic patients if the dose is increased gradually and if concomitant anticonvulsant medication is maintained.

SEDATION

This may be particularly noticeable over the first few days of treatment with agents such as chlorpromazine and thioridazine. Tolerance develops fairly rapidly to this effect.

PARADOXICAL WORSENING OF PSYCHOTIC SYMPTOMS

These may occasionally occur at relatively high doses. This is a phenomenon quite distinct from akathisia or toxic confusion.

TOXIC CONFUSIONAL STATES

These states, with typical clouding of consciousness, can occur particularly in the elderly and with the highly atropinic agents such as thioridazine. The confusion usually resolves rapidly after withdrawal or dose reduction.

Autonomic effects

These are due to the anticholinergic and antinoradrenergic actions of the drugs and are expressed in a wide range of troublesome signs and symptoms, including abnormalities of the ECG.

Atropinic activity can cause dry mouth, inhibition of sweating, blurred vision (mydriasis), constipation (even paralytic ileus), inhibition of ejaculation and urinary retention. Antinoradrenergic effects include cutaneous flushes, blurred vision (miosis) and postural hypotension. The blurring of vision caused by chlorpromazine is due to miosis (anti-NA effects outweigh anti-ACh effects) whereas with thioridazine the reverse is true and blurring is due to mydriasis. Postural hypotension is most commonly associated with suddenly high plasma concentrations resulting from systemic administration. Tolerance to this side-effect develops after a few days. The ECG may show broadening and flattening of T waves and increased QRS intervals. T-wave changes are commonest with thioridazine and least common with drugs of high potency. Sudden death, presumed to be of cardiovascular origin, has very occasionally been reported in phenothiazine-treated patients.

Endocrine effects

Antischizophrenic agents may cause a variety of endocrinological abnormalities due to their interaction with central DA receptors, and probably to a lesser extent with NA and 5-HT receptors. The sites of these actions lie mainly in the hypothalamus and pituitary. The clinically important effects are irregular menstruation, lactation and male impotence.

Drug-induced hyperprolactinaemia seems to underly most of these problems. Through antagonistic action at DA receptors in the anterior pituitary, antischizophrenic drugs induce substantial rises in circulating prolactin concentrations. The ability of these drugs to do this is related to their potency as DA receptor antagonists, there is a low ceiling to this effect (maximal hyperprolactinaemia can occur at subtherapeutic doses of drug) and no tolerance occurs with chronic treatment (Gruen et al., 1978). High circulating prolactin concentrations may interfere with the actions of gonadotrophins at their end organs, resulting in hypogonadism in males and amenorrhoea in females (Thorner and Besser, 1976). Impotence and anovulatory bleeding may also occur. Breast engorgement is not uncommon and lactation can be evoked by gentle pressure on the breast. Male gynaecomastia has also been reported. Phenothiazine-induced male impotence may have two sources; hyperprolactinaemia and inhibition of ejaculation with eventual loss of erectile ability due to autonomic interference (especially with thioridazine). There is no clear evidence that prolonged drug-induced hyperprolactinaemia causes breast cancer, nevertheless any source of hyperprolactinaemia should be avoided in cases of established breast cancer. It is said that glucose tolerance curves may show some shift into the diabetic range. Weight gain on phenothiazine drugs is not unusual and while the effect probably results from a hypothalamic action, it has not yet been clearly explained.

Skin and eye effects

There are three sorts of dermatological complication; allergic (urticarial, maculo-papular, petechial or oedematous), contact dermatitis, and photosensitivity. Urticaria has been reported to occur in approximately 5 per cent of patients receiving chlorpromazine. Contact dermatitis used to be common in ward staff who handled phenothiazine syrups but this is now rare. A phototoxic sensitivity reaction may occur in patients receiving chlorpromazine. It resembles severe sunburn and direct sunlight should be avoided. A very chronic side effect (occurring after 10–15 years) may be blue-grey metallic discoloration of the skin over areas exposed to sunlight. Deposits of melanin-like material may be seen in the dermis after skin biopsy.

Lens and corneal opacities may occur as part of an 'epithelial keratopathy', especially after chronic chlorpromazine treatment. Light brown, granular deposits occur in the anterior lens and posterior cornea and are visible only at slit-lens examination of the eye. The lesions may progress to opaque brown stellate granules found in the lens. Occasionally, the conjunctivae show brown discoloration. Statistically, lens opacities occur more frequently in patients with skin discoloration. Vision is very rarely impaired. The opacities are dose-related and related to chronicity of drug exposure. Sunlight plays a role in both the skin and eye complications of the phenothiazines.

Thioridazine is guilty of a much more serious ophthalmic complication. In doses in excess of $800\ mg \cdot d^{-1}$ a *retinitis pigmentosa* can occur and this is accompanied by substantial visual impairment and even blindness. The retinitis does not remit if the drug is stopped.

Idiosyncratic reactions

These are relatively rare, are not clearly dose-related, and tend to occur early in the course of drug treatment.

JAUNDICE

This can be associated with the use of phenothiazines and in the 1960s the incidence was reported to be as high as 1 per cent. More recently, for reasons unknown, the incidence has fallen to 0.1 per cent at most. Clinical jaundice is preceded by flu-like malaise, abdominal pain, fever, nausea, vomiting and diarrhoea—a picture resembling infectious hepatitis. The biochemical picture is of obstructive jaundice (raised serum bilirubin and alkaline phosphatase) and the pathological picture is one of intrahepatic centralobular cholestasis. There is pericanalicular inflammation with oedema and local infiltration by eosinophils as well as generalized eosinophilia. Most cases have been reported in association with chlorpromazine but it may also occur with thioridazine, promazine, prochlorperazine and, very rarely, fluphenazine.

BLOOD DYSCRASIAS

Agranulocytosis is probably the most serious of all the side effects, but it is luckily very rare, variously quoted as occurring in between 1 in 10 000 and 1 in 500 000 patients treated with phenothiazines such as chlorpromazine and thioridazine. The mortality rate may be as high as 30 per cent. The polymorphonuclear leucocyte count falls rapidly and this is associated with sore throat, ulcerations and fever. Cross-sensitivity between phenothiazines should be assumed.

Phenothiazines quite often reduce the circulating white cell count by 40–80 per cent but this is a temporary and quite innocuous effect. Transient leucocytosis has also been reported. Thrombocytopenic purpura, eosinophilia, haemolytic anaemias and pancytopenia may occur rarely with the phenothiazines.

Drug interactions

Interaction with other drugs may affect the circulating plasma levels of antipsychotic drugs and the possible interaction of antischizophrenic and antiparkinson agents has already been mentioned. Many *hypnotic* and sedative drugs (such as phenobarbitone) are known to induce drug metabolizing enzymes of the hepatic endoplasmic reticulum and so increase the rate of drug metabolism and reduce the plasma concentrations of a wide variety of psychoactive drugs, including most antischizophrenic agents.

Apparent impairment of absorption of chlorpromazine has been reported to occur with concomitant administration of *antacids* such as aluminium hydroxide gels. This effect may be due to delayed emptying and it is thus not desirable to give antacids and chlorpormazine simultaneously, if possible spacing administration a few hours apart.

The metabolism of *tricyclic antidepressants* may be inhibited by various phenothiazines and by haloperidol, and *vice versa*. This suggests the possibility of mutual potentiation but the clinical implications of this remain to be evaluated. The mutual metabolic inhibition between phenothiazines and *propranolol* may render the toxicity of propranolol more likely while increasing the circulating plasma levels of the phenothiazine. Lithium has been shown to lower the plasma concentrations of chlorpromazine, an effect caused by delayed gastric emptying (Rivera-Calimlim, 1976).

Serious doubts about the safety of *haloperidol–lithium* combinations have been raised since the original report by Cohen and Cohen (1974) of four cases of severe extrapyramidal toxicity and irreversible brain damage allegedly due to the combination. However, the results of subsequent systematic investigations and of clinical experience suggest that haloperidol and lithium may be given together at *routine* clinical doses without risk of severe toxicity (Ayd, 1978). There may be an enhanced risk of quick-onset extrapyramidal impairment and, at high dose levels of both drugs, an increased risk of lithium CNS toxicity, and it is therefore prudent to monitor more carefully the patient receiving this combination.

References

ANGRIST, B., SATHANANTHAN, G., WILK, S. and GERSHON, S. Amphetamine psychosis; behavioural and biochemical aspects, *Journal of Psychiatric Research* **11**, 13–23 (1974)

ATSMON, A., BLUM, I., WIJSENBEEK, H., MAOZ, B., STEINER, M. and ZIEGELMAN, G. The short-term effects of adrenergic blocking agents in a small group of psychotic patients, *Psychiatrica, Neurologica and Neurochirgica* **74**, 251–258 (1971)

AYD, F. J. JR. Haloperidol: twenty years' clinical experience, *Journal of Clinical Psychiatry* **39**, 807–814 (1978)

BERGER, P. A. Clinical studies on the role of endorphins in schizophrenia. In *Proceedings of the Third World Congress of Biological Psychiatry*, (Stockholm, 1981), Elsevier/North Holland, Biomedical Press, Amsterdam (1981)

BERGER, P. A., WATSON, S. J., AKIL, H., ELLIOTT, G. R., LUBIN, R. T., PFEFFERBAUM, A., DAVIS, K. L., BARCHAS, J. D. and LI, C. H. β-endorphin and schizophrenia, *Archives of General Psychiatry* **37**, 635–640 (1980)

BORENSTEIN, P. and BLES, G. Effets cliniques et électroencéphalographiques du metroclopramide en psychiatrie, *Thérapie* **20**, 975–995 (1965)

BUCHSBAUM, M. S., DAVIS, G., NABER, D., PICKAS, D., BALLANGER, R., WATERS, R., GOODWIN, F. K., VAN KAMMEN, D., POST, R. and BUNNEY, W. JR. Pain appreciation somatosensory evoked potentials and endorphins in mammals and patients with schizophrenia and affective disorders. In *Proceedings of Third World Congress of Biological Psychiatry*, (Stockholm, 1981), Elsevier/North Holland, Biomedical Press, Amsterdam (1981)

CALDWELL, A. E. History of Psychopharmacology. In *Principles of Psychopharmacology* (Eds. W. G. CLARK and J. DEL GUIDICE), Academic Press, New York (1970)

CARNEY, M. W. P. and SHEFFIELD, B. F. Comparison of antipsychotic depot injections in the maintenance treatment of schizophrenia, *British Journal of Psychiatry* **129**, 476–481 (1976)

CASEY, J. F. BENNETT, I. F., LINDLEY, C. J., HOLLISTER, L. E., GORDON, M. H. and SPRINGER, N. N. Drug therapy in schizophrenia, *American Medical Association of Archives of General Psychiatry* **2**, 210–220 (1960a)

CASEY, J. F., LASKY, J. J., KLETT, C. J., and HOLLISTER, L. E. Treatment of schizophrenic reactions with phenothiazine derivatives, *American Journal of Psychiatry* **117**, 97–105 (1960b)

CHANG, K-J., HAZUM, E. and CUATRECASAS, P. *Trends in Neurosciences*, July, 1980, p. 160 (1980)

CHEUNG, H. K. Schizophrenics fully remitted on neuroleptics for 3–5 years—to stop or continue drugs?, *British Journal of Psychiatry* **138**, 490–494 (1981)

CHOUINARD, G. and JONES, B. D. Neuroleptic-induced supersensitivity psychosis: clinical and pharmacologic characteristics, *American Journal of Psychiatry* **137**, 16–21 (1980)

CIBA FOUNDATION SYMPOSIUM 74 (New Series). *Drug Concentrations in Neuropsychiatry*, Excerpta Medica, Amsterdam (1980)

CIOMPI, L. The natural history of schizophrenia in the long term, *British Journal of Psychiatry* **136**, 413–420 (1980)

COHEN, W. J. and COHEN, N. H. Lithium carbonate, haloperidol and irreversible brain damage, *Journal of the American Medical Association* **230**, 1283–1287 (1974)

CONNELL, P. H. *Amphetamine Psychosis*, Chapman & Hall, London

COOPER, T. B. Plasma level monitoring of anti-psychotic drugs, *Clinical Pharmacokinetics* **3**, 14–38 (1978)

CREESE, I., BURT, D. R. and SNYDER, S. H. Biochemical actions of neuroleptic drugs: focus on the dopamine receptor. In *Handbook of Psychopharmacology* (Eds. L. L. IVERSEN, S. D. IVERSEN and S. H. SNYDER), **10**, 37–89, Plenum Press, New York (1978)

CREESE, I. and SNYDER, S. H. A simple and sensitive radioreceptor assay for antischizophrenic drugs in blood, *Nature* **270**, 180–182 (1977)

CURRY, S. H. Metabolism and kinetics of chlorpromazine in relation to effect. In *Antipsychotic Drugs: Pharmacodynamics and Pharmacokinetics*, 343–352, Pergamon Press, Oxford (1976)

DAVIS, J. M. Efficacy of tranquillizing and antidepressant drugs, *Archives of General Psychiatry* **13**, 552–572 (1965)

DAVIS, J. M. Overview: maintenance therapy in psychiatry: I. Schizophrenia, *American Journal of Psychiatry* **132**, 1237–1245 (1975)

DAVIS, J. M. and COLE, J. O. Antipsychotic drugs. In *Comprehensive Textbook of Psychiatry* (Eds. A. M. FREEDMAN, H. I. KAPLAN and B. J. SADOCK), 2nd edn, **2**, 1921–1941, Williams and Wilkins Co. (1975)

DAVIS, J. M. and GARVER, D. L. Neuroleptics: clinical use in psychiatry. In *Handbook of Psychopharmacology* (Eds. L. L. IVERSEN, S. D. IVERSEN and S. H. SNYDER), **10**, 129–164, Plenum Press, New York (1978)

DENIKER, P. Impact of neuroleptic chemotherapies on schizophrenic psychoses, *American Journal of Psychiatry* **135**, 923–927 (1978)

DE WEID, D., BOHUS, B., VAN REE, J. M., KOVACS, G. L. and GREVEN, H. M. Neuroleptic-like activity of [Des-Tyr^1]—endorphin in rats, *Lancet* **1**, 1046 (1978)

DIAZ-BUXO, J. A., CAUDLE, J. A., CHANDLER, J. T., FARMER, C. D. and HOLBROOK, W. D. Dialysis of schizophrenic patients: a double-blind study, *American Journal of Psychiatry* **137**, 1220–1222 (1980)

DONLON, P. T., HOPKIN, J. T., TUPIN, J. P., WICKS, J. J., WAHBA, M. and MEADOW, A. Haloperidol for acute schizophrenic patients, *Archives of General Psychiatry* **37**, 691–695 (1980)

FALLOON, I., WATT, D. C. and SHEPHERD, M. A comparative controlled trial of pimozide and fluphenazine decanoate in the continuation therapy of schizophrenia, *Psychological Medicine* **8**, 59–70 (1978)

FIELDING, S. and LAL, H. Behavioural actions of neuroleptics. In *Neuroleptics and Schizophrenia: Handbook of Psychopharmacology* (Eds. L. L. IVERSEN, S. D. IVERSEN and S. H. SNYDER), **10**, Plenum Press, New York (1978)

FJALLAND, B., CHRISTENSEN, A. V. and HYTHEL, J. Peripheral and central muscarinic receptor affinity of psychotropic drugs, *Naunyn-Scmiedelberg's Archives of Pharmacology* **301**, 5–9 (1977)

FORSMAN, A., FOLSCH, G., LARSON, M. and OHMAN, R. On the metabolism of haloperidol in man, *Current Therapeutic Research* **21**, 606–617 (1977)

FREEMAN, H. Pimozide as a neuroleptic, *British Journal of Psychiatry* **135**, 82–83 (1979)

FRITH, C. D., STEVENS, M., JOHNSTONE, E. C. and CROW, T. J. Skin conductance responsivity during acute episodes of schizophrenia as a predictor of symptomatic improvement, *Psychological Medicine* **9**, 101–106 (1979)

GARVER, D. L., DEKIRMENJIAN, H., DAVIS, J. M., CASPER, R. and ERICKSEN, S. Neuroleptic drug levels and therapeutic response: preliminary observations with red blood cell bound butaperazine, *American Journal of Psychiatry* **134**, 304–307 (1977)

GERNER, R. H., CATLIN, D. H., GORELICK, D. A., HUI, K. K. and LI, C. H. β-endorphin intravenous infusion causes behavioural change in psychiatric patients, *Archives of General Psychiatry* **37**, 642–647 (1980)

GOLDBERG, S. C., KLERMAN, G. L. and COLE, J. O. Changes in schizophrenic psychopathology and ward behaviour as a function of phenothiazine treatment, *British Journal of Psychiatry* **111**, 120–133 (1965)

GREEN, A. R. and GRAHAME-SMITH, D. G. (−)—Propranolol inhibits the behavioural responses of rats to increased 5-hydroxytryptamine in the central nervous system, *Nature* **262**, 594–596 (1976)

GREENBLATT, D. J., SHADER, R. I. and KOCH-WESER, J. The psychopharmacology of β-adrenergic blockade: pharmacokinetic and epidemiologic aspects. In *Advances in Clinical Pharmacology* (Eds. C. CARLSSON, J. ENGEL and L. HANSSON), **12**, 6–12, Urban and Schwarzenberg, Berlin (1976)

GROVES, J. E. and MANDEL, M. R. The long-acting phenothiazines, *Archives of General Psychiatry* **32**, 893–900 (1975)

GRUEN, P. H., SACHAR, E. J., LANGER, G., ALTMAN, N., LEIFER, M., FRANTZ, A. and HALPERN, F. S. Prolactin responses to neuroleptics in normal and schizophrenic subjects, *Archives of General Psychiatry* **35**, 108–116 (1978)

GRUZELIER, J., CONNOLLY, J., EVES, F., HIRSCH, S., ZAKI, S., WELLER, M. and YORKSTON, N. Effect of propranolol and phenothiazines on electrodermal orienting and habituation in schizophrenia, *Psychological Medicine* **11**, 93–108 (1981)

HASLAM, M. T., BROMHAM, B. M. and SCHIFF, A. A. A comparative trial of fluphenazine decanoate and flupenthixol decanoate, *Acta Psychiatrica Scandinavica* **51**, 92–100 (1975)

HOGARTY, G. E., GOLDBERG, S. C., SCHOOLER, N. R., ULRICH, R. F. and the COLLABORATIVE STUDY GROUP. Drug and sociotherapy in the aftercare of schizophrenic patients; II and III, *Archives of General Psychiatry* **31**, 603–618 (1974)

HOGARTY, G. E. and ULRICH, R. F. Temporal effects of drug and placebo in delaying relapse in schizophrenic outpatients, *Archives of General Psychiatry* **34**, 297–301 (1977)

HOLLISTER, L. E. Antipsychotic medications and the treatment of schizophrenia. In *Psychopharmacology* (Eds. J. D. BARCHAS, P. A. BERGER, R. D. CIARANELLO and G. R. ELLIOTT), Oxford University Press, Oxford (1977)

IVERSEN, L. L. Biochemical and pharmacological studies in schizophrenia: The Dopamine Hypothesis. In *Schizophrenia* (Ed. J. K. WING), Academic Press, London (1979)

IVERSEN, S. D. Brain chemistry and behaviour, *Psychological Medicine* **10**, 527–539 (1980)

JANSSEN, P., BRUGMANS, J., DONY, J. and SCHUERMANS, V. An international double-blind evaluation of pimozide, *Journal of Clinical Pharmacology* **12**, 26–34 (1972)

JESTE, D. V., POTKIN, S. G., SINHA, S., FEDER, S. and WYATT, R. J. Tardive dyskinesia—reversible and persistent, *Archives of General Psychiatry* **36**, 585–590 (1979)

JOHNSON, D. A. W. and FREEMAN, H. Drug defaulting by patients on long-acting phenothiazines, *Psychological Medicine* **5**, 115–119 (1973)

JOHNSTONE, E. C., CROW, T. J., FRITH, C. D., CARNEY, M. W. P. and PRICE, J. S. Mechanism of the antipsychotic effect in the treatment of acute schizophrenia, *Lancet* **1**, 848–851 (1978)

KEBABIAN, J. W., PETZOLD, G. L. and GREENGARD, P. Dopamine-sensitive adenylate cyclase in caudate nucleus of rat brain and its similarity to the 'dopamine receptor', *Proceedings of the National Academy of Science, USA* **69**, 2145–2149 (1972)

KELLY, P. H., SEVIOUR, P. W. and IVERSEN, S. D. Amphetamine and apomorphine responses in the rat following 6-OHDA lesions of the nucleus accumbens septi and corpus striatum, *Brain Research* **94**, 507–522 (1975)

KNIGHTS, A., OKASHA, M. S., SALIH, M. A. and HIRSCH, S. R. Depressive and extrapyramidal symptoms and clinical effects: a trial of fluphenazine versus flupenthixol in maintenance of schizophrenic outpatients, *British Journal of Psychiatry* **135**, 515–523 (1979)

LADER, M. In *Drug Concentrations in Neuropsychiatry*, Ciba Foundation Symposium 74 (New Series), 225–233, Excerpta Medica, Oxford (1980)

LASKY, J. J., KLETT, C. J., COFFEY, E. M., BENNETT, J. L., ROSENBLUM, M. P. and HOLLISTER, L. E. Drug treatment of schizophrenic patients, *Diseases of the Nervous System* **23**, 698–706 (1962)

LINGJAERDE, O. Some pharmacological aspects of depot neuroleptics, *Acta Psychiatrica Scandinavica* (supplement) **246**, 9–14 (1973)

McCREADIE, R. G. and MacDONALD, I. M. High dosage haloperidol in chronic schizophrenia, *British Journal of Psychiatry* **131**, 310–316 (1977)

McCREADIE, R. G., HEYKANTS, J. J. P., CHALMERS, A. and ANDERSON, A. M. Plasma pimozide profiles in chronic schizophrenics, *British Journal of Clinical Pharmacology* **7**, 533–534 (1979)

McGLASHAN, T. H. and CARPENTER, W. T. JR. Post-psychotic depression in schizophrenia, *Archives of General Psychiatry* **33**, 231–239 (1976)

MACKAY, A. V. P. Psychiatric implications of endorphin research, *British Journal of Psychiatry* **135**, 470–473 (1979)

MACKAY, A. V. P. Neurotransmitters in psychiatry, *Medicine* **35**, 1799–1805 (1980)

MACKAY, A. V. P. Controversies in tardive dyskinesia. In *Neurology, Movement Disorders* (Eds. C. D. MARSDEN and S. FAHN) **2**, Butterworths, London (1981a)

MACKAY, A. V. P. Assessment of antipsychotic drugs, *British Journal of Clinical Pharmacology* **11**, 225–236 (1981b)

MACKAY, A. V. P. Endorphins: implications for psychiatry. In *Advanced Medicine* (Ed. D. P. JEWELL), **17**, 180–188, Royal College of Physicians of London, Pitman Medical, London (1981c)

MACKAY, A. V. P. and CROW, T. J. Positive and negative schizophrenic symptoms and the role of dopamine, *British Journal of Psychiatry* **137**, 379–386 (1980)

MACKAY, A. V. P., HEALEY, A. F. and BAKER, J. The relationship of plasma chlorpromazine to its 7-hydroxy and sulphoxide metabolites in a large population of chronic schizophrenics, *British Journal of Clinical Pharmacology* **1**, 425–430 (1974)

MACKAY, A. V. P., BIRD, E. D., SPOKES, E. G., ROSSOR, M., IVERSEN, L. L., CREESE, I. and SNYDER, S. H. Dopamine receptors and schizophrenia: drug effect or illness?, *Lancet* **2**, 915–916 (1980)

MANCHANDA, R. and HIRSCH, S. R. (Des-Tyr')-γ-endorphin in the treatment of schizophrenia, *Psychological Medicine* **11**, 401–404 (1981)

MARCHAND, W. E. Occurrence of painless myocardial infarction in psychotic patients, *New England Journal of Medicine* **253**, 51–55 (1955)

MARSDEN, C. D. and JENNER, P. The pathophysiology of extrapyramidal side-effects of neuroleptic drugs, *Psychological Medicine* **10**, 55–72 (1980)

MARSDEN, C. D., MINDHAM, R. H. S. and MACKAY, A. V. P. Extrapyramidal movement disorders produced by antipsychotic drugs. In *The Pharmacology and Treatment of Schizophrenia* (Eds. P. B. BRADLEY and S. R. HIRSCH), Oxford University Press, London (in Press)

MIDDLEMISS, D. N., BLAKEBOROUGH, L. and LEATHER, S. R. Direct evidence for an interaction of β-adrenergic blockers with the 5-HT receptor, *Nature* **267**, 289–290 (1977)

MINDHAM, R. H. S. Assessment of drug-induced extrapyramidal reactions and of drugs given for their control, *British Journal of Clinical Pharmacology* **3**, 395–400 (1976)

MOUNTAIN, H. E. Crash tranquillization in a milieu therapy setting, *Journal of Logan Mental Health Centre* **1**, 43–44 (1963)

MYERS, D. H., CAMPBELL, P. L., COCKS, N. M., FLOWERDEW, J. A. and MUIR, A. A trial of propranolol in chronic schizophrenia, *British Journal of Psychiatry* **139**, 118–121 (1981)

NEBORSKY, R., JANOWSKY, D., MUNSON, E. and DEPRY, D. Rapid treatment of acute psychotic symptoms with high and low dose haloperidol, *Archives of General Psychiatry* **38**, 195–199 (1981)

NATIONAL INSTITUTE OF MENTAL HEALTH. Psychopharmacology Service Center Collaborative Study Group. Phenothiazine treatment in acute schizophrenia, *Archives of General Psychiatry* **10**, 246–261 (1964)

OLDHAM, A. J. and BOTT, M. The management of excitement in a general hospital psychiatric ward by high-dosage haloperidol, *Acta Psychiatrica Scandinavica* **47**, 369–376 (1971)

PALMOUR, R. M., ERVIN, F. R. and WAGEMAKER, H. Characterisation of a peptide derived from the serum of psychiatric patients, *Abstracts of Social Neurosciences* **7**, 32 (1977)

PEET, M., BETHELL, M. S., COATES, A., KHAMNEE, A. K., HALL, P., COOPER, S. J., KING, D. J. and YATES, R. A. Propranolol in schizophrenia: I. Comparison of propranolol, chlorpromazine and placebo, *British Journal of Psychiatry* **139**, 105–111 (1981a)

PEET, M., MIDDLEMISS, D. N. and YATES, R. A. Propranolol in schizophrenia: II Clinical and biochemical aspects of combining propranolol with chlorpromazine, *British Journal of Psychiatry* **139**, 112–117 (1981b)

PEROUTKA, S. J. and SNYDER, S. H. Differential effects of neuroleptic drugs at brain dopamine, serotonin, alpha-adrenergic and histamine receptors: relationship to clinical potency (1980)

PEROUTKA, S. J., U' PRITCHARD, D. C., GREENBERG, D. A. and SNYDER, S. H. Neuroleptic drug interactions with norepinephrine alpha receptor binding sites in rat brain, *Neuropharmacology* **16**, 549–556 (1977)

PETERSEN, P. V. and NIELSEN, I. M. Thioxanthene derivatives. In *Psychopharmacological Agents* (Ed. M. GORDON), p. 301, Academic Press, New York (1964)

PHILLIPSON, O., BAKER, J., SEBASTIANPILLAI, F., SHEPPARD, G. and BROOK, P. Disappearance of chlorpromazine from plasma following drug withdrawal, *Psychological Medicine* **8**, 331–334 (1978)

PHILLIPSON, O. T., McKEOWN, J. M., BAKER, J. and HEALEY, A. F. Correlation between plasma chlorpromazine and its metabolites and clinical ratings in patients with acute relapse of schizophrenic and paranoid psychosis, *British Journal of Psychiatry* **131**, 172–184 (1977)

PICKAR, D. and BUNNEY, W. E. JR. Acute naloxone in schizophrenic patients: A World Health Organisation Collaborative project. In *Proceedings of the Third World Congress of Biological Psychiatry*, (Stockholm, 1981), Elsevier/North Holland Biomedical Press, Amsterdam (1981)

POST, R. M., JIMERSORI, D. C., BUNNEY, W. E. JR. and GOODWIN, F. K. Dopamine and mania: Behavioural and biochemical effects of the dopamine receptor blocker pimozide, *Psychophamacology* **67**, 297–305 (1980)

QMACH, T. T., DUCHEMIN, A. M., ROSE, C. and SCHWARTZ, J. C. *In vivo* occupation of cerebral histamine H,—receptors evaluated with ^{3}H-mepyramine may predict sedative properties of psychotropic drugs, *European Journal of Pharmacology* **60**, 391–392 (1979)

QUITKIN, F., RIFKIN, A., KANE, J., RAMOS-LORENZI, J. R. and KLEIN, D. F. Long-acting oral versus injectable antipsychotic drugs in schizophrenics, *Archives of General Psychiatry* **35**, 889–892 (1978)

RANDRUP, A. and MUNKVAD, I. Pharmacology and physiology of stereotyped behaviour, *Journal of Psychiatric Research* **11**, 1–10 (1974)

RIVERA-CALIMLIM, L. Impaired absorption of chlorpromazine in rats given trihexyphenidyl, *British Journal of Pharmacology* **56**, 301–305 (1976a)

RIVERA-CALIMLIM, L. Effect of lithium on gastric emptying and absorption of oral chlorpromazine, *Psychopharmacological Communication* **2**, 263–272 (1976b)

RUTHER, E., GERD, J. and NEDOPIL, N. Clinical effects of the synthetic analogue of methionine enkephalin FK-33-824. In *Proceedings of the Third World Congress of Biological Psychiatry*, (Stockholm, 1981), Elsevier/North Holland Biomedical Press, Amsterdam (1982)

SANGIOVANNI, F., TAYLOR, M. A., ABRAMS, R. and GAZTANAGA, P. Rapid control of psychotic excitement states with intramuscular haloperidol, *American Journal of Psychiatry* **130**, 1155–1156 (1973)

SCHONECKER, M. Ein eigenümliches syndrome in oralen bereiches syndrome in oralen bereich bei megaphen applikation, *Nerventartz* **28**, p. 35 (1957)

SEEMAN, P., LEE, T., CHA-WONG, M. and WONG, K. Antipsychotic drug doses and neuroleptic/dopamine receptors, *Nature* **261**, 717–719 (1976)

SHEPHERD, M., LADER, M. and RODNIGHT, R. *Clinical Psychopharmacology*, English Universities Press Ltd., London (1968)

SHEPHERD, M. and WATT, D. C. Long-term treatment with neuroleptics in psychiatry. In *Current Developments in Psychopharmacology* **4**, 217–247, Spectrum Publications Inc., London (1977)

SHEPPARD, G., MACKAY, A. V. P. and KITSON, M. Clonazepam in the treatment of tardive dyskinesia; a controlled study. In *Proceedings of the Third World Congress of Biological Psychiatry*, (Stockholm, 1981), Elsevier/North Holland Biomedical Press, Amsterdam (1982)

SNYDER, S. H. Amphetamine psychosis; a 'model' schizophrenia mediated by catecholamines, *American Journal of Psychiatry* **130**, 61–67 (1973)

SNYDER, S. H. Dopamine receptors, neuroleptics and schizophrenia, *American Journal of Psychiatry* **138**, 460–464 (1981)

SNYDER, S., GREENBERG, D. and YAMAMURA, H. I. Antischizophrenic drugs and brain cholinergic receptors, *Archives of General Psychiatry* **31**, 58–61 (1974)

STANLEY, M. and WILKS, S. Striatal DOPAC elevation predicts antipsychotic efficacy of metoclopramide, *Life Sciences* **24**, 1907–1912 (1979)

STURGEON, D., KUIPERS, L., BERKOWITZ, R., TURPIN, G. and LEFF, J. Psychophysiological responses of schizophrenic patients to high and low expressed emotion relatives, *British Journal of Psychiatry* **138**, 40–45 (1981)

TARRIER, N., VAUGHAN, C., LADER, M. H. and LEFF, J. P. Bodily reactions to people and events in schizophrenics, *Archives of General Psychiatry* **36**, 311–315 (1979)

THORVER, M. O. and BESSER, G. M. Bromocriptine. In *Proceedings of a Symposium at the Royal College of Physicians*, London. (Eds. R. I. S. BAYLISS, P. TURNER and W. P. MACLAY), MCS Consultants, Kent (1976)

TYRER, P. J. Use of β-blocking drugs in psychiatry and neurology, *Drugs* **20**, 300–308 (1980)

UHRBRAND, L. and FAURBYE, A. Reversible and irreversible dyskinesia after treatment with perphenazine, chlorpromazine, reserpine and electoconvulsive therapy, *Psychopharmacologia* **1**, 408–419 (1960)

VAN PUTTEN, T. Why do schizophrenic patients refuse to take their drugs?, *Archives of General Psychiatry* **31**, 67–72 (1974)

VAN PUTTEN, T. The many faces of akathisia, *Comprehensive Psychiatry* **16**, 43–47 (1975)

VAN PUTTEN, T. and MAY, P. R. A. Akinetic depression in schizophrenia, *Archives of General Psychiatry* **35**, 1101–1107 (1978)

VAUGHN, C. E. and LEFF, J. P. The influence of family and social factors on the course of psychiatric illness, *British Journal of Psychiatry* **129**, 125–137 (1976)

VENABLES, P. H. and WING, J. K. Level of arousal and the subclassification of schizophrenia, *Archives of General Psychiatry* **7**, 114–119 (1962)

WATSON, G. D., CHANDARANA, P. C. and MERSKEY, H. Relationships between pain and schizophrenia, *British Journal of Psychiatry* **138**, 33–36 (1981)

WESTLAKE, R. J. and RASTEGAR, A. Hyperpyrexia from drug combinations, *Journal of the American Medical Association* **225**, p. 1250 (1973)

WING, J. K., COOPER, J. E. and SARTORIUS, N. *The Measurement and Classification of Psychiatric Symptoms*, Cambridge University Press, London (1974)

WISTEDT, B., WILES, D. and KOLAKOWSKA, T. Slow decline of plasma drug and prolactin levels after discontinuation of chronic treatment with depot neuroleptics, *Lancet* **i**, p. 1163 (1981)

YORKSTON, N. J., GRUZELIER, J. H., ZAKI, S. A., HOLLANDER, D., PITCHER, D. R. and SERGEANT, H. G. S. Propranolol as an adjunct to the treatment of schizophrenia, *Lancet* **2**, 575–578 (1977)

YORKSTON, N. J., ZAKI, S. A., WELLER, M. P., GRUZELIER, J. H. and HIRSCH, S. R. DL—propranolol and chlorpromazine following admission for schizophrenia, *Acta Psychiatrica Scandinavica* **63**, 13–27 (1981)

Chapter 5

Antiparkinsonian and antidyskinetic drugs

P. Jenner and C. D. Marsden

Introduction

The introduction of neuroleptic drugs into clinical practice and their subsequent development has been examined in detail by MacKay in the previous chapter. The revolution caused by the introduction of chlorpromazine by Delay and colleagues in the early 1950s (Delay, Deniker and Harl, 1952) provided the first of a range of compounds that have become the mainstay of the management of acute toxic confusional states and of patients with acute or chronic schizophrenia (Meyer, 1956; NIMH, 1964; Grinspoon, Ewalt and Shader, 1968; Leff and Wing, 1971; Hirsch *et al.*, 1973; Hogarty, Goldberg and Schooler, 1974). Their clinical impact has been dramatic but, as is nature's way, a price was paid for this success. Thus, almost immediately after the introduction of neuroleptic drugs it was found that they could produce a range of extrapyramidal side effects. Broadly these fall into four categories:

(1) Drug-induced parkinsonism which mirrors idiopathic Parkinson's disease in practically all clinical aspects (Steck, 1954).
(2) Akathisia, a peculiar state of mental and motor restlessness characterized by an intense desire to move in order to gain respite from overwhelming feelings of distress (Steck, 1954).
(3) Acute dystonic reactions which may resemble naturally-occurring dystonic dyskinesias, such as torticollis and other fragments of torsion dystonia, and which are similar to some levodopa-induced dyskinesias (Delay and Deniker, 1957).
(4) Chronic tardive dyskinesias which become recognized after months or years of treatment, and which persist even though the offending neuroleptic agent may be withdrawn (Sigwald *et al.*, 1959; Uhrbrand and Faurbye, 1960).

The drug treatment of these neuroleptic-induced movement disorders represents a major clinical problem. In the main treatment is based on the therapy utilized for idiopathic Parkinson's disease and for a variety of spontaneously occurring dyskinesias. In general the drug control of these disorders is poor and this reflects the paucity of our knowledge concerning their pathophysiology. However, before proceeding to discuss drug treatment it is necessary to describe the characteristics of these syndromes and to outline current concepts of their cause.

Pathophysiology of neuroleptic-induced movement disorders

Parkinsonism

Neuroleptic-induced parkinsonism may be associated with each of the major symptoms of the idiopathic disorder, including akinesia, rigidity, postural abnormalities and tremor (Marsden, Tarsy and Baldessarini, 1975). Akinesia is the earliest and often the only symptom of neuroleptic-induced parkinsonism. Rigidity of the extremities, neck or trunk appear some time after the onset of akinesia. Characteristic postural abnormalities are common, including flexed posture, impairment of righting responses, and a propulsive or retropulsive gait. The characteristic tremor of Parkinson's diseases occurs still later in the course of drug-induced parkinsonism, but is relatively uncommon (Schwab and England, 1968).

Drug-induced parkinsonism may commence within a few days of drug treatment; 50–75 per cent of cases have appeared by one month, and 90 per cent of cases within three months (Ayd, 1961; Freyhan, 1957). Following administration of piperazine-containing phenothiazine drugs, the progression of signs is often condensed such that acute akinesia with mutism may appear within 48 h, followed within days by rigidity and a typical akinetic-rigid syndrome (Delay and Deniker, 1968).

The majority of patients are free of extrapyramidal signs within a few weeks of discontinuation of neuroleptic therapy, but in some instances signs may persist for months, weeks or even years (Hall, Jackson and Swain, 1956; Hershon, Kennedy and McGuire, 1972). The question is whether the small minority that do not recover have subclinical idiopathic Parkinson's disease before starting treatment, or whether the drugs themselves can promote permanent parkinsonism. The incidence of idiopathic Parkinson's disease in the population at large is of the order of 1 in 200 in those over the age of 50. It is likely that the small proportion of patients in whom parkinsonism persists for years after neuroleptic administration and withdrawal indeed did have the idiopathic disease (Marsden and Jenner, 1980). The fact that the age incidence of drug-induced parkinsonism parallels that of idiopathic Parkinson's disease strongly hints that a propensity for the latter may determine the incidence of the former. The implication of this observation is that there must be a large pool of individuals with subclinical degrees of striatal dopamine depletion without overt evidence of parkinsonism. Such patients would be more susceptible to the influence of administration of neuroleptic drugs.

Parkinsonism can be provoked by the use of drugs acting pre-synaptically, such as reserpine or tetrabenazine, or by drugs acting predominantly post-synaptically such as the phenothiazine, thioxanthene, butyrophenone and substituted benzamide classes of neuroleptic drugs.

The incidence of parkinsonism following reserpine therapy given in high doses as an antipsychotic has ranged from 5–29 per cent (Barsa and Kline, 1956; Freyhan, 1957; Goldman, 1961). Following neuroleptic agents, the incidence has varied between 5 and 60 per cent (Freyhan, 1957; 1959; Goldman, 1961; Sheppard and Merlis, 1967). In routine clinical practice some 20–40 per cent of all patients treated with these drugs are reported to exhibit obvious clinical signs of parkinsonism (Marsden, Tarsy and Baldessarini, 1975) It is clear that there is an individual susceptibility to the development of parkinsonism in response to a given dose of neuroleptics. Factors determining such individual susceptibility have not been established, but may well include their pre-existing state of dopamine reserve in the brain.

Idiopathic Parkinson's disease and post-encephalitic parkinsonism both show a common pathophysiology, namely a loss of pigmented brainstem neurons, particularly those of the substantia nigra in the midbrain. This causes a profound depletion of cerebral catecholamines, particularly of dopamine in the caudate nucleus and putamen (corpus striatum), as a result of degeneration of the nigrostriatal dopamine pathway. The main clinical features of Parkinson's disease are due to this severe dopamine depletion in the brain (Ehringer and Hornykiewicz, 1960), for they can be reversed (at least partially and initially) by restoring brain dopamine action, either by oral feeding of the precursor amino acid levodopa (Birkmayer and Hornykiewicz, 1961; Barbeau, 1962; Cotzias, van Woert and Schiffer, 1967), or by directly acting dopamine agonists such as bromocriptine (Calne et al., 1974) or pergolide (Liebermann et al. 1981).

Drug-induced parkinsonism also is due to dopamine deficiency in the brain. Reserpine, and its short-acting analogue, tetrabenzazine, prevent dopamine storage by disrupting intraneuronal granules containing the amine (Bertler, 1961; Glowinski, Iversen and Axelrod, 1966); neuroleptic drugs antagonize cerebral dopamine action by blocking dopamine receptors in the brain (Carlsson and Lindquist, 1963; Janssen, Niemegeers and Schellekens, 1965; van Rossum, 1966). All neuroleptics are dopamine receptor antagonists, at least on acute administration; the evidence that neuroleptic drugs antagonize cerebral dopamine action comes from a variety of animal experimental data which have been discussed in the previous chapters.

There often is delay in the appearance of drug-induced parkinsonism after starting treatment. Mostly it appears within a few weeks or months of starting treatment, rather than after a few days. This may be due, in part, to the accumulation of drug. The pharmacokinetics of most neuroleptic agents are characterized by a long half-life and accumulation in tissue stores (Salzman and Brodie, 1956). However whether this is the only explanation remains to be established. Equally apparent clinically is that drug-induced parkinsonism, once having appeared, may gradually disappear despite continuing drug therapy. Pharmacokinetic causes might explain this observation for there is evidence of increased neuroleptic metabolism with chronic administration of the drugs (Sakalis et al., 1972; Loga, Curry and Lader, 1975), but many neuroleptics accumulate during chronic therapy. A more rational explanation is that dopamine receptor blockade gradually decreases with time and very recent experiments indicate that this is exactly what happens (see below).

Akathisia

Akathisia is a state of motor restlessness that occurs following administration of all classes of neuroleptic drug. Since it occurs also in post-encephalitic and idiopathic Parkinson's disease, and since it occasionally responds to antiparkinsonian medication, it is often assumed to be a basal ganglia disturbance, although there is little compelling evidence to support this concept (Marsden, Tarsy and Baldessarini, 1975).

Akathisia leads to striking complaints of motor tension, of being driven to move, and of an inability to tolerate inactivity (Sarwer-Foner, 1960). The objective manifestations include a variety of patterns of restless motor activity such as shuffling or tapping movements of the feet, continuous shifting of weight and rocking of the trunk while standing and, in more severe cases, an inability to sit, stand or lie still; such patients may pace or run incessantly. The syndrome should not be confused with psychotic agitation or anxiety.

Akathisia may begin within several days after the start of drug treatment, but usually does not occur within the first 48 h. Drug-induced parkinsonism and akathisia commonly occur only after some weeks or months of starting on neuroleptic drugs. Unlike acute dyskinesias, the incidence of akathisia continues to increase with time (Ayd, 1961). The duration of akathisia is extremely variable. Symptoms may spontaneously appear and disappear. Although akathisia may subside within several days or weeks during continuous drug administration, it frequently can persist. Drug withdrawal may result in improvement, although the symptoms may persist unchanged for several months or may even worsen (Kruse, 1960; Hershon, Kennedy and McGuire, 1972). The occurrence of akathisia simultaneously with other extrapyramidal syndromes has complicated its clinical description.

Akathisia probably is the most common reaction to antipsychotic drugs and occurs following administration of reserpine, tetrabenazine, phenothiazines, butyrophenones, thioxanthenes and substituted benzamides. The incidence of akathisia following reserpine has ranged between 0.5–8 per cent (Freyhan, 1957; Goldman, 1961). As in other drug-induced syndromes, the reported incidence with neuroleptics varies according to their potency but ranges between 5 and 50 per cent (Denham and Carrick, 1961; Freyhan, 1959; Goldman, 1961); in routine clinical use the incidence is about 20 per cent (Ayd, 1961). Factors that might account for differences in individual susceptibility are not known. Unlike the other drug-induced syndromes no specific age predisposition has been noted, so that incidence is uniform between the ages of 12 and 65 years (Ayd, 1961).

Akathisia is a paradox. Neuroleptics cause calm, producing mental quiet and motor immobility. Akathisia is manifest by mental unease and motor restlessness. Two hypotheses can be put forward to explain its occurrence. A neuroleptic drug that preferentially blocks pre-synaptic dopamine receptors in concentrations less than those required to antagonize the post-synaptic receptor will have unexpected effects (see Carlsson, 1977). Its pre-synaptic action would lead to increased dopamine synthesis and release of dopamine onto post-synaptic dopamine receptors not antagonized by the drug. As a consequence the functional and behavioural effects of such a drug would be to increase dopaminergic action rather than decrease it, despite the fact that its main effect was to block dopamine receptors. Selective pre-synaptic dopamine receptor antagonism might be invoked to explain drug-induced akathisia, but there are reasons to dismiss this hypothesis. Firstly, reserpine and tetrabenazine, both of which deplete dopamine stores and therefore cannot increase dopamine action may cause obvious akathisia. Secondly, akathisia and drug-induced parkinsonism commonly co-exist (Marsden, Tarsy and Baldessarini, 1975). It is difficult to see how the same drug could simultaneously block pre-synaptic dopamine receptors to produce akathisia and post-synaptic dopamine receptors to produce drug-induced parkinsonism.

An alternative hypothesis is that akathisia is the result of post-synaptic dopamine receptor blockade in cerebral dopamine-containing areas other than the corpus striatum. While blockade of dopamine receptors in the striatum and in mesolimbic areas such as nucleus accumbens produces inhibition of locomotion in the form of akinesia or catalepsy, the reverse occurs on blockade of mesocortical dopamine systems. Destruction of these pathways alone, or of their terminal projection areas in the medial, frontal and cingulate areas, causes locomotor hyperactivity in rodents (Iversen, 1971; Tassin et al., 1978; Carter and Pycock, 1978). If it is assumed that this has a conscious equivalent in man, then both the mental and physical manifestations of akathisia might be attributed to blockade of dopamine receptors in these specific cortical areas. Further work is required to confirm this hypothesis.

Acute dystonic reactions

Acute dystonic reactions occur soon after the commencement of neuroleptic therapy and consist primarily of intermittent or sustained muscular spasms and abnormal postures. Involvement of the muscles of the eyes, face, neck and throat and trunk occur. Continuous slow writhing movements of the extremities with exaggerated postures complete the clinical picture.

Acute dystonic reactions are the earliest of the neuroleptic-induced syndromes to appear and may begin within hours of a single administration. Approximately 50 per cent occur within 48 h and perhaps 90 per cent within 5 d of starting drug therapy (Ayd, 1961; Deniker, 1960). The movements may either remit or fluctuate simultaneously over several hours or days after drug withdrawal, but often re-appear on re-introduction of other drugs of equal potency.

There appear to be no well-documented cases of acute dystonic reactions following the use of reserpine or its analogues. In normal clinical use, the overall incidence of acute dystonic reactions is approximately 2.5–5 per cent of patients, so this is the least frequent drug-induced extrapyramidal syndrome (Ayd, 1961; Chase, 1972). As in the case of parkinsonism, however, the more potent neuroleptic agents are particularly likely to produce acute dystonic reactions. Virtually nothing is known about the factors that predispose this small group of patients to develop the problem. Until recently little was known about their pathophysiology, but new data derived from both animal experiments and human observations have begun to shed light on the matter.

Acute dystonic reactions have been observed in animals treated with neuroleptics, particularly in several species of primates (Deneau and Crane, 1968; Gunne and Barany, 1976; Bedard *et al.*, 1977; Weiss, Santelli and Lusink, 1977). The administration of haloperidol to baboons produced a typical acute dystonic reaction with features such as trismus, forced jaw opening, spasms of tongue with occlusion, gnawing, arching of the back and torticollis, as well as biazarre posturing of the limbs (Meldrum, Anlezark and Meldrum, 1977). A range of neuroleptics produced this response in susceptible animals, including haloperidol, chlorpromazine, pimozide and oxypertine, but thioridazine (a neuroleptic with inherent anticholinergic activity) was ineffective. As in man, anticholinergic drugs abolished the acute dystonic reactions while cholinergic agents intensified haloperidol-induced dystonia.

Further pharmacological exploration in the primate model of neuroleptic-induced dystonic reactions led to the critical observation that disrupting pre-synaptic dopamine mechanisms can prevent the phenomenon. Pre-treatment of monkeys with reserpine (to disrupt granular storage of catecholamines) reduced, but did not abolish, dystonia produced by haloperidol. A combination of reserpine with α-methyl-*p*-tyrosine (which itself was ineffective) abolished or greatly reduced haloperidol-induced dystonia. These results indicated that acute dystonic reactions to neuroleptic drugs are dependent on some pre-synaptic event mediated by both the storage and synthesis of catecholamines. The overall conclusion is that acute dystonic reactions are produced as the result of some effect of neuroleptic drugs on pre-synaptic dopamine mechanisms.

The obvious candidate for such a mechanism is the compensatory increase in dopamine synthesis and release provoked by acute administration of neuroleptic drugs. Like acute dystonic reactions themselves, this increased dopamine release is apparent only on acute administration of a neuroleptic agent. Repeated administration is associated with a decline and eventual disappearance of evidence of increased dopamine turnover (Asper *et al.*, 1973; Scatton, 1977). In addition, administration of anticholinergic drugs not only prevents acute dystonic reactions but also diminishes the increased dopamine release provoked by neuroleptic drugs (O'Keefe, Sharman and Vogt, 1970; Anden, 1972; Corrodi, Fuxe and Lidbrink, 1972). There is, indeed, some evidence to suggest that dopamine release can provoke dystonia. A proportion of patients with Parkinson's disease treated with levodopa develop abnormal movements identical to those of dystonia (Parkes, Bedard and Marsden, 1976). Administration of even larger doses of levodopa combined with a peripheral decarboxylase inhibitor to normal monkeys also can induce dystonic abnormal movements (Paulson, 1973; Mones, 1973; Sassin, 1975). All this evidence, therefore, suggests that acute dystonic reactions in man and animals may be due to increased dopamine release resulting from the acute administration of a neuroleptic drug.

It is difficult, however, to see how the dopamine released by acute neuroleptic administration can stimulate post-synaptic dopamine receptors for these are blocked by the neuroleptic. It could be argued that the doses of the drug invoking acute dystonic reactions act preferentially on pre-synaptic dopamine receptors to cause increased dopamine release, but without blocking the post-synaptic receptor. Alternatively one could invoke the existence of multiple forms of dopamine receptors, only one of which is blocked by the neuroleptic agent (Skirboll and Bunney, 1979).

There is, however, another phenomenon which must be taken into account. Not only are there compensatory changes in the activity of pre-synaptic dopamine neurons in response to acute neuroleptic administration, but it has been established that changes also occur in sensitivity of the post-synaptic receptor. Acute adminis-tration of a single dose of any neuroleptic has been found to lead to a delayed appearance of post-synaptic dopamine receptor supersensitivity (Moller-Nielsen and Christensen, 1975; Martres et al., 1977). Twenty-four hours or so after the acute administration of even a single dose of a neuroleptic agent, mice show enhanced stereotypy or climbing behaviour in response to dopamine agonists, lasting for a matter of a few days to a week. The implication of this finding in relation to acute dystonic reactions is that as the neuroleptic concentration decreases after acute administration, it will leave exposed supersensitive post-synaptic dopamine receptors. At this point in time, persisting increased dopamine release, or even perhaps normal or reduced concentrations of dopamine, may provoke an enhanced dopaminergic response. In other words, the final functional effect of a complex series of changes that occur after the acute administration of a neuroleptic must take into account not only changes in pre-synaptic dopamine release but also changes in post-synaptic dopamine receptor supersensitivity.

Chronic tardive dyskinesias

Of all the extrapyramidal complications of chronic neuroleptic treatment tardive dyskinesias potentially are the most serious. These abnormal movements appear after many months or even years of drug treatment (Crane, 1968; 1973; Marsden, Tarsy and Baldessarini, 1975; Tarsy and Baldessarini, 1976). Characteristically, they affect the face, causing the typical oro-bucco-lingual dyskinesia, but often they may involve the limbs and trunk. The movements typically are choreiform in the elderly, but may be dystonic in the young. Tardive dyskinesia may co-exist with drug-induced parkin-sonism. The same patient may have typical oro-facial movements with distal chorea of the digits co-existent with a blank face, a stooped posture and a slow shuffling gait (Gerlach, 1977a,b). Likewise, tardive dyskinesia may be accompanied by profound akathisia causing both motor distress and overt restlessness.

The abnormal movements that characterize tardive dyskinesia may occur spontaneously without prior drug intake. The evidence incriminating chronic neuroleptic drug intake as the common cause of these abnormal movements is epidemiological. The incidence of tardive dyskinesia in those on chronic neuroleptics is believed to be greatly in excess of that of spontaneous oro-facial dyskinesias. The latter occur in something of the order of less than 1 per cent of the population, while chronic tardive dyskinesias occur in between 20–40 per cent of those on long-term neuroleptic drugs (Degkvitz, 1967; Jus *et al.*, 1976a,b).

The most worrying feature of tardive dyskinesia is that it frequently persists, or even may appear for the first time, when the offending neuroleptic drug is stopped (Degkvitz and Wenzel, 1967; Crane, 1968). Indeed, it is believed that this extrapyramidal complication of neuroleptic therapy may be permanent despite withdrawal of the drug (Crane, 1973). There is debate as to how frequently this occurs, but the risk of permanent tardive dyskinesias has been estimated to be somewhere around 30 per cent of those who develop the problem (Marsden, Tarsy and Baldessarini, 1975).

The clinical pharmacology of tardive dyskinesias indicates that they are due to over-stimulation of dopamine mechanisms in the brain (Klawans, 1973a,b). The movements themselves resemble those produced by levodopa in patients with Parkinson's disease. They can be suppressed, at least partially and temporarily, by drugs that interfere with dopaminergic neurotransmission (Kazamatsuri, Chien and Cole, 1972a,b; Chase, 1972; Gerlach, Reisby and Randrup, 1974). The appearance of tardive dyskinesia on neuroleptic drug withdrawal is another illustration of the influence of dopamine antagonists on the condition. Finally, there is general agreement that the movements of tardive dyskinesias are enhanced by administration of high doses of dopamine agonists (Chase, 1972; Gerlach, Reisby and Randrup, 1974).

Again a paradox immediately is apparent for it would appear that tardive dyskinesia exhibits the pharmacological sensitivity characteristic of dopaminergic over-activity, yet it is produced by drugs whose prime mode of action is to antagonize dopamine receptors. For this reason the development of neuroleptic-induced post-synaptic dopamine receptor supersensitivity has been invoked to explain the occurrence of this disorder (Carlsson, 1970; Klawans, 1973a,b).

The concept of development of post-synaptic receptor supersensitivity as a result of disuse or denervation has been established by peripheral pharmacological studies (Axelsson and Thesleff, 1959; Trendelenberg, 1963a,b). The same phenomenon appears to occur in the central nervous system. Subacute administration of neuroleptic drugs for a matter of weeks leads to the development of pharmacological super-sensitivity when the animals are tested to dopamine agonists some days or weeks after drug withdrawal (Schelkunov, 1967; Tarsy and Baldessarini, 1973, 1974). Such behavioural supersensitivity is accompanied by an appropriate increase in the number of dopamine receptors present in the brain as measured using ligand binding assays (Burt, Creese and Snyder, 1977).

Such studies indicate that short-term neuroleptic administration produces supersensitivity of cerebral dopamine mechanisms which is only evident after drug withdrawal. During the short period of drug administration, however, the neuroleptics still effectively block dopaminergic activity. This leaves the question of the cause of tardive dyskinsia unresolved, for in most cases the abnormal movements appear while the patient is still taking drugs. However, in long-term studies of neuroleptic administration to rodents for periods up to one year, we have demonstrated that, functional dopamine receptor supersensitivity may develop despite continued neuroleptic intake (Clow, Jenner and Marsden, 1978; Clow *et al.*, 1979a,b).

The continuous administration of neuroleptic drugs such as trifluoperazine, thioridazine or *cis*-flupenthixol, to rats in their drinking water produces initial dopamine receptor blockade during the first month of treatment. Thereafter, however, behavioural and biochemical responses return to normal, and by six months of continuous drug intake these animals have become supersensitive to the administration of dopamine agonists such as apomorphine, and show increased numbers of dopamine receptors within the brain.

These results show that the initial inhibition of dopamine action on acute administration of neuroleptic drugs disappears with chronic treatment to be replaced by dopamine receptor supersensitivity, at least as regards behavioural and biochemical indices attributed to striatal dopamine function. Obviously this is of significance in regard to tardive dyskinesias, which can be attributed to striatal dysfunction. The results support the hypothesis that striatal dopamine receptor supersensitivity provoked by chronic neuroleptic administration may be the pathophysiological mechanism responsible for tardive dyskinesia.

Conclusion

Explanations of the mechanisms responsible for the production of extrapyramidal side effects of neuroleptic drugs for the most part have been based on experimental data in animals, but they are to some extent supported by clinical observation. Drug-induced parkinsonism is thought to be due to the post-synaptic dopamine receptor blockade in the striatum, while akathisia may be due to similar blockade of dopamine receptors in mesocortical areas. Acute dystonic reactions may be due to the interaction between the development of acute post-synaptic dopamine receptor supersensitivity with increased dopamine turnover and release provoked by the acute administration of these drugs. Chronic tardive dyskinesias appear to result from gradual disappearance of dopamine receptor blockade in the striatum and the emergence of striatal dopamine receptor supersensitivity, despite continuation of drug intake. It is hoped that these hypotheses will help in the understanding of the basis of the treatment of these disorders now to be discussed.

Drug treatment of neuroleptic-induced movement disorders

The drugs used to treat neuroleptic-induced movement disorders can be divided into two categories, the antiparkinsonian and the antidyskinetic agents (*Table 5.1*). The major approaches used to treat drug-induced parkinsonism are either to increase cerebral dopamine function to overcome the neuroleptic-induced blockade of cerebral dopamine receptors using dopamine agonists, or to functionally restore the normal dopaminergic–cholinergic balance (Bartholini, Stadler and Lloyd, 1973; Duvoisin, 1967; Klawans, 1973b) which exists in striatum by decreasing cholinergic tone with anticholinergics. On the other hand, the treatment of neuroleptic-induced dyskinesias is mainly directed towards reducing cerebral dopamine function utilizing dopamine antagonists, or towards the neuronal events initiated by activation of cerebral dopamine receptors using drugs acting on cholinergic or GABA systems. In the treatment of both parkinsonism and dyskinesias a wide variety of drugs is employed which does not fall into clearly defined pharmacological categories. In the case of the dyskinesias this seems to highlight the inadequacy of therapy and the paucity of knowledge on the underlying pathophysiology of these disorders. We will deal therefore with each group of drugs in turn to summarize the major therapeutic approaches employed.

TABLE 5.1 Drugs in current use as antiparkinsonian and antidyskinetic agent

| Drug | Antiparkinsonian drugs | | | |
| | Clinical efficacy | | | Duration of action |
	Akinesia	Rigidity	Tremor	
Dopamine agonists				
Levodopa	+ + +	+ + +	+ +	2–4 h
Bromocriptine	+ + +	+ + +	+ +	6–8 h
Amantadine	+	+ +	+/−	6–8 h
Anticholinergics	+/−	+	+/−	6–8 h

| Drug | Antidyskinetic drugs | | |
	Acute dystonia	Akathesia	Tardive dyskinesia
Dopamine antagonists			
Neuroleptics	?	+/−	+
Tiapride	?	+/−	+
Oxiperomide	?	?	+
Pre-synaptic agents			
Apomorphine	+/−	?	+/−
Tetrabenazine	?	−	+
Cholinergic agents			
Physostigmine	?	?	−
Deanol	?	?	+/−
Choline	?	?	+/−
Lecithin	?	?	+/−
Anticholinergic agents	+	+	−
GABA active drugs			
Baclofen	?	?	+/−
Sodium valproate	?	?	+/−
Clonazepam	+	+/−	+/−

+   = improve
+/− = uncertain, but benefit claimed or slight effect
−   = worsen

Drugs used in the treatment of neuroleptic-induced parkinsonism

To present the full spectrum of currently available antiparkinsonian therapy we will concentrate initially on the drugs used to treat the idiopathic condition, and will then comment on their application to the treatment of neuroleptic-induced parkinsonism.

LEVODOPA

Cotzias and colleagues (1967) demonstrated that small gradual increments of dosage of D,L-dopa given by mouth were beneficial in the treatment of Parkinson's disease without producing pronounced side effects. These clinical findings were confirmed and further trials showed the active isomer, levodopa, to be more effective. The introduction of high dose oral levodopa therapy was a critical finding in the treatment of Parkinson's disease and, for the first time, showed that there could be successful drug treatment of chronic degenerative neurological disease (Birkmayer and Hornykiewicz, 1961; Barbeau, 1962; Cotzias, van Woert and Schiffer, 1967). The successful use of levodopa to treat Parkinson's disease also confirmed the post-mortem observation that the disease is due to striatal dopamine deficiency (Ehringer and Hornykiewicz, 1960).

Levodopa (L-3,4-dihydroxyphenylalanine; levodopa) (I) is converted to dopamine (II) by L-aromatic amino acid decarboxylase which is located within a variety of nerve endings throughout the periphery and brain. The dopamine formed subsequently is metabolized mainly by the actions of monoamine oxidase and catechol-O-methyl transferase to homovanillic acid (HVA) (III) and 3,4-dihydroxyphenylacetic acid (DOPAC) (IV).

Most actions of levodopa are attributed to formation of dopamine. Most (95 per cent or more) orally administered levodopa is decarboxylated in the periphery but the dopamine formed is too highly polar to penetrate the blood–brain barrier. It is necessary therefore to administer large quantities of levodopa to ensure adequate elevation of cerebral dopamine content.

In animals the peripheral administration of levodopa produces behavioural changes associated with increased cerebral dopamine function, such as locomotion and stereotyped behaviour, and causes a marked elevation of brain dopamine, HVA and DOPAC.

Not all actions of levodopa are due to activation of dopamine receptors for the drug also accumulates in noradrenaline and 5-HT neurons and is decarboxylated to dopamine by L-aromatic amino acid decarboxylase located at these sites. This serves to elevate the cerebral noradrenaline content, since dopamine is a precursor of noradrenaline, which may facilitate cerebral dopamine function. Accumulation of dopamine in 5-HT terminals displaces 5-HT, which may then exert pharmacological effects on its post-synaptic receptor. Additionally, levodopa may be decarboxylated in cerebral capillaries and this may contribute to its pharmacological actions. Indeed, the site of decarboxylation of levodopa in Parkinson's disease is uncertain. It is difficult to envisage how the drug may be adequately decarboxylated in remaining dopamine neurons but the importance of decarboxylation at other sites presently is disputed (*see* Hefti and Melamed, 1980 *versus* Marsden and Jenner, 1981).

The administration of levodopa to patients with Parkinson's disease controls akinesia and rigidity more effectively than tremor. Speech and swallowing are improved and salivation considerably reduced. The improvement is maintained only while treatment is continued. Both post-encephalitic and idiopathic Parkinson's disease respond to levodopa. Lower doses are effective in post-encephalitic parkinsonism but there is a higher incidence of side effects.

Concurrent administration of levodopa with an inhibitor of aromatic L-amino acid decarboxylase that itself is unable to penetrate into the brain, decreases the decarboxylation of levodopa in the periphery (*see* Marsden, 1976). Consequently, a greater proportion of levodopa reaches receptor sites within basal ganglia and the absolute dose of levodopa may be reduced. In the presence of a peripheral decarboxylase inhibitor concentrations of levodopa in plasma are higher and the half-life of the drug is longer than following administration of levodopa alone. At present only two such compounds are available, namely carbidopa and benserazide. There are a number of advantages to such combined therapy (Bianchine, 1980):

(1) The optimal therapeutic dose of levodopa can be reduced to one-quarter of that given alone.
(2) Nausea and vomiting are largely eliminated.
(3) An effective dose of levodopa can be reached more rapidly during initial therapy as it is not necessary to induce tolerance to the initial side effects of levodopa action.
(4) Fluctuations in clinical response to levodopa are reduced, since the concentration of dopamine within the brain does not change so dramatically as a function of time.
(5) The number of patients benefiting from levodopa and the degree of improvement appear greater than with levodopa alone.

In recommended doses the peripheral decarboxylase inhibitors currently employed, when administered alone, are essentially devoid of pharmacological activity, and toxic effects have not been observed. However, when administered in combination with levodopa, they quantitatively enhance the pharmacological action of levodopa. Consequently, the side effects of peripheral decarboxylase inhibitors when administered with levodopa are associated with increased effect of levodopa.

Most patients treated with levodopa experience side effects, the intensity and type of which vary greatly at different stages of treatment. Side effects generally are dose-dependent and reversible. Nausea and anorexia commonly occur during the initial phases of treatment with levodopa, and may be accompanied by vomiting early in treatment, particularly if dosage is increased too rapidly. The commonest cardiovascular effect is postural hypotension with faintness and dizziness. Psychiatric disturbances are produced by levodopa in a significant proportion of patients and frequently limit the dose that can be tolerated. They include agitation, anxiety, elation and insomnia and sometimes drowsiness and depression. More severe effects include aggression, paranoid delusions, hallucinations, suicidal behaviour, and a frank toxic confusional state. The majority of patients on long-term therapy of a year or longer develop abnormal involuntary movements, which vary considerably in pattern and severity, and which often limit the tolerated dose of levodopa (Marsden, 1980). They appear with increasing frequency as drug administration continues and are directly related to the dose of levodopa and to the extent of clinical improvement. These abnormal involuntary movements are the most important side effect of levodopa to limit the dose that can be given. No satisfactory means, pharmacological or otherwise, have yet been found to selectively antagonize these dyskinesias.

The actions of levodopa are diminished by neuroleptics, and by reserpine or tetrabenazine, but are enhanced by administration of amantadine and by the decarboxylase inhibitors, benzerazide and carbidopa. The actions of levodopa may be enhanced also by anticholinergic agents such as benztropine, and also by amphetamine. Non-selective monoamine oxidase inhibitors such as phenelzine and isocarboxazid, which inhibit both the A and B isoenzymes, interfere with inactivation of dopamine, noradrenaline and other catecholamines and exaggerate unpredictably the effects of levodopa and the derived catecholamines. Hypertensive crisis and hyperpyrexia are very real and dangerous sequelae of concurrent administration of non-selective monoamine oxidase inhibitors with levodopa. However, it is interesting to note that a selective inhibitor of monoamine oxidase B, deprenyl, is now under investigation as a drug for Parkinson's disease (*see below*).

Concurrent administration of levodopa with guanethidine, methyldopa, and other antihypertensive agents may cause increased hypotension. α-Adrenergic blocking agents, including propranolol, may enhance the action of levodopa on tremor and diminish cardiac side effects. The concurrent administration of antacids with levodopa may enhance gastrointestinal absorption of the drug and increase its pharmacological actions.

Levodopa is rapidly absorbed from the gastrointestinal tract and peak plasma levels are reached within 0.5–2 h following oral administration. The plasma half-life however, is short, being approximately 1 h. More than 90 per cent of levodopa is decarboxylated in the periphery, due to the wide distribution of L-aromatic amino acid decarboxylase activity, and this occurs extensively during the first pass through the liver. Little unchanged drug reaches the cerebral circulation and probably less than 1 per cent penetrates into brain. Inhibition of peripheral decarboxylase activity markedly increases the fraction of administered levodopa available to pass into the brain.

Most levodopa is converted to dopamine, some of which is in turn transformed into noradrenaline and adrenaline. Methylation to 3-*O*-methyldopa (V) also occurs and this product accumulates in the brain due to its long biological half-life. The dopamine formed from levodopa is rapidly metabolized to produce DOPAC and HVA, but numerous other metabolites of levodopa have been identified. A number of these may possess pharmacological activity that contributes to the actions of levodopa.

V

Dopamine metabolites are rapidly excreted in urine, most of the dose being recovered within 24 h. DOPAC and HVA are the principal acidic metabolites, and they account for approximately half of the administered dose. Negligible amounts of levodopa or its metabolites are found in faeces. After prolonged therapy with levodopa the ratio of DOPAC to HVA excreted may increase reflecting the depletion of methyl donors necessary for metabolism of dopamine by catechol-*O*-methyltransferase. Indeed, most of the dietary intake of methionine can be used for the metabolism of large doses of levodopa.

No clear relationship exists between the therapeutic effects of levodopa and its plasma concentrations in parkinsonian patients (Bergmann *et al.*, 1975). There may, however, be a closer relationship between the concentrations of dopamine (Rossor *et al.*, 1980), but this remains to be further evaluated. Changes in pharmacokinetic handling of levodopa may be responsible for some of the chronic changes which occur during its prolonged use, namely the on–off effect, swinging, and end-of-dose deterioration, but this remains to be established (*see* Marsden and Parkes, 1976; 1977; Marsden, 1980).

OTHER MEANS OF INCREASING CEREBRAL DOPAMINE FUNCTION

Synthetic dopamine agonists have been introduced in attempts to replace levodopa in the treatment of idiopathic Parkinson's disease. Most attempts have met with limited success. ET 495 (piribedil) (VI) was effective only against parkinsonian tremor and not against other primary symptoms. Lisuride (VII) was too short acting and lergotrile (VIII) too toxic. Only bromocriptine has made any impact on current therapy. The other approach adopted has been to potentiate the effects of endogenous dopamine using selective monoamine oxidase inhibitors, such as deprenyl.

Bromocriptine

Bromocriptine mesylate (CB 154; 2-bromo-α-ergocriptine) (IX) is a substituted ergoline derivative now widely used in the treatment of idiopathic Parkinson's disease (Calne *et al.*, 1974a,b; Parkes, Debono and Marsden, 1976; Parkes *et al.*, 1976). It is a potent synthetic post-synaptic dopamine receptor agonist which therefore overcomes the deficiency of dopamine within the striatum and other dopamine containing areas of the brain in this illness.

Bromocriptine is an ergot derivative originally developed approximately ten years ago as an inhibitor of prolactin secretion, bromocriptine was found to possess dopamine agonist activity which led to its investigation for the treatment of Parkinson's disease. Directly acting dopamine agonists might be expected to have advantages over the use of levodopa in the treatment of Parkinson's disease. Unlike levodopa, bromocriptine does not depend on decarboxylase for conversion to its active form, nor on release of dopamine from pre-synaptic terminals onto the receptor site, which presumably is defective Parkinson's disease. Indeed, in very severe cases it might be expected that a synthetic dopamine agonist would be more effective than dopamine itself, and might have a more selective action on those supersensitive receptors affected by the disease, thereby avoiding some of the adverse reactions caused by stimulation of other synapses.

Dopamine agonist properties of bromocriptine are apparent in animal experiments (*see* Parkes, 1978; Reavill, Jenner and Marsden, 1981). Bromocriptine increases locomotor activity in rodents, although this is only apparent after an initial dose-dependent lag phase during which time the motor activity is inhibited. Bromocriptine induces stereotyped behaviour in rats similar to that provoked by apomorphine (Johnson, Loew and Vigouret, 1976). However, the stereotyped response consists mainly of sniffing and licking, while gnawing and biting do not occur. Perhaps the best evidence for a direct activation of post-synaptic dopamine receptors by bromocriptine comes from studies in animals with unilateral 6-hydroxydopamine lesions of the nigrostriatal pathway. Bromocriptine, like apomorphine, induces contraversive rotation in such animals, an effect which is blocked by haloperidol (Corrodi *et al.*, 1973; Reavill, Jenner and Marsden, 1980). Bromocriptine also exhibits the biochemical properties in animals that one expects from a dopamine agonist causing a decrease in dopamine turnover in various brain areas. This is seen as a decrease in the concentration of the dopamine metabolites, HVA and DOPAC, a decrease in dopamine depletion following blockade of tyrosine hydroxylase activity using α-methyl-p-tyrosine, and a decreased accumulation of dopa following blockade of dopa decarboxylase activity (Corrodi *et al.*, 1973; Dolphin *et al.*, 1977; Bannon *et al.*, 1980). Bromocriptine also has the ability to displace radioactive ligands from their specific binding sites to dopamine receptors *in vitro* (*see* Reavill, Jenner and Marsden, 1981). For example, it displaces ^{3}H-dopamine, ^{3}H spiperone and ^{3}H-apomorphine from their specific binding sites in rat striatal preparations. When given peripherally, bromocriptine inhibits the firing of nigrostriatal neurons, an effect which can be reversed by administration of haloperidol, by stimulation of dopamine autoreceptors (Bannon *et al.*, 1980).

Bromocriptine, however, differs from dopamine in one important respect. While dopamine will stimulate the enzyme adenylate cyclase in rat striatal preparations to form cyclic AMP, bromocriptine not only is unable to stimulate this enzyme, but also can inhibit the stimulation induced by dopamine (Markstein *et al.*, 1978,. These data can be interpreted in a number of ways. Based on the currently topical idea that there is more than one type of dopamine receptor in the brain, bromocriptine could selectively act on dopamine receptors which are not linked to the enzyme adenylate cyclase (D-2 receptors) (Kebabian and Calne, 1979). On the other hand, it might be argued that bromocriptine inhibits the dopamine stimulation of adenylate cyclase because it acts as a partial agonist rather than a full dopamine agonist.

Bromocriptine differs from most other post-synaptic dopamine agonists because many of its actions are reduced or prevented by disruption of pre-synaptic dopaminergic neuronal events. Inhibition of the synthesis of dopamine in the pre-synaptic terminals by α-methyl-p-tyrosine, a tyrosine hydroxylase inhibitor, or disruption of storage of dopamine in the pre-synaptic terminals by reserpine, can inhibit the actions of bromocriptine on motor activity (Johnson, Loew and Vigouret, 1976; Dolphin *et al.*, 1977; Reavill, Jenner and Marsden, 1980). Pre-treatment of rats with α-methyl-p-tyrosine, or with α-methyl-p-tyrosine plus reserpine, markedly reduces circling behaviour to bromocriptine in animals with a prior unilateral 6-hydroxydopamine induced destruction of the nigrostriatal pathway. In addition, locomotor acivity induced by bromocriptine in mice is reduced by reserpine or AMPT and these pre-treatments markedly reduce the ability of bromocriptine to induce stereotyped behaviour in rats. The hypothermia produced by administration of bromocriptine also is prevented by administration of α-methyl-*p*-tyrosine (Horowski, 1978). These data strongly suggest that the motor activating effects of bromocriptine are critically dependent on intact pre-synaptic events in dopamine neurons. This distinguishes bromocriptine from apomorphine, whose motor actions are not affected by α-methyl-*p*-tyrosine or reserpine. An obvious explanation for this difference would be that bromocriptine exerts an amphetamine-like action in causing release of dopamine onto post-synaptic receptors. However, this cannot be so since, in the circling rodent model, bromocriptine like apomorphine, induces contraversive rotation indicating a direct action of both drugs on supersensitive denervated post-synaptic receptors. It must be concluded that bromocriptine exerts dopaminergic effects by both a direct action on post-synaptic receptors, and by an action which depends on intact pre-synaptic dopaminergic mechanisms.

The usefulness of bromocriptine in Parkinson's disease may be related to another aspect of its pharmacology, namely that the drug appears to be more effective in activating supersensitive dopamine receptors (in models such as the turning rodent model) rather than stimulating normal dopamine receptors (in producing stereotyped and locomotor changes in otherwise naive animals). The reason why bromocriptine should preferentially work on denervated receptors is unknown, but it would be an obvious advantage in the treatment of Parkinson's disease.

Bromocriptine cannot be looked upon as being a selective dopamine agonist for it also exerts actions on other neuronal pathways (*see* Reavill, Jenner and Marsden, 1981). For example, bromocriptine increases noradrenaline turnover and will displace ^{3}H-dihydroergocriptine, ^{3}H-WB 4101, or ^{3}H-clonidine from α-adrenergic receptors. In addition, many ergot derivatives including bromocriptine also are known to inhibit the noradrenaline sensitive adenylate cyclase system. Bromocriptine also exerts actions on central 5-HT systems, although whether these are direct or indirect is not clear. Bromocriptine causes an increase in brain 5-HT and a decrease in brain 5-HIAA concentrations. Since there are only slight changes in 5-HT synthesis, it has been concluded that bromocriptine reduces 5-HT release *in vivo*, possibly by a direct effect on 5-HT neurons as well as indirectly by an effect on dopamine receptors.

There is evidence also to suggest that an active metabolite may be involved in the actions of bromocriptine. The mono-oxygenase inhibitor SKF 525A inhibits the ability of bromocriptine, but not that of apomorphine, to induce circling behaviour in 6-hydroxydopamine lesioned rodents (Reavill, Jenner and Marsden, 1980). Similarly, others have shown that the hyperthermia induced in cold acclimatized rats by bromocriptine also is prevented by SKF 525A (Silbergeld *et al.*, 1977). There is some controversy, however, concerning the role of active metabolites and the action of bromocriptine for, in other work, the ability of bromocriptine to cause hypothermia in room temperature acclimatized animals (Keller and Da Prada, 1979) and its ability to cause a decrease in striatal homovanillic acid levels, were unaffected by SKF 525A (Enz, Jaton and Vigouret, 1981). In addition, others have shown that SKF 525A does not prevent the bromocriptine-induced reduction of striatal dopa accumulation caused by gamma-butyrolactone (Enz, Jaton and Vigouret, 1981). The effect of SKF 525A cannot be merely attributed to the sedation induced by this agent but no definite conclusion can be reached on the basis of such indirect experiments. The major metabolites of bromocriptine must be examined for their involvement in the motor actions of bromocriptine.

Bromocriptine is as potent as levodopa in relieving the disability of Parkinson's disease, but has the theoretical advantage of having a longer biological half-life (greater than 12 h compared to 2 h for levodopa) (Aellig and Nuesch, 1977). Bromocriptine does not, however, appear to be of greater benefit in those patients where levodopa never produced, or no longer produces, a sufficient clinical response (*see* Godwin-Austen, 1981). This suggests that levodopa failure is due to alteration in post-synaptic receptor sensitivity rather than to loss of pre-synaptic neurons.

The relatively long biological half-life of bromocriptine may, however, be an advantage in the management of some of the chronic problems of levodopa therapy. The addition of bromocriptine tends to smooth out the peaks and troughs of levodopa therapy, and may go some way to alleviating end-of-dose deterioration.

Nausea is the most common side effect of bromocriptine therapy but vomiting, dizziness and postural hypertension also may occur. Other side effects reported include headache, leg cramps, nasal congestion, sedation, hallucinations, dryness of the mouth, constipation, palpitations, and prolonged severe hypotension. Symptomatic hypotension may be more common with bromocriptine than with levodopa. Visual and auditory hallucinations also are more frequent with bromocriptine than with levodopa, though bromocriptine induces less dyskinesia than does levodopa. Reduction of the dosage of bromocriptine leads to disappearance of most of these side effects. Nausea may be diminished by taking bromocriptine with food or by co-administration of an antiemetic agent such as metoclopramide or domperidone.

Bromocriptine has been administered concurrently to patients receiving phenothiazines, and has lowered plasma prolactin concentrations apparently without interfering with psychotropic effect. However, the antiparkinsonian effect of dopaminergic agents can be antagonized by reserpine, phenothiazines and the butyrophenones. High doses of bromocriptine also may result in increased psychotic behaviour.

Bromocriptine is rapidly absorbed after oral administration and concentrations of the drug usually peak in plasma in 2 h (*see* Parkes, 1978). Therapeutic concentrations for the treatment of Parkinson's disease persists three to four times longer than do those of levodopa. The major route of elimination of bromocriptine is biliary. The metabolic pattern of drug excretion in bile is extremely complex, with at least 30 partially or completely characterized metabolites in the rat and monkey.

At least ten different metabolites of bromocriptine have been identified in human urine, whilst only a very small proportion of unchanged bromocriptine is present (*see* Parkes, 1978). Bromolysergic acid is the main metabolite accounting for approximately half the excreted radioactivity. In the rat and rhesus monkey, as well as in man, 2-bromolysergic acid and 2-bromoisolysergic acid are the main urinary metabolites. Accumulative urinary excretion of radioactivity in the urine of man is approximately 6 per cent of the dose after oral administration and 7 per cent after intravenous administration whereas 70 per cent appears in the faeces over 120 h following a single oral dose of bromocriptine. Estimation of bromocriptine levels in human plasma by radio-immunoassay has shown peak levels to occur 2–3 h after drug administration at approximately the same time as the peak antiparkinsonian action and the maximum severity of dyskinesias, and shortly after peak growth hormone levels are achieved.

Deprenyl
Another approach to increasing cerebral dopamine function is to prevent the breakdown of endogenous dopamine by the use of monoamine oxidase inhibitors. However, the combination of levodopa with most available conventional monoamine oxidase inhibitors may cause severe hypertensive crises. Two types of monoamine

oxidase are now recognized (Johnston, 1968). In animal experiments, the type A form of monoamine oxidase deaminates 5-HT and noradrenaline, while dopamine is a substrate for both the A and B subtypes. However, in human brain dopamine is a preferred substrate for monoamine oxidase type B (Glover et al., 1977), so its metabolism may be selectively altered without changing the brain content of 5-HT or noradrenaline. This contrasts with the actions of non-selective inhibitors which will increase the cerebral concentration of all monoamines. L-Deprenyl (phenylisopropylmethylpropinylamine hydrochloride) (X) selectively inhibits monoamine oxidase type B (Knoll, 1976), which is the predominant type in human brain (Glover et al., 1977). The administration of L-deprenyl, given without levodopa, has been shown to increase cerebral dopamine levels, with minimal effects on other transmitter amines (Riederer et al., 1978). It does not cause dangerous hypertensive reactions with levodopa or with tyramine containing foods (Sandler et al., 1978). In addition to its action as a monoamine oxidase inhibitor, L-deprenyl also may cause the release, and block the re-uptake, of catecholamines in the brain (Knoll, 1978; Simpson, 1978).

$$\langle \text{ring} \rangle CH_2CHN \begin{smallmatrix} CH_3 \\ | \\ \end{smallmatrix} \begin{smallmatrix} CH_3 \\ \nearrow \\ \searrow CH_2C \equiv CH \end{smallmatrix}$$

X

There have been several clinical studies of the combined use of levodopa and deprenyl in Parkinson's disease (Birkmayer et al., 1975, 1977; Birkmayer, 1978; Lees et al., 1977; Schachter et al., 1980). Deprenyl appears to enhance and prolong the antiparkinsonian effect of levodopa, while aggravating dopaminergic side effects. Deprenyl alleviates symptom fluctuations in some patients with dose-related swings on levodopa (with or without a decarboxylase inhibitor), although the extent of the benefit varies considerably. Deprenyl, however, appears to be of little benefit in patients with random response swings, and even may cause deterioration in such cases.

No serious side effects have been encountered during the use of deprenyl and no systemic toxicity has been observed. Nausea, postural hypotension and dryness of the mouth, anxiety, insomnia and hallucinations have been described during prolonged deprenyl administration with levodopa.

The mode of action of deprenyl is complex. As far as the drug's antiparkinsonian action is concerned it is probable that its role as a selective monoamine oxidase B inhibitor is of greater importance than effects on dopamine release and re-uptake, which may be due to metabolites of deprenyl. There is no doubt that there is substantial conversion of deprenyl to amphetamine and methylamphetamine (Reynolds et al., 1978), although these are the (−)-isomers (Schachter et al., 1980) which exert little antiparkinsonian effect. The site of metabolism is probably the liver but any amphetamine formed there will readily cross the blood–brain barrier.

Deprenyl appears to be a useful adjunct in the management of dose-related response swings in patients already on optimal levodopa therapy.

Amantadine
Amantadine was introduced as an antiviral agent which probably inhibits penetration of virus into host cells. It is used prophylactically against infection of influenza type A2 virus but, unexpectedly, was found to cause improvement of parkinsonian syndromes. Amantadine probably acts by releasing dopamine (Scatton et al., 1970; Farnebo et al.,

1971; Stone, 1976) from intact dopaminergic terminals that remain in the degenerating striatum of patients with Parkinson's disease. Since it facilitates the release of dopamine, amantadine is of most benefit during concurrent administration of levodopa. Amantadine is known to improve akinesia and rigidity, but usually has a lesser effect on parkinsonian tremor (Schwab *et al.*, 1969). Amantadine is clearly less effective that levodopa, but exerts greater therapeutic activity than anticholinergic drugs (Parkes *et al.*, 1970; Mawdsley *et al.*, 1972). Amantadine acts maximally within a few days, but may lose a portion of its efficacy within 6–8 weeks of continuous treatment. Amantadine is readily absorbed from the gastrointestinal tract and has a relatively long duration of action. It is excreted unchanged in urine and therefore, can accumulate when renal function is inadequate. Compared with levodopa or anticholinergic agents, amantadine is relatively free of side effects, which generally are mild, often transient, and always reversible. Their incidence and severity increases markedly when the daily dosage exceeds 200–300 mg. The most common side effects are livido reticularis and ankle oedema. Orthostatic hypotension, urinary retention, ataxia, hallucinations, a toxic confusional state, and seizures also may occur.

ANTICHOLINERGIC AGENTS

The rationale for using anticholinergic drugs in the treatment of parkinsonism lies in the evidence for a reciprocal balance between dopaminergic and cholinergic activity in the striatum. The deficiency of dopamine in the striatum in Parkinson's disease results in a state of apparent relative cholinergic overactivity. Physostigmine, a centrally active anticholinesterase agent, which increases the striatal concentration of acetylcholine, dramatically worsens parkinsonism, while anticholinergic drugs improve Parkinson's disease (Duvoisin, 1967). In drug-induced parkinsonism there also appears to be a reciprocal cholinergic–dopaminergic balance. Cholinergic drugs cause a worsening of phenothiazine-induced parkinsonism, while anticholinergic agents improve this disorder.

The neuronal basis of the inter-relationship between dopaminergic and cholinergic neuronal systems in the striatum is complex. Neuroleptic drugs increase the rate of synthesis (Sethy and van Woert, 1974) and the neuronal release (Stadler *et al.*, 1973) of acetylcholine in the striatum, while administration of dopamine agonists has the opposite effect. These findings suggest that there may be inhibitory dopamine receptors located on striatal cholinergic neurons that can modulate cholinergic activity. Blockade of post-synaptic dopamine receptors by neuroleptic agents increases the activity of striatal cholinergic systems (Trabucchi *et al.*, 1974). The effect of anticholinergic drugs is to reverse the effects of dopamine receptor blockade. Additionally, cholinergic interneurons in the striatum may exert an action on presynaptic dopamine function so as to reverse the compensatory increases in dopamine turnover caused by the administration of neuroleptic compounds. This mechanism may be of importance in understanding how such agents can be used to control acute dystonic reactions (*see* p. 115).

Anticholinergic drugs were the mainstay of the treatment of Parkinson's disease for more than a century prior to the introduction of levodopa. They are now used more in a supportive role in the treatment of this disorder but, nonetheless, are still very useful in patients with minimal symptoms, or in those unable to tolerate or who do not benefit from levodopa. Furthermore, over half of the patients who show a therapeutic response to levodopa experience further benefit after supplementary treatment with anticholinergic agents.

TABLE 5.2 Currently used anticholinergic drugs in the treatment of parkinsonism

Drug	Structure	Dosage range $(mg \cdot d^{-1})$
Benztropine	(XI)	1–6 mg
Benzhexol	(XII)	2–15 mg
Procyclidine	(XIII)	6–20 mg
Biperiden	(XIV)	2–10 mg
Orphenadrine	(XV)	50–250 mg

A range of anticholinergic drugs, and certain antihistamines possessing anti-cholinergic activity, are used for the treatment of parkinsonism (*Table 5.2*). Although there are essentially no pharmacological differences among the anticholinergic agents commonly used in parkinsonism, certain patients may tolerate one preparation better than another. However, there is little to choose between many of these drugs.

Side effects due to the central anticholinergic activity include mental confusion, delirium, somnolence and hallucinations which may limit their use. All the other common anticholinergic side effects also are observed including dryness of the mouth, difficulty in swallowing, thirst, dilatation of the pupils (which may provoke glaucoma in those with narrow anterior chambers), flushing and dryness of the skin, bradycardia followed by tachycardia with palpitations and even arrhythmias. Reduction of tone and motility of the gastrointestinal tract commonly leads to constipation, and sometimes to gastric stasis and even to intestinal obstruction. Urinary disturbances are common, particularly amongst elderly men who already have prostate enlargement. There is a desire to urinate with hesitancy and a poor stream, and urinary retention may occur. In severe intoxication depression of the central nervous system occurs with hypertension or circulatory failure and respiratory depression. The effects of the anticholinergic drugs may be enhanced by the simultaneous administration of other drugs with anticholinergic properties such as amantadine, some antihistamines, and certain neuroleptics and tricyclic antidepressants.

Little is known of the pharmacokinetic properties of the commonly employed anticholinergic agents, due partly to the lack of suitable analytical techniques and partly to the lack of need for such data in the era in which they were introduced into therapy. Benzhexol is well absorbed from the gastrointestinal tract and peak plasma levels are achieved after 1 h, but it has not been possible to calculate the biological half-life (information supplied by Lederle Laboratories). Benztropine also is well absorbed and is effective for between 3–5 h, but no technique for its estimation in biological fluids has been developed (information supplied by Merck, Sharp and Dohme Ltd). Procyclidine appears to be rapidly absorbed from the gastrointestinal tract, peak plasma levels being achieved after some 2 h, with initial experiments indicating a plasma half-life of about 12 h (Dean, Land and Bye, 1981). Orphenadrine is well absorbed but blood levels are very low as a result of rapid and extensive tissue distribution. The drug is extensively metabolized, only 8 per cent being excreted unchanged. The plasma half-life has not been determined, but only 60 per cent of the drug is eliminated in urine in 72 h (Ellison *et al.*, 1971). Eight metabolites have been identified involving *N*-demethylation and ether cleavage, and subsequent conjugation.

Drug treatment of neuroleptic-induced parkinsonism

Neuroleptic-induced parkinsonism, like idiopathic Parkinson's disease, is due to a functional loss of cerebral dopaminergic activity. Accordingly the drugs used to treat Parkinson's disease have been employed in the management of neuroleptic-induced parkinsonism. The use of dopamine agonists, and in particular levodopa, to overcome the neuroleptic-induced blockade of dopamine receptors might appear a rational therapy. However, the use of levodopa as treatment for neuroleptic-induced parkinsonism generally has been reported to be ineffective or to increase psychiatric symptoms (Fleming, Makar and Hunter, 1970; Yaryura-Tobias *et al.*, 1970), although more recent reports have suggested that the use of relatively low doses of levodopa can reverse neuroleptic-induced parkinsonism in schizophrenic patients without serious psychiatric complications (Inanga *et al.*, 1972; Ogura, Kishimoto and Nakao, 1976; Garfinkel and Stancer, 1976). In addition, there are also reports of the use of higher levodopa dosage in an attempt to reverse tardive dyskinesia, apparently without provoking recurrence of psychotic behaviour (*see below*).

Whether other synthetic dopamine agonists have similar effects is unknown. Piribedil has been shown to be ineffective in the treatment of drug-induced parkinsonism (Mindham, Lamb and Bradley, 1977), but other drugs which either enhance endogenous cerebral dopamine function, such as nomifensine and deprenyl, or act as direct dopamine receptor agonists, such as bromocriptine, do not appear to have been explored in the treatment of the neuroleptic-induced disease. Indeed, of all the antiparkinsonian agents, other than anticholinergic drugs, only amantadine has undergone any serious clinical examination. The results of these trials on amantadine, however, are conflicting.

In an open trial, where the effectiveness of the drug was examined in patients receiving a variety of neuroleptic agents with anticholinergic drugs, amantadine was claimed to control drug-induced parkinsonism (Pacifici *et al.*, 1976). But in a double-blind study comparing amantadine, placebo or orphenadrine on neuroleptic-induced parkinsonism, neither of the active drugs was found to exert any therapeutic action superior to placebo (Mindham *et al.*, 1972).

The limited knowledge available of the effect of dopamine active drugs in the treatment of drug-induced parkinsonism is rather surprising. Perhaps the fear of exacerbation of the underlying psychotic illness has deterred many from attempting trials of such substances. In addition, the use of relatively weak agonist compounds in an attempt to overcome the blockade of dopamine receptors caused by potent neuroleptic drugs does not make pharmacological sense.

The mainstay of treatment of neuroleptic-induced parkinsonism has been the use of anticholinergic agents. Two major therapeutic approaches have been employed:

(1) to treat the symptoms of parkinsonism with anticholinergics once they have appeared;
(2) to co-administer anticholinergic drugs with neuroleptics from the onset of drug treatment, to try to prevent the emergence of acute dystonic reactions and parkinsonism.

The routine use of anticholinergic drugs in an attempt to avoid early extrapyramidal reactions usually is unnecessary. The use of such drugs should be reserved for cases of overt extrapyramidal reactions that respond favourably to such intervention. When given after the appearance of parkinsonian signs anticholinergic drugs are usually of some benefit, but when given prophylactically, the frequency of parkinsonism may not be affected, although the severity of the condition probably is reduced.

However, Mindham (1976) has presented evidence that the effectiveness of anticholinergic drugs is less convincing than might be expected. Many of the drugs employed have never been fully examined in the treatment of idiopathic Parkinson's disease, and most have not been shown to be effective in comparison to placebo in double-blind clinical trials. Those studies comparing anticholinergic compounds to placebo, in general have been unable to show any marked therapeutic effect of these compounds on neuroleptic-induced parkinsonism. Thus, in a double-blind cross-over trial of amantadine, orphenadrine and placebo on parkinsonism induced by fluphenazine, no difference was found between the effect of the treatments (Mindham et al., 1972). In a similar trial, however, procyclidine was found to be beneficial (Mindham, Lamb and Bradley, 1977). In trials comparing the effectiveness of various anticholinergic compounds on drug-induced parkinsonism, no difference was found between individual compounds, but all appeared to reduce symptomatology, although without abolishing parkinsonism (Table 5.3).

When anticholinergic drugs have been administered prophylactically, the results have depended upon the length of treatment. In patients who received anticholinergic therapy for only one month, drug withdrawal caused the appearance of severe parkinsonism and a variety of other symptoms in two-thirds (Orlov et al., 1971). But when anticholinergics are withdrawn after many months of use, a much smaller proportion of patients relapse. Thus, when prophylactic anticholinergic treatment was stopped after 3 to 12 months' treatment, only 8 per cent of patients on chronic neuroleptic therapy developed signs of parkinsonism (McClelland et al., 1974). In general, it seems that the incidence of parkinsonism is higher when anticholinergics are discontinued within three months of the start of neuroleptic therapy than when the drugs are stopped at later times. The conclusion from this would be that tolerance to the extrapyramidal effects of neuroleptic agents develops within three months.

Most studies of preventive therapy with anticholinergic drugs have shown that the majority of patients do not require such medication. Furthermore, many of those who do show drug-induced parkinsonism respond better to a reduction in neuroleptic dosage, or substitution of the drug they are receiving for one with high inherent

TABLE 5.3 Comparison between anticholinergic drugs in the treatment of neuroleptic-induced parkinsonism

Treatment (mg daily dose)	Design	Result	Authors
Promethazine (10) Ethopropazine (25) Benzhexol (2) Placebo	Double-blind randomized cross-over	All drugs superior to placebo; no difference between drugs	St Jean, Donald and Bann (1964)
Methixene (15 or 20) Procyclidine (15 or 20) Orphenadrine (150–200)	?Blind cross-over	No difference between drugs	Ekdawi and Fowke (1966)
		Both drugs superior to placebo	
Benztropine (2) Biperiden (2.5–7.5) Placebo	Double-blind randomized cross-over		Simpson (1970)
Orphenadrine (150) Placebo	Double-randomized cross-over	No difference between drugs	Mindham et al. (1972)
Procyclidine (20) Placebo	Double-blind randomized cross-over	Superior to placebo	Mindham, Lamb and Bradley (1977)

Abridged from Marsden. Mindham and MacKay (1981).

anticholinergic activity such as thioridazine. Different neuroleptic drugs cause varying incidences of parkinsonism. This can be attributed, at least in part, to variations in their own inherent anticholinergic properties (Miller and Hiley, 1974). Drugs with relatively strong anticholinergic properties, such as thioridazine or clozapine, are associated with a lower incidence of parkinsonism than drugs such as trifluoperazine or fluphenazine, which possess little inherent anticholinergic activity. However, although such drugs may be advantageous in the short term, the effect of inherent anticholinergic activity on the propensity to develop tardive dyskinesia must be borne in mind.

There is a strong concern that concurrent administration of anticholinergic agents with neuroleptic drugs may increase the risk of developing tardive dyskinesia (Klawans, 1973; Klawans and Rubovits, 1974). The administration of anticholinergic drugs to patients with tardive dyskinesia exacerbates the movement disorder (Turek et al., 1972; Chouinard, de Moutigny and Annable, 1979). Indeed, the administration of anticholinergic drugs to patients receiving chronic neuroleptic therapy may serve as an aid to the early detection of tardive dyskinesias. Clearly, since the occurrence and intensity of tardive dyskinesias is sensitive to manipulation of cholinergic function, the use of anticholinergic drugs for the treatment of neuroleptic-induced parkinsonism should be avoided where possible.

The potential complications arising from the use of anticholinergic agents in the treatment of neuroleptic-induced parkinsonism has led to a cautious approach to their use. A detailed examination of the present data available has led to the development of the following guidelines (Marsden, Mindham and MacKay, 1981):

(1) The routine therapeutic use of anticholinergic drugs in combination with neuroleptic agents should be avoided since this practice results in many patients receiving unnecessary therapy.
(2) When the occurrence of neuroleptic-induced parkinsonism gives rise to distress, a reduction in dosage of the offending neuroleptic should be considered where this will not prejudice the treatment of the underlying psychotic illness.
(3) Where the dosage of neuroleptic drug cannot be reduced, substitution with an equivalent neuroleptic possessing a lesser propensity to induce parkinsonism should be attempted.
(4) When anticholinergic medication has to be given the drug should be administered only until the symptoms have abated to an acceptable level.
(5) Anticholinergic drugs should not be given for periods greater than three months as longer periods of administration are neither necessary nor effective.
(6) If neuroleptic-induced parkinsonism reappears after withdrawal of anticholinergic medication the drug should only be re-administered for a limited period.

The application of these principles would appear to provide a sensible approach to the treatment of parkinsonism with anticholinergic drugs in patients undergoing neuroleptic therapy and their application should minimize the unwanted side effects of anticholinergic drugs in both the short and long term.

Finally, it is necessary to consider the effect of adding an anticholinergic drug on the antipsychotic action of the neuroleptics. The suggestion has been made that the use of anticholinergic drugs to control drug-induced parkinsonism may reduce the therapeutic activity of the neuroleptic agents (Haase, 1965; Singh and Smith, 1973; Singh and Kay, 1975a,b). Anticholinergic drugs reverse the dopaminergic-cholinergic balance which exists within the striatum and thereby might cause a functional increase in cerebral dopamine activity. This might reverse the effects initiated by the blockade of cerebral dopamine receptors caused by neuroleptic therapy, in the same way as levodopa and other dopamine agonists may exacerbate psychotic symptomatology. Indeed, it has been demonstrated that the administration of anticholinergic agents can cause a decrease in the antischizophrenic activity of neuroleptic drugs.

Such an adverse interaction may be due to changes in plasma concentrations of neuroleptic drugs induced by concomitant anticholinergic therapy. Orphenadrine has been shown to reduce the plasma levels of chlorpromazine when the drugs are given together for a period of weeks (Loga, Curry and Lader, 1975); chlorpromazine levels were greatest in the first week of treatment but then gradually fell. Induction of hepatic monoxygenase activity causing increased drug metabolism represents the most likely explanation. Similarly, chlorpromazine levels fell following introduction of benzhexol therapy but rose following anticholinergic withdrawal (Rivera-Calimlim et al., 1976). In this case impaired absorption of chlorpromazine from the gut due to decreased intestinal motility appears involved. In summary, the use of anticholinergic drugs to control neuroleptic-induced parkinsonism is fraught with difficulties and these drugs should be used for short-term treatment only where other effective measures have failed.

The treatment of drug-induced dyskinesias

The drug treatment of neuroleptic-induced dyskinesias is difficult, and the underlying pathophysiology of these disorders is obscure. Although acute dystonic reactions can be dramatically relieved by anticholinergic and other drugs, the rationale for their use is unclear. Although akathisia is the most common of the drug-induced dyskinesias, its treatment is least well-documented. The therapy of tardive dyskinesia is entirely unsatisfactory; a vast array of drugs has been employed, but none have been found to be reliably effective.

The drugs used against neuroleptic-induced dyskinesias do not fall into well-defined categories. Many have been considered in detail in the previous chapter. We will only deal in detail with those agents which have not received sufficient cover by other authors. Since tardive dyskinesias represent the most serious neuroleptic-induced dyskinesia, and the most difficult therapeutic problem, its drug treatment will be considered first.

TARDIVE DYSKINESIA

The treatment of this condition at the present time is unsatisfactory. Therapy is based on the hypothesis that tardive dyskinesias are due to overactivity of dopaminergic transmission within the brain (Klawans, 1973a,b). The most widely used approaches have been to inhibit dopaminergic transmission by the use of drugs which

(1) block the post-synaptic dopamine receptor,
(2) inhibit dopaminergic function by actions on pre-synaptic dopamine receptors, or
(3) prevent synthesis or deplete pre-synaptic stores of dopamine.

Attempts also have been made to desensitize the post-synaptic dopamine receptor by the administration of high doses of dopamine agonists. The dopamine receptor over-activity hypothesis has been extended to include changes in functional balance which might occur between transmitters within basal ganglia. Thus altering both cholinergic and GABA function within basal ganglia have been assessed for their effects in tardive dyskinesia. In addition, many other compounds have been tried empirically in the hope that they may help tardive dyskinesia.

Drugs decreasing dopaminergic function
From a theoretical viewpoint, increasing the dose of the neuroleptic that was responsible for the tardive dyskinesia, or adding a larger dose of another neuroleptic, should suppress neuroleptic-induced tardive dyskinesias caused by dopamine receptor over-activity. Obviously this is irrational, and such a therapeutic action often is only temporary; the movements may break through neuroleptic therapy, and even may be more intense than initially. Although there seems little point in using neuroleptic drugs to induce more of the same, a number of dopamine receptor blocking neuroleptics (thiopropazate, haloperidol, pimozide, metoclopramide and sulpiride; XVI–XX) have been reported to be effective in double-blind control studies in the treatment of tardive dyskinesias (*Table 5.4*).

It is probable that any of the neuroleptic agents presently available, if given in sufficient dosage will control tardive dyskinesias, albeit temporarily. Pimozide and sulpiride, however, may differ from the other neuroleptics for they exert a more selective action on dopamine receptors than most other neuroleptic compounds. Most neuroleptics act not only as antagonists of cerebral dopamine function, but can act as well on noradrenaline, 5-HT and histamine receptors, and even on cholinergic receptors in the case of drugs such as thioridazine. In contrast, pimozide exhibits a very much higher affinity for dopamine receptors than for other neuronal system, and in low doses can be considered as a selective dopamine antagonist. Sulpiride is without effect on cerebral transmitter systems other than dopamine; it is selective for that population of cerebral dopamine receptors acting independently of adenylate cyclase (Jenner and Marsden, 1981).

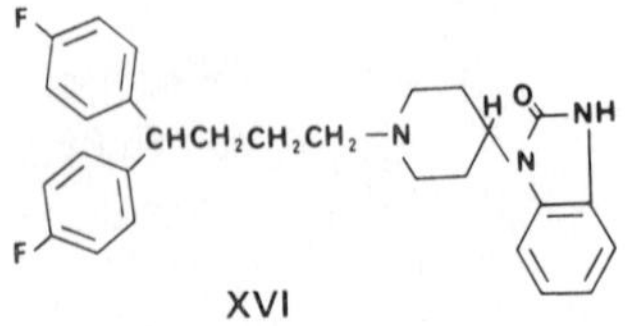

XVI

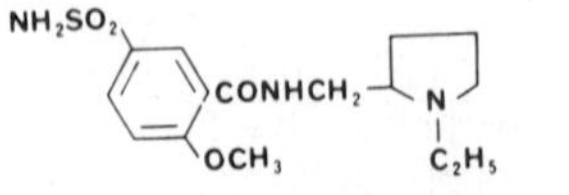

XVII

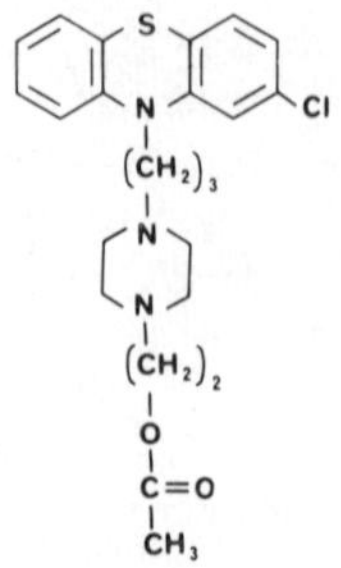

XVIII

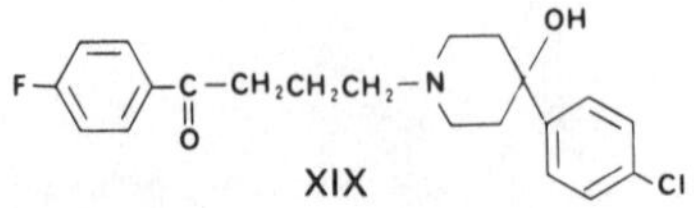

XIX

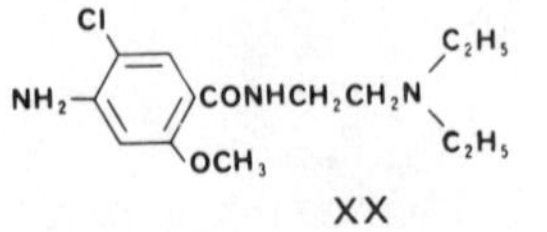

XX

TABLE 5.4 Neuroleptics shown to be effective in the treatment of tardive dyskinesias in placebo-controlled studies

Treatment (mg daily dose)	Design	Authors
Thiopropazate (45)	Double-blind randomized cross-over	Singer and Cheng (1971)
Thiopropazate (10–80)	Double-blind	Kazamatsuri, Chen and Cole (1972b)
Pimozide (6–28)	Double-blind	Claveria et al. (1975)
Haloperidol (2–16)	Double-blind	Kazamatsuri, Chen and Cole (1972b)
Haloperidol (8–16)	Double-blind randomized cross-over	Bateman et al. (1979)
Metoclopramide (40)	Double-blind randomized cross-over	Bateman et al. (1979)
Sulpiride (400–2100)	Single-blind randomized cross-over	Casey, Gerlach and Simmelsgaard (1979)

Adapted from MacKay and Sheppard (1979).

It may be possible to produce a selective dopamine antagonist that can control tardive dyskinesias without causing either an exacerbation of the underlying condition or other extrapyramidal disturbances. Two such compounds have been used experimentally, namely tiapride (XXI) and oxiperomide (XXII), both of which have a pharmacological profile which differs from that of more typical neuroleptic agents. For example, the bilateral injection of dopamine agonists into the striatum of guinea pigs induces a combination of locomotor hyperactivity and peri-oral biting movements (Costall and Naylor, 1975; Costall, Naylor and Owen, 1977). The locomotor hyperactivity can be prevented by the administration of classic neuroleptic compounds, but oxiperomide and tiapride only weakly inhibit this behaviour. In contrast,

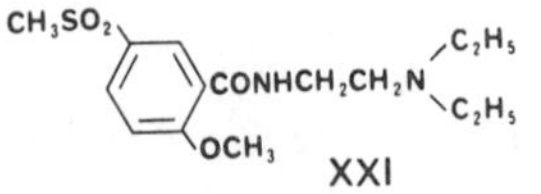

XXI

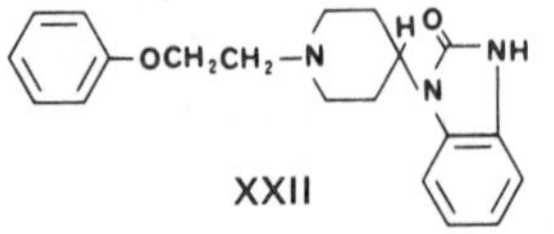

XXII

most classic neuroleptic compounds have limited actions against peri-oral movements, but tiapride and oxiperomide potently inhibit this phenomenon. These data suggest that the compounds act on a set of dopamine receptors responsible for mouthing movements rather than those controlling locomotor activity. Tiapride and oxip-eromide also act preferentially on supersensitive dopamine receptors rather than on normally innervated receptors. Thus in circling rodent models they are four to eight times more effective in blocking rotation due to activation of supersensitive post-synaptic dopamine receptors than in inhibiting circling due to actions of dopamine agonists at normal synapses (Costall et al., 1979). But this is only a relative phenomenon for more typical neuroleptics, such as haloperidol, are also twice as effective in blocking supersensitive dopamine receptors than innervated receptors. In clinical trial both oxiperomide and tiapride have been found effective in controlling levodopa induced dyskinesias (Bedard, Parkes and Marsden, 1978; Price, Parkes and Marsden, 1978). Their ability to prevent or reverse tardive dyskinesia, however, remains uncertain.

Drugs acting on pre-synaptic dopamine receptors
Dopamine agonist compounds have been used to treat tardive dyskinesia. This form of therapy is based on the idea that low doses of dopamine agonists may act preferentially on pre-synaptic dopamine receptors. By this means they might prevent synthesis and release of endogenous dopamine onto the post-synaptic receptors, thereby func-tionally decreasing dopaminergic transmission. Apomorphine (XXIII) has been reported to be of limited benefit (Tolosa, 1974; 1978; Smith et al., 1977), although further study is required to evaluate the full potential of this treatment, particularly when combined with an anti-emetic agent, such as domperidone or metoclopramide.

HO
HO
N—CH₃   XXIII

Indirectly-acting dopamine agonists which release dopamine, such as methylphenidate and amphetamine, in general have been found to have no effect or to exacerbate this disorder, as might be expected (Fann, Davis and Wilson, 1973; Smith et al., 1977). Similarly, worsening of tardive dyskinesia also has been reported with levodopa (Hippius and Longemann, 1970; Gerlach, Reisby and Randrup, 1974), although on occasions, in low oral dosage, it has been claimed to cause improvement (Carroll, Curtis and Kormen, 1977). Of the newer dopamine agonists only bromocriptine has been employed in the treatment of tardive dyskinesia and the results of these studies are conflicting (Barnes, Kidger and Taylor, 1978; Chase and Tamminga, 1979; Tamminga and Chase, 1981).

The place of low dose dopamine agonist therapy in the treatment of tardive dyskinesia is uncertain. Further work must be carried out before it can be considered useful in the treatment of the disorder.

However, before dismissing dopamine agonist therapy, it must be noted that levodopa has been employed in another way to treat tardive dyskinesia. Friedhoff (1977) has argued that since tardive dyskinesia appears due to dopamine receptor overactivity, sustained administration of dopamine agonists should cause a decrease in sensitivity of the post-synaptic dopamine receptor so as to diminish abnormal movements. He and his colleagues have shown that the dopamine receptor super-sensitivity induced in rats by repeated haloperidol administration, and subsequent withdrawal, can be reversed by administration of levodopa (Friedhoff, Bonnet and Rosengarten, 1977). Subsequently, Friedhoff has demonstrated that some weeks of high dose levodopa therapy may improve tardive dyskinesia in man, although initially it makes it worse (Alpert and Friedhoff, 1979).

Drugs depleting pre-synaptic stores of dopamine
Agents that reduce pre-synaptic synthesis or stores of dopamine have been evaluated extensively in the treatment of tardive dyskinesia. The compounds used include tetrabenazine, reserpine, α-methyldopa, α-methyl-*p*-tyrosine, and oxypertine. Most have been reported to be of some benefit in some patients, but relatively few have been subjected to full clinical trial. The only compound which at present has any established use is tetrabenazine (XXIV) which, in most studies, appears effective. Two major advantages of this therapeutic approach are immediately obvious. Firstly, amine depletors such as tetrabenazine have not been reported to cause tardive dyskinesias themselves and, secondly, the benefit derived may be more long lasting than that produced by the administration of higher doses of post-synaptically acting neuroleptic agents.

Tetrabenazine   Tetrabenazine (XXIV), a benzoquinolizine drug, acts by disruption of amine storage granules in brain. Originally introduced as a reserpine-like compound for use in the treatment of psychoses and psychoneuroses, it was subsequently shown to be of value in the management of tardive dyskinesias and other movement disorders, including chorea and dystonia.

Neurotransmitter depleting agents, such as reserpine and tetrabenazine, cause a depletion of brain monoamines (Quinn, Shore and Brodie, 1959) by disruption of storage mechanisms in amine storage granules located in pre-synaptic nerve terminals (Iversen, 1967). The effects of tetrabenazine, however, differ from those of reserpine. Reserpine causes destruction of storage granules such that normal neuronal function is not restored until newly formed amine storage granules are transported to nerve terminals, which takes some days (Haggendal and Dahlstrom, 1977). In contrast, tetrabenazine's effects are short lasting and reversible (Quinn, Shore and Brodie, 1959). Tetrabenazine and reserpine also may show differential effects on the functional pool of amines located in the nerve terminals (Kuczenski, 1977). Thus, tetrabenazine, but not reserpine, antagonizes the action of amphetamine, which acts through release of newly formed amines from this pool, suggesting that it may disrupt the small functional pool of dopamine. Tetrabenazine, like reserpine, does not specifically act on dopamine neurons, but also inhibits the storage of transmitter in 5-HT and noradrenaline terminals, although its effect on 5-HT is less marked than that of reserpine. In complete contrast to reserpine, however, tetrabenazine does not disrupt the storage of amines in peripheral tissues, so it is a selective centrally-acting drug (Quinn, Shore and Brodie, 1959).

Although tetrabenazine was originally introduced as an antipsychotic agent, it was soon reported to be of use in decreasing the symptoms of a variety of movement disorders, including those of Huntington's disease (Brandrup, 1961; Pakkenberg, 1968). For almost a decade these initial reports went unnoticed until the problem of

XXIV   XXV

tardive dyskinesia became of such importance that many drugs underwent clinical investigation. Subsequently, tetrabenazine has been shown to be effective in many patients in double-blind clinical trials in neuroleptic-induced tardive dyskinesias, Huntington's chorea and spontaneous dystonia (Godwin-Austen and Clark, 1971; Swash et al., 1972; Kazamatsuri, Chen and Cole, 1972; Pakkenberg and Fog, 1974; McLellan, Chalmers and Johnson, 1974; Toglia, McGlamery and Sambandham, 1978; Asher and Aminoff, 1981). Some studies have suggested that tolerance develops to the beneficial effects of tetrabenazine, but this is not usual. Co-administration of neuroleptic drugs, such as pimozide, has been suggested to provide greater benefit, but there can be no long-term rationale for using a combination that might serve to enhance the underlying disorder.

Drowsiness is the most frequent side effect of tetrabenazine therapy, although individual susceptibility differs. Depression also is frequent, and akathisia and parkinsonian symptoms may be observed at high doses. Most side effects tend to be dose-related, but resolve when drug dosage is reduced. Peripheral side effects generally are not observed and hypotension usually does not occur. However, overdosage has produced hypotension, sedation, sweating and hypothermia. Tetrabenazine has been reported to reduce the actions of both levodopa and reserpine.

Drugs altering cholinergic function

If tardive dyskinesias are due to an overactivity of cerebral dopamine function then restoration of the dopaminergic-cholinergic balance within basal ganglia by cholinergic agonist drugs might alleviate the condition. Anticholinergic drugs, such as benztropine, worsen tardive dyskinesia similarly to their effect in Huntington's chorea (Tarsy and Bralower, 1977).

The principal drugs used to augment cholinergic activity in tardive dyskinesia have been physostigmine, deanol, choline and lecithin. Of these compounds only physostigmine has been claimed to be effective in substantial double-blind studies (Tamminga et al., 1977), and even this has been disputed since, in other trials, physostigmine has been shown either to have no effect (Gerlach, Reisby and Randrup, 1974) or to increase dyskinetic movements (Tarsy, Leopold and Sax, 1974). Deanol (2-dimethyl-aminoethanol) at first was thought to be effective, but subsequent double-blind examination in larger studies has been less encouraging. Choline has been reported to be of value in uncontrolled trials and in a single double-blind trial. More recently, lecithin (phosphatidylcholine) has been claimed to improve tardive dyskinesia in uncontrolled studies.

Physostigmine   Physostigmine (eserine) (XXV) is a reversible anticholinesterase drug extracted from the Calibar bean. It was first used in 1877 by Laquer in the treatment of glaucoma. Physostigmine, like all anticholinesterase agents, can produce an enhancement of cholinergic function throughout the body. Unlike some other cholinesterase inhibitors such as neostigmine, physostigmine crosses the blood–brain barrier and can reverse the central as well as the peripheral effects of anticholinergic agents such as atropine.

The side effects of physostigmine therapy include salivation, anorexia, nausea, vomiting, abdominal cramps and diarrhoea. Symptoms of overdosage include sweating, lacrimation, involuntary defaecation and urination, flushing, myosis, conjunctival congestion, ciliary spasm, nystagmus, restlessness, agitation, fear, excessive dreaming, hallucinations, bradycardia, hypotension and eventually severe weakness and paralysis, convulsions and coma. Its use may be limited by the large number of side effects it produces, but the peripheral effects can be prevented by the co-administration of a peripheral anticholinergic agent, such as methylscopolamine bromide, which does not penetrate into the brain.

Physostigmine is rapidly absorbed from the gut, and is largely destroyed in the body by hydrolysis of the ester linkage by cholinesterases. It is rapidly removed, little remaining within 2 h of administration, so must be given parenterally if it is to be effective in the treatment of tardive dyskinesia.

Deanol   Deanol (2-dimethylaminoethanol) (XXVI) has been employed as a central stimulant in the treatment of general debility, mild depression, chronic headache and some behavioural disorders in children. In theory it is a precursor of choline which is transformed to acetylcholine in the brain.

$$CH_3 \diagdown \hspace{-1mm} N-CH_2CH_2OH$$
$$CH_3 \diagup$$

XXVI

Deanol enters the brain after intraperitoneal administration but does not appear to raise brain choline levels (Zahniser, Chou and Hanin, 1977). Rapid phosphorylation occurs in brain to produce phosphatidyldimethylaminoethanol, a naturally occurring phospholipid, but which is not normally found in brain (*see* Ansell and Spanner, 1979). Conversion of dimethylaminoethanol to choline only occurs in organs such as the liver, where methylation of the lipid-bound base can occur. So although deanol increases plasma choline concentrations, evidence for alteration of central acetylcholine formation is poor. Indeed deanol can inhibit choline transport into brain and so might inhibit acetylcholine formation (Millington, McCall and Wurtman, 1978).

Initial open clinical trials suggested that deanol therapy reduced or abolished tardive dyskinesia, Huntington's chorea and levodopa induced dyskinesia (Walker, Hoehn and Sears, 1973; Miller, 1974; Casey and Deney, 1975). However, subsequent double-blind studies in larger groups of patients have been unable to confirm these findings in a variety of movement disorders (Tarsy and Bralower, 1977; Simpson *et al.*, 1977; Tamminga *et al.*, 1977).

Deanol therapy causes headache, muscle tension, insomnia, pruritus and postural hypotension. In general, it would not appear to be a treatment of benefit to patients with tardive dyskinesia.

Choline   Choline (XXVII) is the immediate precursor of acetylcholine and so is potentially able to elevate brain acetylcholine content. Choline therapy may be of some value in the treatment of tardive dyskinesias but the amounts of choline required to elevate brain acetylcholine levels and to provide clinical benefit are large.

$$CH_3-\overset{\overset{\displaystyle CH_3}{|}}{\underset{\underset{\displaystyle CH_3}{|}}{N}}-CH_2CH_2OH$$

XXVII

Choline is converted into acetylcholine by choline acetyl transferase, which is located in cholinergic nerve terminals. Some choline is generated within brain but most is obtained from the periphery, either by means of a low affinity choline uptake mechanism that normally is saturated, or by uptake of choline-containing phospholipids (*see* Ansell and Spanner, 1979; Haubrich, Gerber and Pflueger, 1979). Present evidence would suggest that choline can be a rate limiting substrate in the synthesis of acetylcholine. The concentration of choline in brain is below Km for choline acetyltransferase, so that raising the extracellular choline concentration increases the acetylcholine content of brain and peripheral tissues. Large doses of choline do raise the free choline content and acetylcholine concentration of brain (Cohen and Wurtman, 1975; 1976; Haubrich et al., 1975). However, the amount of the administered choline utilized in this manner is minute, for usually there is more than adequate choline available for acetylcholine synthesis. However, the increased acetylcholine in brain induced by massive doses of choline is functionally active in animals, for it causes an increase in brain tyrosine hydroxylase activity (Ulus and Wurtman, 1976) and inhibits stereotyped behaviour induced by apomorphine (Davis et al., 1978a). Indeed administration of choline has been shown to reduce the enhancement of apomorphine-induced stereotyped behaviour induced by prior neuroleptic treatment of rats (Davis et al., 1978b).

Choline therapy has been shown to be of little benefit in the treatment of Huntington's chorea (Fann et al., 1974; Aquilonius and Eckernas, 1977; Growdon, Cohen and Wurtman, 1977a,b), but has been reported to improve memory (Sitaram, Weingarten and Gillin, 1978) and to benefit those with Alzheimer's disease (Boyd et al., 1977; Etienne et al., 1978), where choline acetyl transferase activity may be decreased. The claims that choline benefits tardive dyskinesia are not yet substantial (Davis, Berger and Hollister, 1975; Davis et al., 1976; Growdon, Cohen and Wurtman, 1977; Barbeau, 1978). In double-blind controlled studies, choline chloride therapy caused improvement in approximately 50 per cent of patients with tardive dyskinesia (Davis et al., 1976; Growdon, Cohen and Wurtman, 1977). However, since no relapse was observed in some patients during placebo substitution, possible spontaneous remission cannot be ignored. The effect of choline therapy was not observed after acute administration, and approximately 7 d of treatment with up to 20 g of choline chloride daily is required to obtain a clinically beneficial effect (see Davis, Berger and Hollister, 1979).

Side effects of choline therapy include dizziness, nausea, increased salivation and diarrhoea, but these may respond to treatment with a peripheral anticholinergic agent. Unfortunately, patients develop a fishy odour due to degradation of choline to trimethylamine in the gut (Lee et al., 1976).

Lecithin   The phospholipid lecithin (phosphatidylcholine) (XXVIII) is the major phospholipid in brain, liver, plasma and most other tissues. It is an important structural component of membranes, and also is a source of fatty acids and choline.

$$
\begin{array}{l}
\quad\ \ CH_2O-\underset{\underset{O}{\|}}{C}-R_1 \\
R_2-\underset{\underset{O}{\|}}{C}-OCH \qquad\quad CH_3 \\
\quad\ \ CH_2O-\underset{\underset{O}{\|}}{\overset{OH}{P}}-OCH_2CH_2-\underset{\underset{CH_3}{\|}}{\overset{+}{N}}-CH_3
\end{array}
$$

XXVIII

Lecithin in the diet also forms the major source of choline, so lecithin consumption will increase plasma and brain choline levels and elevate brain acetylcholine content (Hirsch and Wurtman, 1978). Commercial lecithin is a mixture of phosphatides and other substances that contain phosphatidylcholine. It is extracted from a variety of sources including the fat or oil of the soyabean or rapeseed, bovine brain, or egg (see Wurtman, 1979). The phosphatidylcholine content of commercial lecithin products varies between 20–70 per cent depending on source, but purified products containing more than 99 per cent phosphotidylcholine are available.

The mechanism by which phosphatidylcholine gives rise to choline is unresolved (*see* Ansell and Spanner, 1979). It seems likely that the major degradative pathway involves phospholipases A1 and A2, lysophospholipase and glycerophosphocholine diesterase. However, whatever the mechanism, it is clear that administration of lecithin eventually increases acetylcholine levels in brain and peripheral tissues and that it is more effective in elevating choline concentrations than choline itself (Hirsch, Growdon and Wurtman, 1978; Wurtman, Hirsch and Growdon, 1977). Endogenous phosphatidyl-choline concentrations in plasma are high, so it remains a mystery why administration of large doses of exogenous lecithin should enhance choline and acetylcholine concentrations.

Administration of lecithin has been claimed to suppress tardive dyskinesia, and to be of benefit in Friedreich's ataxia but not in Huntington's chorea (Growdon *et al.*, 1978; Gelenberg, Wojcik and Growdon, 1979; Barbeau, 1979). Lecithin also has been used in Alzeheimer's disease, and has been suggested to reduce dyskinesias in parkinsonian patients receiving levodopa therapy (Perry, Perry and Tomlinson, 1977; Barbeau, 1979). Apparently it makes Gilles de la Tourette's disease worse.

In tardive dyskinesia, lecithin therapy is said to reduce, but not abolish, abnormal movements. The improvement is accompanied by substantial increases in serum choline levels. Following withdrawal of lecithin, deterioration occurs within several days and a return to the baseline state occurs within one to two weeks (*see* Gelenberg, Wojcik and Growdon, 1979). The overall impression is that lecithin is at least effective as choline in treating tardive dyskinesia, but with fewer side effects and greater acceptability to patients.

Lecithin therapy results in some diarrhoea and mild nausea and dizziness. Patients do not, however, develop the fishy odour accompanying choline therapy and lecithin does not possess the bitter taste of choline, so it is more palatable. Weight gain occurs during lecithin therapy. A few patients have been reported to develop parkinsonian symptoms during lecithin therapy.

Lecithin is well absorbed from the gut, little appearing in faeces (*see* Fox, Betzing and Lekim, 1979). The plasma half-life is approximately 30 h and due to tissue incorporation only 50 per cent is excreted in urine or expired air 120 h after a single administration. The elevation of plasma choline following lecithin administration is greater and longer lasting than after equivalent choline chloride therapy.

Drugs altering GABA function
Attempts to correct basal ganglia function also have focused on altering the activity of the GABA systems which form the major inhibitory pathways in this area of the brain. Baclofen (XXIX), sodium valproate (XXX) and benzodiazepines have been used in an attempt to potentiate GABA action. The effectiveness of baclofen has been confirmed in three controlled studies (Gerlach, Rye and Kristjansen, 1978; Korsgaard, 1976; Gerlach, 1977), although one other was unable to detect any effect (Vasavan-Nair *et al.*, 1978). The use of sodium valproate is more controversial; it has been reported to be effective in a single controlled trial in tardive dyskinesia (Linnoila, Viukari and Hietala, 1976), but this has not been confirmed in other studies (*see for example* Gibson, 1978). Benzodiazepines, such as clonazepam (XXXI), have some use in controlling a range of dyskinetic movements, including those of tardive dyskinesia. More recently, a novel GABA prodrug, progabide (XXXII), also has been claimed to be effective in the treatment of tardive dyskinesias, but this has not been introduced into clinical practice.

Cl—⟨ ⟩—CHCH₂COOH
           |
           CH₂NH₂

XXIX

CH₃CH₂CH₂
              ⟩CHCOOH
CH₃CH₂CH₂

XXX

XXXI

XXXII

Baclofen Baclofen (4-chlorophenyl GABA) produces biochemical changes in rodents similar to GABA agonists, but electrophysiologically and in other test its actions are not identical to those of a GABA agonist. Its exact mechanism of action is not known.

The drug is used widely for the treatment of spasticity in patients with multiple sclerosis, and may be of some value in patients with spasticity due to spinal cord injury or other disease. It has been claimed also to be effective in the control of tardive dyskinesias in some patients. The effect on the oral movement pattern has been reported to be characterized by a reduced frequency, an unchanged or slightly reduced amplitude, and an increased duration of each separate mouth opening and tongue protrusion, a response pattern very similar to that seen with α-methyl-*p*-tyrosine (Gerlach, Rye and Kristjansen, 1978).

The use of baclofen in tardive dyskinesia is associated with sedation, muscle weakness and confusion in up to half the patients. These side effects appear mainly in elderly patients, sometimes occurring before the antidyskinetic effect, thus limiting the practical usefulness of baclofen in the treatment of tardive dyskinesia. Similar to other muscle relaxants, it may also impair the ability of patients to walk or stand, and may on occasion also cause a severe toxic confusional state.

Sodium valproate The use of sodium valproate in the treatment of tardive dyskinesia has met with limited success. Critical examination of the only beneficial trial (Linnoila, Viukari and Hietala, 1976) revealed little effect on the oro-buccal facial movements (*see* MacKay and Sheppard, 1979). Sodium valproate has antiepileptic activity against a variety of types of seizures while causing only a minimal sedation and other central side effects. The mechanism of action of valproate is unknown, although it has been suggested that selective increases in concentrations of GABA in synaptic regions may be prompted by inhibition of GABA transaminase or succinic semialdehyde dehydrogenase, inhibition of re-uptake by glial cells and nerve endings, or some combination of these actions.

Valproate is rapidly and almost completely absorbed on oral administration. Peak concentrations in plasma are observed in 1–4 h although this can be delayed if the drug is taken with food. The drug binds strongly plasma proteins, and is extensively metabolized so that more than 70 per cent is excreted as various metabolites. The half-life of valproate in epileptic patients is approximately 15 h.

The use of valproate is associated with limited toxicity, the most common side effect being gastrointestinal irritation and CNS effects such as sedation, ataxia and incoordination which occur only infrequently. However, there have been reports that sodium valproate occasionally may cause hepatotoxicity, which can be lethal, especially in children.

Benzodiazepines   Only two common benzodiazepines are of use in controlling dyskinesias, namely diazepam and clonazepam. The clinical use and pharmacology of these compounds is extensively discussed in Chapter 6. Only a brief description of the actions of clonazepam will be given here.

Benzodiazepines are, of course, employed primarily as sedative and antianxiety drugs, but a large number also possess broad antiepileptic properties. Of these, clonazepam is the most commonly used. The pharmacology of all benzodiazepines suggests that they interact in the brain with a specific benzodiazepine receptor, which facilitates activation of the GABA receptor complex (p. 137). Clonazepam, in particular, also is thought to exert actions on cerebral 5-HT mechanisms, although whether this is a direct action, or is mediated indirectly via benzodiazepine or GABA receptor systems is not clear.

Clonazepam has been administered to patients with neuroleptic-induced dyskinesias with consistent improvement (O'Flanagan, 1975). It is effective also in suppressing some of the choreiform movements observed in patients with Huntington's chorea (Peiris, Boralessa and Lionel, 1976). The other uses of clonazepam are in the treatment of myoclonus, in particular post-anoxic action myoclonus, and in the treatment of status epilepticus.

The most common side effects of clonazepam therapy are drowsiness and dizziness. Other side effects that may occur include fatigue, muscular hypotonia, lack of coordination, ataxia, aggression, irritability, and mental changes. The principal side effects of oral medication namely drowsiness, somnolence, fatigue and lethargy, although occurring in up to 50 per cent of patients initially, tend to subside during continued administration. Gradual tolerance to the beneficial effects of the drug may also be observed such that dosage has to be increased at intervals.

Clonazepam is well absorbed following oral administration and concentrations in plasma are maximal within 2–4 h. Approximately half of the drug in plasma is bound to circulating protein. Clonazepam is metabolized principally by reduction of the nitro function to produce the inactive 4-amino derivative. Less than 1 per cent of the drug is recovered unchanged in urine and the rest is excreted as conjugated or free metabolites. The plasma half-life is long, being of the order of 1–2 d.

Other therapeutic approaches to tardive dyskinesia

A large number of other compounds have been investigated as treatments of tardive dyskinesia (*see* MacKay and Sheppard, 1979; Baldessarini and Tarsy, 1978; Jeste and Wyatt, 1979). Lithium, papaverine, pyridoxine, barbiturates, oestrogens, progestogens, clozapine, imipramine, isocarboxyzid, L-tryptophan, disulfiram, fusaric acid, propranolol, cyproheptadine and manganese have all been employed. In open clinical trials the majority of these compounds have been reported to be successful in the treatment of tardive dyskinesia in some patients. Few have been properly evaluated. In the case of lithium, for example, numerous early reports were not confirmed when the drug was subjected to double-blind control study. Indeed, there is little to suggest that any of these compounds are effective in tardive dyskinesia. It may be that tardive dyskinesia is not a single entity. If different subtypes exist, they may respond in different ways to pharmacological manipulation.

ACUTE DYSTONIC REACTIONS

Neuroleptic-induced acute dystonic reactions are the most dramatic of the movement disorders caused by neuroleptic therapy. Stopping the offending drugs allows the dystonic symptoms to disappear as drug levels decline. However, the distress caused by an acute dystonic reaction often requires more positive drug treatment. Acute dystonic reactions respond dramatically to standard anticholinergic drug therapy, given intravenously or intramuscularly (*see above*). In patients with a known propensity for the development of acute dystonic reactions, further episodes can be avoided either by reduction of neuroleptic therapy, where possible, or by prophylactic co-administration of anticholinergic drugs.

Many other drugs have been found to abort acute dystonic reactions. Since acute neuroleptic-induced dystonia appears to be due to some form of functional dopamine overactivity, then decreasing dopaminergic transmission should be effective. Low doses of dopamine agonists such as apomorphine and methylphenidate have been reported to reverse acute dystonic reactions. A number of other drugs with various actions (*Table 5.5*) also have been found to abolish neuroleptic-induced acute dystonic reactions. The mechanism by which these compounds produce their effects in this situation is not known.

TABLE 5.5 Drugs used occasionally to treat neuroleptic-induced acute dystonia

Drugs	Authors
Barbiturates	Gailitis, Knowles and Longobardi (1960)
Caffeine	Sarwer-Foner (1960)
Diazepam	Korczyn and Goldberg (1972)
Pethidine	Perez (1961)
Apomorphine	Gessa, Tagliamonte and Gessa (1972)
Methylphenidate	Fann (1966)

Akathisia

The treatment of neuroleptic-induced akathisia has been hampered by the present poor understanding of the pathophysiology of this disorder. The clinical definition of the disorder also is vague so that akathisia often is confused with persistent movements of the limbs observed in tardive dyskinesia, or with exacerbation of the underlying psychotic state. As a result of these confusions, the clinical pharmacology of akathisia is very uncertain.

Akathisia apparently is relatively resistant to treatment with anticholinergic and antihistaminergic drugs, and is said to show no response to physostigmine. This suggests that either its pathophysiology is not related to the same type of dopamine receptor blockade as observed in neuroleptic-induced parkinsonism, or that the inter-relationship between dopamine and acetycholine is different in that area of the brain where akathisia is produced, for example in the cerebral cortex. The effect of most dopamine agonist compounds on this condition does not appear to have been reported, although this may be due to fears that they would exacerbate the underlying schizophrenia. Reduction of neuroleptic dosage is an effective form of management of akathisia, but on occasions the syndrome may persist or become worse. Probably, the use of benzodiazepines, such as clonazepam or diazepam, to suppress the motor restlessness and mental distress, represents the most common form of drug treatment of this disorder.

References

AELLIG, W. H. and NUESCH, E. Comparative pharmacokinetic investigation with tritium-labelled ergot alkaloids after oral and intravenous administration to man, *International Journal of Clinical Pharmacology* **115**, 106-112 (1977)

ALPERT, M. and FRIEDHOFF, A. J. Clinical trials of dopamine receptor supersensitivity modification. In *Catecholamine: Basic and Clinical Frontiers* (Eds. E. USDIN, I. J. KOPIN and J. BARCHAS), 1590–1592, Pergamon Press, New York (1979)

ANDEN, N. E. Dopamine turnover in the corpus striatum and the limbic system after treatment with neuroleptic and anti-acetylcholine drugs, *Journal of Pharmacy and Pharmacology* **24**, 905–906 (1972)

ANSELL, G. B. and SPANNER, S. Sources of choline for acetylcholine synthesis in the brain. In *Nutrition and the Brain* (Eds. A. BARBEAU, J. H. GROWDON and R. J. WURTMAN), **5**, 35–46, Raven Press, New York (1979)

AQUILONIUS, S. M. and ECKERNAS, S. A. Choline therapy in Huntington's chorea, *Neurology* **27**, 887–889 (1977)

ASHER, S. W. and AMINOFF, M. J. Tetrabenazine and movement disorders, *Neurology (NY)* **31**, 1051–1054 (1981)

ASPER, H., BAGGIOLINI, M., BURKI, H. R., LAUENER, H., RUCH, W. and STILLE, G. Tolerance phenomena with neuroleptics: catalepsy, apomorphine stereotypies and striatal dopamine metabolism in the rat after single and repeated administration of loxapine and haloperidol, *European Journal of Pharmacology* **22**, 287–294 (1973)

AXELSSON, J. and THESLEFF, S. A study of supersensitivity in denervated mammalian skeletal muscle. *Journal of Physiology (London)* **147**, 178–193 (1959)

AYD, F. J. A survey of drug-induced extrapyramidal reactions, *Journal of the American Medical Association* **175**, 1054–1060 (1961)

BALDESSARINI, R. J. and TARSY, D. Tardive dyskinesia. In *Psychopharmacology: A Generation of Progress* (Eds. M. A. LIPTON, A. DI MASCIO and K. F. KILLAM), 993–1004, Raven Press, New York (1978)

BANNON, M. J., GRACE, A. A., BUNNEY, B. S. and ROTH, R. H. Evidence for an irreversible interaction of bromocriptine with central dopamine receptors, *Naunyn-Schmiedeberg's Archives of Pharmacology* **312**, 37–41 (1980)

BARBEAU, A. The pathogenesis of Parkinson's disease: A new hypothesis, *Canadian Medical Association Journal* **87**, 802–807 (1962)

BARBEAU, A. Emerging treatments: replacement therapy with choline or lecithin in neurological diseases, *Canadian Journal of Neurological Sciences* **5**, 157–161 (1978)

BARBEAU, A. Lecithin in movement disorders. In *Nutrition and the Brain* (Eds. A. BARBEAU, J. H. GROWDON and R. J. WURTMAN), **5**, 263–271, Raven Press, New York (1979)

BARNES, T., KIDGER, T. and TAYLOR, P. On the use of dopamine agonists in tardive dyskinesia, *American Journal of Psychiatry* **135**, 132–133 (1978)

BARSA, J. A. and KLINE, N.S. Use of reserpine in disturbed patients, *American Journal of Psychiatry* **112**, 684–691 (1956)

BARTHOLINI, G., STADLER, H. and LLOYD, K. G. Cholinergic-dopaminergic interactions in the extrapyramidal system. In *Progress in the Treatment of Parkinsonism* (Ed. D. B. CALNE), 233–241, Raven Press, New York (1973)

BATEMAN, D. N., DUTTA, D. K., McCLELLAND, H. A. and RAWLINS, M. D. Metoclopramide and haloperidol in tardive dyskinesia, *British Journal of Psychiatry* **135**, 505–508 (1979)

BEDARD, P., DELEAN, J., LAFLEUR, J. and LAROCHELLE, L. Haloperidol-induced dyskinesias in the monkey, *Le Journal Canadien des Sciences Neurologique* **4**, 197–201 (1977)

BEDARD, P., PARKES, J. D. and MARSDEN, C. D. Effect of new dopamine-blocking agent (oxiperomide) on drug-induced dyskinesias in Parkinson's disease and spontaneous dyskinesias, *British Medical Journal* **1**, 954–956 (1978)

BERGMAN, S., CURZON, G., FRIEDEL, J., GODWIN-AUSTEN, R. B. MARSDEN, C. D. and PARKES, J. D. The absorption and metabolism of a standard dose of levodopa in patients with parkinsonism, *British Journal of Clinical Pharmacology* **1**, 417–424 (1975)

BERTLER, A. Effect of reserpine on the storage of catecholamines in brain and other issues, *Acta Physiologica Scandinavica* **51**, 75–83 (1961)

BIANCHINE, J. R. Drugs for Parkinson's disease; centrally acting muscle relaxants. In *The Pharmacological Basis of Therapeutics*, 6th edn (Eds. A. GOODMAN GILMAN, A. S. GOODMAN and A. GILMAN), 475–493, MacMillan, New York (1980)

BIRKMAYER, W. Long-term treatment with L-deprenyl, *Journal of Neural Transmission* **43**, 239–244 (1978)

BIRKMAYER, W. and HORNYKIEWICZ, O. Der L-Dioxyphenylalanin (= dopa)–Effekt bei der Parkinson-Akinese, *Wiener Klinische Wochenschrift* **73**, 787–788 (1961)

BIRKMAYER, W., RIEDERER, P., YOUDIM, M. B. H. and LINAUER, W. The potentiation of the anti-akinetic effect after L-dopa treatment by an inhibitor of MAO-B, deprenyl, *Journal of Neural Transmission* **36**, 303–326 (1975)

BIRKMAYER, W., RIEDERER, P., AMBROZI, L. and YOUDIM, M. B. H. Implications of combined treatment with Madopar and L-Deprenyl in Parkinson's disease, *Lancet* **2**, 439–443 (1977)

BOYD, W. D., GRAHAME-WHITE, J., BLACKWOOD, G., GLEN, I. and McQUEEN, J. Clinical effects of choline in Alzheimer's senile dementia, *Lancet* **2**, 711 (1977)

BRANDRUP, C. Tetrabenazine treatment in persisting dyskinesia caused by psychopharma, *American Journal of Psychiatry* **118**, 551–552 (1961)

BURT, D. R., CREESE, I. and SNYDER, S. H. Antischizophrenic drugs: chronic treatment elevates dopamine receptor binding in brain, *Science* **196**, 326–328 (1977)

CALNE, D. B., TEYCHENNE, P. F., LEIGH, P. N., BAMJI, A. N. and GREEN, J. K. Treatment of parkinsonism with bromocriptine, *Lancet* **2**, 1335–1356 (1974a)

CALNE, D. B., TEYCHENNE, P. F., CLAVERIA, L. E., EASTMAN, R., GREENACRE, J. K. and PETRIE, A. Bromocriptine in parkinsonism, *British Medical Journal* **4**, 442–444 (1974b)

CARLSSON, A. Biochemical implications of dopa-induced actions on the central nervous system with particular references to abnormal movements. In *L-dopa and Parkinsonism* (Eds. A. BARBEAU and F. H. McDOWELL), 205–213, Davis, Philadelphia (1970)

CARLSSON, A. Does dopamine play a role in schizophrenia? *Psychological Medicine* **7**, 583–597 (1977)

CARLSSON, A. and LINDQVIST, M. Effect of chlorpromazine or haloperidol on formation of 3-methoxytyramine and normetanephrine in mouse brain, *Acta Pharmacologica et Toxicologica* **20**, 140–144 (1963)

CARROLL, B., CURTIS, G. and KORMEN, E. Paradoxical response to dopamine agonists in tardive dyskinesia, *American Journal of Psychiatry* **134**, (7) 785–789 (1977)

CARTER, C. J. and PYCOCK, C. J. Studies on the role of catecholamines in the frontal cortex, *British Journal of Pharmacology* **42**, p. 402 (1978)

CASEY, D. E. and DENNY, D. Deanol in the treatment of tardive dyskinesia, *American Journal of Psychiatry* **132**, 864–867 (1975)

CASEY, D. E., GERLACH, J. and SIMMELSGAARD, H. Sulpiride in tardive dyskinesia, *Psychopharmacology* **66**, 73–77 (1979)

CHASE, T. N. Drug-induced extrapyramidal disorders, *Research Publications of the Association of Nervous and Mental Diseases* **50**, 448–471 (1972)

CHASE, T. N. and TAMMINGA, C. A. Pharmacological studies of tardive dyskinesia. In *Long-Term Effects of Neuroleptics* Eds. F. CATTABENI, G. RACAGNI, P. F. SPANO and E. COSTA, *Advances in Psychopharmacology* **24**, 457–461, Raven Press, New York (1979)

CHOUINARD, G., DE MONTIGNY, C. and ANNABLE, L. Tardive dyskinesia and anti-parkinson medication, *American Journal of Psychiatry* **136**, 228–229 (1979)

CLAVERIA, L., TEYCHENNE, P., CALNE, D., HASKAYNE, L., PETRIE, A., PALLIS, C. and LODGE-PATCH, I. Tardive dyskinesia treated with pimozide, *Journal of the Neurological Sciences* **24**, 393–340 (1975)

CLOW, A., JENNER, P. and MARSDEN, C. D. An experimental model of tardive dyskinesias, *Life Sciences* **23**, 421–424 (1978)

CLOW, A., JENNER, P., THEODOROU, A. and MARSDEN, C. D. Striatal dopamine receptors become supersensitive while rats are given trifluoperazine for six months, *Nature* **278**, 59–61 (1979a)

CLOW, A., JENNER, P. and MARSDEN, C. D. Changes in dopamine mediated behaviour during one year's neuroleptic administration, *European Journal of Pharmacology* **57**, 365–375 (1979b)

COHEN, E. L. and WURTMAN, R. J. Brain acetylcholine: Increase after systemic choline administration, *Life Science* **16**, 1095–1102 (1975)

COHEN, E. L. and WURTMAN, R. J. Brain acetylcholine: Control by dietary choline, *Science* **19**, 561–562 (1976)

CORRODI, H., FUXE, K. and LIDBRINK, P. Interaction between cholinergic and catecholaminergic neurons in rat brain, *Brain Research* **43**, 397–416 (1972)

CORRODI, H., FUXE, K., HOKFELT, T., LIDBRINK, P. and UNGERSTEDT, U. Effect of ergot drugs on central catecholamine neurons: evidence for a stimulation of central dopamine neurons, *Journal of Pharmacy and Pharmacology* **25**, 409–410 (1973)

COSTALL, B. and NAYLOR R. J. Neuroleptic antagonism of dyskinetic phenomena, *European Journal of Pharmacology* **33**, 301–312 (1975)

COSTALL, B., FORTUNE, D. H., NAYLOR, R. J. and NOHRIA, V. A study of drug action on normal and denervated striatal mechanisms, *European Journal of Pharmacology* **56**, 207–216 (1979)

COSTALL, B., NAYLOR, R. J. and OWEN, R. T. Investigation into the nature of the peri-oral movements induced by 2-(N, N-dipropyl)-amino-5, 6-dihydroxytetralin, *European Journal of Pharmacology* **45**, 357–367 (1977)

COTZIAS, G. C., VAN WOERT, M. H. and SCHIFFER, L. M. Aromatic amino acids and modification of parkinsonism. *New England Journal of Medicine* **276**, 374 (1967)

CRANE, G. E. Tardive dyskinesia in patients treated with major neuroleptics: a review of the literature, *American Journal of Psychiatry* **124**, 40–48 (1968)

CRANE, G. E. Persistent dyskinesia, *British Journal of Psychiatry* **122**, 395–405 (1973)

DAVIS, K. L., BERGER, P. A. and HOLLISTER, L. E. Choline for tardive dyskinesia, *New England Journal of Medicine* **293**, 152 (1975)

DAVIS, K. L., BERGER, P. A. and HOLLISTER, L. E. Clinical and pre-clinical experience with choline chloride in Huntington's disease and tardive dyskinesia: Unanswered questions. In *Nutrition and the Brain* (Eds. A. BARBEAU, J. H. GROWDON and R. J. WURTMAN), **5**, 305–315, Raven Press, New York (1979)

DAVIS, K. L., HOLLISTER, L. E., BARCHAS, J. D. and BERGER, P. A. Choline in tardive dyskinesia and Huntington's disease, *Life Science* **19**, 1507–1516 (1976)

DAVIS, K. L., HOLLISTER, L. E., VENTO, A. L. and SIMONTON, S. Chlorine chloride in animal modals of tardive dyskinesia, *Life Science* **22**, 1699–1708 (1978b)

DAVIS, K. L., HOLLISTER, L. E., VENTO, A. L. and SIMONTON, S. Chlorine chloride in methylphenidate and apomorphine-induced stereotypy, *Life Science* **22**, 2171–2178 (1978a)

DEAN, K., LAND, G. and BYE, A. Analysis of procyclidine in human plasma and urine by gas–liquid chromatography, *Journal of Chromatography* **221**, 408–413 (1981)

DEGKVITZ, R. Uber die Ursachen der persisteirenden extrapyramidalen Hyperkineser nach langfristiger. Anwendung von Neuroleptika, *Activitas Nervosa Superior (Praha)* **12**, 67–68 (1967)

DEGKVITZ, R. and WENZEL, W. Persistent extrapyramidal side effects after long-term application of neuroleptics. In *Neuropsychopharmacology. International Congress series. No. 129* (Ed. H. BRILL), 608–615, Excerpta Medica, Amsterdam (1967)

DELAY, J. and DENIKER, P. Characteristiques neurophysiologiques des medicaments neuroleptiques. Rapport Symposium Intenationale Medicaments Psychotropies, Milan 1957. In *Psychotropic Drugs* (Eds. S. GARRATINI and V. GHETTI), 485–501, Elsevier, Amsterdam (1957)

DELAY, J. and DENIKER, P. Drug-induced extrapyramidal syndromes. In *Handbook of Clinical Neurology*, Diseases of the Basal Ganglia (Eds. P. J. VINKEN and G. K. BRUYN), **56**, 248–266, North-Holland, Amsterdam (1968)

DELAY, J., DENIKER, P. and HARL, J. M. Utilisation en therapeutique psychiatrique d'une phenothiazine d'action centrale elective (4560 RP), *Annales Medico-Psychologiques* **110**, 112-117 (1952)

DENEAU, G. A. and CRANE, G. E. Dyskinesia in rhesus monkeys tested with high doses of chlorpromazine. In *Psychotropic Drugs and Dysfunctions of the Basal Ganglia* (Eds. G. E. CRANE and J. R. GARDNER), 12–14, US Public Health Service Publication. No. 938, Washington, DC (1968)

DENHAM, J. and CARRICK, D. J. Therapeutic value of thioproperazine and the importance of the associated neurological disturbances, *Journal of Mental Science* **107**, 326–345 (1961)

DENIKER, P. Experimental neurological syndromes and the new drug therapies in psychiatry, *Comprehensive Psychiatry* **1**, 92–102 (1960)

DOLPHIN, A. C., JENNER, P., SAWAYA, M. C. B., MARSDEN, C. D. and TESTA, B. The effect of bromocriptine on locomotor activity and cerebral catecholamines in rodents, *Journal of Pharmacy and Pharmacology* **29**, 727–734 (1977)

DUVOISIN, R. C. Cholinergic-anticholinergic antagonism in parkinsonism, *Archives of Neurology* **17**, 124–136 (1967)

EHRINGER, H. and HORNYKIEWICZ, O. Verteilung von Noradrenalin und Dopamine im Gehirn des Menschen und ihr Verhalten bei Erkrankungen des extrapyramidalen Systems, *Klinische Wochenschrift* **38**, 1236–1239 (1960)

EKDAWI, M. Y. and FOWKE, R. A controlled trial of antiparkinson drugs in drug-induced Parkinsonism, *British Journal of Psychiatry* **112**, 633–636 (1966)

ELLISON, T., SNYDER, A., BOLGER, J. and OKUN, R. Metabolism of orphenadrine citrate in man, *Journal of Pharmacology and Experimental Therapeutics* **176**, 289–295 (1971)

ETIENNE, P., GAUTHIER, S., JOHNSON, G., COLLIER, B. MENDIS, T., DASTOOR, D., COLE, M. and MULLER, H. F. Clinical effects of choline in Alzheimer's disease, *Lancet* **1**, 508–509 (1978)

ENZ, A., JATON, A. L., and VIGOURET, J. M. Time of onset of dopaminergic (DP) action of bromocriptine (BR) in biochemical and behavioural tests, *Union of Swiss Societies of Experimental Biology*, Abstracts of the 13th Annual Meeting, p. 66 (1981)

FANN, W. E. Use of methylphenidate to counteract acute dystonic effects of phenothiazine, *American Journal of Psychiatry* **122**, 1293–1294 (1966)

FANN, W., DAVIS, J. and WILSON, I. Methylphenidate in tardive diskinesia, *American Journal of Psychiatry* **130**, 922–924 (1973)

FANN, W. E., LAKE, C. R., GERBER, C. J. and McKENZIE, G. Cholinergic suppression of tardive dyskinesia, *Psychopharmacology* **37**, 101–107 (1974)

FARNEBO, L., FUXE, K., GOLDSTEIN, M., HAMBERGER, B. and UNGERSTEDT, U. Dopamine and noradrenaline releasing action of amantadine in the central and peripheral nervous system: A possible mode of action in Parkinson's disease, *European Journal of Pharmacology* **16**, 27–38 (1971)

FLEMING, P., MAKAR, H. and HUNTER, K. R. Levodopa in drug-induced extrapyramidal disorders, *Lancet* **2**, 1186 (1970)

FOX, J. M., BETZING, H. and LEKIM, D. Pharmacokinetics of orally injested phosphatidylcholine. In *Nutrition and the Brain* (Eds. A. BARBEAU, J. H. GROWDON and R. J. WURTMAN), **5**, 95–108, Raven Press, New York (1979)

FREYHAN, F. A. Psychomotility and parkinsonism in treatment with neuroleptic drugs, *Archives of Neurology and Psychiatry* **78**, 465–472 (1957)

FREYHAN, F. A. Therapeutic implications of differential effects of new phenothiazine compounds, *American Journal of Psychiatry* **115**, 577–585 (1959)

FRIEDHOFF, A. Receptor sensitivity modification (RSM) – a new paradigm for the potential treatment of some hormonal and transmitter disturbances, *Comprehensive Psychiatry* **18**, 309–317 (1977)

FRIEDHOFF, A. J., BONNETT, K. and ROSENGARTEN, H. Reversal of two manifestations of dopamine receptor supersensitivity by administration of L-dopa, *Research Communication of Clinical Pathology and Pharmacy* **16**, 411–423 (1977)

GAILITIS, J., KNOWLES, R. R. and LONGOBARDI, A. Alarming neuromuscular reactions due to prochlorperazine, *Annals of Internal Medicine* **52**, 538–542 (1960)

GARFINKEL, P. E. and STANCER, H. C. L-Dopa and schizophrenia, *Canadian Psychiatric Association Journal* **21**, 27–29 (1976)

GELENBERG, A. J., WOJCIK, J. D. and GROWDON, J. H. Lecithin for the treatment of tardive dyskinesia. In *Nutrition and the Brain* (Eds. A. BARBEAU, J. H. GROWDON and R. J. WURTMAN), **5**, 285–303, Raven Press, New York (1979)

GERLACH, J. Relationship between tardive dyskinesia, L-dopa-induced hyperkinesia and parkinsonism, *Psychopharmacology* **51**, 259–263 (1977a)

GERLACH, J. The relationship between parkinsonism and tardive dyskinesia, *American Journal of Psychiatry* **134**, 781–784 (1977b)

GERLACH, J., REISBY, N. and RANDRUP, A. Dopaminergic hypersensitivity and cholinergic hypofunction in the pathophysiology of tardive dyskinesia, *Psychopharmacologia (Berlin)* **34**, 21–35 (1974)

GERLACH, J., RYE, T. and KRISTJANSEN, P. Effect of baclofen on tardive dyskinesia, *Psychopharmacology* **56**, 145–151 (1978)

GESSA, R., TAGLIAMONTE, A. and GESSA, G. L. Blockade by apomorphine of haloperidol-induced dyskinesia in schizophrenic patients, *Lancet* **2**, 981–982 (1972)

GIBSON, A. C. Sodium valproate and tardive dyskinesia, *British Journal of Psychiatry* **133**, 82 (1978)

GLOVER, V., SANDLER, M., OWEN, F. and RILEY, G. J. Dopamine is a monoamine oxidase B substrate in man, *Nature* **265**, 80–81 (1977)

GLOWINSKI, J., IVERSEN, L. L. and AXELROD, J. Storage and synthesis of norepinephrine in the reserpine-treated rat brain, *Journal of Pharmacology and Experimental Therapeutics* **151**, 385–399 (1966)

GODWIN-AUSTEN, R. B. Aspects of bromocriptine therapy in Parkinson's disease, *Research and Clinical Forums* **3**, 19–23 (1981)

GODWIN-AUSTEN, R. and CLARK, T. Persistent phenothiazine dyskinesia treated with tetrabenazine, *British Medical Journal* **4**, 25–26 (1971)

GOLDMAN, D. Parkinsonism and related phenomena from administration of drugs: Their production and control under clinical conditions and possible relation to therapeutic effect, *Review of Canadian Biology* **20**, 549–560 (1961)

GRINSPOON, L., EWALT, J. R. and SHADER, R. Psychotherapy and pharmacotherapy in chronic schizophrenia, *American Journal of Psychiatry* **124**, 1645–1652 (1968)

GROWDON, J. H., COHEN, E. L. and WURTMAN, R. J. Effects of oral choline administration on serum and CSF choline levels in patients with Huntington's disease, *Journal of Neurochemistry* **28**, 229–232 (1977a)

GROWDON, J. H., COHEN, E. L. and WURTMAN, R. J. Clinical and chemical effects of choline administration, *Annals of Neurology* **1**, 418–422 (1977b)

GROWDON, J. H., GELENBERG, A. J., DOLLER, J., HIRSCH, M. J., and WURTMAN, R. J. Lecithin can suppress tardive dyskinesia, *New England Journal of Medicine* **298**, 1029–1030 (1978)

GROWDON, J. H., HIRSCH, M. J., WURTMAN, R. J. and WIENER, W. Oral choline administration to patients with tardive dyskinesia, *New England Journal of Medicine* **297**, 524–527 (1977)

GUNNE, L. M. and BARANY, S. Haloperidol-induced tardive dyskinesia in monkeys, *Psychopharmacology* **50**, 237–240 (1976)

HAASE, H. J. Clinical observations on the actions of neuroleptics. In *The Action of Neuroleptic Drugs. A Psychiatric, Neurological and Pharmacological Investigation* (Eds. H. J. HAASE and JANSSEN), 1–118, North-Holland, Amsterdam (1965)

HAGGENDALE, J. and DAHLSTROM, A. The recovery of noradrenaline in adrenergic nerve terminals of the rat after reserpine treatment, *Journal of Pharmacy and Pharmacology* **23**, 81–89 (1971)

HALL, R. A., JACKSON, R. B. and SWAIN, J. M. Neurotoxic reactions resulting from chlorpromazine administration, *Journal of the American Medical Association* **161**, 214–218 (1956)

HAUBRICH, D. R., GERBER, N. H. and PFLUEGER, A. B. Choline availability and the synthesis of acetylcholine. In *Nutrition and the Brain* (Eds. A. BARBEAU, J. H. GROWDON and R. J. WURTMAN), **5**, 57–71, Raven Press, New York (1979)

HAUBRICH, D. R., WANG, P. F. L., CLODY, D. E. and WEDEKING, P. W. Increase in rat brain acetylcholine concentration induced by choline and deanol, *Life Science* **17**, 975–980 (1975)

HEFTI, F. and MELAMED, E. L-Dopa's mechanism of action in Parkinson's disease, *Trends in Neurosciences* **3**, 229–231 (1980)

HERSHON, H. I., KENNEDY, P. F. and McGUIRE, R. J. Persistence of extrapyramidal disorders and psychiatric relapse after withdrawal of long-term phenothiazine therapy, *British Journal of Psychiatry* **120**, 41–50 (1972)

HIPPIUS, H. and LONGEMANN, G. Zur wirkung von dioxyphenylalanin (L-dopa) auf extrapyramidal motorische hyperkinesen nach langfristiger neuroleptische therapie, *Arzneimittel Forschung* **20**, 894–896 (1970)

HIRSCH, M. J. and WURTMAN, R. J. Lecithin consumption elevates acetylcholine concentrations in rat brain and adrenal gland, *Science* **202**, 223–225 (1978)

HIRSCH, M. J., GROWDON, J. H. and WURTMAN, R. J. Relations between dietary choline or lecithin intake, serum choline levels and various metabolic indices, *Metabolism* **27**, 953–960 (1978)

HIRSCH, S. R., GAIND, R., ROHDE, P. D., STEVENS, B. C. and WING, J. K. Outpatient maintenance of chronic schizophrenic patients with long-acting fluphenazine: double blind placebo trial. Report to MRC Committee on Clinical Trials in Psychiatry, *British Medical Journal* **1**, 633–637 (1973)

HOGARTY, G. C., GOLDBERG, S. L. and SCHOOLER, N. R. Drug and sociotherapy in the aftercare of schizophrenic patients, II. Two year relapse rates, *Archives of General Psychiatry* **31**, 603–608 (1974)

HAROWSKI, R. Differences in the dopaminergic effects of the ergot derivatives bromocriptine and d-LSD as compared with apomorphine, *European Journal of Pharmacology* **51**, 157–166 (1978)

INANGA, K., INOUE, K., TACHIBANA, H., OSHIMA, M. and KOTORII, T. Effects of L-dopa in schizophrenia, *Folia Psychiatrica et Neurologica* **26**, 145–157 (1972)

IVERSEN, L. L. *Uptake and Storage of Noradrenaline in Sympathetic and Adrenergic Nerves*, Cambridge University Press, London (1967)

IVERSEN, S. D. The effect of surgical lesions to frontal cortex and substantia nigra on amphetamine responses in rats, *Brain Research* **31**, 295–311 (1971)

JANSSEN, P. A. J., NIEMEGEERS, C. J. F. and SCHELLEKENS, K. H. L. Is it possible to predict the clinical effects of neuroleptic drugs (major tranquillizers) from animal data? I. Neuroleptic activity spectra for rats, *Arzneimittel Forschung* **15**, 104–112 (1965)

JENNER, P. and MARSDEN, C. D. Substituted benzamide drugs as selective neuroleptic agents, *Neuropharmacology*, (In press) (1981)

JESTE, D. V. and WYATT, R. J. In search of treatment for tardive dyskinesia. Review of the literature, *Schizophrenia Bulletin* **5**, 251–293 (1979)

JOHNSON, A. M., LOEW, D. M. and VIGOURET, J. M. Stimulant properties of bromocriptine on dopamine receptors in comparison to apomorphine. (+) – amphetamine and L-dopa, *British Journal of Pharmacology* **56**, 59–68 (1976)

JOHNSON, J. P. Some observations upon a new inhibitor of monoamine oxidase in brain tissue, *Biochemical Pharmacology* **17**, 1285–1297 (1968)

JUS, A., PINEAU, R., LACHANCE, R., PELCHAT, G., JUS, K., PIRES, P. and VILLENEUVE, R. Epidemiology of tardive dyskinesia. Part I, *Diseases of the Nervous System* **37**, 210–214 (1976a)

JUS, A., PINEAU, R., LACHANCE, R., PELCHAT, G., JUS, K., PIRES, P. and VILLENEUVE, R. Epidemiology of tardive dyskinesia. Part II, *Diseases of the Nervous System* **37**, 257–261 (1976b)

KAZAMATSURI, H., CHEN, C. and COLE, J. Treatment of tardive dyskinesia: clinical efficacy of a dopamine-depleting agent, tetrabenazine, *Archives of General Psychiatry* **27**, 95–99 (1972a)

KAZAMATSURI, H., CHEN, C. and COLE, J. Treatment of tardive dyskinesia; short term efficacy of dopamine blocking agents haloperidol and thiopropazate, *Archives of General Psychiatry* **27**, 100–106 (1972b)

KAZAMATSURI, H., CHEN, C. and COLE, J. Long-term treatment of tardive dyskinesia with haloperidol and tetrabenazine, *American Journal of Psychiatry* **130**, 479–483 (1973)

KEBABIAN, J. W. and CALNE, D. B. Multiple receptors for dopamine, *Nature* **277**, 93–96 (1979)

KELLER, H. H. and DA PRADA, M. Central dopamine agonists activity and microsomal biotransformation of lisuride, lergotrile and bromocriptine, *Life Science* **24**, 1211–1222 (1979)

KLAWANS, H. L. The pharmacology of extrapyramidal movement disorders. In *Monograph in Neural Science* (Ed. M. M. Cohen), S. Karger, Basel (1973a)

KLAWANS, H. L. The pharmacology of tardive dyskinesias, *American Journal of Psychiatry* **130**, 82–86 (1973b)

KLAWANS, H. L. and RUBOVITS, R. Effect of cholinergic and anticholinergic agents on tardive dyskinesias, *Journal of Neurology, Neurosurgery and Psychiatry* **27**, 941–947 (1974)

KNOLL, A. J. Analysis of the pharmacological effect of selective monoamine oxidase inhibitors. In *Monoamine Oxidase and its Inhibition* (Eds. G. E. W. Wolstenholme and T. J. Knight), 135–162, Elsevier, Amsterdam (1976)

KNOLL, A. J. The possible mechanism of action of (−) – deprenyl in Parkinson's disease, *Journal of Neural Transmission* **43**, 177–198 (1978)

KORCZYN, A. D. and GOLDBERG, G. J. Intravenous diazepam in drug-induced dystonic reactions, *British Journal of Psychiatry* **121**, 75–77 (1972)

KORSGAARD, S. Baclofen (Lioresal) in the treatment of neuroleptic-induced tardive dyskinesia. *Acta Psychiatrica Scandinavica* **54**, 17–24 (1976)

KRUSE, W. Persistent muscular restlessness after phenothiazine treatment : Report of three cases, *American Journal of Psychiatry* **117**, 152–153 (1960)

KUCZENSKI, R. Differential effects of reserpine and tetrabenazine on rat striatal synaptosomal dopamine biosynthesis and synaptosomal dopamine posts, *Journal of Pharmacology and Experimental Therapeutics* **201**, 357–367 (1977)

LEE, C. W. G., YU, J. S., TURNER, B.B. and MURRAY, K. G. Trimethylaminuria : fishy odours in children, *New England Journal of Medicine* **295**, 937–938 (1976)

LEES, A. J., SHAW, K. M., KOHOUT, L. J., STERN, G. M., ELSWORTH, J. D., SANDLER, M. and YOUDIM, M. B. H. Deprenyl in Parkinson's disease, *Lancet* **2**, 791–796 (1977)

LEFF, J. P. and WING, J. K. Trials of maintenance therapy in schizophrenia, *British Medical Journal* **3**, 599–604 (1971)

LIEBERMANN, A., GOLDSTEIN, M., LEIBOWITZ, M., NEOPHYTIDES, A., KUPERSMITH, M., PACT, V. and KLEINBERG, D. Treatment of advanced Parkinson's disease with pergolide, *Neurology (NY)* **31**, 675–682 (1981)

LINNOILA, M., VIUKARI, M. and HIETALA, O. Effects of sodium valproate on tardive dyskinesia, *British Journal of Psychiatry* **129**, 114–119 (1976)

LOGA, S., CURRY, S. and LADER, M. Interactions of orphenadrine and phenobarbitone with chlorpromazine ; plasma concentrations and effects in man, *British Journal of Clinical Pharmacology* **2**, 197–208 (1975)

McCLELLAND, H. A., BLESSED, G., BHATE, S., ALI, N. and CLARKE, P. A. The abrupt withdrawal of antiparkinson drugs in schizophrenic patients, *British Journal of Psychiatry* **124**, 151–159 (1974)

MACKAY, A. V. P. and SHEPHERD, G. P. Pharmacotherapeutic trials in tardive dyskinesia, *British Journal of Psychiatry* **135**, 489–499 (1979)

McLELLAN, D. L., CHALMERS, R. J. and JOHNSON, R. W. A double-blind trial of tetrabenazine, thiopropazate and placebo in patients with chorea, *Lancet* **1**, 104–107 (1974)

MARKSTEIN, P., HERRING, P. L., BUEKI, H. R., ASPER, H. and RUCH, W. The effect of bromocriptine on rat striatal adenylate cyclase and rat brain monoamine metabolism, *Journal of Neurochemistry* **31**, 1163–1172 (1978)

MARSDEN, C. D. Combined treatment with selective decarboxylase inhibitors. In *The Clinical Uses of Levodopa* (Ed. G. STEIN), 107–126, Media Technical Publication (1976)

MARSDEN, C. D. 'On–off' phenomena in Parkinson's disease. In *Parkinson's Disease – Current Progress, Problems and Management* (Eds. U. K. RINNE, M. KLINGER and G. STAM), 241–254, Elsevier-North Holland Biomedical Press, Amsterdam (1980)

MARSDEN, C. D. and JENNER, P. The pathophysiology of extrapyramidal side-effects of neuroleptic drugs, *Psychological Medicine* **10**, 55–72 (1980)

MARSDEN, C. D. and JENNER, P. L-Dopa's mechanism of action in Parkinson's disease, *Trends in Neuroscience* **4**, 148–150 (1981)

MARSDEN, C. D. and PARKES, J. D. 'On–off' effects in patients with Parkinson's disease on chronic levodopa therapy, *Lancet* **1**, 292–296 (1976)

MARSDEN, C. D. and PARKES, J. D. Success and problems of long-term levodopa therapy in Parkinson's disease, *Lancet* **1**, 345–349 (1977)

MARSDEN, C. D., MINDHAM, R. H. S. and MACKAY, A. V. P. Extrapyramidal movement disorders produced by antipsychotic drugs, (In press) (1981)

MARSDEN, C. D., TARSY, D. and BALDESSARINI, R. J. Spontaneous and drug induced movement disorders in psychotic patients. In *Psychiatry Aspects of Neurologic Disease* (Eds. D. F. Benson and D. Blumer), 219–266, Grune & Stratton, New York (1975)

MARTRES, M. P., COSTENTIN, J., BAUDRY, M., MARCAIS, H., PROTAIS, P. and SCHWARTZ, J. C. Long-term changes in the sensitivity of pre-and post-synaptic dopamine receptors in mouse striatum evidence by behavioural and biochemical studies, *Brain Research* **136**, 319–337 (1977)

MAWDSLEY, C., WILLIAMS, I. R., PULLAR, I. A., DAVIDSON, D. L. and KINLOCH, N. E. Treatment of parkinsonism by amatadine and levodopa, *Clinical Pharmacology & Therapeutics* **13**, 575–583 (1972)

MELDRUM, B. S., ANLEZARK, G. M. and MARSDEN, C. D. Acute dystonia as an idiosyncratic response to neuroleptic drugs in baboons, *Brain* **100**, 313–326 (1977)

MEYER, H. H. Die Behandlung exogener Psychosen mit Phenothiazenderivaten, *L'Encephale* **45**, 524–527 (1956)

MILLER, E. M. Deanol in the treatment of levodopa-induced dyskinesias, *Neurology* **24**, 116–119 (1974)

MILLER, E. M. Deanol: a solution for tardive dyskinesia, *New England Journal of Medicine* **91**, 796–797 (1974)

MILLER, R. and HILEY, R. Antimuscarinic properties of neuroleptics and drug-induced parkinsonism. *Nature* **248**, 596–597 (1974)

MILLINGTON, W. R., McCALL, A. L. and WURTMAN, R. J. Deanol acetamidobenzoate inhibits the blood-brain barrier transport of choline, *Annals of Neurology* **4**, 302–306 (1978)

MINDHAM, R. H. S. Assessment of drug-induced extrapyramidal reactions and of drugs given for their control, *British Journal of Clinical Pharmacology* **3**, 395–400 (1976)

MINDHAM, R. H. S., GAIND, R., ANSTEE, B. H. and RIMMER, L. Comparison of amantadine, orphenadrine and placebo in the control of phenothiazine-induced parkinsonism, *Psychological Medicine* **2**, 406–413 (1972)

MINDHAM, R. H. S., LAMB, P. and BRADLEY, R. A comparison of piribedil, procyclidine and placebo in the control of phenothiazine-induced parkinsonism, *British Journal of Psychiatry* **130**, 581–585 (1977)

MOLLER-NIELSEN, I. and CHRISTENSEN, A. V. Long-term effects of neuroleptic drugs, *Journal of Pharmacology (Paris)* **6**, 277–282 (1975)

MONES, R. J. Experimental dyskinesia in normal rhesus monkeys. In *Advances in Neurology* (Eds. A. BARBEAU, T. N. CHASE and G. W. PAULSON), **1**, 665–670, Raven Press, New York (1973)

NATIONAL INSTITUTE OF MENTAL HEALTH. Phenothiazine treatment in acute schizophrenia: effectiveness, *Archives of General Psychiatry* **10**, 246–261 (1964)

O'FLANAGAN, P. M. Clonazepam in the treatment of drug-induced dyskinesia, *British Medical Journal* **1**, 269 (1975)

OGURA, C., KISHIMOTO, A. and HAKAO, T. Clinical effect of L-dopa on schizophrenia, *Current Therapeutic Research* **20**, 308–318 (1976)

O'KEEFE, R., SHARMAN, D. F. and VOGT, M. Effect of drugs used in psychoses on cerebral dopamine metabolism, *British Journal of Pharmacology* **38**, 287–304 (1970)

ORLOV, P., KASPORIAN, G., DIMASCIO, A. and COLE, N. O. Withdrawal of antiparkinson drugs, *Archives of General Psychiatry* **25**, 410–412 (1971)

PACIFICI, G. M., NARDINI, M., FERRARI, P., LATINI, R., FIESCHI, C. and MORSELLI, P. L. Effect of amantadine on drug-induced Parkinsonism: relationship between plasma levels and effect, *British Journal of Clinical Pharmacology* **3**, 883–889 (1976)

PAKKENBERG, H. The effect of tetrabenazine in some hyperkinetic syndromes, *Acta Neurologica Scandinavica* **44**, 391–393 (1968)

PAKKENBERG, H. and FOG, R. Spontaneous oral dyskinesia: results of tetrabenazine, pimozide, or both, *Archives of Neurology* **31**, 352–353 (1974)

PARKES, J. D. Bromocriptine, *Advances in Drug Research* **12**, 247–344 (1978)

PARKES, J. D., BEDARD, P. and MARSDEN, C. D. Chorea and torsion in parkinsonism, *Lancet* **2**, 155 (1976)

PARKES, J. D., DEBONO, A. G. and MARSDEN, C. D. Bromocriptine in Parkinsonism: long-term treatment, dose response and comparison with levodopa, *Journal of Neurology, Neurosurgery and Psychiatry* **39**, 1101–1108 (1976)

PARKES, J. D., MARSDEN, C. D., DONALDSON, I., GALEA-DEBONO, A., WALTERS, J., KENNEDY, G. and ASSELMAN, P. Bromocriptine treatment in Parkinson's disease, *Journal of Neurology, Neurosurgery and Psychiatry* **39**, 184–193 (1976)

PARKES, J. D., ZILKHA, K. J., CALVER, D. M. and KNILL-JONES, R. P. Controlled trial of amantadine hydrochloride in Parkinson's disease, *Lancet* **1**, 259–262 (1970)

PAULSON, G. W. Dyskinesia in monkeys. In *Advances in Neurology* (Eds. A. BARBEAU, T. N. CHASE and G. W. PAULSON), **1**, 647–650, Raven Press, New York (1973)

PEIRIS, J. B., BORALESSA, H. and LIONEL, N. D. Clonazepam in the treatment of choreiform activity, *Medical Journal of Australia* **1**, 225–227 (1976)

PEREZ, L. M. Treatment of extrapyramidal symptoms, *New England Journal of Medicine* **264**, 1269 (1961)

PERRY, E. K., PERRY, R. H. and TOMLINSON, B. E. Dietary lecithin supplement in dementia of Alzheimer type, *Lancet* **2**, 242–243 (1977)

PRICE, P., PARKES, J. D. and MARSDEN, C. D. Tiapride in Parkinson's disease, *Lancet* **2**, 1106 (1978)

QUINN, Z. P., SHORE, P. A. and BRODIE, B. E. Studies of Ro 1–9569 (tetrabenazine), a non-indole tranquillizing agent with reserpine-like effects, *Journal of Pharmacology and Experimental Therapeutics* **127**, 103–109 (1959)

REAVILL, C., JENNER, P. and MARSDEN, C. D. Metabolite involvement in bromocriptine-induced circling behaviour in rodents, *Journal of Pharmacy and Pharmacology* **32**, 278–284 (1980)

REAVILL, C., JENNER, P. and MARSDEN, C. D. Pharmacological and biochemical aspects of the mechanisms of action of bromocriptine, *Research and Clinical Forum* **3**, 7–17 (1981)

REIDERER, P., YOUDIM, M. B. H., BIRKMEYER, W. and JELLINGER, K. Monoamine oxidase activity during (−)–deprenyl therapy: human post-mortem studies. In *Advances in Biochemical Psychopharmacology* (Eds. P. J. ROBERTS, G. N. WOODRUFF and L. L. IVERSEN), **19**, 377–382, Raven Press, New York (1978)

REYNOLDS, G. P., ELSWORTH, J. D., BLAU, K., SANDLER, M., LEES, A. J. and STERN, G. M. Deprenyl is metabolised to methamphetamine and amphetamine in man, *British Journal of Clinical Pharmacology* **6**, 542–544 (1978)

RIVERA-CALIMLIM, L., NARALLAH, H., STRAUSS, J. and LASAGNA, L. Clinical response and plasma levels: effect of dose, dosage schedules, and drug interactions on plasma chlorpromazine levels, *American Journal of Psychiatry* **133**, 646–652 (1976)

ROSSOR, M. N., WATKINS, J., BROWN, M. J., REID, J. L. and DOLBERG, C. T. Plasma levodopa, dopamine and therapeutic response following levodopa therapy of parkinsonian patients, *Journal of Neurological Sciences* **46**, 385–392 (1980)

St JEAN, A., DONALD, M. and BANN, T. A. Interchangeability of antiparkinson medication, *American Journal of Psychiatry* **120**, 1189–1190 (1964)

SAKALIS, G., CURRY, S. H., MOULD, G. P. and LADER, M. H. Physiological and clinical effects of chlorpromazine and their relationship to plasma level, *Clinical Pharmacology and Therapeutics* **13**, 931–946 (1972)

SALZMAN, N. P. and BRODIE, B. B. Physiological disposition and fate of chlorpromazine and a method for its estimation in biological materials, *Journal of Pharmacology and Experimental Therapeutics* **118**, 46–54 (1956)

SANDLER, M., GLOVER, V., ASHFORD, A. and STERN, G. M. Absence of 'cheese effect' during deprenyl therapy: some recent studies, *Journal of Neural Transmission* **43**, 209–215 (1978)

SARWER-FONER, G. J. Recognition and management of drug-induced extrapyramidal reactions and 'paradoxical' behavioural reactions in psychiatry, *Canadian Medical Association Journal* **83**, 312–318 (1960)

SASSIN, J. F. Drug-induced dyskinesia in monkeys. In *Advances in Neurology* (Eds. B. S. MELDRUM and C. D. MARSDEN), **10**, 47–54, Raven Press, New York (1975)

SCATTON, B. Differential regional development of tolerance to increase in dopamine turnover upon repeated neuroleptic administration, *European Journal of Pharmacology* **46**, 363–369 (1977)

SCATTON, B., CHERAMY, A., BESSON, M. J. and GLOWINSKI, J. Increased synthesis and release of dopamine in the striatum of the rat after amantadine treatment. *European Journal of Pharmacology* **13**, 131–133 (1970)

SCHACHTER, M., MARSDEN, C. D., PARKES, J. D., JENNER, P. and TESTA, B. Deprenyl in the management of response fluctuations in patients with Parkinson's disease on levodopa, *Journal of Neurology, Neurosurgery and Psychiatry* **43**, 1016–1021 (1980)

SCHELKUNOV, E. L. Adrenergic effect of chronic administration of neuroleptics, *Nature* **214**, 1210–1212 (1967)

SCHWAB, R. S. and ENGLAND, A. C. Parkinson syndromes due to various causes. In *Handbook of Clinical Neurology*, Diseases of the Basal Ganglia (Eds. P. J. VINKEN and G. W. BRUYN), **6**, 227–247, North Holland, Amsterdam (1968)

SCHWAB, R. S., ENGLAND, A. C., POSKANZER, D. and YOUNG, R. R. Amantadine in the treatment of Parkinson's disease, *Journal of the American Medical Association* **208**, 1168–1170 (1969)

SCHWAB, R. S., POSKANZER, D. C., ENGLAND A. C. and YOUNG, R. R. Amantadine in Parkinson's disease. Review of more than two years' experience, *Journal of the American Medical Association* **222**, 792–795 (1972)

SETHY, V. M. and VAN WOERT, M. H. Modification of striatal acetylcholine concentration by dopamine receptor agonists and antagonists, *Research Communication in Chemical Pathology and Pharmacology* **8**, 13–28 (1974)

SHEPPARD, C. and MERLIS, S. Drug-induced extrapyramidal symptoms: Their incidence and treatment, *American Journal of Psychiatry* **123**, 886–889 (1967)

SIGWALD, J., BOUTIER, D., RAYMONDEAUD, C. and PIOT, C. Quatre cas de dyskinesia facio-bucco-linguo-masticatrice a evolution prolongee secondaire a un traitment pars les neuroleptiques, *Revue Neurologie* **100**, 751–755 (1959)

SILBERGELD, E. K., ALDER, H., KENNEDY, S. and CALNE, D. B. The roles of pre-synaptic function and hepatic drug metabolism in the hypothermic action of two novel dopaminergic agonists, *Journal of Pharmacy and Pharmacology* **29**, 632–635 (1977)

SIMPSON, G. M. Controlled studies of antiparkinson agents in the treatment of drug-induced extrapyramidal symptoms, *Acta Psychiatrica Scandinavica*, Suppl. **212**, 44–51 (1970)

SIMPSON, G. M. and LASKA, E. Sensitivity to a phenothiazine (butaperazine), *Canadian Psychiatric Association Journal* **13**, 499–506 (1968)

SIMPSON, G. M., BOITASHEVSKY, A., YOUNG, M. A. and LEE, H. J. Deanol in the treatment of tardive dyskinesia, *Psychopharmacology* **52**, 257–261 (1977)

SIMPSON, L. L. Evidence that deprenyl, a type B monoamine oxidase inhibitor, is an indirectly acting sympathomimetic amine, *Biochemical Pharmacology* **27**, 1591–1595 (1978)

SINGER, K. and CHENG, M. Thioipropazate hydrochloride in persistent dyskinesia, *British Medical Journal* **4**, 22–25 (1971)

SINGH, M. M. and SMITH J. M. Reversal of some therapeutic effects of an antipsychotic agent by an antiparkinsonism agent, *Journal of Nervous and Mental Disease* **157**, 50–58 (1973)

SINGH, M. M. and KAY, S. R. A comparative study of haloperidol and chlorpromazine in terms of clinical effect and therapeutic reversal with benztropine in schizophrenia. Theoretical implications for potency differences among neuroleptics, *Psychopharmacologia (Berlin)* **43**, 103–113 (1975a)

SINGH, M. M. and KAY, S. R. A longitudinal therapeutic comparison between two prototypic neuroleptics (haloperidol and chlorpromazine) in matched groups of schizophrenics. Non-therapeutic interactions with trihexyphenidyl. Theoretical implications for potency differences, *Psychopharmacologia (Berlin)* **43**, 115–123 (1975b)

SITARAM, N., WEINGARTNER, H. and GILLIN J. C. Human serial learning: enhancement with arecoline and choline and impairment with scopolamine, *Science* **201**, 274–276 (1978)

SKIRBOLL, L. R. and BUNNEY, B. S. Effects of chronic haloperidol treatment of spontaneous activity in the caudate nucleus. In *Catecholamines: Basic and Clinical Frontiers* (Eds. E. USDIN, I. J. KOPIN and J. BARCHAS), 634–636, Pergamon Press, New York (1979)

SMITH, R., TAMMINGA, C., HARASZJI, J., PANDEY, G. and DAVIS, J. Effects of dopamine agonists in tardive dyskinesia, *American Journal of Psychiatry* **134**, 765–768 (1977)

STADLER, H., LLOYD, K. G., GADEA-CIRIA, M. and BARTHOLINI, G. Enhanced striatal acetylcholine release by chlorpromazine and its reversal by apomorphine, *Brain Research* **55**, 476–480 (1973)

STECK, H. Le syndrome extrapyramidal et diencephlique au cours des traitements au Largactil et au Serpasil, *Annales Medico-Psychologiques* **112**, 737–743 (1954)

STONE, T. W. Responses of neurons in the cerebral cortex and caudate nucleus to amantadine, amphetamine and dopamine, *British Journal of Pharmacology* **56**, 101–110 (1976)

SWASH, M., ROBERTS, A. K., ZAKKS, H. and HEATHFIELD, K. W. G. Treatment of involuntary movement disorders with tetrabenazine, *Journal of Neurology, Neurosurgery and Psychiatry* **35**, 186–191 (1972)

TAMMINGA, C. A. and CHASE, T. N. Bromocriptine and CF 25–397 in the treatment of tardive dyskinesia, *Archives of Neurology* **37**, 204–205 (1981)

TAMMINGA, C. S., SMITH, R. C., ERICKSON, S. E., CHANG, S. and DAVIS, J. M. Cholinergic influences in tardive dyskinesia, *American Journal of Psychiatry* **134**, 769–774 (1977)

TARSY, D. and BALDESSARINI, R. J. Pharmacologically-induced behavioural supersensitivity to apomorphine, *Nature* **245**, 262–263 (1973)

TARSY, D. and BALDESSARINI, R. J. Behavioural supersensitivity to apomorphine following chronic treatment with drugs which interfere with the synaptic function of catecholamines, *Neuropharmacology* **13**, 927–940 (1974)

TARSY, D. and BALDESSARINI, R. J. The tardive dyskinesia syndrome. In *Clinical Neuropharmacology* (Ed. H. L. KLAWANS), **1**, 29–61, Raven Press, New York (1976)

TARSY, D. and BRALOWER, M. Deanol acetamidobenzoate treatment in choreiform movement disorders, *Archives of Neurology* **34**, 756–758 (1977)

TARSY, D., LEOPOLD, N. and SAX, D. Physostigmine in choreiform movement disorder, *Neurology* **24**, 28–33 (1974)

TASSIN, J. P., STINUS, L., SIMON, M., BLANC, G., THIERRY, A. M., LE MOAL, M., CARDO, B. and GLOWINSKI, J. Relationship between the locomotor hyperactivity induced by A10 lesions and the destruction of the fronto-cortical dopaminergic innervation in the rat, *Brain Research* **141**, 267–281 (1978)

TOGLIA, J. U., McGLAMERY, M. and SAMBANDHAM, R. R. Tetrabenazine in the treatment of Huntington's chorea and other hyperkinetic movement disorders, *Journal of Clinical Psychiatry* **39**, 81–87 (1978)

TOLOSA, E. Paradoxical suppression of chorea by apomorphine, *Journal of the American Medical Association* **229**, 1579–1580 (1974)

TOLOSA, E. S. Modification of tardive dyskinesia and spasmodic torticollis by apomorphine, *Archives of Neurology* **35**, 459–462 (1978)

TRABUCCHI, M., CHENEY, D., RACAGNI, G. and COSTA, E. Involvement of brain cholinergic mechanisms in the action of chlorpromazine, *Nature* **249**, 664–666 (1974)

TRENDELENBURG, U. Supersensitivity and subsensitivity to sympathomimetic amines, *Pharmacological Reviews* **15**, 225–276 (1963a)

TRENDELENBURG, U. Time course of changes in sensitivity after denervation of the nictitating membrane of the spinal cat. *Journal of Pharmacology* **142**, 335–342 (1963b)

TUREK, I., KURLAND, A., HANLON, T. and BOHM, M. Tardive dyskinesia: its relation to neuroleptic and antiparkinson drugs, *British Journal of Psychiatry* **121**, 605–612 (1972)

UHRBRAND, L. and FAURBYE, A. Reversible and irreversible dyskinesia after treatment with perphenazine chlorpromazine, reserpine and electroconvulsive therapy, *Psychopharmalogia (Berlin)* **1**, 408–419 (1960)

ULUS, I. H. and WURTMAN, R. J. Choline administration: activation of tyrosine hydroxylase in dopaminergic neurons of rat brain, *Science* **194**, 1060–1061 (1976)

VAN ROSSUM, J. M. Significance of dopamine-receptor blockade for mechanism of action of neuroleptic drugs, *Archives Internationales de Pharmacodynamie et de Therapie* **160**, 492–494 (1966)

VASAVAN-NAIR, N. P., YASSA, R., RUIS-NAVARRO, J. and SCHWARTZ, G. Baclofen in the treatment of tardive dyskinesia, *American Journal of Psychiatry* **135**, 1562–1563 (1978)

WALKER, J. E., HOEHN, M. and SEARS, E. Dimethylaminoethanol in Huntington's chorea, *Lancet* **1**, 1512–1513 (1973)

WEISS, B., SANTELLI, S. and LUSINK, G. Movement disorders induced in monkeys by chronic haloperidol treatment, *Psychopharmacology* **53**, 289–293 (1977)

WURTMAN, J. J. Sources of choline and lecithin in the diet. In *Nutrition and the Brain* (Eds. A. BARBEAU, J. H. GROWDON and R. J. WURTMAN), **5**, 73–81, Raven Press, New York (1979)

WURTMAN, R. J., HIRSCH, M. J. and GROWDON, J. H. Lecithin consumption elevates serum free choline levels, *Lancet* **2**, 68–69 (1977)

YARYURA-TOBIAS, J. A., WOLPERT, A., DANA, L. and MERLIS, J. Action of L-dopa in drug-induced extrapyramidalism, *Diseases of the Nervous System* **31**, 60–61 (1970)

ZAHNISER, N. R., CHOU, D. and HANIN, I. Is 2-dimethylaminoethanol (deanol) indeed a precursor of brain acetylcholine? A gas chromotographic evaluation, *Journal of Pharmacology and Experimental Therapeutics* **200**, 545–559 (1977)

Chapter 6

Antianxiety drugs

P. J. Tyrer

The drugs described in this chapter are those that are primarily prescribed in psychiatry for the relief of anxiety and induction of sleep. The list of drugs with anxiety relieving properties is a long one and some drugs with proven antianxiety effects have had to be omitted. These include the monoamine oxidase inhibitors, neuroleptics, tricyclic and tricyclic-like antidepressants, which are dealt with in separate chapters. The nomenclature of antianxiety drugs is a confusing one, much of which has been generated by the indiscriminate use of the word 'tranquillizer'. Anxiety is a mood state with unpleasant symptoms which can be clearly separated into somatic and psychological components (Hamilton, 1959; Tyrer, 1979). Relief of anxiety can be achieved by suppression or attenuation of the symptoms and need not necessarily be accompanied by sedation or tranquillization, features which only concern the psychological aspects of anxiety. The ideal antianxiety drug would suppress or remove the symptoms of anxiety entirely without producing any effects on higher cortical function so sedation would not be shown. Some antianxiety drugs, although far from ideal in their anxiety-relieving effects, have no effects on cortical function and never produce sedation. For this reason the words 'sedative' and 'tranquillizer' will be mentioned infrequently and then only for comparative purposes. In this chapter the drugs are described according to the classification given in Chapter 1 (*Table 1.2*):

(1) general central anxiolytics,
(2) specific central anxiolytics, and
(3) peripheral anxiolytic drugs.

Generalized central anxiolytics (sedative drugs)

These drugs reduce anxiety by generalized depression of cortical and subcortical neurons and are therefore non-specific in their antianxiety effects. Because they are non-specific they also depress the activity of the major regulatory centres in the brainstem, particularly the vasomotor and cardiorespiratory centres. This makes the drugs dangerous in overdosage and when taken with other central depressant compounds. Many of the drugs also carry the major disadvantage of tolerance and habituation in chronic dosage. True pharmacological dependence is a common problem in such cases and serious withdrawal syndromes follow cessation of treatment. Most of these drugs belong to the nineteenth century when they were the

126

TABLE 6.1 Classification of antianxiety drugs

Classification	Group	Date of introduction to medicine	Current use in psychiatry
Generalized central anxiolytics	Alcohol	Not known	Very little
	Barbiturates	1862	Very little
	Paraldehyde	1882	Very little
Specific central anxiolytics	Propanediols	1955	Occasional
	Benzodiazepines	1959	Very great
Peripheral anxiolytics	Beta-adrenoceptor blocking drugs	1959	Occasional

only antianxiety drugs available (*Table 6.1*). Their major disadvantages have led to most of them being superseded by newer, safer and more effective agents and many of the drugs are only mentioned for historical reasons.

Alcohol

The use of alcohol as an antianxiety agent is discussed in more detail in Chapter 13. Although for practical reasons alcohol may be considered with the barbiturates, as it has similar effects and carries similar risks, it is sometimes still recommended for treatment of anxiety. Because of the obvious danger of symptomatic drinking foreshadowing alcohol addiction it is very difficult to recommend alcohol for this purpose under any circumstances. The best case has been made out in psychogeriatrics. Alcohol in the form of beer and wine is more socially acceptable than other drugs with this population and there are some reports that it reduces anxiety and agitated behaviour without much risk of dependence (Chien, Stotsky and Cole, 1973; Mishara and Kastenbaum, 1974). These reports refer to treatment of elderly people in institutions where control of treatment can be carefully monitored. It is only in such situations that alcohol should ever be considered as therapy.

Barbiturates

INTRODUCTION

All barbiturates are derivatives of barbituric acid, a relatively simple drug first synthesized by von Bayer in 1862. All barbiturates possess the basic barbituric acid nucleus and most of their structural differences are relatively minor (*Figure 6.1*).

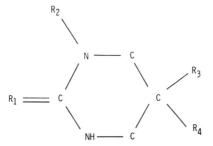

Figure 6.1 Basic structure of barbiturates

Barbiturates are among the oldest psychiatric drugs and the first member of the series, barbitone (Veronal) was introduced to medicine in 1903. From then until the mid 1960s they were the most popular antianxiety drugs and hypnotics used in psychiatry. Because they have been superseded by more selective compounds they are now mainly of historical interest and only mentioned briefly in this review.

PHARMACOLOGY

The barbiturates are general depressants of all living tissues but the central nervous system is especially sensitive. The mechanism of action is almost certainly related to the ability of barbiturates to facilitate γ-aminobutyric acid (GABA) transmission (Barker and Ransom, 1978). GABA is an inhibitory neurotransmitter that is widely distributed throughout the brain and it is predictable that facilitation of its transmission will lead to reduced anxiety and arousal. Because barbiturates do not bind to benzodiazepine receptors the specific antianxiety effects of GABA–benzodiazepine receptor stimulation are lacking (Braestrup and Nielsen, 1980). Thus barbiturates also depress activity in other parts of the central nervous system, and this becomes dangerous when it affects the cardiorespiratory and vasomotor centres. At high dosage, cardiac output falls, respiratory drive becomes sluggish and less responsive to hypoxia and hypercapnia. Soon death from cardiorespiratory failure follows. The toxic doses of barbiturates are not much higher than therapeutic ones, which makes them so dangerous in overdosage.

PHARMACOKINETICS

Barbiturates are readily absorbed after oral administration and rapidly cross the blood–brain barrier. The biological half-lives of barbiturates vary considerably and this fact has led to their separation into short-, medium- and long-acting groups (*Table 6.2*). The most short-acting (e.g. methohexitone sodium) have biological half-lives of less than an hour, and because of their rapid onset and short duration of action are mainly used as intravenous anaesthetics. The long-acting barbiturates (e.g. phenobarbitone) have half-lives of 72 h or more. The intermediate or medium-acting group of barbiturates have half-lives ranging from 5 to 60 h.

The liver is the main organ involved in the metabolism of barbiturates. Barbiturates

TABLE 6.2 Classification of barbiturates

Class	Approved name	Trade name	Dosage (mg)	Comments
Short-acting	Methohexitone sodium	Brietal	50–120 IV	Used for induction of anaesthesia
	Thiopentone sodium	Intraval		
Medium acting (intermediate)	Pentobarbitone sodium	Nembutal	100–200	Little clinical difference
	Quinalbarbitone	Seconal	50–200	between these
	Amylobarbitone	Amytal	30–200	compounds
Long-acting	Phenobarbitone	Luminal	90–300	Usually used as anticonvulsants but in lower dosage have mild sedative action
	Methylphenobarbitone	Prominal	100–600	
	Primidone	Mysoline	125–1000	

stimulate the activity of the liver microsomal enzymes concerned with their meta-bolism. This phenomenon, which appears to represent an increase in the concentration of enzyme protein, is called 'enzyme induction' (Conney, 1967). This is important for two reasons. It leads to the development of tolerance in that a greater drug dose is required to produce the same plasma level (and clinical effect) and it also leads to important drug interactions. Other drugs which do not themselves stimulate their own metabolism but use the same microsomal enzymes, have their metabolism stimulated by barbiturates so that tolerance develops and an increase in the dosage of the second drug is required to produce the same pharmacodynamic effect.

CLINICAL USE

Acute therapy
There is no indication for acute therapy with barbiturates for the treatment of anxiety. Safer and more effective drugs are available and widely used. Barbiturates are less expensive than most of the alternatives but this factor alone cannot justify their use. Prescription of barbiturates as hypnotics can be justified for very short periods only, rarely longer than a week. These strictures apply to the medium-acting group of barbiturates which are mainly used for psychiatric disorders. Short-acting barbiturates have an important place in anaesthesia and also may be used for abreactive purposes (narcoanalysis) in somewhat lower dosages. Care must be taken even with these drugs as frequent use can lead to tolerance and dependence. Long-acting barbiturates such as phenobarbitone and primidone have an important place in the treatment of epilepsy and, possibly because of their long half-lives, rarely lead to abuse or dependence.

Maintenance therapy
A certain number of individuals who were prescribed barbiturates regularly, usually as a hypnotic, before there were more effective drugs available, have continued to take the barbiturate without increasing the dose. There are no figures available of the proportion that such patients make to the total of barbiturate prescriptions but there is evidence that much barbiturate prescription is long term (Tyrer, 1978). Although it is difficult to justify this continued prescription of barbiturates many doctors defend it by pointing out that such patients have taken the same dose for many years, are in no danger of addiction and have failed to respond to other forms of treatment. Nevertheless, wherever possible it is advisable to replace the barbiturate with another drug or to phase out treatment altogether. If maintenance therapy is chosen it is important to keep a check on the prescriptions to make certain that the dosage is not gradually increased. This procedure can only be permitted for hypnotics at night; regular day time use of barbiturates is almost certainly going to lead to tolerance and dependence and cannot be justified under any circumstances.

Several methods of weaning patients off barbiturates have been prescribed. Smith and Wesson (1970) suggested replacing the medium-acting barbiturate with the long-acting barbiturate, phenobarbitone, which carries virtually no risk of dependence. They suggest that for each 400 mg of the medium-acting barbiturate 30 mg of phenobarbitone should be prescribed and the change made over several weeks. The barbiturate may also be replaced gradually with a benzodiazepine such as diazepam in a step-wise manner (*Drug and Therapeutics Bulletin*, 1976). Each 100 mg of barbiturate is replaced by 5 mg of diazepam and the rate of substitution can be as little as one dose per week. The changeover takes between 6 and 12 weeks to complete and because it is so gradual withdrawal symptoms are avoided.

ADVERSE EFFECTS

Acute unwanted effects
The margin between therapeutic effects and toxicity with barbiturates is small. Because of this they are dangerous in overdosage, and particularly when taken with alcohol. Cardiorespiratory collapse is the commonest cause of death following overdosage. Severe respiratory depression through the effects of the barbiturates on the respiratory centre is the main cause of this collapse and reduced cardiac output and cardiac arrhythmias occur as secondary phenomena (Shubin and Weil, 1971). Skin eruptions are common with barbiturates (Almeyda and Levantine, 1972) and bullous lesions are more frequent than with other drugs. Confusion is a common problem with barbiturates in the elderly; another reason for avoiding their use. Falls during confusional episodes may lead to serious sequelae such as fractures and dislocations (McDonald and McDonald, 1977). When barbiturates are used as hypnotics they may be effective in inducing sleep but on waking they produce unpleasant hangover effects. Hangover is an appropriate word as the symptoms—muzziness, headache, difficulty in concentration and a general feeling of discontent (Haider, 1968)—are very like those produced by alcohol, a similar central depressant drug.

Teratogenesis
Although there is little evidence that specific malformations occur in infants born of mothers taking barbiturates there is a higher than expected incidence of malformation in babies born of mothers who ingest barbiturate drugs (Greenberg *et al.*, 1977). Quite apart from other considerations it is wise not to prescribe barbiturates during the first trimester of pregnancy.

Long-term adverse effects
The major adverse effect of long-term prescription of barbiturates is drug dependence. This is a true pharmacological dependence and is described in more detail in Chapter 12. The withdrawal syndrome includes restlessness and confusion, with somatic symptoms such as shaking, nausea and stomach cramps, together with a high incidence of epileptic seizures (Isbell *et al.*, 1950). Patients dependent on barbiturates should not be withdrawn abruptly without other pharmacological cover.

DRUG INTERACTIONS

Many drug interactions occur between barbiturates and other compounds. Several of these are due to enzyme induction, discussed earlier. In all these instances the barbiturate induces its own metabolism and also that of other drugs. The dosage of the other drugs has to be increased to produce the effect that was achieved before prescription of the barbiturate. Initially by increasing the dose equilibrium is again attained but if the barbiturate drug is suddenly withdrawn the enzyme induction stops and the effects of unnecessarily high dosage of the other drug become apparent. The main drugs which interact with barbiturates in this way are:

(1) coumarin anticoagulants (e.g. warfarin),
(2) chlorpromazine,
(3) chloramphenicol,
(4) phenytoin,
(5) griseofulvin,
(6) androgens, oestrogens and corticosteroids.

The most dramatic effects of this interaction are found with the anticoagulants when barbiturates are withdrawn. The higher dose of anticoagulant needed to overcome the enzyme induction is no longer compensated and greater anticoagulant activity is shown, so there is a risk of haemorrhage (Breckenridge and Orme, 1971). Barbiturates reduce the antibiotic effect of chloramphenicol and griseofulvin and thereby may cause undertreatment of the bacterial and fungal infections for which those drugs are prescribed. Interaction with steroids is usually only significant when exogenous steroids are being prescribed for an appropriate physical condition (e.g. lupus erythematosus). The interaction with chlorpromazine and other phenothiazines is often difficult to interpret as chlorpromazine also induces the metabolism of barbiturates (Conney, 1967), so it is almost impossible to predict the effects of the combination. In all other cases the effect of the other drugs can usually be restored to their former level by increasing the dosage but this is not always predictable, particularly after chronic therapy. It is preferable not to prescribe barbiturates with any of these other drugs with the exception of phenytoin in the treatment of epilepsy, and when phenytoin is prescribed with a barbiturate as an anticonvulsant a check on serum levels is a wise precaution when the dose of barbiturate is altered.

Barbiturates may also precipitate attacks of acute intermittent porphyria. In former days when barbiturates were prescribed in hospital regularly as hypnotics it was sometimes the cause of diagnostic puzzlement to find patients admitted for minor conditions developing acute abdominal pain and bizarre neurological symptoms. In many instances they were described as 'hysterical' before the diagnosis of acute intermittent porphyria was eventually made.

COMPARISON WITH OTHER FORMS OF TREATMENT

There is abundant evidence that barbiturates are less safe and less easily tolerated than other antianxiety drugs and are much more likely to lead to drug dependence. Of all the generalized central depressant drugs used for treating anxiety barbiturates appear to be the most prone to dependence. These factors alone would make their prescription ill advised but there is still a strong feeling among physicians that they are more potent than the benzodiazepines and other antianxiety drugs and therefore may be used in 'resistant cases'. This view is mistaken as there is good evidence that barbiturates are less effective than benzodiazepines in the treatment of anxiety even when a flexible dosage regimen allows patients to chose their own levels of treatment (Lader, Bond and James, 1974). There is no doubt that barbiturates are effective hypnotics but the severity and duration of hangover effects are greater than with the benzodiazepines (Haider, 1968; Bond and Lader, 1973). Barbiturates suppress rapid eye movement (REM) sleep and there is a 'rebound' phenomenon after the drugs are stopped during which there is an increase in the proportion of REM sleep. This lasts for several weeks after withdrawal (Oswald and Priest, 1965). Its clinical significance is not fully clear but may explain the excessive dreaming that often follows withdrawal, which can be unpleasant if experienced as nightmares.

COMBINATIONS OF BARBITURATES AND OTHER THERAPY

In the past several drugs have been marketed which contain barbiturates in combination with other compounds, although it is gratifying that the number is steadily falling. The most well known of these the now obsolete barbiturate–amphetamine mixture (Drinamyl). This combination has both stimulant and sedative properties and was formerly used for treating reactive (neurotic) depression. Although they were relatively effective treatments in the short term the rapid development of tolerance and addiction have made their continued prescription unacceptable. Because of the risks of overdosage barbiturates have sometimes been combined with emetic drugs (e.g. amylobarbitone and emetine, Amylomet). In normal dosage the combination does not lead to vomiting and may be taken with impunity, but after overdose the drugs are vomited before absorption into the body. This combination has not proved popular in clinical practice. Barbiturates are also marketed in combination with analgesics (e.g. butobarbitone, codeine phosphate and paracetamol, Sonalgin; aspirin and butobarbitone, Tercin), with antihistamines (butobarbitone and promethazine, Sönergan) and with belladonna alkaloids (belladonna, ergotamine and phenobarbitone, Bellergal). These combination drugs confer no special advantages over their parent compounds and the chief danger is that doctors may prescribe them without knowing they are barbiturates.

No comparisons have been made between the effectiveness of different drugs for abreactive purposes and it is difficult to know whether barbiturates are superior in any way to other agents. Their occasional use for this purpose can nonetheless be justified.

Barbiturate-like drugs

There are several drugs which, although not barbiturates, are so similar in their clinical and pharmacological effects that they can be considered with them. Glutethimide (Doriden) and methaqualone (Revonal) (also marketed as Mandrax in combination with the antihistamine diphenhydramine) are not barbiturates but the implication that they are safer is untrue. They have similar effects to barbiturates in overdosage and are particularly prone to tolerance and dependence. This has led to their becoming drugs of abuse. Both were originally marketed as hypnotics (glutethimide 250–500 mg at night; methaqualone 200–250 mg at night) but when dependence develops they are taken most frequently during the day. Tolerance develops through enzyme induction (Conney et al., 1960) and the hypnotic effect is reduced after only a few weeks of regular dosage (Kales et al., 1970a). Methyprylone (Noludar) is also marketed as a hypnotic in a dose of 200–400 mg at night. It is related to glutethimide but is not quite so prone to tolerance and dependence.

Chloral and its derivatives

These compounds are chemically similar to ethyl alcohol but although, like alcohol, they are generalized central depressant drugs, they are better for use in psychiatry. Paraldehyde and chloral hydrate have been in clinical use for over a century, and perhaps because they have been sitting so long at the tranquillizer table, their merits have been overlooked in favour of the flashy new arrivals.

STRUCTURE AND PHARMACOLOGY

Chloral hydrate and paraldehyde are simple aliphatic compounds (*Figure 6.2a* and *b*). Paraldehyde is a polymer of acetaldehyde and chloral hydrate a substituted alcohol. They depress neuronal function generally but have a wider safety margin than barbiturates. Paraldehyde is excreted through the lungs as well as the liver and can be

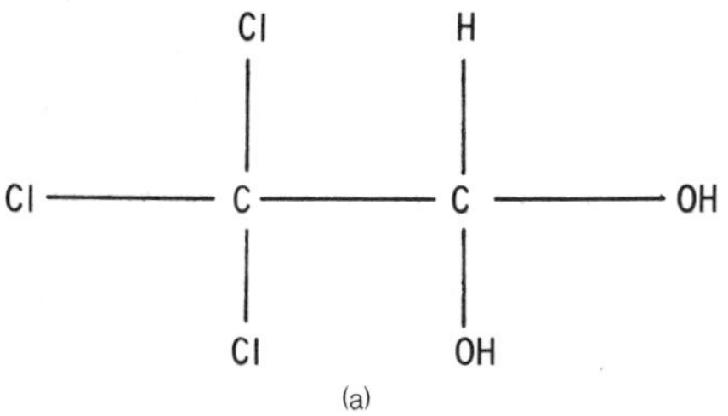

Figure 6.2a Chloral hydrate

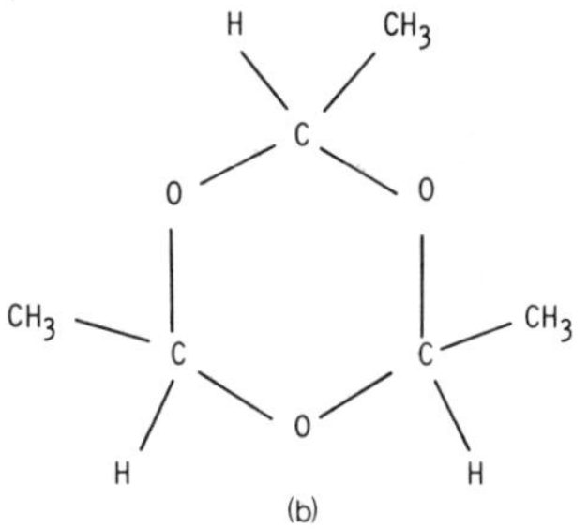

Figure 6.2b Paraldehyde

recognized by its characteristic smell in the expired air. Chloral hydrate may cause gastric irritation and also has a slightly unpleasant smell. When made up in appropriate compound elixirs this smell is counteracted.

CLINICAL USE

Both paraldehyde and chloral hydrate are effective hypnotics for short-term use. Paraldehyde in a dose of 2–5 g and chloral hydrate, 1–3 g at night, are adequate for induction of sleep and do not lead to pronounced hangover effects the next day. Both have the advantage that they can be given as suppositories as well as by mouth. They tend to be used more frequently among the elderly but there is no reason why they should not be used in younger age groups. They produce much less suppression of REM sleep than barbiturates and pharmacological dependence is also much less common. However, in chronic dosage the hypnotic effect of chloral hydrate is reduced (Kales *et al.*, 1970b) and the same is likely to be true of paraldehyde.

The unpleasant smell of chloral hydrate can be avoided by giving closely related drugs that have identical clinical effects. The two most commonly used are dichloralphenazone (Welldorm, 650–1950 mg at night, and triclofos (Tricloryl) 500–2000 mg at night. Both these compounds are also available as elixirs and may be given in lower dosage to children. Because these compounds have good safety margins they are also sometimes used in continuous narcosis therapy. None of these compounds should be given for the relief of anxiety and they are rarely indicated during the day. Paraldehyde in a dose of 2.5–10 g intramuscularly is sometimes given to control acute behaviour disturbance.

DRUG INTERACTIONS

Because these compounds are generalized central depressant drugs they have an additive effect with other central depressant drugs, including ethyl alcohol. Care should therefore be taken when they are prescribed together. Chloral hydrate may produce enzyme induction in the same way as barbiturates leading to increased warfarin metabolism (Cucinell *et al.*, 1966) but others have claimed that active blood warfarin levels can be increased as the trichloracetic acid metabolite of chloral displaces warfarin from plasma proteins (Sellers and Koch-Weser, 1970). Chloral should not be prescribed together with coumarin anticoagulants because of these possible interactions.

In appropriate dosage both paraldehyde and chloral hydrate are equivalent in efficacy to other hypnotic drugs but in chronic dosage are less effective than benzodiazepines such as flurazepam (Kales *et al.*, 1970a). Because of their wide safety margin and low risk dependence they are superior to barbiturates and barbiturate-like drugs. There is insufficient evidence to decide whether they are less likely to produce dependence than benzodiazepine hypnotics.

Specific central anxiolytics (ataractic drugs)

These drugs are more selective than the generalized central anxiolytics and act preferentially on the functional systems of the brain concerned with anxiety. In anatomical terms they have their major action on the limbic system, particularly the hypothalamus and associated structures, and their pharmacological effects are achieved through specific inhibition of the neurotransmitter systems concerned with generating anxiety. They reduce anxious behaviour and aggression and to varying degrees are anticonvulsant muscle relaxants. These pharmacological effects are achieved with little influence on cortical function. The benzodiazepines constitute the largest group of these compounds and their advantages over the generalized central anxiolytics are such that they have largely replaced the latter in the treatment of anxiety (*Table 6.1*). The propanediols constitute the important group.

Propanediols

For a short period between 1955 and 1960 the propanediols were the most widely used antianxiety drugs in the USA and to a lesser extent were popular in other countries. They represented the first of the selective antianxiety drugs but because their clinical effects are less specific than the benzodiazepines that followed them they have rapidly fallen in popularity.

STRUCTURE AND PHARMACOLOGY

Only two of the propanediols have achieved widespread use, meprobamate and tybamate. They are relatively simple aliphatic compounds (*Figure 6.3*), and were synthesized after modification to the structure of mephenesin, a muscle relaxant drug

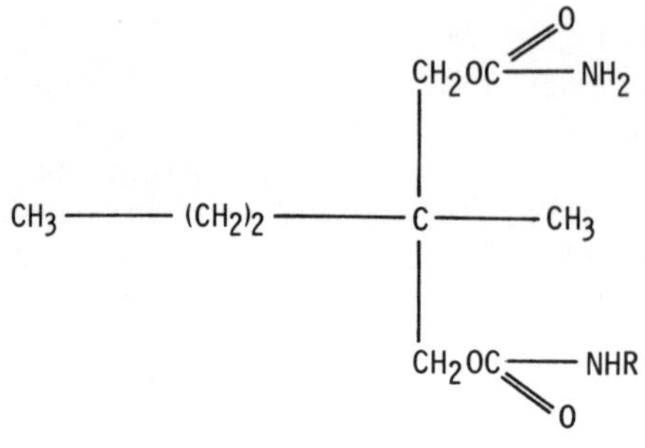

$$CH_3 \longrightarrow (CH_2)_2 \longrightarrow C \longrightarrow CH_3$$

with $CH_2OC \overset{O}{\underset{}{\diagup}} NH_2$ above and $CH_2OC \underset{O}{\diagdown} NHR$ below the central carbon.

Figure 6.3 Basic structure of propanediols

used for the relief of spasticity. Pharmacologically the propanediols have two main effects; they show relative specificity in acting on the thalamus and limbic system (Kletzkin and Berger, 1959) and have muscle relaxing effects on skeletal muscles (Berger, 1954). They also show some anticonvulsant activity but this has seldom been employed clinically.

Both meprobamate and tybamate are rapidly absorbed after oral administration and peak plasma concentrations are reached in about 1 h. Meprobamate has inactive metabolites and is rapidly excreted through the kidneys within 48 h. Tybamate is excreted more rapidly and has a plasma half-life of only 4 h (Shelton and Hollister, 1967).

CLINICAL USE

It is the unfortunate lot of the propanediols to be pale imitators of the benzodiazepines in almost all their pharmacological and clinical effects. Thus, whilst meprobamate in particular is known to be an effective antianxiety drug from clinical trials (Raymond et al., 1957; Rickels et al., 1959), the propanediols are generally inferior to benzodiazepines in the treatment of anxiety, insomnia, muscular disorders and epilepsy. However, in no clinical trials have benzodiazepines been markedly superior to propanediols and several studies have shown no clinical differences (Greenblatt and Shader, 1974, p.76). Because propanediols are not so specific in their anxiolytic action as the benzodiazepines, drowsiness, lack of concentration and other central depressive effects occur more commonly. In maintenance therapy pharmacological dependence has also been described as a potential problem (Swanson et al., 1973) amd may be a serious risk in those with a history of dependence (e.g. drinking problems). Tolerance and dependence are frequently found and withdrawal symptoms develop after suddenly stopping meprobamate in moderately high dosage (Hollister and Glazener, 1960). Tybamate is unusual in that withdrawal reactions do not develop after patients are suddenly withdrawn from high dosage (Shelton and Hollister, 1967).

DRUG INTERACTIONS

There are no specific drug interactions with propanediols although their effects are additive to the central effects of other depressant drugs. Like barbiturates, propanediols may precipitate attacks of acute intermittent porphyria.

CHOICE OF PROPANEDIOL

There is little to choose between the two chief members of the propanediol family. Meprobamate (Equanil, Miltown, Milonorm) is marketed in dosages of 400–3200 mg daily. Tybamate is no longer available in some countries although it has certain merits, particularly with regard to pharmacological dependence. Mephenesin has now no place in psychiatry and other members of the group, such as mebutamate and carisoprodol, have no special advantages. Comparisons between meprobamate and tybamate in the treatment of anxiety and insomnia have yielded conflicting results and there is no clear evidence that the shorter duration of action of tybamate confers any clinical advantages (Barsa and Saunders, 1963; Rickels et al., 1968). Other drugs have been combined with meprobamate in a number of preparations, notably analgesics (e.g. Equagesic, a combination of meprobamate, aspirin, ethoheptazine and calcium carbonate). Such combinations have no particular merit.

The propanediols have no special properties that make them superior to other antianxiety agents. Although they are effective antianxiety compounds they are not superior to the benzodiazepines and confer no special advantages. Despite this, they still have a place in the treatment of anxiety states, particularly when muscular tension is an important symptom.

Benzodiazepines

Although the first benzodiazepine was synthesized in 1955 by Sternbach the essential precursors had been studied by him more than 20 years earlier when he was working in Cracow, Poland. 1955 saw the advent of the first true benzodiazepine, chlordiazepoxide. It was hardly an auspicious beginning because the drug was expected to have little pharmacological activity and was not tested until 1957. Then Lowell Randall of Roche noted unexpected sedative effects similar to meprobamate but with much higher potency. Soon afterwards its striking ability to make aggressive animals calm suggested its use as an antianxiety drug. This set off a flurry of open clinical investigations in 1959 and 1960 which strongly supported anxiety-relieving properties (Randall, 1960; 1961). Pharmacological analysis had shown chlordiazepoxide to be a 1,4-benzodiazepine and a search for further compounds was started immediately. Not surprisingly, Roche were ahead of their competitors. Sternbach synthesized diazepam in 1959 and this was marketed under the trade name of Valium in 1962. Nitrazepam, another Roche product, was introduced soon afterwards, and oxazepam, the first of a number of benzodiazepines synthesized at Wyeth Laboratories, appeared at about the same time. Thus the benzodiazepine era was well established by 1963.

CHEMISTRY, PHARMACOLOGY AND TOXICOLOGY

The basic benzodiazepine nucleus is illustrated (*Figure 6.4*). Its key feature is a seven-membered ring of nitrogen and carbon atoms, the diazepine ring. It is this ring that gives the benzodiazepine group of drugs their particular chemical properties although it is also clear from the pharmacology of the latest benzodiazepine, clobazam, that the structurally related 1,5-benzodiazepines have similar pharmacological properties. The structural formulae of the commonly used benzodiazepines are shown in *Table 6.3*. Most of the modifications to the basic structure are minor ones and do not fundamentally change their pharmacological properties.

For this reason (and pharmacokinetic ones that are discussed later) the benzodiazepines can be considered as a homogeneous drug group although there is some variation in potency between different members. Their actions may be grouped into four sections; antianxiety, antiaggressive, muscle relaxant and anticonvulsant. Antianxiety effects were discovered early on in animal studies and alerted interest to their therapeutic potential. Benzodiazepines differ from barbiturates and to a lesser extent, from the propanediols, in their ability to reduce anxiety without significant impairment of consciousness. Benzodiazepines have selective effects in the limbic system, the area of the brain most intimately concerned with the experience of anxiety (Olds and Olds, 1969). More recent research has shown that the specific effects of benzodiazepines have a neurochemical basis. In 1976 benzodiazepine receptors were discovered in the central nervous system (Möhler and Okada, 1977) and high concentrations of these receptors are found in the limbic system, cerebral cortex and cerebellum (possibly explaining their anticonvulsant as well as anxiolytic effects and

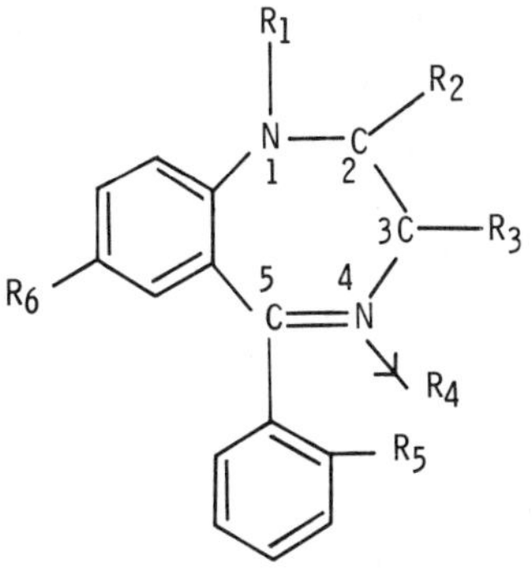

Figure 6.4 Basic 1,4-benzodiazepine nucleus

TABLE 6.3 Structural formulae of the commonly used benzodiazepines

	R_1	R_2	R_3	R_4	R_5	R_6
Chlordiazepoxide	—	$NHCH_3$	—	O	—	Cl
Diazepam	CH_3	O	—	—	—	Cl
Desmethyldiazepam	—	O	—	—	—	Cl
Nitrazepam	—	O	—	—	—	NO_2
Oxazepam	—	O	OH	—	—	Cl
Lorazepam	—	O	OH	—	Cl	Cl
Flurazepam	$CH_2CH_2N(C_2H_5)_2$	O	—	—	F	Cl
Clonazepam	—	O	—	—	Cl	NO_2
Medazepam	CH_3	—				Cl
Chlorazepate	—	OH	COOK	—	—	Cl
Triazolam	$C(CH_3)NN$(ring)	OK	—	—	Cl	Cl
Ketazolam	CH_3	O	—	COCH $(CCH_3)O$(ring)	—	Cl

their tendency to produce ataxia). Benzodiazepines also facilitate GABA transmission in the central nervous system (Haefely, 1978) but, unlike the barbiturates and other antianxiety drugs, benzodiazepines specifically bind to a special recognition site on the GABA receptor that itself is functionally linked to the benzodiazepine receptor (Braestrup and Nielsen, 1980). This is probably why the benzodiazepines have such selectivity in reducing anxiety. It also suggests that a naturally occurring substance (an endogenous ligand) is present in the brain and is concerned with the physiological control of anxiety, but its isolation is still awaited. The recent discovery of at least two types of benzodiazepine receptor, which explain the muscle relaxing and anticonvulsant effects of benzodiazepines as well as the anxiolytic ones (Squires *et al.*, 1979; Young *et al.*, 1981) suggests that further understanding of the mode of action of the benzodiazepines is likely in the near future.

Linked to the antianxiety actions of benzodiazepines are their effects on aggression. Early on in the studies with chlordiazepoxide it was noted that aggressive monkeys were calmed by doses much lower than the hypnotic ones (Randall *et al.*, 1960). Studies since then have been to some extent contradictory. In some cases benzodiazepines have shown a pronounced calming influence and in others have made apparently calm animals aggressive. The explanation for this paradoxical change is that anxious animals tend to inhibit their aggression and if this anxiety is relieved the aggression may show itself. This has led to the phenomenon of 'releasing aggression' which also has its counterpart in man. There is no real evidence that benzodiazepines actually create aggression and hostility occurring as a consequence of anxiety (a common association) is improved by benzodiazepines. Skeletal muscle relaxation is also a common property of the benzodiazepines which is independent of antianxiety effects. Although both central and peripheral actions are involved the central ones are far the most important (Hudson and Wolpert, 1970; Crankshaw and Raper, 1970), and there js no direct relaxing action on muscle fibres themselves (Crankshaw and Raper, 1968). The muscle relaxing effect is of value in treating spasticity and other disorders in which muscle tone is increased (Matthews, 1966). Clinical studies have shown that cerebral palsy (Griffiths and Sylvester, 1964), tetanus (when very high doses may be used) (Femi-Pearse, 1966) and spasticity in adults due to disease or injury (McFarland, 1963) may all be helped by benzodiazepines.

There are some differences in the anticonvulsant activity of different benzo-diazepines. Although all are anticonvulsant, lorazepam, clonazepam, nitrazepam and diazepam are more potent than desmethyldiazepam and chlordiazepoxide. Clonazepam (Rivotril) is specifically marketed as an anticonvulsant drug although there is little evidence that it is superior in anticonvulsant activity to some of the other benzodiazepines. The benzodiazepines all produce an increase in fast activity in the electroencephalogram, usually recorded as an increase in the proportion of beta activity (greater than 13 Hz) (Oswald and Priest, 1965; Montagu, 1972; Bond and Lader, 1973). The clinical significance of this increase in fast activity, which is also shown by barbiturates and propanediols, is not known.

TOXICOLOGY

Benzodiazepines are remarkably free of serious toxic effects and even if they were only of equivalent efficacy to barbiturates and propanediols they would always be preferred on grounds of safety. If given in excessive dosage they produce drowsiness and 'woolly headed' feelings, as a consequence of their depressant effects on the cortex, but little in the way of other side effects. The adjective 'excessive' should not be rigidly attached to quantity of dosage; there is great variation in dosage requirements between patients and within individuals, dosage needs are also dependent on the stage of the disorder. One of the first signs that an episode of pathological anxiety is naturally coming to an end is awareness by the patient that a dose of benzodiazepine which formerly just took the edge off of his anxiety now creates drowsiness. At dosages which produce drowsiness concentration and vigilance are often impaired and so workers engaged in intermittent repetitive tasks may be less effective when taking benzodiazepines. Even in doses that cause no symptoms benzodiazepines impair reaction time and affect driving performance (Betts, Clayton and Mackay, 1972) and may be responsible for the increased number of patients on benzodiazepines involved in road accidents (Skegg, Richards and Doll, 1979). In higher dosage benzodiazepines can cause dizziness and, in some cases, ataxia, with a characteristic staggering gait and impaired coordination. Most side effects are uncommon, ranging from 0.2 per cent for ataxia to 5.7 per cent for drowsiness (Miller, 1973), and are more than twice as common in the elderly than in patients under 40 (Boston Collaborative Drug Surveillance Program, 1973).

When benzodiazepines are used as hypnotics there is inevitably a 'hangover' effect the following morning. This is usually less unpleasant than with the barbiturates (Haider, 1968; Bond and Lader, 1972) but can be important clinically. Subjective feelings of muzziness, difficulty in concentration and drowsiness may persist up to 12 h after taking the drug. There have been claims that some of the newer benzodiazepines with short half-lives are less prone to hangover effects; this is discussed below.

Benzodiazepines have no toxic effects on the hepatic, haemopoetic or renal systems and are remarkably safe in overdosage; no fatalities have been reported when a benzodiazepine alone has been taken. Death may occur when a benzodiazepine is taken with another central depressive drug (particularly alcohol), when potentiation (or more usually, addition) of cerebral depressive effects occur. Although no unequivocal teratogenic effects have been reported with benzodiazepines, a high incidence of cleft lip and palate in infants of mothers taking benzodiazepines during the first trimester of pregnancy has been reported (Safra and Oakley, 1975), and it is wise to avoid prescription of benzodiazepines early in pregnancy wherever possible. Horrobin and his colleagues (1979) have suggested that diazepam, whilst not causing carcinoma may promote tumour growth. These effects have not been replicated by others (Jackson and Harris, 1981) and at present the evidence is too tenuous to affect clinical practice.

Occasionally intravenous benzodiazepines can cause thrombophlebitis, particularly if small veins are used for injections. The danger can be minimized by using the larger veins in the antecubital fossa, diluting the drug with the patients' blood, and by using lorazepam rather than diazepam for intravenous use (*Drug and Therapeutics Bulletin*, 1981a).

Unlike many other psychotropic drugs which secondarily increase appetite and thereby tend to put on weight, benzodiazepines have little or no appetite stimulant properties.

PHARMACOKINETICS

Absorption
All the benzodiazepines are rapidly absorbed by mouth and clinical effects are normally noted within 1 h, and peak plasma levels within 2 h. Surprisingly, intramuscular injection of chlordiazepoxide and diazepam produces a delay in the absorption of the parent drug and a similar delay in the production of its active metabolites, but intravenous injection leads to an almost immediate response. Lorazepam is preferred for intramuscular and intravenous use because of its more rapid absorption (Greenblatt *et al.*, 1979).

Distribution
Benzodiazepines are rapidly distributed throughout the body. There is considerable binding of benzodiazepines to plasma proteins and this may be clinically important as it is only unbound benzodiazepines that penetrate the blood–brain barrier. To date there are no clinical studies relating the proportion of bound and unbound benzodiazepine to its pharmacological effects.

Metabolism
Much the most important clinical aspect of the pharmacokinetics of benzodiazepines is their duration of pharmacological action and that of their active metabolites. Although there are between 6 and 15 benzodiazepines in clinical use (the number

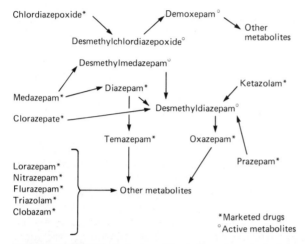

Figure 6.5 Metabolic pathways of benzodiazepines. A small percentage of chlordiazepoxide is also metabolized to desmethyldiazepam

varies from country to country) their similarities far outweigh their differences. One reason for this is that so many compounds marketed as new drugs are metabolites or precursors of other marketed compounds (*Figure 6.5*). This is a practice that may lead to commercial success but cannot be justified pharmacologically and clinically.

Although important pharmacological differences may sometimes be produced by minor structural alterations in a compound this can hardly be the case when it is known that the drug will produce an active metabolite which is itself another marketed drug. In pharmacokinetic terms the benzodiazepines can be divided into two main groups on the basis of their duration of action; long-acting and short-acting benzodiazepines (Committee on the Review of Medicines, 1980). The long-acting group contains compounds which have a half-life of over 30 h or are themselves metabolized to active compounds which have a similarly long half-life. The key to the metabolic pathway of many of the benzodiazepines is the drug desmethyldiazepam (*Figure 6.5*). This has a half-life of between 50 and 180 h (Hillestad, Hansen and Melsom, 1974; Klotz *et al.*, 1977) and so all compounds metabolized to desmethyldiazepam are in the long-acting group. The different members of the two groups are illustrated in *Table 6.4*.

Excretion
Benzodiazepines are excreted through the liver and in hepatic disease excretion is delayed (Klotz *et al.*, 1975). Older patients are more sensitive to the effects of benzodiazepines (Castleden *et al.*, 1977), but this is not due to greater absorption or higher plasma levels, although there is an increased half-life of the parent benzodiazepine drug in such patients (Klotz *et al.*, 1975). In fact older patients have lower plasma benzodiazepine levels for a given dose than younger ones (Rutherford, Okoko and Tyrer, 1978), and the increased pharmacological effects are probably related to the greater sensitivity of the ageing brain (*see* p. 389). Findings such as these illustrate that too much should not be inferred from a simple pharmacokinetic measurement such as a half-life when taken in isolation. Although there have been suggestions that benzodiazepines may induce their own metabolism, thereby leading to tolerance and dependence (Kanto *et al.*, 1974) there is no evidence that plasma levels of one benzodiazepine, diazepam, are reduced after chronic therapy (Rutherford, Okoko and

TABLE 6.4 Classification of benzodiazepines

Group	Approved name	Trade name	Dose equivalent to 5 mg diazepam	Active metabolites
Short-acting (half-life of 10 h or less)	Triazolam	Halcion	0.1	
	Temazepam	Euhypnos Normison	5	Oxazepam
	Oxazepam	Serenid-D Serenid-Forte	15	—
	Lormetazepam	Noctamid	0.5	
Medium-acting (half-life 11-30 h)	Lorazepam	Ativan	1.2	—
	Bromazepam	Lexotanil*	—	Hydrocyl metabolite
	Flunitrazepam	Rohypnol*	—	Desmethylflu-nitrazepam
Long-acting (half-life more than 30 h)	Diazepam	Valium Atensine	5	Desmethyldiazepam
	Clobazam	Frisium	10	Desmethylclobazam
	Chlordiazepoxide	Librium Tropium	10	Desmethylchlor-diazepoxide Demoxepam
	Ketazolam	Anxon	15	Desmethyldiazepam
	Medazepam	Nobrium	7.5	Diazepam Desmethyldiazepam
	Prazepam	Vesstran* Centrax	—	Desmethylmedazepam Desmethyldiazepam
	Chlorazepate	Tranxene	10	Desmethyldiazepam
	Desmethyldiazepam (nordiazepam)	Madar*	—	—
	Clonazepam	Rivotril	N/A	—
	Flurazepam	Dalmane	10	Desalkylflurazepam
	Nitrazepam	Mogadon Remnos	5	

*Not available in the UK

Tyrer, 1978; Greenblatt *et al.*, 1981). As yet there is no proven relationship between the pharmacokinetics of benzodiazepines and the occurrence of pharmacological dependence.

Most published studies of the pharmacokinetics of benzodiazepines are single dose studies or multiple dose studies spread over several days. These may sometimes mislead, as many benzodiazepines accumulate in chronic dosage and lead to different pharmacological effects. This is most evident with the long-acting benzodiazepines metabolized to desmethyldiazepam. After as little as 4 d of therapy with diazepam plasma desmethyldiazepam levels rise above that of diazepam because of the difference in the half-lives (Kaplan *et al.*, 1973; Tyrer *et al.*, 1982) (*see* p. 152). As des-methyldiazepam is an active metabolite the antianxiety effects of a regular dosage of diazepam after 7 d of continuous therapy last at least 24 h, whereas they would last only

4 h in single dose studies. Even an alleged short-acting benzodiazepine such as temazepam with a half-life of only 8 h is not without problems in chronic dosage. Temazepam is a highly effective hypnotic with little or no hangover effects in acute dosage (Briggs, Castleden and Kraft, 1980). However, in elderly patients it does accumulate after regular therapy (Huggett *et al.*, 1981) and then is more likely to produce hangover effects. As Dr Boulenger and Professor Lader have shown in Chapter 3, a simple relationship between the elimination half-life of a compound and duration of clinical response is seldom shown; it is well illustrated by the pharmacokinetics of benzodiazepines.

RELATIONSHIP BETWEEN PLASMA LEVELS OF BENZODIAZEPINES AND CLINICAL RESPONSE

Although there are reliable and relatively easy methods of measuring benzodiazepines in plasma and serum they have not been used much in clinical practice because a consistent relationship between plasma levels and clinical response has not been established. Most studies have reported no significant correlations between the plasma levels of the active compounds or their metabolites and their antianxiety effects (Kanto *et al.*, 1974; Tansella *et al.*, 1975; Bond, Hailey and Lader, 1977), although a significant relationship has been reported within individuals only (Robin, Curry and Whelpton, 1974). One study has shown a significant correlation between one of the metabolites of chlordiazepoxide, desmethylchlordiazepoxide and clinical response (Lin and Friedel, 1979) and a weak relationship for plasma diazepam and desmethyldiazepam has been reported in a study of anxious in-patients (Tyrer *et al.*, 1982). In neither study has the relationship been sufficiently strong to recommend that the measuring of plasma levels would be helpful in determining clinical response. In both of the latter studies (plasma or serum) levels were correlated with the change in rated anxiety scores rather than the raw scores themselves and this may account for some of the disparity between these and other studies.

The consensus of evidence from the studies as a whole is that plasma levels are not of particular value in monitoring clinical response although they may be useful in testing compliance or abuse as immediate past dosage is closely related to plasma levels (Rutherford, Okoko and Tyrer, 1978). As the clinical effects of benzodiazepines are experienced so rapidly after dosage it is not surprising that they, rather than pharmacokinetic variables, are likely to be most important in determining dosage.

DEPENDENCE ON BENZODIAZEPINES

Although benzodiazepines carry a much lower risk of dependence than either the propanediols or the barbiturates there has been increasing evidence that they can lead to a form of true pharmacological dependence in many patients. An early study by Hollister and his colleagues (1961) indicated that taking benzodiazepines in higher than normal therapeutic dosage was likely to be followed by an acute abstinence syndrome on sudden withdrawal, and later reports suggested that tolerance and active drug-seeking behaviour could occur after high dosage as well as being associated with severe withdrawal reactions after stopping the drug (Gordon, 1967; Clare, 1971; Fruensgaard, 1976; Preskorn and Denner, 1977). In the withdrawal period epileptic seizures and psychotic features, particularly paranoid ideas and hallucinations, were described. Reports of these cases were relatively uncommon considering the widespread use of benzodiazepines, and, on the basis of published evidence, Marks (1978) concluded that the risk of developing benzodiazepine dependence was 1 in 5 million months of all patient use and 1 in 50 million months of patients in therapeutic use.

Marks made valid criticism of some of the published case reports as other drugs and alcohol were frequently abused with the benzodiazepine. As almost all benzodiazepines are prescribed in therapeutic dosage the risks of pharmacological dependence, if confirmed by other data, would be too infinitesimal to justify clinical concern. However, a small number of published reports does not necessarily indicate that dependence is not a serious problem; it may be just under-reported. In recent years there has been increasing evidence that therapeutic use of benzodiazepines can be associated with withdrawal reactions if medication is suddenly stopped after long-term therapy. Minor withdrawal reactions after stopping chlordiazepoxide were noted after four months of therapy but not after two months (Covi et al., 1973), and clear-cut withdrawal phenomena, including epileptic seizures, have been reported by a number of authors in patients stopping benzodiazepines after continuous treatment ranging from six months to many years (Rifkin, Quitkin and Klein, 1976; Mendelson, 1978; Pevnick, Jasinski and Haertzen, 1978; Winokur et al., 1980; Howe, 1980). There is recent evidence that withdrawal reactions are more severe after stopping a short-acting benzodiazepine (lorazepam) than a long-acting one (diazepam) and that with diazepam reactions only occur when serum levels of the long-acting metabolite, desmethyldiazepam, fall rapidly (Tyrer, Rutherford and Huggett, 1981). A similar phenomenon described as 'rebound insomnia' has been noted with benzodiazepine hypnotics by Kales and his colleagues (1978) who have suggested that it is caused by a relative deficiency of endogenous benzodiazepine-like molecules in the brain when (exogenous) benzodiazepine levels fall rapidly.

The symptoms of the benzodiazepine withdrawal syndrome usually begin within 3 d of stopping a short-acting benzodiazepine and between 4 and 8 d after stopping a long-acting member of the series. They are probably more common with higher dosage and longer duration of therapy (Ayd, 1979). There is sometimes difficulty in distinguishing withdrawal effects from a return of pre-existing anxiety and in minor manifestations of the syndrome such a distinction may be impossible. Insomnia, muscle tension, headache and panic attacks come into this category. In more severe cases withdrawal symptoms include perceptual changes such as hypersensitivity to sound, sight, smell and touch, awareness of rocking or oscillating movements of the immediate environment ('perceptual ataxia'), extreme irritability, dysphoria and, rarely, epileptic seizures and paranoid symptoms (Fruensgaard, 1976; Pevnick, Jasinski and Haertzen, 1978; Lader, 1981). If the symptoms are truly those of withdrawal they usually begin to subside after an interval of days although sometimes they may last several weeks.

A great deal more needs to be done to establish the risk factor for developing benzodiazepine dependence. Unfortunately animal studies are of little help as pharmacological dependence has never been established in any animal species with low dosage of benzodiazepines although after suddenly stopping benzodiazepines taken in high chronic dosage in monkeys withdrawal symptoms are shown (Yanagita and Takahashi, 1973). In man the dosage level and duration of treatment necessary before dependence becomes a serious risk is still not known. It is also not clear whether there are any differences between the benzodiazepines in their potential to produce dependence although the evidence cited above suggests greater risk for short-acting benzodiazepines.

CLINICAL USE

The primary use of benzodiazepines is for the relief of pathological anxiety. As anxiety is such a common component of medical and psychiatric illness it might be thought that the use of benzodiazepines would be the same in all these conditions. This is not so, mainly because the period of anxiety relief required varies considerably. This will affect the choice of benzodiazepine, the route by which it is administered, and the frequency of prescription.

The other non-psychiatric uses of benzodiazepines will only be mentioned briefly. The anticonvulsant activity of most benzodiazepines is sufficiently great for them to be used in the treatment of epilepsy and clonazepam (Rivotril) is used solely for this purpose. Benzodiazepines are particularly effective in treating epilepsy characterized by myoclonic jerks or tonic–clonic seizures (Nanda *et al.*, 1977) and, given intravenously, in the treatment of status epilepticus (Parsonage and Norris, 1967). Lorazepam and diazepam may both be given intravenously and are invaluable in resistant cases. Benzodiazepines do not have any significant interactions with other

TABLE 6.5 Clinical indications for benzodiazepines
(For convenience the dosage of diazepam alone is given for all indications)

Disorder	Usual daily dosage	Recommended duration	Comments
Stress reactions	5–10	1–3 d	May be used in IF dosage for up to 2 weeks
Insomnia	5–10	IF	—
Anxiety states (neuroses)	5–20	IF	Similar dosage used for treatment of secondary anxiety in other psychiatric disorders
Agoraphobia and social phobias	2–20	IF	To be taken before exposure to phobic situations
Hypochondriacal states	5–15	IF	Use only when symptoms clearly related to anxiety
Neuromuscular disorders	5–30	For duration of disorder	Dependence may be a necessary evil if control of the disorder is successfully achieved by drugs
Epilepsy	10–30	Variable, depending on control of seizures	Best used for short periods, particularly valuable in status epilepticus
Drug and alcohol withdrawal	5–40	7 d	*See* Chapter 12 for further details
Anaesthesia premedication	5–20	Pre-operatively	Produces anterograde amnesia, thereby giving special advantages (*see* text)

IF = intermittent flexible dosage determined by patient up to an agreed maximum anticonvulsants (Nanda et al., 1977) and, as their central depressant effects are less than with the barbiturates, a combination of a barbiturate and a benzodiazepine is preferable to two barbiturate anticonvulsants.

Benzodiazepines are also useful in anaesthesia, both as premedication before surgical and dental operations, and sometimes intravenously to induce anaesthesia. The benzodiazepines have the advantage of producing anterograde amnesia in moderate dosage (e.g. 20 mg of diazepam, 4 mg of lorazepam) and this may be useful when there is a special anxiety about an operation (e.g. prior to ECT). Lorazepam may be superior to diazepam in producing amnesia when given by mouth as premedication (Wilson, 1973), but if diazepam is given intravenously amnesia for the immediate following events is virtually complete (Dundee and Pandit, 1972).

The muscle relaxant properties of benzodiazepines have already been mentioned (p. 138). As many neurological and muscular disorders suitable for treatment with benzodiazepines are chronic ones a decision has to be made as to whether it is safe to continue long-term therapy. Despite the risk of dependence the decision is seldom a difficult one. The benefits of continued treatment are usually much greater than the handicap of dependence and long-term therapy is justified provided the clinical indications for therapy continue (Table 6.5).

USE OF BENZODIAZEPINES IN PSYCHIATRY

Acute use
Stress and adjustment reactions   Acute reactions to stress are now accepted as a diagnostic term (WHO, 1978), and are described as 'very transient disorders of any severity or nature which occur in individuals without any apparent mental disorder in response to exceptional physical and mental stress'. Many instances of normal anxiety can be included in this group and it is quite appropriate to take one or more doses of a benzodiazepine to alleviate the unpleasantness of these feelings. There is seldom any need to continue treatment for more than 2–3 d. Short-term use of benzodiazepines as hypnotics also comes under this category. Often the reactions to acute stress are not immediate and tend to run a fluctuating course. If they continue for several weeks and are associated with stresses such as bereavement or separation they are described as 'adjustment reactions' (WHO, 1978). Symptoms of anxiety and depression are common in adjustment reactions. Benzodiazepines may sometimes be appropriate treatment but prescription should be kept to a minimum to avoid habitual use. The use of an intermittent flexible dosage regimen is the most economical in terms of total dosage (Winstead et al., 1974) and is clinically more appropriate than fixed dosage determined by the calendar. All anxiety, no matter how persistent or severe, fluctuates greatly from hour to hour and from day to day (Tyrer, 1976) and it is therefore pointless to prescribe a regular fixed dose for a prolonged period. Intermittent flexible dosage also has the advantage of detecting the natural improvement that almost invariably follows stressful reactions; if the drugs are taken only in response to symptoms their administration will cease when the symptoms disappear.

Insomnia   All good antianxiety drugs are good hypnotics and benzodiazepines are no exception. The ideal hypnotic induces sleep rapidly and has a duration of action of up to 8 h. There should be no hangover or other unwanted effects on waking and the drug should not impair judgement or other aspects of higher mental function. Benzodiazepine drugs with a short duration of action (Table 6.4) would therefore be preferable as hypnotics. Unfortunately, the marketing policies of the pharmaceutical firms are not always based on pharmacological considerations. Lorazepam, oxazepam, temazepam and triazolam all have half-lives of 12 h or less but only two, temazepam and triazolam, are recommended as hypnotics. Flurazepam and nitrazepam are the most commonly prescribed benzodiazepine hypnotics in the UK and both lead to marked hangover effects with impairment of psychomotor function up to 18 h after taking the drug (Malpas *et al.*, 1970; Bond and Lader, 1973). Desmethyldiazepam, as noted earlier, is a common metabolite of six benzodiazepines and has a very long half-life of up to 210 h. Despite this in some countries it is marketed as a hypnotic. Not surprisingly, although it is effective it carries marked residual effects (Tansella *et al.*, 1975).

These differences in duration of action may sometimes be used to positive effect. For example, if insomnia is associated with marked day time anxiety it may be more appropriate to prescribe a long-acting benzodiazepine, such as diazepam. In choosing a benzodiazepine for treating insomnia it is often best to ignore the official labels attached to the drugs and pick on the basis of required duration of action. As a general rule the hypnotic dose is about twice the dose required for alleviation of anxiety (*Table 6.4*).

Tolerance tends not to develop to any serious extent with short-term prescription of benzodiazepines as hypnotics (Kales *et al.*, 1970a), but because of the problems of cumulation and dependence it is best to avoid regular fixed dosages, which are perhaps more likely to develop in insomnia as the consumption of a sleeping tablet is a common night time ritual.

Anxiety states Anxiety states (used synonymously with anxiety neuroses) are common psychiatric disorders and account for the largest proportion of benzodiazepine prescription. In general practice they tend to be short-lived but in psychiatric practice they frequently become chronic and have a poor outcome compared with depressive disorders (Schapira *et al.*, 1972). Chronically anxious patients almost invariably have insomnia as well and depression is also a common accompaniment.

There is ample evidence that benzodiazepines are effective in anxiety states (Greenblatt and Shader, 1974), and anxiety states are one of their specific indications. There is considerable variation in the presentation of anxiety states. Some patients have relatively mild symptoms but change gradually, if at all, whereas others have rapid fluctuations in the form of panic attacks. In such states the normal effect changes within seconds to acute distress with marked somatic symptoms of anxiety such as shaking, palpitations, sweating, churning stomach movements, nausea, giddiness and muscular tension. Such states are sometimes accorded a separate diagnostic label as panic anxiety.

Variations between anxiety states will determine the choice of benzodiazepine. Unfortunately there is no 'instant benzodiazepine' that can reduce anxiety within minutes and even intravenous benzodiazepines given in low dosage for the treatment of anxiety take up to 30 min to produce their full effect (Kelly, Pik and Chen, 1973). Because episodes of panic are short lasting it is preferable to use a short-acting benzodiazepine such as lorazepam unless the panic attacks are very frequent. For patients with longer periods of anxiety, particularly when associated with insomnia, it is better to use a long-acting benzodiazepine. This may often be given in a single daily dose. Intermittent flexible dosage is also recommended to keep dosage requirements to a minimum. Sometimes the opposite view may be taken that acute anxiety is so unpleasant and tends to reinforce further anxiety, that it must be treated vigorously with regular benzodiazepines for a short period. There is no evidence to suggest which of the procedures is superior in relieving anxiety but on *a priori* grounds it is reasonable to expect that some patients treated with fixed regular dosage will receive much more benzodiazepine than they need to control their symptoms. This will inevitably lead to impairment of psychomotor function with adverse sequelae such as road accidents (Skegg, Richards and Doll, 1979). There are reports that the new 1,5-benzodiazepine, clobazam, does not impair psychomotor performance and car driving skills (Hindmarch and Gudgeon, 1980) and may therefore be preferred.

Agoraphobia and social phobias   Phobic anxiety has the same clinical characteristics as anxiety states, but the anxiety is more predictable as it is bound to certain situations. The most 'pure' phobias are the so called mono-symptomatic phobias of insects, heights, thunder, blood and other clearly identifiable stimuli. Benzodiazepines are rarely indicated in such disorders. Agoraphobia and social phobias are more complex (Marks, 1969) and other anxiety and depressive symptoms frequently co-exist with them. Benzodiazepines are frequently prescribed for these disorders but intermittent flexible dosage is the exception rather than the rule. Phobic disorders represent *par excellence* the conditions that lend themselves to intermittent treatment because they are so predictable. There is some uncertainty about the best time of taking a benzodiazepine before exposure to the phobic situation. An early report suggested that if the benzodiazepine was taken 4 h before exposure its effect was greater than if it were given much later (Marks *et al.*, 1972). This would suggest that benzodiazepines have their major effect on anticipatory anxiety, which often reinforces phobic fears and avoidance. However, a later study showed no evidence of this 'waning effect' (Hafner and Marks, 1976) and it is probably best for patients to experiment with the timing of their dosage to see which produces the greatest effect. In most cases a short-acting benzodiazepine is recommended unless there are concomitant 'free-floating' anxiety symptoms.

Hypochondriacal states   These include a mixed group of disorders, ranging from dysmorphophobia and accident neurosis to depressive illness and socially acceptable illness behaviour (Snaith, 1981). Benzodiazepines may be of some value in these disorders when the hypochondriasis is concentrated on somatic symptoms of anxiety. Such patients usually consult many other doctors before arriving at the psychiatrists and will have received many therapies, both medical and non-medical, for their symptoms. A benzodiazepine may often be helpful if the major symptom is within the range of somatic symptoms of anxiety and it often has greater effect if the patient does not know that it is a psychotropic drug. Unfortunately, hypochondriacal states tend to be long-lasting and it may be difficult to avoid long-term prescription.

Tardive dyskinesia (*See* p. 114.)

Drug and alcohol withdrawal   This subject is dealt with extensively in Chapters 12 and 13. The use of benzodiazepines in these disorders represents an important short-term use of these compounds. Long-term prescription should be avoided because of the major risks of pharmacological dependence.

Maintenance therapy
Although short-term use of benzodiazepines is recommended in psychiatry (Committee on the Review of Medicines, 1980) many patients find themselves

receiving maintenance therapy. Unless treatment is with triazolam or, possibly temazepam, some cumulation is liable to occur. This might be expected to lead to increased tranquillizing effects but this rarely happens. After high dosage of benzodiazepines there is considerable tolerance to their clinical effects (Greenblatt *et al.*, 1979) and this may account for the lack of progressive tranquillization. Although patients may not notice any handicap on regular benzodiazepine dosage they are likely to suffer some psychomotor impairment. Wherever possible it is best to revert to intermittent flexible dosage with the option of effecting withdrawal at a later stage. It is best to explain to the patient the reasons for giving flexible dosage and to show him how his symptoms can determine his dosage requirements. Most patients taking maintenance benzodiazepines are unhappy about their regular consumption and cooperate in this sort of exercise.

For patients taking benzodiazepines for other medical disorders it is not possible to use their symptoms as a means of determining their dosage in the same way and regular maintenance treatment may be unavoidable.

WITHDRAWAL OF BENZODIAZEPINES

There are no specific problems from withdrawing benzodiazepines after short-term use except for a return of the symptoms for which they were originally prescribed. There is also little problem in withdrawing from intermittent flexible dosage, even when it has been taken for many months, provided there have been periods of up to several days during which medication has not been taken. The main difficulty is withdrawing benzodiazepines when they have been taken in regular dosage. Although obvious pharmacological dependence is rare, dependence in the form of withdrawal reactions after stopping drug therapy is relatively common. On present evidence it appears that dependence can develop in some patients taking regular benzodiazepines for three months or more and the problem is clinically significant after six months' continuous therapy. A tendency for patients to take high doses of the drug is also a serious warning sign (Lapierre, 1981).

Withdrawal is best accomplished in three stages. Initially the drug continues to be prescribed in regular dosage but the total daily dosage is reduced gradually. Many dependent patients can reduce their dosage significantly in this way before stopping their drug. The second stage is instituted when patients cannot reduce any further without a return of symptoms. As noted earlier these symptoms are as likely to be the early withdrawal symptoms of stopping benzodiazepines as a return of the symptoms for which the benzodiazepine was originally prescribed. In the second stage patients taking a short-acting benzodiazepine are changed to an equivalent dose of long-acting benzodiazepine. This is because a gradual fall in circulating benzodiazepines is more easy to achieve with compounds with a long duration of action that are slowly eliminated from the body. The long-acting benzodiazepine is given as a single dose (most commonly at night) and further gradual reduction is attempted. If it is not successful a beta-adrenoceptor blocking drug such as propranolol may be added. There is some evidence that this reduces the severity of withdrawal reactions (Tyrer, Rutherford and Huggett, 1981) and in the low dosage used (60–120 mg daily) there is no danger of any form of withdrawal reaction when this itself is stopped. Further withdrawal can be achieved by taking the benzodiazepine on alternate days or on every third day.

The final stage involves assessment of the patient after he has not taken any benzodiazepines for at least 10 d and preferably 3–4 weeks. This is because withdrawal symptoms may take several weeks to be overcome and it is only after this time that assessment of 'baseline' symptoms can be made. If the patient continues to have some anxiety symptoms at this stage the doctor has a choice of

(1) alternative non-pharmacological treatment,
(2) benzodiazepines in intermittent flexible dosage with an agreed maximum of less than 10 mg of diazepam daily (or equivalent dose of another benzodiazepine), or
(3) the prescription of an alternative antianxiety drug.

It is a matter of clinical judgement which option is chosen; as yet there is no indication which is best.

DRUG INTERACTIONS

Benzodiazepines are remarkably free of adverse drug interactions. In animal studies the effects of benzodiazepines are additive to those of other central depressive drugs such as alcohol and barbiturates (Fujimori, 1965) but in man, using relatively low dosage of both alcohol and benzodiazepine drug, no significant potentiation of alcohol-induced psychomotor impairment has been demonstrated (Lawton and Cahn, 1963; Betts, Clayton and Mackay, 1972). Interaction with high dosages has not been studied under controlled conditions but, in view of the information derived from animal work, it seems likely that there are some additive central depressive effects. For this reason it is recommended that great care should be taken when combining benzodiazepines and central depressant agents, particularly under circumstances when good psychomotor coordination is needed.

There have been isolated reports of benzodiazepines interacting with levodopa (diminution of antiparkinsonian activity), coumarin anticoagulants (enhanced anti-coagulant effect) and phenytoin (increasing plasma phenytoin levels and predisposing to toxicity) but there is no independent confirmation of these findings (Greenblatt and Shader, 1974). Benzodiazepines are potentiated to some degree by cimetidine. In one study in which the side effects of benzodiazepines were evaluated it was found that cigarette smokers had a lower incidence of side effects than non-smokers (Boston Collaborative Drug Surveillance Program, 1973). This implies an interaction between nicotine and benzodiazepines but this remains to be demonstrated.

DIFFERENCES BETWEEN BENZODIAZEPINES

It is reasonable for the clinician to ask whether there is any point in knowing all the benzodiazepines on the market and whether the new agents introduced each year represent any real advance. Although there are some clear differences (mainly pharmacokinetic ones) between the benzodiazepines (Garattini, Mussini and Randall, 1973; Shader and Greenblatt, 1980; Ameer and Greenblatt, 1981) these are of no significance to the clinician unless they represent differences in clinical effects. In general the differences between benzodiazepines have turned out to be of little clinical importance and make the introduction of new benzodiazepines very hard to justify except on commercial grounds (Tyrer, 1974; *Drug and Therapeutics Bulletin*, 1978). Like rows of brand detergents fighting for the housewife's attention each benzodiazepine stridently proclaims its so-called advantages over its competitors. But the consumers are presented with a false choice; it is the packaging that sells the

TABLE 6.6 Differences between benzodiazepines

Property	Anti-anxiety	Hypnotic	Muscle relaxant	Anti-convulsant	Speed of action	Duration of action	Risk of dependence	Safety	Psychomotor impairment
Chlordiazepoxide				Less than other benzodiazepines	Rapid	Long	Low		
Diazepam					Rapid	Long	Low		
Desmethyldiazepam					Slow	Long	Low		
Clorazepate					Slow	Long	Low		
Prazepam	Equal when equivalent dosage used[a]	Equal when equivalent dosage used[a]	Equal when equivalent dosage used[a]	Equal when equivalent dosage used[a]	Slow	Long	Low	All compounds have a very wide safety margin	All compounds produce mild psychomotor impairment with the possible exception of Clobazam
Ketazolam					Slow	Long	Low		
Medazepam					Rapid	Long	Low		
Oxazepam					Rapid	Short	Moderate		
Lorazepam					Rapid	Medium	Moderate		
Nitrazepam					Rapid	Long	Low		
Flurazepam					Rapid	Long	Low		
Temazepam					Rapid	Short	Moderate		
Triazolam					Rapid	Short	Moderate		
Clonazepam					Rapid	Long	Low		
Clobazam					Rapid	Long	Low		

[a] See Table 6.4 for details of equivalent dosage

product, not its specific content, as all are basically similar. By being diverted into pharmacokinetic niceties in marketing the benzodiazepines the pharmaceutical industry is making the error of assuming that all pharmacokinetic differences are necessarily pharmacodynamic ones. Until pharmacokinetic factors have been shown to correlate with clinical ones they must remain suspect and clinical observations given primary importance (Dollery, 1973). It is easy for the practitioner to take at face value the plausible argument that because a benzodiazepine has a short elimination half-life it necessarily has a short duration of action. Dr Boulenger and Professor Lader have shown in Chapter 2 that pharmacokinetics is a dynamic process in which different processes are constantly changing. The elimination (β) phase appears to have taken precedence over the distribution (α) phase in promoting the benzo- diazepines and insufficient attention has been given in advertisements to the relationship between the parent benzodiazepine and its active metabolites. No-one expects the ordinary clinician to be thoroughly familiar with the complexities of the two or three compartment models of benzodiazepine pharmacokinetics, and to justify the introduction of a new compound with deceptively simple pharmacokinetic arguments alone will only mislead. In discussion of the differences between the benzodiazepines, pharmacokinetic differences will therefore be mentioned only where they are of confirmed clinical importance.

The clinical variations between benzodiazepines are shown in *Table 6.6* and from this it is clear that their similarities far outweigh their differences. In particular there is no evidence that antianxiety or hypnotic effects differ from one benzodiazepine to another, provided that they are given in equivalent dosage. Of course there are now so many benzodiazepines available that no one study can compare all of them, but similar efficacy is repeatedly found, particularly in studies where equivalent dosage is assured by patients taking the drug in flexible dosage (Lader, Bond and James, 1974; Kanto *et al.*, 1979). Similarly, all benzodiazepines are equally safe in overdosage and carry the same low risk of interaction. These are the major factors determining the choice of a drug and differences in other clinical effects are correspondingly less important. Each individual benzodiazepine is described below but only those features that distinguish it from other benzodiazepines are mentioned.

CHLORDIAZEPOXIDE

Chlordiazepoxide is the oldest marketed benzodiazepine and is a useful yardstick by which to compare the others. It is rapidly absorbed after oral administration and after a single dose is eliminated quickly from the body with a half-life of about 14 h. With repeated dosage the active metabolites, demoxepam, desmethylchlordiazepoxide and desmethyldiazepam accumulate and contribute to clinical effects. As these drugs have a long duration of action, with half-lives of up to 200 h, chlordiazepoxide comes into the long-acting group of benzodiazepines. In general parenteral administration of chlordiazepoxide should be avoided as the drug tends to precipitate at the injection site giving poor and erratic absorption (Greenblatt, Shader and Koch-Weser, 1974). For this reason it is less often given than lorazepam, clonazepam and diazepam in the treatment of epilepsy although it has some anticonvulsant properties.

Although chlordiazepoxide now tends to be prescribed less often than other benzodiazepines it is a sound, reliable compound that is just as good as the newer ones and considerably cheaper than most. It is particularly popular for the management of alcohol withdrawal symptoms, and in one recent study of American physicians was the drug of first choice in 60 per cent of respondents (Favazza and Martin, 1974).

DIAZEPAM

Diazepam is the most commonly prescribed drug in the UK (Skegg, Doll and Perry, 1977) and probably in the world. It is a very similar in its general clinical properties to chlordiazepoxide, having a relatively short duration of effect when given in a single dose but after regular dosage clinical effects are prolonged mainly because of accumulation of its major metabolite, desmethyldiazepam (also called nordiazepam). If diazepam is given in regular dosage once daily (e.g. at night) it will therefore have hypnotic effects immediately and antianxiety effects for most of the following day. It is rapidly absorbed by mouth and the onset of antianxiety effects is 30–60 min, lasting for 3–4 h after a single dose. Intravenous diazepam is given frequently in anaesthesia and in the treatment of epilepsy and has a shorter duration of action (less than 2 h) because it is so rapidly distributed throughout the body. Pain may be noticed at the injection site when intravenous diazepam is given; this can be reduced by withdrawing the syringe so that the injection is diluted with the patient's blood (Mitchell Heggs, quoted by Kelly, Pik and Chen, 1973); and thereby minimizes the risks of thrombophlebitis. A new preparation of diazepam, Diazemuls (Kabivitrum), has recently been marketed, in which diazepam is prepared in an oil-in-water emulsion that is less likely to cause endothelial damage.

   When diazepam is given in regular dosage (or after a single overdose) its active metabolite, desmethyldiazepam, becomes progressively more important in determining the clinical effects. As desmethyldiazepam has a much longer half-life than diazepam its blood levels rise steadily and after a few days exceed those of diazepam (Kaplan *et al.*, 1973). When diazepam is stopped the plasma desmethyldiazepam levels fall more slowly than those of diazepam and significant amounts are still circulating up

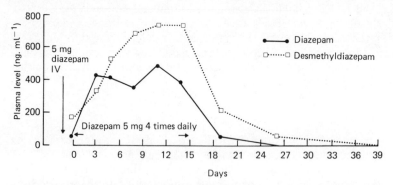

Figure 6.6 Cumulation of plasma desmethyldiazepam in an anxious patient on regular dosage of diazepam for two weeks

to two weeks afterwards (*Figure 6.6*). This accounts for the 'honeymoon period' experienced by patients who stop diazepam after regular dosage and feel well for several days. After this time circulating desmethldiazepam levels fall, withdrawal reactions may be shown or original anxiety symptoms re-emerge.

DESMETHYLDIAZEPAM

Although N-desmethyldiazepam is not marketed in the UK it is described here because of its importance in the metabolic pathways of benzodiazepines. It is available as a hypnotic (Madar) in some European countries and, although effective, can produce marked hangover effects (Tansella *et al.*, 1975). This is not surprising as the drug has the longest duration of action of all the benzodiazepines with a half-life ranging from 30–210 h. In regular dosage the drug therefore accumulates and after about two weeks of treatment steady state levels are usually achieved. Its chief significance is that it is a major contributor to the clinical effects of the drugs described below. Because of its long duration of action there is no point in prescribing desmethyldiazepam more than once a day.

PRAZEPAM, CLORAZEPATE AND KETAZOLAM

These three drugs are 'prodrugs', as the parent compounds have no significant pharmacological action but are all metabolized to desmethyldiazepam. The only variation between them is in the rate at which this process takes place. Clorazepate is rapidly converted to desmethyldiazepam by hydrolysis and decarboxylation in the stomach after contact with gastric hydrochloric acid. Almost all the drug absorbed in the small bowel is desmethyldiazepam, not clorazepate, and patients will have the same response as if they had taken the equivalent dose of desmethyldiazepam (unless they happen to have achlorhydria). Prazepam and ketazolam take a little longer to be metabolized to desmethyldiazepam. Prazepam is almost completely dealkylated by first past metabolism (*see* Chapter 2, p. 23) in the liver but peak desmethyldiazepam levels take up to 48 h to be achieved. Ketazolam is also metabolized to desmethyldiazepam in the liver and its smooth transformation is alleged to improve its anxiolytic effect. There is no evidence that its clinical effects differ from diazepam and desmethyldiazepam (*Drug and Therapeutics Bulletin*, 1980) although in one study it was found that more drowsiness occurred with diazepam than ketazolam (Fabre, McLendon and Gainey, 1978). As the difference was small and the overall incidence of side effects the same with both diazepam and ketazolam, this evidence is not adequate to claim that ketazolam is superior to diazepam with respect to side effects.

The clinical significance of the differences in the rates of distribution and metabolism of clorazepate, prazepam and ketazolam has yet to be established. Although there is clear evidence that all three drugs are effective in once daily dosage (Robin, Curry and Whelpton, 1974; Greenblatt and Shader, 1978; Fabre, McLendon and Gainey, 1978) no studies have compared the clinical effects of these three prodrugs, and it seems very likely that in all clinical respects their effects would be identical.

MEDAZEPAM

Medazepam has some of the qualities of the three prodrugs as it too is metabolized to desmethyldiazepam. It is also metabolized to diazepam and desmethyldiazepam, both of which are clinically active, and as medazepam itself is an antianxiety drug, all five drugs (including the two active metabolites of desmethyldiazepam) contribute to clinical response after regular dosage. In short-term or occasional dosage medazepam and diazepam have the main pharmacological action and prescription two or three times daily could be justified. Once the drug has been taken regularly for a week or more there is little point in prescribing it more than once daily, as after this period it is a long-acting benzodiazepine and best given at night. A controlled study comparing medazepam with diazepam, chlordiazepoxide and amylobarbitone sodium showed it to be of equivalent efficacy to the two benzodiazepines and superior to amylobarbitone sodium and placebo (Lader, Bond and James, 1974). This result is predictable because of the pharmacokinetics of medazepam.

OXAZEPAM

Oxazepam is the final active metabolite in the breakdown of many benzodiazepines (*Figure 6.5*). It has no active metabolites (being mainly metabolized to inactive glucuronide) and its relatively short elimination half-life (about 10 h) makes it more suitable as a hypnotic than as an antianxiety drug. Nevertheless it is only marketed as an anxiolytic and there are no formal studies of its use as a hypnotic. Because of its short half-life accumulation does not occur in regular dosage and steady state levels are achieved in a few days. For reasons mentioned earlier regular dosage is more likely to lead to dependence than with long-acting benzodiazepines such as diazepam and flurazepam and if the drug is withdrawn rapidly after regular dosage withdrawal reactions may be shown (Mendelson, 1978).

Oxazepam has no particular advantages over other benzodiazepines although the absence of major adverse reactions over its long period of use (18 years) emphasize its reliability and safety.

LORAZEPAM

Lorazepam is virtually identical to oxazepam, having a relatively short duration of action (half-life of 10–20 h) and inactive glucuronide metabolites. It is also rapidly absorbed by oral administration. Lorazepam is also marketed as an antianxiety drug although, like oxazepam, it would be more appropriately prescribed as a hypnotic. Lorazepam is one of the benzodiazepines available in an injectable form. Intravenous lorazepam is less likely to cause endothelial damage than intravenous diazepam and may be preferred in anaesthesia. Intramuscular lorazepam is also more rapidly absorbed than diazepam and chlordiazepoxide by the intramuscular route (Greenblatt *et al.*, 1979) and may therefore offer advantages when it is necessary to give a benzodiazepine by this route. Although the pharmacodynamics and pharmacokinetics of lorazepam have been studied intensively (Ameer and Greenblatt, 1981) the findings are generally typical of all short-acting benzodiazepines. Withdrawal symptoms after stopping regular lorazepam dosage are more severe than with diazepam (Tyrer, Rutherford and Huggett, 1981) and epileptic seizures have been reported (Einarson, 1980; Howe, 1980).

NITRAZEPAM

Nitrazepam is the most frequently prescribed benzodiazepine hypnotic in Europe although surprisingly, it is not marketed in the USA. Its relatively long duration of action (half-life 27 h) makes it a little unsatisfactory for this purpose as cumulation occurs in regular dosage (Breimer, Jochemsen and von Albert, 1980) and hangover effects are common (Malpas *et al.*, 1970; Bond and Lader, 1972). If, however, the insomniac is also anxious by day the longer duration of action will be beneficial. Nitrazepam has no active metabolites.

It is an effective antianxiety and hypnotic drug and is very similar to diazepam. The common practice of giving two or more benzodiazepines simultaneously (Tyrer, 1978), diazepam by day and nitrazepam at night being the most favoured combination, is therefore quite unnecessary. It merely reflects the success of advertising in separating hypnotics from antianxiety effects.

FLURAZEPAM

Flurazepam is marketed only as a hypnotic but as it has a duration of action of well over 24 h it is hardly ideal for this purpose. It is metabolized to desalkylflurazepam, an active metabolite with a half-life of up to 100 h, and this is primarily responsible for its prolonged clinical effects. Clinical studies confirm that it is an effective hypnotic with the same predilection to hangover effects as other benzodiazepine hypnotics (Kales *et al.*, 1971; Bond and Lader, 1973). The long duration of action accounts for the continuing hypnotic effects for several days after the drug is stopped. After this period 'rebound insomnia' occurs (Kales, Scharf and Kales, 1978). As this reaction is temporary it is best construed as a withdrawal reaction.

TEMAZEPAM

Temazepam is involved in the metabolic pathway of diazepam and other benzo-diazepines that are metabolized to desmethyldiazepam, although it is not produced in clinically significant quantities. Temazepam itself is partly metabolized to oxazepam although this probably plays little part in its clinical activity. Its half-life of between 8 and 10 h makes it most suitable for prescription as a hypnotic and indeed it is used almost exclusively for this purpose. There is good evidence that it is a highly effective hypnotic (Briggs, Castleden and Kraft, 1980). Because of its relatively short half-life one would expect that it was less likely to produce residual effects than long-acting benzodiazepines. Clinical studies have not shown that temazepam offers significant advantages over these other benzodiazepines in this respect. Although it has relatively few hangover effects (Harry and Latham, 1980) long-acting benzodiazepines such as diazepam produce similarly low hangover effects when used in equivalent dosage (Hindmarch, 1979; Nicholson, 1979). However, these studies have been carried out in volunteers rather than in clinical patients and are not necessarily conclusive. They were also carried out with single dosage and under these circumstances significant amounts of desmethyldiazepam and other long-acting metabolites are not produced. Other studies have shown that temazepam is superior to nitrazepam and flurazepam in producing fewer residual effects on waking (Nicholson, 1981).

The evidence of studies with temazepam in patients or volunteers suggest that it is an effective hypnotic that is not likely to accumulate on repeated dosage, except possibly in the elderly (Huggett *et al.*, 1981). If repeated dosages are given it is probably superior to long-acting benzodiazepines (Lader, 1979).

As temazepam is a short-acting benzodiazepine long-term therapy might be associated with the development of dependence, and a case has recently been reported (Ratna, 1981).

TRIAZOLAM

Triazolam has the shortest half-life of benzodiazepines currently marketed and has a duration of action of only about 4 h. It too is marketed as a hypnotic and as it is more potent than other benzodiazepines significantly lower doses are required. Clinical studies have shown that triazolam in a dose of only 0.25 mg at night is similar in efficacy to other benzodiazepine hypnotics (Bowen, 1978), and has little in the way of residual effects on waking (Mendelson *et al.*, 1976; Bowen, 1978). In geriatric patients the lower dose of 0.125 mg at night is often adequate (Lipani, 1978).

Because of its short duration of action triazolam appeared to be an improvement on the existing benzodiazepines and might have been expected to take its place quietly together with other compounds. However, a curious controversy developed in Holland in 1979 which led to the banning of the drug in that country. This followed allegations that the drug was responsible for a series of unusual side effects which were quite different from those of other benzodiazepines. Much of the debate for and against this hypothesis took place in the glare of publicity and has been criticized by Lasagna as an example of 'trial by media' (Lasagna, 1980). There is no other evidence, either before or since this episode, that suggests triazolam has a greater tendency to produce adverse effects than other benzodiazepines. For reasons already discussed it might be more likely to produce pharmacological dependence than longer acting benzodiazepines but many of the adverse reactions reported in Holland occurred after a few days of therapy.

CLOBAZAM

Clobazam differs from all other benzodiazepines in clinical use in that it is a 1,5-benzodiazepine (*Figure 6.7*). The structural change appears to be a relatively small one, with just a change in the positions of the carbon and nitrogen atoms in the seven-membered diazepine ring, but it leads to differences in its chemical and pharmacological properties (Kuch, 1979). Clinical studies of the compound show that it has similar properties to other benzodiazepines but that doses required to produce tranquillization and reduced aggression were lower than those that impaired psychomotor activity. Clobazam is also similar in anticonvulsant activity to diazepam.

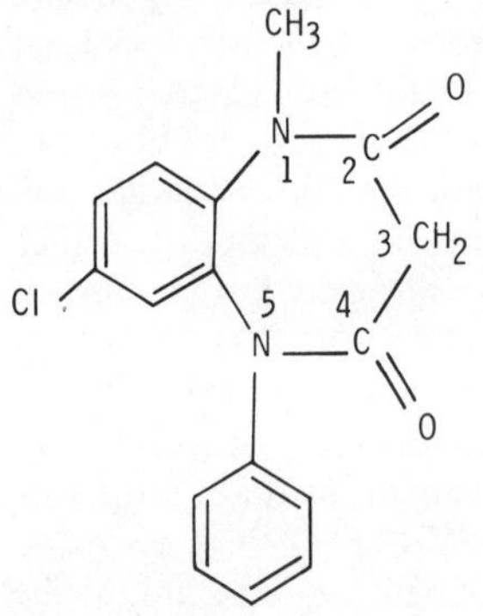

Figure 6.7 Clobazam (a 1,5-benzodiazepine)

The clinical effects of clobazam are partly due to the parent compound but are contributed to significantly by its major metabolite, N-desmethylclobazam, after regular dosage. N-desmethylclobazam has a half-life of up to 50 h and takes considerably longer than clobazam to reach steady state levels after regular dosage (Rupp *et al.*, 1979). For this reason clobazam is regarded as a long-acting benzodiazepine.

The evidence that clobazam has less effect on psychomotor performance than equivalent doses of other benzodiazepines is supported by a number of studies in different experimental situations (Doongaji *et al.*, 1978; Salkind, Hanks and Silverstone, 1979; Biehl, 1979) and implies that the antianxiety effects of clobazam are more 'pure' than those of other benzodiazepines as they can reduce anxiety without sedation. Despite these encouraging findings more evidence is needed from clinical studies in anxious patients that it is safe to take clobazam when operating machinery or engaged in other tasks that require fine coordination or a rapid reaction time.

LORMETAZEPAM

Lormetazepam is a recently introduced benzodiazepine marketed specifically for the treatment of insomnia. It has a short elimination half-life (10 h) and is metabolized mainly to inactive glucuronides, although more than 5 per cent is metabolized to lorazepam. It produces fewer hangover effects than flurazepam but more rebound insomnia on withdrawal (Oswald *et al.*, 1978), suggesting that it is as prone to dependence as other short-acting benzodiazepines. In other respects it behaves as other benzodiazepines and cannot be considered a therapeutic advance (*Drug and Therapeutics Bulletin*, 1981b).

CHOICE OF BENZODIAZEPINES

Between two and three benzodiazepines are introduced throughout the world each year. With such a number to choose from it might appear a particularly difficult task to decide which is most appropriate for a specific problem. In fact the choice is easy. Because so many benzodiazepines are pharmacodynamic replicas of other benzodiazepines they can be regarded as identical for all important clinical purposes. The 'benzodiazepine bonanza' (Tyrer, 1974) has continued unabated and has been replaced by the 'benzodiazepine bamboozle' (Lader, 1980) in that the justifications for introducing each new benzodiazepine become progressively more devious and abstruse. This makes it difficult to recognize a genuinely new benzodiazepine, such as clobazam.

For most psychiatric purposes it is only necessary to use two benzodiazepines, one with a long duration of action and one with a short one. In general, phobic disorders, 'pure' insomnia and acute stressful situations (e.g. public speaking) require a short-acting benzodiazepine and most other psychiatric disorders require a long-acting compound. Because there are personal idiosyncrasies in response to different benzodiazepines it is reasonable to have a third benzodiazepine available also; this might be one of the medium-acting ones. If further work shows clobazam to be consistently superior to other benzodiazepines in its effect on psychomotor function then clobazam may be the benzodiazepine of choice in the long-acting group. Until then, it is reasonable to choose one of the older compounds such as diazepam, because it is well tried and reliable, and also cheap. For the short-acting benzodiazepine there is little to choose between triazolam, temazepam and oxazepam, except that the potency of triazolam is such that it would be difficult to achieve dosages suitable for treating moderate or mild anxiety with the strength of tablet currently available. Oxazepam is considerably cheaper than the other two short-acting compounds.

There may be many other factors leading to the choice of another benzodiazepine in a specific instance. Anxious patients are notoriously fickle with regard to drug therapy; many have difficulty in swallowing tablets and prefer capsules, and some develop severe side effects with one compound only to have none at all when this is changed to a new compound that is virtually identical. It is important to realize that many of these apparent differences are psychological rather than pharmacological. For example, in one study in which chlordiazepoxide was given in the same strength but in different coloured capsules, it was found that the best response was achieved with green capsules and the worst response with yellow ones (Schapira *et al.*, 1970). One newspaper could not resist the obvious headline that 'yellows gave you the blues'. It is not uncommon to see psychiatric patients who have taken many different benzodiazepines during the course of a chronic anxiety state. Each time a change is made they appear to be improved but before long they are asking for a change as they 'seem to have got used to the tablets'. In most such cases the expected improvement that follows a change is entirely of psychological origin.

Lorazepam and diazepam are similar in efficacy when given intravenously in equivalent dosage but lorazepam may be preferred because of the lower risk of endothelial damage unless a special preparation of diazepam (e.g. Diazemuls) is chosen.

There is considerable variation in the recommended frequency of dosage and strength of tablet prescribed. This may be relevant when reducing a benzodiazepine after a long course of treatment. For reasons already discussed, a gradual reduction of tablets is recommended, but this is difficult with some benzodiazepines which only exist in a single dosage strength (e.g. clorazepate). In such cases benzodiazepines, such as diazepam or chlordiazepoxide, which exist in several dosage strengths may be preferable.

Other antianxiety drugs

There are several antianxiety drugs that are not benzodiazepines but which have a similar selectivity of action. Although they are pharmacologically different and have been introduced into antianxiety therapy independently they can usefully be considered together.

CHLORMETHIAZOLE

Structure and pharmacology
Chlormethiazole has a relatively simple structure developed from part of the vitamin B molecule (*Figure 6.8*). It is available in capsule form and also a syrup and for intravenous injection in the form of chlormethiazole edisylate. Pharmacologically chlormethiazole has similar properties to the benzodiazepines. It is markedly anticonvulsant and is an effective antianxiety drug and hypnotic. Its mode of action is uncertain but probably involves stimulation of GABA transmission in the brain. The pharmacokinetics of chlormethiazole are unusual. It is absorbed extremely rapidly by mouth, and when given in syrup form peak concentrations are achieved after only 20 min (Jostell *et al.*, 1978). It is rapidly metabolized to at

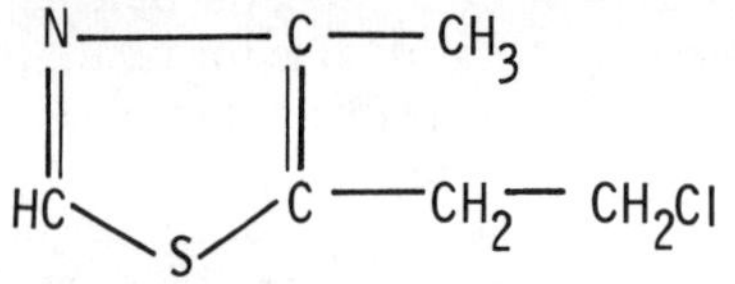

Figure 6.8 Chlormethiazole

least five metabolites and these probably play little part in the pharmacological activity of chlormethiazole. It has a mean elimination half-life of between 3–5 h and this has even been found in elderly subjects (Briggs, Castleden and Kraft, 1980).

Chlormethiazole is excreted very rapidly, even in patients with hepatic disease, and although the liver is the main route of excretion it is likely that extrahepatic routes are also involved. It has relatively few toxic effects and in this respect is similar to the benzodiazepines. Drowsiness, conjunctival and nasal irritation are the most common side effects. There is an additive effect with other central depressant drugs (including alcohol) and the patient should be warned about this. There are no other significant drug interactions.

Clinical studies have shown chlormethiazole to be an effective antianxiety drug and hypnotic (Middleton, 1978; Castleden, George and Sedgwick, 1979). As a hypnotic it compares favourably with temazepam, with 384 mg of chlormethiazole equivalent to 20 mg of temazepam (Briggs, Castleden and Kraft, 1980). Because of its short half-life no cumulation occurs with chlormethiazole after repeated dosage.

The major criticism of chlormethiazole is its capacity to produce pharmacological dependence. One influential report describing the danger of dependence with the drug (Hession, Verma and Mohan Bhakta, 1979) was criticized by others as overstating the dangers (Exton-Smith and McLean, 1979), as other addictive drugs, particularly alcohol, were taken with chlormethiazole. Whilst there is no doubt that chlormethiazole is potentially addictive, its frequently recommended use in the treatment of alcohol withdrawal (see Chapter 13) has involved a population that is particularly prone to addiction and may therefore be unrepresentative. Nevertheless, the potential for pharmacological dependence is such that it is best to avoid day time prescription of chlormethiazole for anxiety and to follow a rigid stepwise reduction of dosage in the treatment of alcoholism and drug withdrawal, so that therapy is completed within 10 d. Escalation of dosage does not appear to be a problem in elderly patients but mild dependence of the type seen with benzodiazepines may develop. This may be considered to be an acceptable risk in such patients, for whom chlormethiazole may be the preferred treatment because of its short duration of action, rapid metabolism and excretion.

BENZOCTAMINE

Benzoctamine is an unusual antianxiety agent that is unrelated to any other commercially available drugs. It is structurally a dibenzobicyclo-octadiene (*Figure 6.9*)

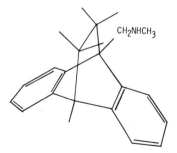

Figure 6.9 Benzoctamine

(Wilhelm and Schmidt, 1969) and its effects on animals include reduction of aggression and muscle tension. It has few toxic effects and is unusual amongst antianxiety drugs in that overdosage does not depress activity in the respiratory centre; it has the opposite effect of stimulating respiratory drive. Drug interactions are also few.

Although several studies show benzoctamine to be an effective antianxiety drug (Goldstein and Weiner, 1970; Lo and Lo, 1973) this holds no particular advantages except in patients with poor respiratory function. Although it has relatively few side effects these may still be a greater problem than with the benzodiazepines (Lo and Lo, 1973). The average daily consumption is 30–60 mg in divided dosage. There is no published evidence that it produces dependence but the drug has not been widely prescribed and it is unwise to be firm on this issue.

OXYPERTINE

Oxypertine is a neuroleptic drug and was originally introduced as a treatment for schizophrenia in the 1960s. It was not very successful, except in Japan (*see* p. 64), and in 1971 was marketed in much lower dosage as an antianxiety agent. It is mentioned here because although it has similar antianxiety effects to other neuroleptic drugs its main clinical use is in the treatment of anxiety and so it may appear to be different from other neuroleptic drugs. There is no evidence that it is superior to other neuroleptic drugs given in low dosage, despite optimistic claims soon after it was introduced (*Drug and Therapeutics Bulletin*, 1971).

CHLORMEZANONE

Chlormezanone is also a novel antianxiety drug that is said to be effective in patients who may not respond to other antianxiety agents. In many ways it is similar to meprobamate in its clinical effects (Friedman, Moskowitz and Rosen, 1966), but if a higher dosage is used (e.g. 800 mg daily) it is similar in efficacy to the benzodiazepines. Unfortunately at this dosage it produces significantly more sedation (Rickels *et al.*, 1974). The drug has been available in clinical practice for over 20 years and there are no reports of serious dangers. It may be regarded as an alternative to the benzodiazepines if there are particular reasons for not prescribing the latter.

Antipsychotic drugs

PHARMACOLOGY

In his review of antischizophrenic drugs in Chapter 4 Dr Mackay described the sedative properties of these compounds which occur largely as a result of their blockade of central α-noradrenergic receptors. Drugs that strongly block central α-noradrenergic receptors such as chlorpromazine, thioridazine and droperidol therefore produce more sedation than drugs that only have weak α-blocking activity. The antihistaminic activity of these drugs also contributes to their sedative effects. These properties are manifest in lower dosage than are required to achieve dopamine blockade.

CLINICAL USE

The sedative properties of antischizophrenic drugs have led to their marketing in two different dosage regimens; in high dosage for their antipsychotic effects, and in low dosage (about one-fifth of the high dosage) for the relief of anxiety and insomnia. The practitioner should therefore be very conscious of dosage when using these drugs. For example, the indole antipsychotic drug, oxypertine, was introduced as an anti-schizophrenic drug over 20 years ago with a recommended dosage of 100–300 mg. It was not particularly successful and ten years ago was re-introduced in the UK as an antianxiety drug (Integrin) with a recommended daily dosage of 20–60 mg.

All the antischizophrenic drugs can perform this dual role and those which are strongly sedative (e.g. thioridazine) given more often at night. The older drugs, chlorpromazine, trifluoperazine, prochlorperazine, perphenazine, fluphenazine, halo-peridol and flupenthixol are most frequently used for the treatment of anxiety in low dosage and there is no reason to choose one of the newer preparations. Prochlorperazine may also be particularly useful if nausea, giddiness and vertigo are associated with the anxiety because of the drug's central vestibular effects. Flupenthixol also has energizing and antidepressant effects (p. 231).

It is difficult to place the antipsychotic drugs in rank order of efficacy of anxiolytic action. They are clearly not specific antianxiety drugs and therefore cannot be superior to the benzodiazepines in this respect. Nevertheless the results of clinical trials comparing benzodiazepines with antischizophrenic drugs show no special superiority of the benzodiazepines. Greenblatt and Shader (1974), in reviewing the clinical trials of benzodiazepines published at that time, describe the results of 12 trials comparing a benzodiazepine with an antischizophrenic drug. In nine of these there was no difference in efficacy, in one the antischizophrenic drug was superior and in only two was the benzodiazepine superior. Comparison has not been made between antischizophrenic drugs and benzodiazepines as hypnotics and for this purpose benzodiazepines are almost certainly superior.

Antipsychotic drugs have relatively few unwanted effects in low dosage. In a few patients extrapyramidal symptoms such as tremor and rigidity may occur but other dystonic reactions are rare. Dizziness due to postural hypotension (another α-adrenergic blocking effect) and symptoms due to anticholinergic effects (dry mouth, constipation, etc.) are also possible but uncommon in low dosage. Other unwanted effects due to drug idiosyncrasy such as cholestatic jaundice and skin rashes occur in similar frequency no matter what dosage is given. Tardive dyskinesia has been discussed earlier. Although it is very rare with antischizophrenic drugs in low dosage its resistance to treatment makes it the most serious unwanted effect. For this reason treatment with antipsychotic drugs for anxiety should rarely be long term.

Pharmacological dependence with antipsychotic drugs is virtually unknown. Indeed, most patients are only too ready to reduce and stop their drugs as soon as their symptoms are relieved. In this respect antipsychotic drugs are quite different from the benzodiazepines, which tend to lead to demands for further prescription. If antianxiety drugs are required for short-term prescription in patients who are known to be prone to dependence it is reasonable to prescribe one of the antipsychotic drugs in low dosage.

Antidepressants

Antidepressant drugs have been discussed fully in other chapters and their antianxiety effects mentioned. This is not only relevant in treating anxiety associated with depression but also in anxiety states alone. With so many other antianxiety drugs available it is difficult to argue that antidepressants should have a specific place in treating anxiety in the absence of depression. Nevertheless the evidence that antidepressants are so often prescribed in low dosage well below those to relieve depression (Tyrer, 1978) suggests that antidepressants are being used primarily as sedatives. This form of prescription is defensible provided it is understood that any benefit noticed is not a consequence of a specific antidepressant effect. No antidepressant is specifically marketed as a hypnotic or antianxiety drug, although some tricyclic antidepressants, particularly amitriptyline and trimipramine, which frequently cause drowsiness (p. 207) are of equivalent efficacy to most marketed hypnotics when taken at night. Most practising clinicans will be aware of the depressed patient who when seen initially has been taking a hypnotic drug only. When an appropriate antidepressant is prescribed the hypnotic can usually be withdrawn without much difficulty.

Although it is seldom ideal to prescribe any drug primarily for one of its unwanted effects the use of antidepressants as antianxiety and hypnotic drugs is close to becoming an established clinical indication, forcing our attention through usage rather than through drug marketing or the advice of clinical pharmacology.

Combined preparations including antianxiety drugs

There are many combined psychotropic drugs incorporating two or more compounds in one capsule or tablet. Antianxiety drugs are probably the most commonly used in these combinations. They have been combined with antidepressants because of the known association between anxiety and depressive symptoms. The combinations used in the UK are illustrated in *Table 6.7*. Although this may seem rational there are many

TABLE 6.7 Combination drugs used for the treatment of anxiety and depression

Drug type— antianxiety drug	Drug type— other drug	Trade names	Constituent drugs
Benzodiazepines	Tricyclic antidepressants	Limbitrol-5 Limbitrol-10	Chlordiazepoxide Amitriptyline (in different dosage)
Antischizophrenic drug	Tricyclic antidepressant	Triptafen-DA Triptafen-Minor	Perphenazine
		Triptafen-Forte	Amitriptyline (in different dosage)
		Motival	Fluphenazine Nortriptyline
		Motipress	Fluphenazine Nortriptyline
Antischizophrenic drug	MAOI	Parstelin	Tranylcypromine Trifluoperazine

reasons for decrying the use of these combinations. Ignorance of the ingredients is much more common when several drugs are combined under one trade name and exposure to dangerous drug interactions may therefore occur unwittingly. More important criticism comes from the pharmacodynamic differences between antianxiety and antidepressant drugs. Antianxiety drugs act within hours and are best taken in flexible dosage controlled by clinical response, but antidepressants need to be taken regularly for several weeks before the full antidepressant effects are shown. The immediate effects should not influence dosage unless they are negative and unpleasant, in which case change to a different drug or revision of dosage (e.g. to once daily dosage at night) will be necessary.

When both antianxiety and antidepressant drugs are taken in the same tablet it is very difficult to achieve both these requirements. The drugs are given in fixed combination and so make no allowance for pharmacokinetic differences in the absorption and metabolism of each member. If the doctor is very lucky both the antianxiety and antidepressant drugs could be given in the correct dosage but even then the need to maintain regular dosage for the antidepressants will lead to the incorrect use of the antianxiety component.

In practice most patients take a relatively low dose which is inadequate to produce true antidepressant effects. The combination drug then becomes a combination of two antianxiety drugs and offers no advantages over one drug alone. If antianxiety and antidepressant effects are both required it is best to prescribe the drugs separately in appropriate dosage or to give an antidepressant such as doxepin or flupenthixol which has both antidepressant and anxiolytic actions.

Peripheral anxiolytics

Beta-adrenoceptor blocking drugs

INTRODUCTION

Beta-adrenoceptor blocking drugs were introduced to medicine 20 years ago and their main clinical use has been in cardiovascular disorders, particularly in the treatment of angina and hypotension. Their antianxiety effects were first suspected in 1965 when it was noted that propranolol reduced the pulse rate of anxious patients to a significantly greater extent than in control subjects (Turner, Granville-Grossman and Smart, 1965). These marked physiological changes suggested that anxious patients might benefit from receiving a beta-blocking drug and in 1966 Granville-Grossman and Turner reported the results of a clinical trial in which propranolol was compared with placebo in a cross-over design. After both drugs had been taken under double-blind conditions a choice was made between the two agents. Propranolol proved to be significantly superior to placebo. Later studies have confirmed that other beta-blocking drugs, including practolol (Bonn, Turner and Hicks, 1972), sotalol (Tyrer and Lader, 1973) and oxprenolol (McMillin, 1973) all have similar antianxiety effects and are superior to placebo. This work established that beta-blocking drugs were definitely efficacious in the treatment of anxiety but did not establish whether they were superior to other antianxiety treatment.

PHARMACOLOGY AND TOXICOLOGY

The structure of the most commonly used beta-adrenoceptor blocking drug, propranolol is illustrated (*Figure 6.10a*). The literature on the pharmacology of beta-blockade is an extensive one but most of it is beyond the scope of psychiatry. In summary, catecholamines, which are structurally similar to the beta-blocking drugs (*Figure 6.10b*), have been shown to act on two types of receptors, alpha- and beta-receptors, which are present in the effector organs. In general, the alpha-agonist effects are inhibitory and the beta-agonist ones excitatory (*Table 6.8*). Because of this the beta-blocking drugs have received the most attention in the treatment of anxiety, as it has been

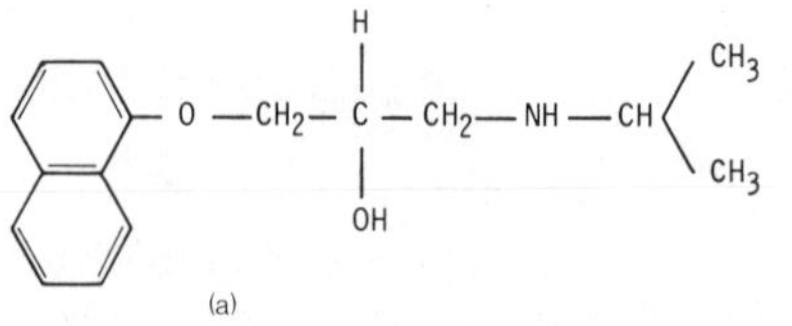

Figure 6.10a Propranolol

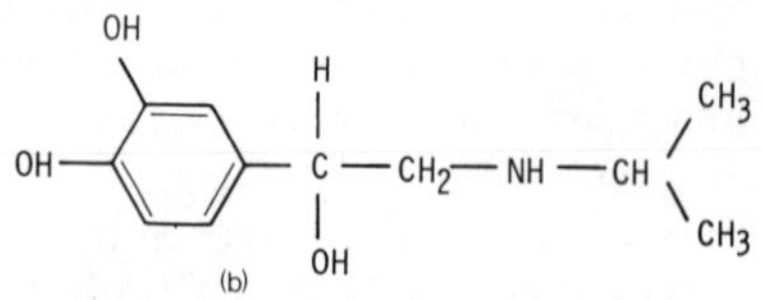

Figure 6.10b Isoprenaline

known for many years that excess catecholamine secretion accompanies anxious disorders (von Euler and Lundberg, 1954).

There has been argument whether or not the mechanism of antianxiety action of beta-blocking drugs in anxiety is due to a central or peripheral effect. In general, the evidence favours a predominantly peripheral mechanism as

(1) beta-blocking drugs that do not pass the blood–brain barrier, such as practolol, are similar in their antianxiety effects to other beta-blockers that readily enter the brain (Bonn, Turner and Hicks, 1972),
(2) the dextroisomers of beta-blocking drugs have no beta-blocking activity and also no antianxiety effects (Bonn and Turner, 1971),
(3) the dosage used to alleviate anxiety is relatively low and in this dosage no central effects can be detected (Lader and Tyrer, 1972).

The mechanism by which beta-blocking drugs alleviate anxiety through peripheral blockade is thought to be through interruption of the feedback loop between perception of autonomic and somatic symptoms of anxiety and the reinforcement of centrally produced anxiety because of this awareness (Breggin, 1964; Granville-Grossman and Turner, 1966). This does not necessarily explain why some patients

TABLE 6.8. Classification of adrenergic receptors

Effector organ	Response to stimulation	Receptor type
Arteries	Vasoconstriction	alpha
Arteries	Vasodilatation	beta
Heart–sino-auricular node	Increased frequency of firing	beta
Heart–atrio-ventricular node	Increased frequency of firing	beta
Heart–ventricle	Increased force of contraction	beta
Bronchial muscle	Relaxation	beta
Gastrointestinal sphincters	Contraction	alpha
Urethral sphincters	Contraction	alpha
Uterus	Contraction (usually)	alpha
Stomach	Relaxation	alpha and beta
Intestine	Relaxation	alpha and beta
Radial muscle of iris	Contraction	alpha
Ciliary muscle	Relaxation	beta
Submaxillary gland	Secretion	alpha

NB Metabolic effects are not included as it is doubtful whether these are true alpha or beta effects persistently express their anxiety in a somatic manner, often picking out one of the bodily channels of anxious expression to the exclusion of all others. It is when these channels are those affected by beta-stimulation, particularly cardiac symptoms and tremor, that treatment with beta-blocking drugs is so effective (Tyrer, 1976). What is against the 'feedback hypothesis' is that patients who express their anxiety somatically and improve with beta-blocking drugs often relapse when the drug is withdrawn, even though the feedback loop has been broken (*Lancet*, 1981).

An alternative view is that beta-blocking drugs act centrally by reducing basal levels of anxiety independently of aroused anxiety (Gottschalk, Stone and Gleser, 1974). Although there are beta-adrenergic receptors in the brain their relationship to anxiety is far from clear. As it is still not known how beta-blocking drugs exert their hypotensive effects it is unlikely that receptor theory will provide an early answer to the antianxiety effects. What is undoubtedly clear is that the antianxiety effects are not just sedative ones. There can be impairment of central nervous function after beta-blockade but this is dose-related, with only one positive central effect (impaired reaction time) reported in the dosage range used to treat anxiety (i.e. propranolol 40–120 mg daily or equivalent dosage of other beta-blockers) (Turner, 1977).

PHARMACOKINETICS

Beta-blocking drugs are readily absorbed by mouth and produce physiological evidence of beta-blockade within 1 h of administration. They are metabolized mainly in the liver and as their elimination half-lives are short there is no significant cumulation in chronic dosage. Plasma levels are generally correlated with beta-blocking effects but in the only anxiety study which recorded plasma levels there was no apparent relationship although relief of anxiety occurred with plasma concentrations between 5 and 56 ng·ml^{-1} (Tyrer, 1976, p. 84). Studies on patients with essential tremor have suggested that satisfactory reduction of tremor is achieved with plasma levels of less than 40 mg·ml^{-1} and that there is nothing to be gained by exceeding this level (Jefferson, Jenner and Marsden, 1979a).

CLINICAL USE

The place of beta-blocking drugs in the treatment of anxiety is still not clear. Although there are now many studies that demonstrate that beta-blockers are more effective than placebo in relieving anxiety (Jefferson, 1974; Tyrer, 1980; Noyes *et al.*, 1981), this is itself not an adequate reason to prescribe them, particularly when alternatives such as the benzodiazepines are available. Comparisons between beta-blocking drugs and benzodiazepines are relatively few. For most anxious patients benzodiazepines are superior in efficacy (Tyrer and Lader, 1974a; Hallstrom *et al.*, 1981) or, if equivalent, offer no particular advantages to the beta-blocking drug (Jefferson, 1974; Wheatley, 1969).

Beta-blocking drugs have been reported as having differential effects in somatic and psychic anxiety (Tyrer and Lader, 1974a), with somatically anxious patients showing a superior response equivalent to that of diazepam. Other studies have also shown that somatic complaints, particularly tremor, cardiac and respiratory symptoms, are preferentially helped by beta-blockade (Hartvig and Fjerdingstad, 1974; Kathol *et al.*, 1980). This concept of somatic anxiety is different from mere somatic symptoms, and is better termed somatosthenic anxiety, as the patients regard their major problems as somatic in nature, often denying anxiety altogether. This explains why many patients with diagnostic labels such as neurocirculatory asthenia, hyperventilation syndrome, hyperdynamic circulatory state and effort syndrome do so well when treated with beta-blocking drugs (Marsden, 1971). Their symptoms represent the extreme of somatic anxiety (Tyrer, 1976). From our knowledge of the physiological effects of beta-blockade, cardiac, respiratory and tremor symptoms should be those most helped by beta-blockade and this is confirmed in clinical practice (Tyrer and Lader, 1974b). Somatic symptoms such as sweating, nausea, dizziness and bowel disturbance are not helped by beta-blockade. The benefit of beta-blocking drugs for treating drug and alcohol withdrawal (pp. 148 and 361) is also likely to be mediated through somatic and autonomic pathways.

If somatic symptoms are associated with high levels of anxiety and not perceived to be primary problems then beta-blocking drugs are relatively ineffective (Hallstrom *et al.*, 1981). The same has been found with clinical phobic disorder such as agoraphobia, in which reduction of somatic symptoms appears to confer no beneficial effects (Hafner and Milton, 1977). If, however, the somatic symptoms in the phobic situation are the sole complaint, such as the trembling of the musician in an orchestra or the palpitations of the public speaker, beta-blocking drugs are beneficial (Taggart, Carruthers and Somerville, 1973; James *et al.*, 1977).

The length of therapy with beta-blocking drugs is uncertain. In patients who derive benefit treatment is usually needed for at least six months and if reduced too early relapse may occur. Dosage is considerably lower than that used to treat schizophrenia (Chapter 4) and usually lower than is used in treating hypertension. Approximate dosages for treating anxiety are propranolol $(40–120 \, mg \cdot d^{-1})$, oxprenolol $(80–240 \, mg \cdot d^{-1})$, sotalol $(60–80 \, mg \cdot d^{-1})$ and acebutolol $(100–300 \, mg \cdot d^{-1})$. Because the symptoms are intermittent it is best to take the drugs in flexible dosage between one and three times daily.

DIFFERENCES BETWEEN BETA-BLOCKING DRUGS

The beta-blockers are divided into those with partial agonist activity, which have intrinsic sympathomimetic effects, and those without this property, and can also be separated into cardioselective drugs, which have a selective action on $\beta 1$ receptors in the heart, and non-selective drugs which block $\beta 1$ and $\beta 2$ receptors. $\beta 2$ receptors are present in the respiratory tract and in patients prone to asthma non-selective beta-blockers may precipitate attacks. These differences are of little importance in psychiatric disorders, although there is some evidence that cardioselective beta-blocking drugs are less effective in reducing abnormal tremor than non-selective ones (Jefferson, Jenner and Marsden, 1979b).

UNWANTED EFFECTS

Although in high dosage beta-blocking drugs may produce drowsiness, light-headedness and, in rare instances, visual hallucinations (Stephen, 1966; Tyrer and Lader, 1973), these are not found in the low dosage used to treat anxiety. Depression has been reported as an unwanted effect in hypertensive patients treated with propranolol (Waal, 1967) but the relationship of this to drug treatment is disputed (Fitzgerald, 1967). Because asthma may be precipitated in susceptible subjects a cardioselective beta-blocker is preferable in patients with a past history of asthma.

The major concern with chronic use of beta-blocking drugs is the risk of idiosyncratic drug reactions, particularly sclerosing inflammatory disease in the eye, peritoneum and other mucous membranes, and neurovascular disorders such as Raynaud's phenomenon. These disorders have occasionally been reported in long-term treatment of cardiac patients (*Lancet*, 1978) and are more common with practolol, which is now rarely prescribed. Practolol cannot be recommended for use in psychiatry for this reason. The risk with other beta-blockers is small but should be taken into account in long-term therapy.

DRUG INTERACTIONS AND COMBINATION THERAPY

Beta-blocking drugs are generally safe and there are no absolute contraindications to their use with other drugs, although care must be taken when they are combined with sympathomimetic amines (e.g. ephedrine) and cimetidine because of potentiation of their effects. Beta-blocking drugs and clonidine are best avoided in combination because of the risk of hypertension following clonidine withdrawal. Occasionally hypoglycaemia may occur and diabetic patients may need a revised dosage of insulin or oral hypoglycaemic drugs.

Because beta-blocking drugs are most commonly used in the treatment of anxiety they are often combined with benzodiazepines in clinical practice. A recent study showed combined diazepam and propranolol treatment of chronic anxiety to be more effective than either drug alone (Hallstrom *et al.*, 1981), supporting a synergistic action of the two drugs.

SUMMARY

Beta-blocking drugs are effective in reducing anxiety and the somatic symptoms associated with cardiac functional disorders and minor phobias. They do not produce pharmacological dependence or impair cerebral function in the low dosage need to treat these disorders and thereby offer advantages over the benzodiazepines. However, they are generally less effective than the benzodiazepines and will seldom be preferred for the treatment of severe anxiety. Combination therapy with benzodiazepines is highly effective and may be particularly useful when patients taking a benzodiazepine alone are unable to keep their dosage within the therapeutic range.

Other peripheral anxiolytics

There are no other peripheral anxiolytics currently used to any extent in psychiatry. The combination of alpha- and beta-blocking activity might be thought valuable in reducing the bodily symptoms of anxiety but the only drug available with these properties, labetalol, has not been used for this purpose. Alpha-blockers such as phentolamine and phenoxybenzamine, have too many side effects to justify their use, but a recent introduction, indoramin, may be worthy of study. Antihistamines such as promethazine, cyclizine, mepyramine and chlorpheniramine, may be highly effective in treating nausea and other gastrointestinal symptoms but they act centrally. As they also produce sedation they could be regarded as antianxiety drugs and are often used as hypnotics in young children.

One of the first drug treatments of anxiety was intravenous acetylcholine, given in an attempt to 'neutralize' the sympathetic arousal of anxiety. Good results were reported (Phillips and Hutchinson, 1954) and later studies were carried out in patients with agoraphobia, again with encouraging results (Sim and Houghton, 1966). As these studies were not controlled trials and as the enthusiasm of the therapists is clear from

TABLE 6.9 Comparison of antianxiety drugs

	Barbiturates	Propanediols	Chloral derivatives	Neuroleptic drugs	Benzodiazepines	Beta-adrenoceptor blocking drugs	Chlormethiazole
Antianxiety efficacy	Fair	Fair	Fair	Good	Excellent	Fair	Good
Hypnotic efficacy	Good	Fair	Good	Fair	Excellent	None	Excellent
Safety	Very poor	Good	Good	Fair	Excellent	Good	Good
Unwanted effects	Common	Occasional	Occasional	Occasional	Rare	Rare	Rare
Risk of dependence	High	Moderate	Low	Very low	Moderate	None	Moderate
Drug interactions	Common	Occasional	Occasional	Occasional	Rare	Occasional	Occasional

their published reports it is usually assumed that the improvement shown by the patient was independent of acetylcholine. However, no-one has repeated this work and the possibility that intravenous acetylcholine has anxiolytic effects should not be discounted.

Comparison of antianxiety drugs

It is difficult to condense the details of antianxiety drug therapy in a way that makes comparison possible but in *Table 6.9* their main therapeutic and unwanted effects are shown. The choice of drug will depend on many considerations and general guidelines oversimplify the issues, so the prescriber has to make his own decision. It will depend on his experience of the drugs, the likely duration of treatment, the age of the patient and response to previous therapy, among many other factors. Good therapy will rarely involve the drug alone and the doctor can only compliment himself that a satisfactory response has been made to treatment when the patient has stopped therapy and remained well.

References

AHLQUIST, R. P. A study of the adrenotropic receptors, *American Journal of Physiology* **153**, 586–600 (1948)

ALMEYDA, J and LEVANTINE, A. Drug Reactions. XVII. Cutaneous reactions to barbiturates, chloral hydrate and its derivatives, *British Journal of Dermatology* **86**, 313–316 (1972)

AMEER, B. and GREENBLATT, D. J. Lorazepam: a review of its clinical pharmacological properties and therapeutic uses, *Drugs* **21**, 161–200 (1981)

AYD, F. J. Benzodiazepines: dependance and withdrawal, *Journal of the American Medical Association* **242**, 1401–1402 (1979)

BALTER, M. B. and LEVINE, J. O. The nature and extent of psychotropic drug usage in the United States, *Psychopharmacological Bulletin* **5**, 3–13 (1969)

BARKER, J. C. and RANSOM, B. R. Pentobarbitone pharmacology of mammalian central neurons grown in tissue culture, *Journal of Physiology* **280**, 355–372 (1978)

BARSA, J. A. and SAUNDERS, J. C. Tybamate, a new tranquilizer, *American Journal of Psychiatry* **120**, 492–493 (1963)

BERGER, F. M. The pharmacological properties of 2-methyl-2-*n*-propyl-1, 3-propanediol dicarbonate ('Milton'), a new interneuronal blocking agent, *Journal of Pharmacological and Experimental Therapy* **112**, 413–423 (1954)

BETTS, T. A., CLAYTON, A. S. and MACKAY, G. M. Effects of four commonly used tranquillisers on low-speed driving performance tests, *British Medical Journal* **4**, 580–584 (1972)

BIEHL, B. Studies of clobazam and car-driving, *British Journal of Clinical Pharmacology* **7**, 85s–90s (1979)

BOND, A. J. and LADER, M. H. Residual effects of hypnotics, *Psychopharmacologia* **25**, 117–132 (1972)

BOND, A. J. and LADER, M. H. The residual effects of flurazepam, *Psychopharmacologia* **32**, 223–235 (1973)

BOND, A. J., HAILEY, D. M. and LADER, M. H. Plasma concentrations of benzodiazepines, *British Journal of Clinical Pharmacology* **4**, 51–56 (1977)

BONN, J. A. and TURNER, P. D-Propranolol and anxiety, *Lancet* **1**, 1355–1356 (1971)

BONN, J. A., TURNER, P. and HICKS, D. C. Beta-adrenergic-receptor blockade with practolol in treatment of anxiety, *Lancet* **1**, 814–815 (1972)

BOSTON COLLABORATIVE DRUG SURVEILLANCE PROGRAM. Clinical depression of the central nervous system due to diazepam and chlodiazepoxide in relation to cigarette smoking and age, *New England Journal of Medicine* **288**, 277–280 (1973)

BOWEN, A. J. Comparative efficacy of triazolam, flurazepam and placebo in out-patient insomniacs, *Journal of International Medical Research* **6**, 337–342 (1978)

BRAESTRUP, C. and NIELSEN, M. Benzodiazepine receptors, *Arzneimiltel-Forschung* **30**, 852–857 (1980)

BRECKENRIDGE, A. and ORME, M. Clinical implications of enzyme induction, *Annals of the New York Academy of Science* **179**, 421–431 (1971)

BREGGIN, P. The psychophysiology of anxiety with a review of the literature concerning adrenaline, *Journal of Nervous and Mental Diseases* **139**, 558–568 (1964)

BREIMER, D. D., JOCHEMSEN, R. and VON ALBERT, H. H. Pharmacokinetics of benzodiazepines: short-acting versus long-acting. *Arzneimittel-Forschung* **30**, 875–881 (1980)

BRIGGS, R. S., CASTLEDEN, C. M. and KRAFT, C. A. Improved hypnotic treatment using chlormethiazole and temazepam, *British Medical Journal* **280**, 601–604 (1980)

CAMERON, J. M. Advances in toxicology, *Practitioner* **207**, 543–548 (1971)

CASTLEDEN, C. M., GEORGE, C. F. and SEDGWICK, E. M. Chlormethiazole – no hangover effect but not an ideal hypnotic for the young, *Postgraduate Medical Journal* **55**, 159–160 (1979)

CASTLEDEN, C. M., GEORGE, C. F., MARCER, D. and HALLETT, C. Increased sensitivity to nitrazepam in old age, *British Medical Journal* **1**, 10–12 (1977)

CHIEN, C. P., STOTSKY, B. A. and COLE, J. O. Psychiatric treatment for nursing home patients: drug, alcohol and milieu, *American Journal of Psychiatry* **130**, 543–548 (1973)

CLARE, A. W. Diazepam, alcohol, and barbiturate abuse, *British Medical Journal* **4**, 340 (1971)

COMMITTEE ON THE REVIEW OF MEDICINES. Systematic review of the benzodiazepines, *British Medical Journal* **280**, 910–912 (1980)

CONNEY, A. H. Pharmacological implications of microsomal enzyme induction, *Pharmacological Review* **19**, 317–366 (1967)

CONNEY, A. H., DAVISON, C., GASTEL, R. and BURNS, J. J. Adaptive increases in drug-metabolising enzymes induced by phenobarbital and other drugs, *Journal of Pharmacology and Experimental Therapy* **130**, 1–8 (1960)

COVI, L., LIPMAN, R. S., PATTISON, J. H., DEROGATIS, L. R. and UHLENHUTH, E. Length of treatment with anxiolytic sedatives and response to their sudden withdrawal, *Acta Psychiatrica Scandinavica* **49**, 51–64 (1973)

CRANKSHAW, D. P. and RAPER, C. Some studies on peripheral actions of mephenesin, methocarbonal and diazepam, *British Journal of Pharmacology* **34**, 579–590 (1968)

CRANKSHAW, D. P. and RAPER, C. Mephenesin, methocarbanol, chlordiazepoxide and diazepam: actions on spinal reflexes and ventral root potentials, *British Journal of Pharmacology* **38**, 148–156 (1970)

CUCINELL, S. A., ODESSKY, L., WEISS, M. and DAYTON, P. G. The effect of chloral hydrate on bishydroxycoumarin metabolism: a fatal outcome. *Journal of the American Medical Association* **197**, 366–368 (1966)

DOLLERY, C. T. Pharmacokinetics – master or servant, *European Journal of Clinical Pharmacology* **6**, 1-2 (1973)

DOONGAJI, D. R., SHETH, A., APTE, J. S., LAKDAWALA, P. D., KHARE, C. B. and THATTE, S. S. Clobazam versus diazepam – a double-blind study in anxiety neurosis, *Journal of Clinical Pharmacology* **18**, 358–364 (1978)

DRUG AND THERAPEUTICS BULLETIN. Oxypertine **9**, 94–95 (1971)

DRUG AND THERAPEUTICS BULLETIN. How to get patients off barbiturates **14**, 11–12 (1976)

DRUG AND THERAPEUTICS BULLETIN. Therapeutic differences between benzodiazepines **16**, 46–48 (1978)

DRUG AND THERAPEUTICS BULLETIN. Yet another benzodiazepine **18**, 94–95 (1980)

DRUG AND THERAPEUTICS BULLETIN. Local problems of injecting some benzodiazepines **19**, 11–12 (1981a)

DRUG AND THERAPEUTICS BULLETIN, Lormetazepam – another benzodiazepine, (In press) (1981b)

DUNDEE, J. W. and PANDIT, S. K. Anterograde amnesic effects of pethidine, hyoscine and diazepam in adults, *British Journal of Pharmacology* **44**, 140–144 (1972)

EINARSON, T. R. Lorazepam withdrawal seizures, *Lancet* **1**, 151 (1980)

EULER, U. S. VON and LUNDBERG, U. Effect of flying on the epinephrine excretion in airforce personnel, *Journal of Applied Psychology* **6**, 551–555 (1954)

EXTON-SMITH, A. N. and McLEAN, A. E. Uses and abuses of chlormethiazole, *Lancet* **1**, 1093 (1979)

FABRE, L. F., McLENDON, D. M. and GAINEY, A. Double-blind comparison of ketazolam administered once a day with diazepam and placebo in anxious out-patients, *Current Therapeutic Research* **24**, 875–883 (1978)

FAVAZZA, A. R. and MARTIN, P. Chemotherapy of delirium tremens: a survey of physicians' preferences, *American Journal of Psychiatry* **131**, 1030–1033 (1974)

FEMI-PEARSE, D. Experience with diazepam in tetanus, *British Medical Journal* **2**, 862–865 (1966)

FITZGERALD, J. D. Propranolol-induced depression, *British Medical Journal* **2**, 372–373 (1967)

FRIEDMAN, D., MOSKOWITZ, M. D. and ROSEN, M. Effects of chlormezanone on anxiety and tension: a double-blind study, *Current Therapeutic Research* **8**, 7–11 (1966)

FRUENSGAARD, K. Withdrawal psychosis: a study of 30 consecutive cases, *Acta Psychiatrica Scandinavica* **53**, 105–118 (1976)

FUCCELLA, L. M., BOLCIONI, G., TAMASSIA, V., FERRARIO, L. and TOGNONI, G. Human pharmacokinetics and bioavailability of temazepam administered in soft gelatine capsules, *European Journal of Clinical Pharmacology* **12**, 383–386 (1977)

FUJIMORI, H. Potentiation of barbital hypnosis as an evaluation method for central nervous system depressants, *Psychopharmacologica* **7**, 374–378 (1965)

GARATTINI, S., MUSSINI, E. and RANDALL, L. O. *The Benzodiazepines*, Raven Press, New York (1973)

GOLDBERG, H. L. and FINNERTY, R. J. Comparative efficacy of tofisopam and placebo, *American Journal of Psychiatry* **136**, 196–199 (1979)

GOLDSTEIN, B. J. and WEINER, D. M. Comparative evaluation of benzoctamine and diazepam in the treatment of anxiety, *Journal of Clinical Pharmacology* **10**, 194–198 (1970)

GORDON, E. B. Addiction to diazepam (Valium), *British Medical Journal* **1**, 112 (1967)

GOTTSCHALK, L. A., STONE, W. N. and GLESER, G. C. Peripheral versus central mechanisms accounting for antianxiety effect of propranolol, *Psychosomatic Medicine* **36**, 47–56 (1974)

GRANVILLE-GROSSMAN, K. L. and TURNER, P. The effect of propranolol on anxiety, *Lancet* **1**, 788–790 (1966)

GREENBERG, G., INMAN, W. H. W., WEATHERALL, J. A. C., ADELSTEIN, A. M. and HASKEY, J. C. Maternal drug histories and congenital abnormalities, *British Medical Journal* **2**, 853–856 (1977)

GREENBLATT, D. J. and SHADER, R. I. *Benzodiazepines in Clinical Practice*, Raven Press, New York (1974)

GREENBLATT, D. J. and SHADER, R. I. Prazepam and lorazepam, two new benzodiazepines, *New England Journal of Medicine* **299**, 1342–1344 (1978)

GREENBLATT, D. J., ALLEN, M. D. and SHADER, R. I. Toxicity of high dose flurazepam in the elderly, *Clinical Pharmacological Therapy* **21**, 355–361 (1977)

GREENBLATT, D. J., SHADER, R. I. and KOCH-WESER, J. Slow absorption of intramuscular chlordiazepoxide, *New England Journal of Medicine* **291**, 1116–1118 (1974)

GREENBLATT, D. J., SHADER, R. I., FRANKE, K., MACLAUGHLIN, D. S., HARMATZ, J. S., ALLEN, M. D., WERNER, A. and WOO, E. Pharmacokinetics and bioavailability of intravenous, intramuscular and oral lorazepam in humans, *Journal of Pharmaceutical Science* **68**, 57–63 (1979)

GREENBLATT, D. J., LAUGHREN, T. P., ALLEN, M. D., HARMATZ, J. S. and SHADER, R. I. Plazma diazepam and desmethyldiazepam concentrations during long-term diazepam therapy, *British Journal of Clinical Pharmacology* **11**, 35–40 (1981)

GREGG, E. and AKHTER, I. Chlormethiazole abuse, *British Journal of Psychiatry* **134**, 627–629 (1979)

GRIFFITHS, A. P. W. and SYLVESTER, P. E. Clinical trial of diazepam in adult cerebral palsy, *Annals of Physical Medicine*, Suppl. 25–29 (1964)

HAEFELY, W. E. Central actions of benzodiazepines: general introduction, *British Journal of Psychiatry* **133**, 231–238 (1978)

HAFNER, J. and MARKS, I. Exposure *in vivo* of agoraphobics: contributions of diazepam, group exposure and anxiety evocation, *Psychological Medicine* **6**, 71–88 (1976)

HAFNER, J. and MILTON, F. The influence of propranolol on the exposure *in vivo* of agoraphobics, *Psychological Medicine* **7**, 417–425 (1977)

HAIDER, I. A double-blind controlled trial of a non-barbiturate hypnotic – nitrazepam, *British Journal of Psychiatry* **114**, 337–343 (1968)

HALLSTROM, C., TREASADEN, I., EDWARDS, J. G. and LADER, M. Diazepam, propranolol and their combination in the management of chronic anxiety, *British Journal of Psychiatry* **139**, 417–421 (1981)

HAMILTON, M. The assessment of anxiety states by rating, *British Journal of Medical Psychology* **32**, 50–55 (1959)

HARRY, T. V. A. and LATHAM, A. N. Hypnotic and residual effects of temazepam in volunteers, *British Journal of Clinical Pharmacology* **9**, 618–620 (1980)

HARTVIG, P. and FJERDINGSTAD, S. Betablokkere; psykiatrien, *Nordisk Psykiatrisk Tidsskrift* **28**, 547–553 (1974)

HESSION, M. A., VERMA, S. and MOHAN BHAKTA, K. G. Dependence on chlormethiazole and effects of its withdrawal, *Lancet* **1**, 953–954 (1979)

HILLESTAD, L., HANSEN, T. and MELSOM, H. Diazepam metabolism in normal man. Serum concentration and clinical effect after oral administration and cumulation, *Clinical and Pharmacological Therapy* **16**, 485–489 (1974)

HINDMARCH, I. Effects of hypnotic and sleep-inducing drugs on objective assessments of human psychomotor performance and subjective appraisals of sleep and early morning behaviour, *British Journal of Clinical Pharmacology* **8**, Suppl. 1, 43–46 (1979)

HINDMARCH, I. and GUDGEON, A. C. The effects of clobazam and lorazepam on aspects of psychomotor performance and car handling ability, *British Journal of Clinical Pharmacology* **10**, 145–150 (1980)

HOLLISTER, L. E. and GLAZENER, F. S. Withdrawal reactions from meprobamate, alone and combined with promazine: a controlled study, *Psychopharmacologia* **1**, 336–341 (1960)

HOLLISTER, L. E., MOTZENBECKER, F. P. and DEGAN, R. O. Withdrawal reaction from chlordiazepoxide (Librium), *Psychopharmacologia* **2**, 63–68 (1961)

HORROBIN, D. F., GHAYUR, J. and KARMALI, R. A. Mind and cancer, *Lancet* **1**, 978 (1979)

HOWE, J. G. Lorazepam withdrawal seizures, *British Medical Journal* **280**, 1163–1164 (1980)

HUDSON, R. D. and WOLPERT, M. K. Central muscle relaxant effects of diazepam, *Neuropharmacologica* **9**, 481–488 (1970)

HUGGETT, A., FLANAGAN, R. J., COOK, P., CROME, P. and CORLESS, D. Chlormethiazole and temazepam, *British Medical Journal* **282**, 475 (1981)

ISBELL, H., ALTSCHUL, S., KORNETSKY, C. H., EISENMAN, A. J., FLANARY, H. G. and FRASER, H. F. Chronic barbiturate intoxication, *Archives of Neurology and Psychiatry* **64**, 1–16 (1950)

JACKSON, M. R. and HARRIS, P. A. Absence of effect of diazepam on tumours, *Lancet* **1**, 104 (1981)

JAMES, I. M., GRIFFITHS, D. N. W., PEARSON, R. M. and NEWBURY, P. Effect of oxprenolol on stage-fright in musicians, *Lancet* **2**, 952–954 (1977)

JEFFERSON, D., JENNER, P. and MARSDEN, C. D. Relationship between plasma propranolol concentration and relief of essential tremor, *Journal of Neurology, Neurosurgery and Psychiatry* **42**, 831–837 (1979a)

JEFFERSON, D., JENNER, P. and MARSDEN, C. D. Beta-adrenoceptor antagonists in essential tremor, *Journal of Neurology, Neurosurgery and Psychiatry* **42**, 904–909 (1979b)

JEFFERSON, J. W. Beta-adrenergic receptor blocking drugs in psychiatry, *Archives of General Psychiatry* **31**, 681–691 (1974)

JOSTELL, K-G., AGURELL, S., ALLGÉN, L-G., KUYLENSTIERNA, B., LINGREN, J-E., ÅBERG, G. and ÖSTERLÖF, G. Pharmacokinetics of clomethiazole in healthy subjects. *Acta Pharmacology and Toxicology* **43**, 180–189 (1978)

KALES, A., SCHARF, M. B. and KALES J. D. Rebound insomnia: a new clinical syndrome, *Science* **201**, 1039–1041 (1978)

KALES, A., ALLEN, C., SCHARF, M. B. and KALES, J. D. Hypnotic drugs and their effectiveness. All-night E.E.G. studies of insomniac patients, *Archives of General Psychiatry* **23**, 226–232 (1970a)

KALES, A., PRESTON, T. A., TAN, T-L. and ALLEN, C. Hypnotics and altered sleep–dream patterns, *Archives of General Psychiatry* **23**, 211–218 (1970b)

KALES, A., KALES, J., BIXLER, E. O. and SLYE, E. S. Effects of placebo and flurazepam on sleep patterns in insomniac subjects, *Clinical Pharmacology and Therapy* **12**, 691–697 (1971)

KANTO, J., IISALO, E., LEHTINEN, V. and SALMINEN, J. The concentrations of diazepam and its metabolites in the plasma after an acute and chronic administration, *Psychopharmacologia (Berlin)* **36**, 123–131 (1974)

KANTO, J., IISALO, E.U.M., HOVI-VIANDER, M. and KANGAS, L. A comparative study on the clinical effects of oxazepam and diazepam. Relationship between plasma level and effect, *International Journal of Clinical Pharmacology and Biopharmacy* **17**, 26–31 (1979)

KAPLAN, S. A., JACK, M. L., ALEXANDER, K. and WEINFELD, R. W. Pharmacokinetic profile of diazepam in man following single intravenous and oral and chronic oral administration, *Journal of Pharmaceutical Science* **62**, 1789–1796 (1973)

KATHOL, R., NOYES, R. JR., SLYMEN, D. J., CROWE, R. R., CLANCY, J. and KERBER, R. E. Propranolol in chronic anxiety disorders: a controlled study, *Archives of General Psychiatry* **37**, 1361–1367 (1980)

KATO, R. and VASSANELLI, P. Induction of increased meprobamate metabolism in rats pretreated with some neurotropic drugs, *Biochemical Pharmacology* **11**, 779–794 (1962)

KELLY, D., PIK, R. and CHEN, C.-N. A psychological and physiological evaluation of the effects of intravenous diazepam, *Journal of Psychiatry* **122**, 419–426 (1973)

KLETZKIN, M. and BERGER, F. M. Effect of meprobamate on limbic system of the brain. *Proceedings of the Society of Experimental Biology and Medicine* **100**, 681–683 (1959)

KLOTZ, U., ANTONIN, K. H. and BRECK, P. R. Comparison of the pharmacokinetics of diazepam after single and subchronic doses, *Journal of Clinical Pharmacology* **10**, 121–126 (1976)

KLOTZ, U., ANTONIN, K. H., BRUGEL, H. and BIECK, P. R. Disposition of diazepam and its major metabolite desmethyldiazepam in patients with liver disease, *Clinical Pharmacology and Therapeutics* **21**, 430–436 (1977)

KLOTZ, U., AVANT, G. R., HOYUMPA, A., SCHENKER, S. and WILKINSON, G. R. The effects of age and liver disease on the disposition and elimination of diazepam in adult man, *Journal of Clinical Investigation* **55**, 347–359 (1975)

KUCH, H. Clobazam: chemical aspects of the 1,4 and 1,5-benzodiazepines, *British Journal of Clinical Pharmacology* **7**, Suppl. 1, 17–21 (1979)

LADER, M. Symposium summary on temazepam and related 1,4-benzodiazepines, *British Journal of Clinical Pharmacology* **8**, Suppl. 1, 81–83 (1979)

LADER, M. Personal communication (1980)

LADER, M. Benzodiazepine dependence. In *The Misuse of Psychotropic Drugs* (Eds. R. MURRAY, H. GHODSE, C. HARRIS, C. WILLIAMS and P. WILLIAMS), Headly Bros., Kent (1981)

LADER, M. H. and TYRER, P. J. Central and peripheral effects of propranolol and sotalol in normal human subjects, *British Journal of Pharmacology* **45**, 557–560 (1972)

LADER, M. H., BOND, A. J. and JAMES, D. C. Clinical comparison of anxiolytic drug therapy, *Psychological Medicine* **4**, 381–387 (1974)

LANCET. Editorial – long-term safety of beta-blocking drugs, *Lancet* **1**, 1242–1243 (1978)

LANCET. Editorial – the hyperkinetic heart, *Lancet* **2**, 967 (1981)

LAPIERRE, Y. D. Benzodiazepine withdrawal, *Canadian Journal of Psychiatry* **26**, 93–95 (1981)

LASAGNA, L. The Halcion story: trial by media, *Lancet* **i**, 815–816 (1980)

LAWTON, M. P. and CAHN, B. The effects of diazepam (Valium) and alcohol on psychomotor performance, *Journal of Nervous and Mental Diseases* **136**, 550–554 (1963)

LIN, K. M. and FRIEDEL, R. O. Relationship of plasma levels of chlordiazepoxide and metabolites to clinical response, *American Journal of Psychiatry* **136**, 18–23 (1979)

LIPANI, J. A. Preference study of the hypnotic efficacy of triazolam 0.125 mg compared to placebo in geriatric patients with insomnia, *Current Therapeutic Research* **24**, 397–402 (1978)

LO, W. H. and LO, T. Clinical trial of benzoctamine versus chlordiazepoxide in anxiety neurosis, *Journal of Clinical Pharmacology* **13**, 48–53 (1973)

McDONALD, J. B. and McDONALD, E. T. Nocturnal femoral fractures and continuing widespread use of barbiturate hypnotics, *British Medical Journal* **2**, 483–485 (1977)

McFARLAND, H. R. Chloridazepoxide for spasticity, *Diseases of the Nervous System* **24**, 296–298 (1963)

McMILLIN, W. P. Oxprenolol in anxiety, *Lancet* **1**, 1193 (1973)

MALPAS, A., ROWAN, A. J., JOYCE, C. R. B. and SCOTT, D. F. Persistent behavioural and electroencephalographic changes after single doses of nitrazepam and amylobarbitone sodium, *British Medical Journal* **2**, 762–764 (1970)

MARKS, I. *Fears and Phobias*, Heinemann, London (1969)

MARKS, I. M., VISWANATHAN, R., LIPSEDGE, M. S. and GARDNER, R. Enhanced relief of phobias by flooding during waning diazepam effect, *British Journal of Psychiatry* **121**, 493–505 (1972)

MARKS, J. *The Benzodiazepines: Use, Overuse, Misuse, Abuse*, MTP Press, Lancaster (1978)

MARSDEN, C. W. Propranolol in neurocirculatory asthenia and anxiety, *Postgraduate Medical Journal*, Suppl. 47, 100–103 (1971)

MATTHEWS, W. B. Ratio of maximum H reflex to maximum M response as a measure of spasticity, *Journal of Neurology, Neurosurgery and Psychiatry* **29**, 201–204 (1966)

MENDELSON, G. Withdrawal symptoms after oxazepam, *Lancet* **1**, 565 (1978)

MENDELSON, W. P., GOODWIN, D. W., HILL, S. Y. and REICHMAN, J. D. The morning after: residual E.E.G. effects of triazolam and flurazepam, alone and in combination with alcohol, *Current Therapeutic Research* **19**, 155–163 (1976)

MIDDLETON, R. S. W. Temazepam (Euhypnos) and chlormethiazole: a comparative study in geriatric patients *Journal of International Medical Research* **6**, 121–125 (1978)

MILLER, R. R. Drug surveillance utilizing epidemiologic methods: a report from the Boston Collaborative Drug Surveillance Program, *American Journal of Hospital Pharmacy* **30**, 584–592 (1973)

MISHARA, B. L. and KASTENBAUM, R. Wine in the treatment of long-term geriatric patients in mental institutions, *Journal of the American Geriatric Society* **22**, 88–94 (1974)

MÖHLER, H. and OKADA, T. Benzodiazepine receptor: demonstration in the central nervous system, *Science* **198**, 849–851 (1977)

MONTAGU, J. D. Effects of diazepam on the EEG in man, *European Journal of Pharmacology* **17**, 167–170 (1972)

NANDA, R. N., JOHNSON, R. H., KEOGH, H. J., LAMBIE, D. G. and MELVILLE, I. D. Treatment of epilepsy with clonazepam and its effect on other anticonvulsants, *Journal of Neurology, Neurosurgery and Psychiatry* **40**, 538–543 (1977)

NICHOLSON, A. N. Performance studies with diazepam and its hydroxylated metabolites, *British Journal of Clinical Pharmacology* **8**, Suppl. 1, 39–42 (1979)

NICHOLSON, A. N. The use of short- and long-acting hypnotics in clinical medicine, *British Journal of Clinical Pharmacology* **11**, Suppl. 1, 61–69 (1981)

NOYES, R. Jr., KATHOL, R., CLANCY, J. and CROWE, R. R. Antianxiety effects of propranolol: a review of clinical studies. In *Anxiety: New Research and Changing Concepts* (Eds. D. F. KLEIN and J. RABKIN), 81–93, Raven Press, New York (1981)

OLDS, M. E. and OLDS J. Effects of anxiety-relieving drugs on unit discharges in hippocampus, reticular midbrain, and pre-optic area in the freely moving rat, *International Journal of Neuropharmacology* **8**, 87–103 (1969)

OSWALD, I. and PRIEST, R. G. Five weeks to escape the sleeping pill habit, *British Medical Journal* **2**, 1093–1095 (1965)

OSWALD, I., ADAM, K., BORROW, S. and IDZIKOWSKI, C. The effects of two hypnotics on sleep, subjective feelings and skilled performance, *Advances in Biosciences* **12**, 51–64 (1978)

PARSONAGE, M. J. and NORRIS, J. W. Use of diazepam in treatment of severe convulsive status epilepticus, *British Medical Journal* **3**, 85–88 (1967)

PEVNICK, J. S., JASINSKI, D. R. and HAERTZEN, C. A. Abrupt withdrawal from therapeutically administered diazepam, *Archives of General Psychiatry* **35**, 995–998 (1978)

PHILLIPS, R. M. and HUTCHINSON, J. T. Intravenous acetylcholine in the treatment of the neuroses, *British Medical Journal* **1**, 1468–1470 (1954).

PRESKORN, S. H. and DENNER, L. J. Benzodiazepines and withdrawal psychosis: report of three cases, *Journal of the American Medical Association* **237**, 36–38 (1977)

PRIEST, R. G. (1980). The benzodiazepines: a clinical review. In *Benzodiazepines: To-day and Tomorrow* (Eds. R. G. Priest, V. Vianna Filho, R. Amrein and M. Skreta), MTP Press, Lancaster (1980)

RANDALL, L. O. Pharmacology of methaminodiazepoxide, *Diseases of the Nervous System* **21**, March Suppl. 7–12 (1960)

RANDALL, L. O. Pharmacology of chlordiazepoxide ('Librium'), *Diseases of the Nervous System* **22**, July Suppl. 7–15 (1961)

RANDALL, L. O., SCHALLEK, W., HEISE, G. A., KEITH, E. F. and BAGDON, R. E. The psychosedative properties of methaminodiazepoxide, *Journal of Pharmacology and Experimental Therapy* **129**, 163–171 (1960)

RATNA, L. Addiction to temazepam, *British Medical Journal* **282**, 1837–1838 (1981)

RAYMOND, M. J., LUCAS, C. J., BEESLEY, M. L., O'CONNELL, B. A. and ROBERTS, J. A. F. A trial of five tranquillising drugs in psychoneurosis, *British Medical Journal* **2**, 63–66 (1957)

RICKELS, K., CLARK, T. W., EWING, J. H., KLINGENSMITH, W. C., MORRIS, H. M. and SMOCK, C. D. Evaluation of tranquillizing drugs in medical out-patients, *Journal of the American Medical Association* **171**, 1649–1656 (1959)

RICKELS, K., HESBACHER, P., VANDERVORT, W., PHILLIPS, F., HUTCHISON, J., SABLOSKY, L. and LAVAN, D. Tybamate—a perplexing drug, *American Journal of Psychiatry* **125**, 320–326 (1968)

RICKELS, K., PEREIRA-OGAN, J. A., CASE, W. G., CSANALOSI, I., MIRMAN, M. J., NATHANSON, J. E. and PARISH, L. C. Chlormezanone in anxiety: a drug rediscovered? *American Journal of Psychiatry* **131**, 592–595 (1974)

RICKELS, K., DOWNING, R. W. and WINOKUR, A. Anti-anxiety drugs: clinical use in psychiatry. In *Handbook of Psychopharmacology*, Vol. 13, Biology of Mood and Anti-anxiety Drugs (Eds. L. L. IVERSON, S. D. IVERSON and S. H. SNYDER), 395–430, Plenum Press, New York (1978)

RIFKIN, A., QUITKIN, F. and KLEIN, D. F. Withdrawal reaction to diazepam, *Journal of the American Medical Association* **236**, 2172–2173 (1976)

ROBIN, A., CURRY, S. H. and WHELPTON, R. Clinical and biochemical comparison of clorazepate and diazepam, *Psychological Medicine* **4**, 388–392 (1974)

RUPP, W., BADIAN, M., CHRIST, O., HAJDÚ, P., KULKARNI, R. D., TAEUBER, K., UIHLEIN, M., BENDER, R. and VANDERBEKE, O. Pharmacokinetics of single and multiple doses of clobazam in humans, *British Journal of Clinical Pharmacology* **7**, Suppl. 1, 51–57 (1979)

RUTHERFORD, D. M., OKOKO, A. and TYRER, P. J. Plasma concentration of diazepam and desmethyldiazepam during chronic therapy, *British Journal of Clinical Pharmacology* **6**, 69–73 (1978)

SAFRA, M. J. and OAKLEY, G. P. Association between cleft lip with or without cleft palate and prenatal exposure to diazepam, *Lancet* **2**, 478–480 (1975)

SALKIND, M. R., HANKS, G. W. and SILVERSTON, J. T. Evaluation of the effects of clobazam, a 1,5 benzodiazepine, on mood and psychomotor performance in clinically anxious patients in general practice, *British Journal of Clinical Pharmacology* **7**, Suppl. 1, 113–118 (1979)

SCHAPIRA, K., McCLELLAND, H. A., GRIFFITHS, N. R. and NEWELL, D. J. Study on the effects of tablet colour in the treatment of anxiety states, *British Medical Journal* **2**, 446–449 (1970)

SCHAPIRA, K., ROTH, M., KERR, T. A. and GURNEY, C. The prognosis of affective disorders: the differentiation of anxiety states from depressive illnesses, *British Journal of Psychiatry* **121**, 175–183 (1972)

SELLERS, E. M. and KOCH-WESER, J. Potentiation of warfarin-induced hypoprothrombinemia by chloral hydrate, *New England Journal of Medicine* **283**, 827–831 (1970)

SHADER, R. I. and GREENBLATT, D. J. Benzodiazepines: some aspects of their clinical pharmacology. In *Ciba Foundation Symposium 74: Drug Concentrations in Neuropsychiatry*, 141–155, Elsevier, North Holland, Amsterdam (1980)

SHELTON, J. and HOLLISTER, L. E. (1967). Simulated abuse of tybamate in man: failure to demonstrate withdrawal reactions, *Journal of the American Medical Association* **199**, 338–340 (1967)

SHUBIN, H. and WEIL, M. H. Shock associated with barbiturate intoxication, *Journal of the American Medical Association* **215**, 263–268 (1971)

SIM, H. and HOUGHTON, H. Phobic anxiety and its treatment, *Journal of Nervous and Mental Diseases* **143**, 484–491 (1966)

SKEGG, D. C. G., DOLL, R. and PERRY, J. Use of medicines in general practice, *British Medical Journal* **1**, 1561–1563 (1977)

SKEGG, D. C. G., RICHARDS, S. M. and DOLL, R. Minor tranquillisers and road accidents, *British Medical Journal* **1**, 917–919 (1979)

SMITH, D. E. and WESSON, D. R. A new method for treatment of barbiturate dependence, *Journal of the American Medical Association* **213**, 294–295 (1970)

SNAITH, R. *Clinical Neurosis.* Oxford University Press, Oxford (1981)

SQUIRES, R. F., BENSON, D. I., BRAESTRUP, C., COUPET, J., KLEPNER, C. A., MYERS, V. and BEER, B. Some properties of 'brain specific' benzodiazepine receptors: new evidence for multiple receptors, *Pharmacology and Biochemistry of Behaviour* **10**, 825–830 (1979)

STEPHEN, S. A. Unwanted effects of propranolol, *American Journal of Cardiology* **18**, 463–468 (1966)

SWANSON, D. W. WEDDIGE, R. L. and MORSE, R. M. Abuse of prescription drugs, *Mayo Clinics Proceedings* **48**, 359–367 (1973)

TAGGART, P., CARRUTHERS, M. and SOMERVILLE, W. Electrocardiogram, plasma catecholamines and lipids, and their modification by oxprenolol when speaking before an audience, *Lancet* **ii**, 341–346 (1973)

TANSELLA, M., SICILIANI, O., BURTI, L., SCHIAVON, M., ZIMMERMAN TANSELLA, Ch., GERNA, M., TOGNONI, G. and MORSELLI, P. L. N-desmethyldiazepam and amylobarbitone sodium as hypnotics in anxious patients: plasma levels, clinical efficacy and residual effects, *Psychopharmacologia* **41**, 81–85 (1975)

TOGNONI, G., GOMENI, R., DeMAIO, D., ALBERTI, G. D., FRANCIOSI, P. and SCIEGHI, G. Pharmacokinetics of N-desmethyldiazepam in patients suffering from insomnia and treated with nortriptyline, *British Journal of Clinical Pharmacology* **2**, 227–232 (1975)

TURNER, P. Clinical and experimental studies on the central effects of beta-blockade in man. In *Beta-blockers and the Central Nervous System* (Ed. P. KIELHOLZ), 90–108, Huber, Bern (1977)

TURNER, P., GRANVILLE-GROSSMAN, K. L. and SMART, J. V. Effect of adrenergic receptor blockade on the tachycardia of thyrotoxicosis and anxiety state, *Lancet* **2**, 1316–1318 (1965)

TYRER, P. The benzodiazepine bonanza, *Lancet* **ii**, 709–710 (1974)

TYRER, P. *The Role of Bodily Feelings in Anxiety* (Maudsley Monograph No. 23), Oxford University Press, London (1976)

TYRER, P. Drug treatment of psychiatric patients in general practice, *British Medical Journal* **2**, 1008–1010 (1978)

TYRER, P. Anxiety states. In *Recent Advances in Clinical Psychiatry* (Ed. K. GRANVILLE-GROSSMAN), **3**, 161–183, Churchill-Livingstone, Edinburgh (1979)

TYRER, P. J. Beta-blocking drugs in psychiatry and neurology, *Drugs* **20**, 113–121 (1980)

TYRER, P. J. and LADER, M. H. Effects of beta-adrenergic blockade with sotalol in chronic anxiety, *Clinical and Pharmacological Therapeutics* **14**, 418–426 (1973)

TYRER, P. J. and LADER, M. H. Response to propranolol and diazepam in somatic and psychic anxiety, *British Medical Journal* **2**, 14–16 (1974a)

TYRER, P. J. and LADER, M. H. Physiological response to propranolol and diazepam in chronic anxiety, *British Journal of Clinical Pharmacology* **1**, 387–390 (1974b)

TYRER, P., RUTHERFORD, D. and HUGGETT, T. Benzodiazepine withdrawal symptoms and propranolol, *Lancet* **1**, 520–522 (1981)

TYRER, P., TREASADEN, I., MORETON, K., FLANAGAN, R. and RILEY, P. Clinical value of plasma diazepam concentrations (to be published) (1982)

WAAL, H. J. Propranolol-induced depression, *British Medical Journal* **2**, 50 (1967)

WALTERS, A. J. and LADER, M. H. Hangover effect of hypnotics in man, *Nature* **229**, 637–638 (1971)

WHEATLEY, D. Comparative effects of propranolol and chlordiazepoxide, *British Journal of Psychiatry* **115**, 1411–1412 (1969)

WILHELM, M. and SCHMIDT, P. L. Synthese und Eigenschaften von l-aminoalkyl-dibenzo (b,e) bicyclo (2,2,2) octadienen, *Helvetica Chimica Acta* **52**, 1385–1395 (1969)

WILSON, J. Lorazepam as a premedicant for general anaesthesia, *Current Medical Research Opinions* **1**, 308–316 (1973)

WINOKUR, A., RICKELS, K., GREENBLATT, D. J., SNYDER, P. J. and SCHATZ, N. J. Withdrawal reaction from long term, low dosage, administration of diazepam, *Archives of General Psychiatry* **37**, 101–105 (1980)

WINSTEAD, D. K., ANDERSON, A., EILSERS, M. K., BLACKWELL, B. and ZAREMBA, A. L. Diazepam on demand: drug-seeking behavior in psychiatric inpatients, *Archives of General Psychiatry* **30**, 349–351 (1974)

WORLD HEALTH ORGANIZATION. *International Classification of Disease*, 9th Edn, WHO, Geneva (1978)

YANAGITA, T. and TAKAHASHI, S. Dependence liability of several sedative-hypnotic agents evaluated in monkeys, *Journal of Pharmacology and Experimental Therapy* **185**, 307–316 (1973)

YOUNG, W. S., NIEHOFT, D., KUHAR, M. J., BEER, B. and LIPPA, A. S. Multiple benzodiazepine receptor: localisation by light microscopic radiohistochemistry, *Journal of Pharmacology and Experimental Therapy* **216**, 425–430 (1981)

Chapter 7

Tricyclic antidepressants

R. H. Mindham

This chapter deals with the tricyclic antidepressant drugs only; newer, related drugs will be dealt with elsewhere, as will other substances which are used in the treatment of depressive states. The tricyclic drugs have been in widespread clinical use for almost 25 years and this has produced an extensive literature dealing with every aspect of their clinical effects. New antidepressive drugs tend to differ from the tricyclic drugs chemically although often resembling them in their pharmacological effects. As a consequence the tricyclic group of drugs is no longer expanding and the most recent member of the group has been in use for about ten years. For this reason it is timely to assess the tricyclic drugs collectively and individually and to review their place in the evolution of the drug treatment of depressive states.

Introduction

The discovery of the antidepressive properties of imipramine

Thiele and Holzinger synthesized iminodibenzyl in 1889 and described its chemical properties. In the period immediately following the Second World War the possible use of the substituted iminodibenzyls was investigated and they were found to be antihistaminic, anticholinergic, sedative and hypnotic (Haefliger, 1959). The iminodibenzyls resemble the phenothiazine drugs chemically (*Figure 7.1* and *Figure 7.2*). When the pharmacological effects of chlorpromazine and the drug's potential in the treatment of disturbed psychotic patients was recognized in the early 1950s, interest in the

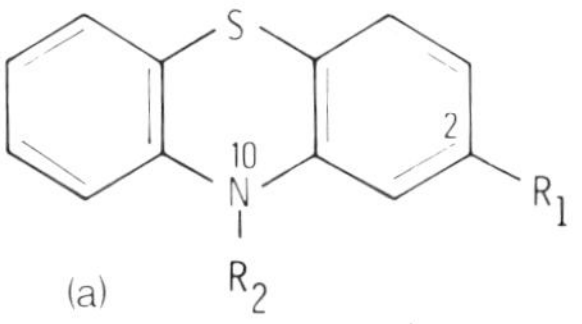

Figure 7.1a General formula of phenothiazines

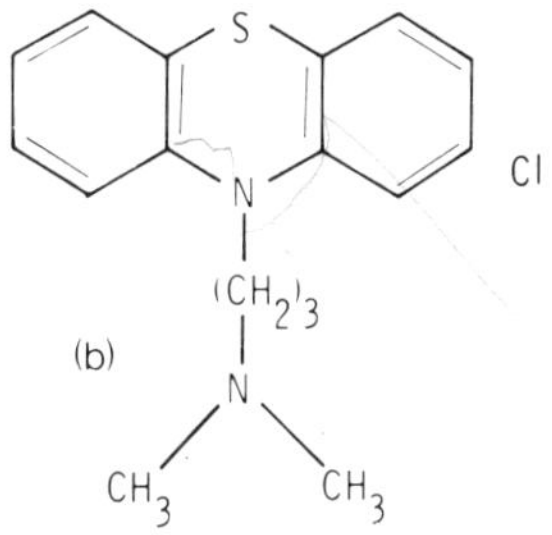

Figure 7.1b Chlorpromazine

177

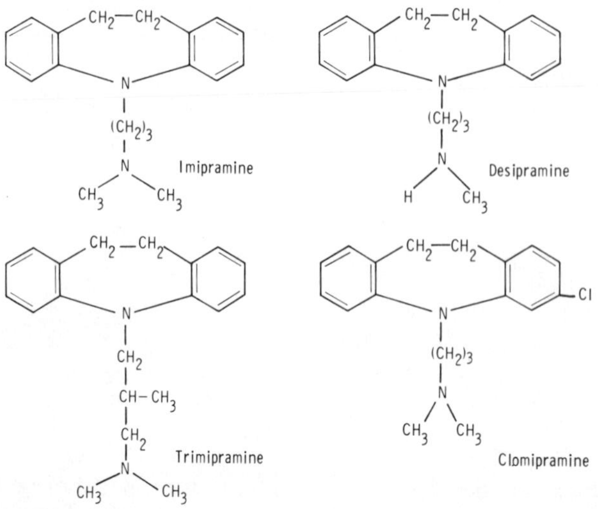

Figure 7.2

pharmacological properties of the iminodibenzyls was renewed. Kuhn (1957) investigated the sedative properties of imipramine in chronic psychotic patients suffering from a variety of psychiatric disorders. Close observation of several hundred patients showed that patients with depressive symptomatology benefited from the drug but other diagnostic groups in general did not; a few showed worsening in their clinical state. Although Kuhn's studies were open, uncontrolled and clinical in type his observations of the clinical and unwanted effects of imipramine have been largely confirmed. There is clearly a place in psychopharmacology for the carefully conducted clinical study of large numbers of patients. The summary from one of Kuhn's earlier papers on imipramine illustrates the comprehensive nature and accuracy of his observations:

'Over a three-year period, more than 500 psychiatric patients of various diagnostic categories were treated with imipramine hydrochloride. It was demonstrated that the compound has potent antidepressant action. Best responses were obtained in cases of endogenous depression showing the typical symptoms of mental and motor retardation, fatigue, feeling of heaviness, hopelessness, guilt and despair. The condition is furthermore characterized by the aggravation of symptoms in the morning with a tendency to improvement during the day. Treatment with imipramine hydrochloride resulted in full or social recovery in a high percentage of the patients. As a rule, the initial response was evident in 2–3 d, while in some cases 1–4 weeks of therapy were required. In view of the symptomatic nature of the action of imipramine hydrochloride therapy must be maintained as long as the illness lasts.' (Kuhn, 1958.)

Kuhn also described most of the unwanted effects of imipramine and the effects seen in other psychiatric conditions such as schizophrenia, dementia and mania.

Since these original observations a very large number of studies of the pharmacological and clinical effects of imipramine have been conducted, providing us with an extensive knowledge of the drug's characteristics. The pharmacological properties of imipramine are essentially the same as those of other tricyclic antidepressants.

Pharmacology

The mood-elevating properties of tricyclic antidepressants are believed to result from their ability to inhibit re-uptake of monoamines from the synaptic cleft into the neurons after central neurotransmission. The important monoamines are noradrenaline (NA), 5-hydroxytryptamine (5-HT) and dopamine (DA), although most tricyclic antidepressants have little effect on dopamine re-uptake. The significance of this ability to block the re-uptake of monoamines derives from the catecholamine hypothesis of affective disorders, which state that depression is a result of relative deficiency of central monoamines at transmitter sites. This developed from the observation that the hypotensive drug, reserpine, occasionally precipitates a severe depressive illness and also severely depletes NA, 5-HT and DA at central nerve terminals as well as peripheral ones. Although the hypothesis is clearly not an adequate explanation of the biochemistry and pharmacology of affective disorders (*see* Chapter 9) it has been of great practical value and is still the most appropriate for explaining the actions of tricyclic antidepressants (Schildkraut, 1969).

The inhibition of re-uptake of NA and 5-HT is illustrated in *Figure 7.3*. The monoamines are stored in granules close to the ends of nerve terminals and are released to enable neurotransmission to take place to the post-synaptic receptor. They are then 'sucked back' from the synaptic cleft into the nerve ending and returned to their storage sites. By inhibiting this re-uptake mechanism the tricyclic antidepressants allow monoamine levels in the synaptic cleft to rise and so counter the deficiency.

When reserpine is administered to rats it produces sedation. If reserpine is administered by injection, to rats which have previously been treated with desipramine, the animals exhibit hyperactivity instead of sedation. This observation suggests that the amines released from the cells following the administration of reserpine are not reabsorbed because of a change in the cell membrane. The effect is not seen if the reserpine is given in small doses over a period of hours, or if the brain stores of amine are depleted before the administration of reserpine. Tricyclic drugs do not appear to cause depletion of the amines in the nerve cells when given alone (Carlsson, 1966).

Tricyclic antidepressants show some selectivity in their ability to inhibit the re-uptake of 5-HT and NA (Glowinski and Axelrod, 1964; Carlsson, 1966).

The tertiary amines, of which imipramine and amitriptyline are examples, predominantly decrease the re-uptake of indole amines (mainly 5-HT) whereas secondary

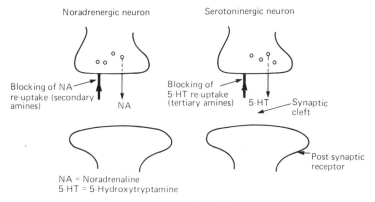

Figure 7.3 Mechanism of action of tricyclic antidepressants

amines such as desipramine and nortriptyline reduce the re-uptake of noradrenaline (*Figure 7.3*). A number of drugs inhibit the re-uptake of both indole and catecholamines more or less equally; this may be because tertiary amine tricyclic drugs are frequently metabolized to secondary amines in the body which are themselves pharmacologically active, with both forms being present in the body in substantial amounts at the same time. Several drugs (e.g. clomipramine) have been developed which selectively inhibit the re-uptake of 5-HT. In addition to a tertiary amine structure, a three-carbon side-chain and a chlorine atom in the 3-position of the tricyclic nucleus also favours a specific 5-HT uptake inhibiting ability (Iversen and MacKay, 1979).

No tricyclic antidepressant is a 'pure' inhibitor of 5-HT or NA re-uptake and their selectivity is only relative. It is reasonable for the clinician to ask about the significance of these differences in re-uptake inhibition and whether it should affect his clinical practice? At present the answer is that no-one knows. There is no apparent difference in the efficacy of the selective 5-HT and NA re-uptake inhibitors although the possibility that there are specific 5-HT and NA-type deficient depressions is still open. The reason why treatment with antidepressants is associated with a long delay before clinical response is also unexplained, as the inhibition of monoamine re-uptake in central neurons appears to be complete within 24 h of administration.

The tricyclic drugs have many properties which they share with the phenothiazines which they so closely resemble chemically. They show mild atropine-like anticholinergic effects, antihistamine effects, local anaesthetic action, cardiovascular effects include hypotension and changes in conduction in the heart, variable sedative actions and are very weak inhibitors of monoamine oxidase. Some of these effects give rise to the many unwanted effects of the tricyclic drugs which are described in detail later. It has sometimes been suggested that the antidepressant effects of the tricylics follows from their anticholinergic actions. This idea was tested experimentally in a study in which 58 depressed patients were treated using two dosage levels of desmethyl imipramine. Measurements of urinary output of desmethyl imipramine, of salivation and of the incidence of side effects were compared in responders and non-responders. No differences were found between the two groups, and it was concluded that the antidepressive effect of the drug was not dependent upon its anticholinergic effects as revealed by its unwanted effects, nor were differences in metabolism, as reflected by urinary excretion of metabolites, associated with response to the drug (Watt, Crammer and Elkes, 1972).

Pharmacokinetics

Absorption

The tricyclic antidepressant drugs are rapidly and completely absorbed when given by mouth. In a study of imipramine the drug was readily detectable in the portal vein within 10 min of administration, and absorption was complete within 80 min (Dencker *et al.*, 1976). There is therefore little point in giving antidepressants intravenously or intramuscularly despite the marketing of such preparations. In the blood the drugs are bound to plasma albumin and in many cases the bound component amounts to 90–95 per cent of the drug administered, at a therapeutic dosage (Borgå *et al.*, 1969). A remarkable twin study showed that plasma binding of drugs is partly determined by genetic factors (Alexanderson, Evans and Sjöqvist, 1969). Twins were invited to take part in a study of the metabolism of nortriptyline. The subjects were asked to take $0.2 \, \mathrm{mg \cdot kg^{-1}}$ of body weight twice daily for 8 d. Blood samples were taken on days 6, 7 and 8 for the estimation of plasma levels of the drug. The results showed that the plasma levels in identical twins were often very similar; a less close relationship was seen in the fraternal twins. The concurrent administration of other drugs led to the disappearance of the close relationship between plasma levels of nortriptyline in both identical and fraternal twins. A series of studies has shown that it is the unbound portion of the drug which is therapeutically active but that binding is readily reversible to make the bound drug available (Borgå et al., 1970).

Distribution

The drugs are rapidly and widely distributed from the blood to the bodily tissues. They are concentrated in the liver and intestines and, to a lesser extent, in the brain. However, brain concentrations in man, following therapeutic dosage, are unknown (Peet and Coppen, 1979).

Metabolism

The drugs are metabolized predominantly in the liver and excreted in the bile and urine. Many of the tricyclics are demethylated and hydroxylated in the body. Some of the metabolites are active antidepressants themselves; for example, desipramine and nortriptyline are demethylated metabolites of imipramine and amitriptyline respectively.

Plasma levels and clinical response

The concentration of tricyclic drugs in the plasma following oral or parenteral administration has been extensively studied (Amsterdam, Brunswick and Mendels, 1980). Following oral administration a peak plasma level is reached after 1–4 h, falling thereafter more slowly. The half-lives of the drugs are generally long: 54–198 h for protriptyline (Moody et al., 1977), 40 h for amitriptyline (Braithwaite and Widdop, 1971), and 7–13 h for imipramine (Gram et al., 1976). If the drugs are given frequently a 'steady-state' plasma level is reached in which absorption and elimination are in equilibrium. Once the steady state is reached, in spite of small fluctuations, it stays fairly constant. There are very large differences between patients in the steady-state levels attained following similar doses of a drug; this difference may be as much as 40-fold (Hammer and Sjöqvist, 1967). These differences are partly due to inherited characteristics (Alexanderson, Evans and Sjöqvist, 1969). Concurrent administration of barbiturates reduces the steady-state levels of many tricyclic drugs probably by induction of relevant enzymes (Alexanderson, Evans and Sjöqvist, 1969). Benzodiazepines do not appear to have this effect (Silverman and Braithwaite, 1973). Some neuroleptics have been shown to inhibit the metabolism of imipramine leading to increased plasma levels (Gram and Overø, 1972). Older patients have been shown to develop higher steady-state plasma levels of some tricyclic drugs and to eliminate these drugs more slowly. These findings are clearly relevant to the increased susceptibility of old people to the effects, both wanted and unwanted, of this group of drugs (Nies et al., 1977).

The effect on steady-state plasma levels of various dosage regimens of tricyclic drugs has been examined. In one study amitriptyline was given to a series of patients either as 25 mg three times a day or as 75 mg at night (Braithwaite, Narra and Gaind, 1974). Plasma levels were very similar with only marginally larger diurnal variations in plasma levels of the drugs in those on the nightly dosage schedule. The authors believe that the degree of change in plasma level seen following nightly dosage would be unlikely to reduce the drug's effectiveness. Further, it is anticipated that once-daily dosage of drugs will lead to greater patient compliance and therapeutic advantage. The advantage of a sustained release preparation is uncertain.

Early studies of the *relationship between plasma levels of tricyclic drugs and therapeutic response* produced varying and contradictory results. The relationship is still unclear, difficult to interpret and not yet widely applicable to clinical practice.

Imipramine was the first tricyclic drug to be investigated in this way. An early study showed a linear relationship between plasma imipramine levels and clinical improvement in patients suffering from 'endogenous depression' (Walter, 1970). In this study plasma levels of imipramine only were estimated and the levels of metabolites ignored. A series of later studies in which the combined plasma levels of both imipramine and desmethylimipramine were measured showed a linear relationship between plasma levels of the drugs and clinical response, with a minimal plasma level below which improvement did not occur (Olivier-Martin *et al.*, 1975; Glassman *et al.*, 1977; Reisby *et al.*, 1977).

Several studies of amitriptyline in which both amitriptyline and its metabolite, nortriptyline, were estimated have shown a linear relationship between plasma levels and therapeutic effect with a lower plasma level below which improvement is not seen (Braithwaite *et al.*, 1972; Montgomery and Braithwaite, 1975; Ziegler *et al.*, 1976; Kupfer *et al.*, 1977). Two studies have found no such relationship (Coppen *et al.*, 1978; Jungkunz and Kuss, 1978).

There have been a relatively large number of investigations of the effects of nortriptyline; it was chosen for study because at the time it was thought to have no active metabolites and, as a consequence, would present fewer problems in interpretation. Early investigations in Sweden suggested a curvilinear relationship between plasma levels of nortriptyline and therapeutic effects with the best results being seen in patients with intermediate plasma levels of the drug, and poorer results in those patients with high or low levels (Åsberg *et al.*, 1971). These findings have been repeated by workers both from this group and from independent departments (Kragh-Sørensen, Åsberg and Eggert-Hansen, 1973; Ziegler *et al.*, 1976; Montgomery *et al.*, 1978). In another study the experimental procedure was reversed: patients were deliberately treated in groups in which the nortriptyline level was controlled at a medium or high level. This study confirmed the therapeutic disadvantage of the high plasma level of the drug (Kragh-Sørensen, Hansen and Baastrup, 1976). Two further studies not only failed to show a curvilinear response pattern but failed to show any relationship between plasma level and therapeutic effect at all (Burrows, Mowbray and Davies, 1972; Lyle *et al.*, 1974).

There have been fewer studies of the clinical significance of plasma levels of other tricyclic drugs. The studies performed on protriptyline and doxepin have yielded conflicting results (Amsterdam, Brunswick and Mendels, 1980). In the case of clomipramine no relationship between plasma level and clinical effect was found but a curvilinear effect was found for its metabolite desmethylclomipramine (Broadhurst, James and Corte, 1977). A pilot study of butriptyline showed no clear pattern (Burrows *et al.*, 1977).

The evidence is difficult to interpret as the results of studies are so much at variance. The findings suggest that a linear relationship exists between plasma levels of drug and therapeutic effects for the tertiary amine tricyclic drugs including imipramine and amitriptyline and possibly clomipramine. A curvilinear relationship has been shown in some centres for the secondary amine tricyclic drug, nortriptyline.

At least one worker has questioned the interpretation of the data of some studies and argues that there is evidence for a curvilinear relationship between therapeutic effect and the plasma levels of amitriptyline and nortriptyline (Åsberg, 1980). This worker supports her contention by five main observations:

(1) where studies concern subjects suffering from 'endogenous depression', strictly defined, a positive relationship between plasma levels of tricyclic drugs and clinical effects is more consistently found;
(2) studies showing no evidence of declining clinical effect with high concentrations of drugs often include few patients in the higher range of plasma levels;
(3) many studies include patients suffering from a wide range of depressive states, many of them secondary;
(4) weak correlations may easily be unnoticed;
(5) a clinically homogeneous group of subjects may be biochemically heterogeneous.

The findings of a poorer response with higher plasma levels of certain tricyclic drugs has been attributed to a blockade of adrenergic receptors by higher drug concentrations; an effect also seen after the administration of phenothiazine drugs (Åsberg et al., 1971; Åsberg and Sjöqvist, 1978). A central anticholinergic effect could also be present but this explanation is regarded as less likely.

Should the evidence which points to a difference between tertiary and secondary amine tricyclics in the relationship between plasma levels and therapeutic effects be confirmed a pharmacological explanation of the observed effect would be required. In the present state of knowledge it is difficult to understand why a tertiary amine drug which is represented in the body partly as its secondary amine metabolite should have very different properties from the secondary amine itself. More information is clearly required in this area.

More recently attention has turned to the pattern of metabolism of tricyclic drugs in different individuals. It has been known for some time that, following oral administration, as much as 60 per cent of imipramine is metabolized during its first passage through the liver. Most of the drug lost in this process is metabolized by demethylation to desipramine (Denker et al., 1976). The extent of demethylation on the first passage through the liver has been shown to vary greatly between individuals. Similarly, clomipramine shows a high but variable degree of demethylation on the first passage through the liver (Nagy and Johansson, 1977). In the cases of both imipramine and clomipramine the plasma concentration of the demethylated metabolites may exceed that of the parent drug as much as seven-fold. The degree of demethylation may offset the therapeutic effect of the drug, and there is some evidence that a low rate of demethylation may be associated with a better therapeutic effect (Muscettola et al., 1978). These findings reflect the early findings that slow metabolizers of imipramine were likely to show greater therapeutic benefit from the drug as compared with those who metabolized the drug more quickly (Haydu, Dhrymiotis and Quinn, 1962). This study was conducted before sophisticated methods of estimating plasma levels of drugs were available.

Findings of this kind have led to suggestions that better therapeutic effects might be obtained by manipulating the rate of demethylation. This may be achieved by giving the drug by intravenous infusion, and this method of administration has been practised in the UK to some extent. Alternatively, imipramine-N-oxide might be given; the drug is inactive itself but is reduced mainly to imipramine. The use of this drug is under investigation (Nagy and Hansen, 1978). The administration of imipramine-N-oxide produces roughly similar levels of imipramine and demethyl imipramine in the tissues

(Nagy, 1980). This finding requires confirmation. The clinical significance of modifying the proportion of metabolites of imipramine or other tricyclic drugs is as yet unknown.

Clinical application of plasma level studies

Estimation of plasma levels of tricyclic drugs has not been widely employed in clinical practice and has remained largely a research procedure. There are differing views as to the extent to which it is desirable to monitor plasma levels in clinical practice in those hospitals where the service is available. Should psychiatric clinics plan to provide this facility in the future? One view is that routine monitoring of plasma levels of tricyclic drugs should always be carried out in certain circumstances:

(1) in patients with co-existing physical disease, particularly heart disease;
(2) in the elderly patients where metabolism of drugs is slower, more variable and likely to produce the more severe unwanted effects;
(3) where the patient is suspected of not taking the drugs as prescribed;
(4) in endogenous depression where an optimum plasma level can be expected to produce a maximal response (Åsberg and Sjöqvist, 1978).

Other workers are more tentative in recommending estimations of plasma levels in clinical practice. Several workers believe that the evidence is not yet sufficiently firm for definite recommendations to be made (Amsterdam, Brunswick and Mendels, 1980). Another recommends the determination of plasma levels in special circumstances: in detecting non-compliance with treatment; in detecting suboptimal dosage; to investigate unexpected effects possibly due to the drug; monitoring progress after overdosage; monitoring levels of drugs in special groups of patients such as children and the elderly (Hollister, 1978). The author is, however, against the widespread use of plasma estimations in clinical practice: 'Arguments for routine plasma monitoring of plasma concentrations of tricyclics are compelling neither clinically nor on the basis of any cost-benefit analysis'.

Although the points made in this argument are of some interest the fact remains that by far the majority of doctors who prescribe tricyclic drugs do not have access to a service for plasma estimation and are unlikely ever to have such a service available to them. A leading article in the *British Medical Journal* regards the relationship between plasma levels of tricyclic drugs and their therapeutic effects as being insufficiently understood to allow definite advice to be given on the use of plasma estimations in clinical practice. A possible exception is in the use of nortriptyline, where a relatively large amount of information is available (*British Medical Journal*, 1978).

On the evidence at present available it is not yet appropriate for plasma estimations of tricyclic drugs to become a required part of clinical practice.

Clinical use

Following the open studies of Kuhn and others, controlled trials of the tricyclic drugs in the treatment of depressive disorders were undertaken in many parts of the world. The circumstances in which these early trials were conducted were very different from those of the present day.

Although early studies of the use of the monoamine oxidase inhibiting drugs were under way there were no treatments of depressive illness of proven efficacy other than electroconvulsive therapy. Amphetamines either alone or in combination with barbiturates had proved to have a purely transient effect on mood and did not relieve the effects of underlying depressive illness. In spite of the use of ECT there were still many chronically depressed patients living in mental hospitals as permanent inmates. Thus there was little doubt in the minds of investigators that rigorous studies involving comparisons with placebo were both scientifically necessary and ethically justifiable. Once initial studies have shown tricyclic drugs to be superior to placebo, further placebo controlled trials in the investigation of drugs developed later, were more difficult to justify, and there was a change to comparisons between drugs, usually involving comparison with drugs used in the earlier studies. For this reason there are relatively few properly controlled studies of the tricyclic drugs, and as a consequence those which were carried out have become the reference points of subsequent studies and are of great importance in the interpretation of the majority of studies of the tricyclic drugs.

A selection of the early studies will be described in detail.

Controlled studies of imipramine

An early controlled clinical trial of imipramine was that of Ball and Kiloh (1959) in which 48 depressed out-patients were given either imipramine 250 mg daily or placebo, and the results compared after four weeks of treatment. The patients were divided into those considered to be suffering from endogenous or reactive depressive illnesses. Amongst those suffering from endogenous depression 74 per cent of those who received imipramine responded as compared with 22 per cent of those receiving placebo; among those suffering from reactive depression 59 per cent on the active drug responded as compared with 20 per cent on placebo. In this study unwanted effects were noted to be severe. A number of further studies varying in detail gave similar results (Kenning, Richardson and Tucker, 1960; Friedman, De Mowbray and Hamilton, 1961). In these studies imipramine was given in a dosage of 200–225 mg daily over a period of four to six weeks and comparison was made by a double-blind method with the effect of placebo.

In a study of depressed in-patients, thought not to require electroconvulsive therapy, the effects of imipramine 150–300 mg daily were compared with the effects of placebo. The patients receiving imipramine showed a greater degree of improvement after two weeks of treatment but at four weeks the differences between the groups were no longer statistically significant. The authors believed that their results suggest that imipramine is less effective in the less severely depressed patient and that the greater part of the improvement observed in their patients was attributable to the effect of admission to hospital and other non-specific effects (Robin and Langley, 1964).

In a study performed in the USA the effects of placebo were compared with those of imipramine, given in flexible dosage, in severely depressed hospital in-patients. The treatments were given for four weeks. No differences were shown in the degree of clinical improvement in the two treatment groups. There was no difference between the groups as regards the numbers of patients who eventually required electroconvulsive therapy or in the number of treatments given. An interesting aspect of the study was that the administration of active drug and placebo followed a similar pattern throughout the trial even though the substances were both given in a flexible way. This observation tends to confirm the validity of the procedure of giving drugs according to flexible schedules in trials and the 'blindness' of assessments in this particular trial (Roulet et al., 1962).

In a trial in which only patients considered sufficiently ill to require electroconvulsive therapy were studied, the effects of imipramine were compared with those of placebo (Rees, Brown and Benaim, 1961). The treatments were allocated at random and each continued for three weeks after which the patients were changed to the alternative treatment. Patients received four 25 mg tablets on the first day; the dosage was increased by two 5 mg tablets to a maximum of 150 mg of imipramine daily. This was continued for 5 d before being reduced to 130 mg daily until 21 d of the study. Placebo tablets were given similarly. The trial showed that patients improved to a greater extent when they were receiving imipramine compared with the period when they were receiving placebo. About 35 per cent of the patients made a full recovery in the three weeks during which imipramine was given. A deficiency of this trial is that the treatments were given for only three weeks, and in relatively small dosage; we now know that more patients respond when drugs are given for longer periods and in higher dosage.

A statistical review of placebo controlled trials of imipramine in the treatment of depressive illness suggests that the effectiveness of imipramine in acute 'endogenous' depressive illness is indisputable, whereas the value of the drug in chronic, atypical and neurotic disorders is less clear (Rogers and Clay, 1975).

A few studies have tried to reduce the risk of the code being broken in double-blind studies of imipramine and a control treatment by using atropine as the control treatment. In these circumstances all patients might be expected to experience similar unwanted effects. In one study imipramine 150 mg daily and atropine were given to 42 depressed out-patients for four weeks each according to a cross-over design. Imipramine was shown to be superior to placebo (Uhlenhuth and Park, 1964). In another study imipramine in variable dosage was compared with atropine in 195 out-patients with various depressive conditions. The drugs were given for eight weeks and imipramine was shown to carry a clear advantage for patients (Daneman, 1961).

Introduction of amitriptyline

Amitriptyline, which closely resembles imipramine chemically, was introduced in the late 1950s, and the first reports of its clinical effects appeared in 1960. The pharmacological effects of amitriptyline closely resemble those of imipramine, except that it is more sedative.

Amitriptyline was compared with placebo in two trials for the treatment of chronically depressed patients and showed itself to be superior (Garry and Leonard, 1963; Skarbek and Smedberg, 1962). In another trial the effect of amitriptyline in the treatment of depressed patients was compared with that of atropine (Hollister et al., 1964). No difference was revealed between the effects of amitriptyline and atropine.

A number of studies have compared the clinical efficacy of amitriptyline with that of imipramine. One of the largest and most thorough was that performed by Burt et al. (1962). In this trial the effects of amitriptyline and imipramine were compared by a double-blind method in 73 female in-patients suffering from depressive disorder. The patient group was stratified with respect to age and severity before random allocation to treatment. Several criteria of improvement were employed, including the Hamilton scale for depression. The drugs were given in a dosage of 150 mg daily for one week, then 200 mg daily for the next three or five weeks, and then 100 mg daily for the next six months. The patients were assessed after four weeks of treatment and either discharged on the lowest dosage of drugs, or given ECT, or a further two weeks on 200 mg of the drug before re-assessment. Overall assessment after one week showed amitriptyline to be superior but at four weeks the apparent superiority of amitriptyline did not reach a level of statistical significance. Amitriptyline was more effective in combating insomnia, anxiety and agitation. There were other differences between the drugs in the way they appeared to affect specific symptoms of depressive illness.

In spite of variations in the results of the studies and the occasional occurrence of conflicting results, there appears to be good evidence that both imipramine and amitriptyline have antidepressant properties and that in many respects their effects are comparable, if qualitatively different in some respects, with that of electroconvulsive therapy.

Other tricyclic antidepressant drugs

Since the introduction of imipramine and amitriptyline to psychiatry a large number of other tricyclic drugs with antidepressive properties have been developed and assessed clinically. These substances include desipramine, trimipramine, nortriptyline, protriptyline, opipramol, dothiepin, doxepin, butriptyline, iprindole and dibenzepin.

Desipramine

Desipramine is of particular interest; it is the demethylated metabolite of imipramine, desmethylimipramine (DMI), and is itself an antidepressant drug. The discovery that desipramine appears in the body following the administration of imipramine prompted the suggestion that desipramine might be the active substance producing the effects which followed the administration of imipramine. It was argued that if this was so, the administration of desipramine might lead to a more rapid and enhanced antidepressant effect than is seen when imipramine is given. Preliminary experiments in rats and in man suggested that desipramine had very similar pharmacological properties to that of imipramine but with a more rapid onset of action and an activating effect more pronounced than that shown by imipramine (Brodie et al., 1961).

A number of studies have compared the efficacy of imipramine and desipramine. Two open uncontrolled studies of the use of desipramine in a dosage of 150 mg daily suggested that the drug was effective and that it began to show its antidepressive effects only three days after administration was started (Ban and Lehmann, 1962; Mann and Heseltine, 1963). Two controlled studies have shown imipramine to be superior to desipramine (Wilson et al., 1963; Edwards, 1965), and a number have shown no difference between them (Waldron and Bates, 1965; Rose and Westhead, 1964; Hargreaves and Maxwell, 1967; Lafave et al., 1965). Some of these investigators found desipramine to have a more rapid effect initially but the difference in the speed of action was not significant statistically and, moreover, there was no advantage to the patients on desipramine over a period of three to four weeks compared with those receiving imipramine. Two placebo controlled studies of the antidepressive effects of desmethylimipramine showed it to have very limited advantages over placebo. In one, DMI or placebo was randomly allocated to 69 newly admitted depressed patients. The mean dosage of DMI over the last two of three weeks' treatment was 100 mg daily. Changes in depressive symptomatology were measured; both groups of patients showed improvement, which was greater amongst those on placebo but the differences between them were insignificant. The failure to show a therapeutic effect of DMI greater than placebo may be attributable to the use of a relatively low dosage for too short a period of time (Hollister *et al.*, 1963). In a similar study 40 depressed patients were allocated to DMI, 100–400 mg daily, or to placebo for one to three weeks. Global assessment of change showed an advantage to the patients on DMI but this finding was not supported by more objective measures. The authors attribute the inconsistency of their results to weaknesses in methodology, especially the inadequacy of the rating scales used, rather than to a lack of efficacy of the drug (Vestre, Janecek and Zimmermann, 1967).

A comparison of DMI and nortriptyline in the treatment of depression showed the drugs to have a similar antidepressive effect overall but with DMI giving more rapid relief from depressed mood and nortriptyline more effective control of anxiety and agitation (Haider, 1968). A similar study showed the drug to be of similar antidepressive effectiveness with nortriptyline improving sleep to a greater extent and DMI leading to reduced anxiety and greater activity (Stewart and Mitchell, 1968).

Trimipramine

Trimipramine has a very similar formula to that of imipramine, the only difference being an additional methyl group attached to the aliphatic side-chain (*Figure 7.2*). The drug is one of the most sedative of the tricyclic group. The effects of trimipramine and imipramine have been compared in a number of studies. A trial using a double-blind design and sequential analysis of results showed trimipramine in a dosage of 150 mg daily to be superior to imipramine 150 mg daily in the treatment of severely depressed in-patients (Burns, 1965). In this study trimipramine produced more unwanted effects than imipramine, drowsiness being particularly troublesome. This finding might be held to suggest that trimipramine is a more potent substance than imipramine and should be given in a proportionately smaller dosage. In a similar study, however, using the same two drugs in the treatment of depressed gynaecological patients, similar therapeutic effects were produced by the drugs in a dosage of 75–100 mg daily, but without severe unwanted effects (Lean and Sidhu, 1972). Somewhat unexpectedly, in this study sedative effects were more marked with imipramine as were most of the unwanted effects. In another trial of trimipramine and imipramine, each given in a dosage of 150 mg daily, therapeutic effects were similar but giddiness was the most common unwanted effect and was more commonly seen in patients on trimipramine (Satija, Advani and Bansal, 1973).

Comparisons between trimipramine and amitriptyline have been made in both general and hospital practice. An early study in general practice showed the drugs to be of similar therapeutic effectiveness. A flexible dosage schedule was used and amitriptyline turned out to have been used in a lower dosage than trimipramine but amitriptyline had produced marginally more unwanted effects. Trimipramine was more effective in relieving accompanying anxiety. An important finding of the study was that improvement between the fourth and sixth weeks of treatment was quite marked (General Practitioner Research Group, 1967). A hospital trial of the two drugs employed the drug in similar dosage throughout; 75 mg daily for one week, 150 mg daily for the fourth week. Therapeutic and unwanted effects were very similar, and there was no difference between the drugs as regards speed of onset of therapeutic effect (Burke, Sainsbury and Mezo, 1967). A combined hospital and general practice study compared the effects of amitriptyline and trimipramine with those of placebo. Amitriptyline was the most effective therapeutically, trimipramine the next and placebo the least. Amitriptyline and imipramine were given in a dosage of 75 mg for the first two weeks and 150 mg for the second two weeks; a very small proportion of the subjects on each drug were unable to take the full dosage. Amitriptyline produced most unwanted effects, slightly more than trimipramine and markedly more than placebo. Although the two drugs appear to be effective antidepressants the results suggest that amitriptyline is the more potent (Rickels *et al.*, 1970).

Clomipramine

Clomipramine is closely related to imipramine structurally, having an additional chlorine atom in position 3 in the molecule (*Figure 7.2*). Clomipramine closely resembles imipramine in its pharmacological properties and clinical effects. It is one of the most specific inhibitors of 5-HT known (Waldmeier *et al.*, 1976).

In an early trial clomipramine was compared with imipramine in the treatment of depressive illness and the two remedies found to have very similar therapeutic and unwanted effects. The drugs were given according to a flexible dosage schedule but most patients received six tablets a day. The tablets of clomipramine contained 12.5 mg of the drug and those of imipramine 25 mg; accordingly the author concludes that clomipramine has twice the potency of imipramine (Symes, 1967).

A study comparing the effects of clomipramine 150 mg daily with imipramine 150 mg daily showed the drugs to be similar both therapeutically and in producing unwanted effects. The control of symptoms of anxiety was also similar (Rack, 1973). A similar study comparing clomipramine with amitriptyline 150 mg daily gave a similar picture. There was an early advantage to amitriptyline in controlling insomnia. Both drugs showed similar unwanted effects but these were marginally more severe with amitriptyline (Hynes, 1973). A study conducted in Jamaica showed amitriptyline 150 mg daily and clomipramine 150 mg daily to have similar therapeutic effects. There was, however, a high incidence of unwanted effects among the patients taking clomipramine and particularly of postural hypotension. These findings led the author to recommend that clomipramine should not be a tricyclic antidepressant of first choice (Harding, 1973). A study in which clomipramine and imipramine were compared with placebo in the treatment of depressed hospital in-patients showed the drugs to have a similar effect and to be clearly superior to placebo. An early advantage to imipramine was not seen after four and eight weeks of treatment. Because of early reports that clomipramine was more potent than imipramine a smaller capsule of clomipramine was used (18.75 mg as compared with 25 mg) and the capsules were given three times a day; the author believes that this was the reason for the differences observed in the severity of unwanted effects (Gore, 1973).

Clomipramine has been claimed to be of value in the treatment of patients suffering from obsessive–compulsive and phobic states. A number of small uncontrolled studies have been reported and these suggested promising results in a previously unpromising area (Rack, 1973; Marshall and Micev, 1973; Walter, 1973). The mechanisms of the effects observed were unclear and were particularly difficult to evaluate in uncontrolled investigations. A more recent study which compared the effects of clomipramine with behavioural treatments showed that the effectiveness of clomipramine in relieving obsessive–compulsive symptoms was dependent upon the concomitant relief of depressive symptoms (Marks *et al.*, 1980). From this study it seems likely that clomipramine has no specific effect upon obsessive–compulsive symptoms and that its effect is dependent upon its antidepressant properties. Thus, the drug is unlikely to be more effective in the treatment of obsessive–compulsive states than other effective antidepressive drugs.

A number of papers have appeared describing the administration of clomipramine by intravenous infusion. Studies have compared the therapeutic effects of the drugs given in this way with those of other drugs given orally. In view of the rapid and complete absorption of tricyclic drugs when given by mouth intravenous infusion appears unlikely to have any particular advantage. A possible effect is that intravenous infusion avoids immediate passage through the liver where tricyclic drugs are metabolized. By-passing the liver could alter the proportions of the drug and its metabolite in the body in the period shortly after administration. Although the demethylated metabolites of tricyclic drugs often have antidepressive properties they may exert different effects on amine metabolism thereby presenting the possibility of somewhat different clinical effects. A clinical study comparing the antidepressive effects of clomipramine given in a daily dosage of 75 mg by the intravenous route with a single daily oral dose of 75–100 mg showed no differences between the treatments. There was an impression that the onset of improvement was earlier with intravenous administration. Unwanted effects were minimal (Aguirre, 1968). This paper cannot be regarded as conclusive as it has important methodological weaknesses. The pattern of plasma levels of the drug and its metabolites produced by various routes of administration do not appear to have been closely studied.

The marketing of clomipramine had been based not on its antidepressant effects alone but on the claims that it could be administered by intravenous infusion with advantages to the patient in speed of action and increased efficacy; and that it is especially effective in the treatment of the symptoms of obsessive–compulsive illness and of phobic states. These claims appear to have been both specious and misleading; in truth it is simply another member of the group of tricyclic antidepressants and with very similar therapeutic and unwanted effects.

Nortriptyline

Nortriptyline is the demethylated metabolite of amitriptyline and is analogous to desipramine (*Figure 7.4*). Nortriptyline was shown to be superior to placebo in the treatment of depressed out-patients using a double-blind cross-over trial design with three weeks on each treatment (MacLean and Rees, 1966). This study cannot be regarded as entirely satisfactory as cross-over studies are only suitable for the assessment of treatments of uniformly persistent disorders. Unwanted effects recorded included: dryness of the mouth, tremulousness, sweating, dizziness, distressing epigastric sensations and headache. Two studies have compared the effects of nortriptyline with amitriptyline. One employed a dosage of 100 mg daily of each drug and showed a marked improvement in depressive symptomatology during treatment with no statistical differences between them (Leahy and Martin, 1967). The other study utilized a double-blind comparison of the effects of nortriptyline and amitriptyline. All

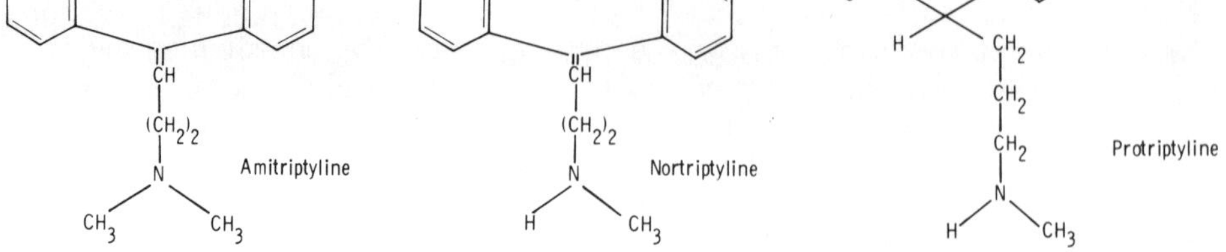

Figure 7.4

patients showed marked improvement; this was more rapid among patients on nortriptyline but at six weeks the results were similar with both drugs (Mendels, 1968). The dosage of drugs used was not given.

Nortriptyline and desipramine have been shown to exert similar antidepressant effects (Stewart and Mitchell, 1968). A double-blind trial in 31 depressed patients compared the effects of nortriptyline 150 mg daily and protriptyline 60 mg daily over a four-week period. The drugs proved to have similar therapeutic effects. Nortriptyline produced more drowsiness and protriptyline more complaints of dry mouth and blurred vision (Priest, 1976). A trial comparing the effects of isocarboxazid 30 mg daily and nortriptyline 100 mg daily in depressed out-patients showed improvement in a substantial proportion with no differences between the treatments (Hays and Steinart, 1969).

The pharmacokinetics of this drug have been extensively studied (p. 108).

Protriptyline

Protriptyline is chemically very similar to nortriptyline (*Figure 7.4*). An early open study suggested the drug to be an active antidepressive substance with relatively little sedative effect. Unwanted effects were similar to those produced by other tricyclic drugs (General Practitioner Research Group, 1968). A double-blind comparison in 156 depressed patients showed the antidepressive effect of imipramine and protriptyline to be similar (Krakowski, 1965). In this study imipramine was given in a dosage of 75–200 mg daily and protriptyline 30–60 mg daily. Unwanted effects were noted in 40 patients on protriptyline and 33 patients on imipramine. The unwanted effects of imipramine were less severe as well as less frequent. Postural hypotension was seen in 20 per cent of the cases on protriptyline and necessitated withdrawal of the drug in two cases. Protriptyline appeared to give a more rapid onset of improvement whereas imipramine was better tolerated. These details suggest that protriptyline may have been administered at a comparatively higher dosage than imipramine.

The speed of action of protriptyline was specifically examined in a later trial (Lewis and Silverstone, 1970). In a double-blind study protriptyline 45 mg daily and imipramine 150 mg daily were randomly allocated to 46 depressed in-patients. The progress of patients was followed over a 17-d period; throughout the administration protriptyline was associated with greater amelioration in depressive symptoms and this effect was particularly marked between 5 and 10 d. As the trial progressed thereafter differences between the treatments diminished. Unwanted effects were of similar frequency and type although anticholinergic effects were marginally more severe with protriptyline. Fewer patients who received protriptyline required other drugs for the control of anxiety. This study tends to confirm claims that protriptyline has a more rapid onset of action but suggests that as treatment progresses this advantage diminishes. The trial was too short to permit full evaluation of this effect.

A detailed study of the effects of amitriptyline and protriptyline in depressed out-patients showed protriptyline to be effective in relieving depression of mood and insomnia but with efficacy bearing no relationship to the control of agitation (McConaghy *et al.*, 1968).

Dothiepin

Dothiepin has a chemical formula resembling that of chlorpromazine but its clinical effects more closely resemble those of the tricyclic antidepressants (*Figure 7.5*). In an

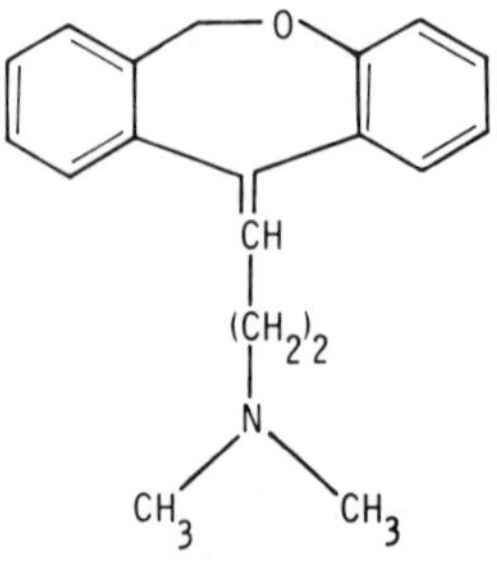

Figure 7.5

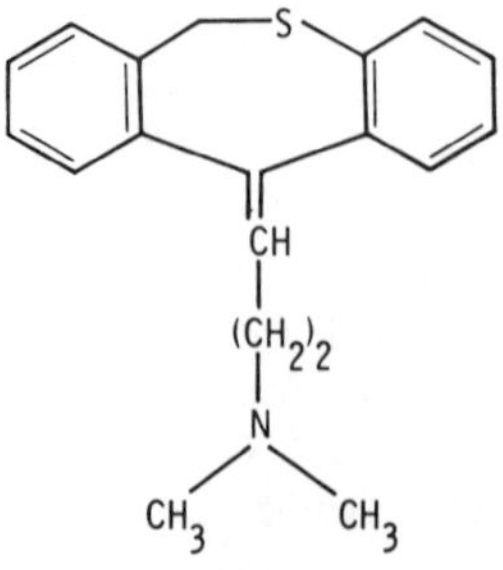

early study of dothiepin the effects of the drug were compared with those of amitriptyline in the treatment of 50 depressed out-patients. Dothiepin proved to be superior to amitriptyline in the relief of symptoms of depression. Relief of anxiety occurred to a similar extent in patients on either drug. There was a close relationship between improvement in these two symptoms; patients showing little improvement in one tending to show little change in the other. Unwanted effects were similar among patients on either drug but dothiepin was better tolerated. A flexible dosage schedule was used; this resulted in an average daily dosage of 150 mg of dothiepin but only 75 mg for amitriptyline; this difference in dosage is important in the interpretation of the results (Lipsedge, Rees and Pike, 1971). A study carried out in general practice compared dothiepin 75 mg daily with chlordiazepoxide 30 mg daily in the treatment of 88 patients suffering from 'tension, anxiety and emotional disturbance' over a three-week period. Dothiepin was found to be superior in the relief of symptoms and to produce a lower incidence of drowsiness (Johnson, Sacco and Yellowley, 1973). A comparison of imipramine and dothiepin in the treatment of depressed patients over a six-week period showed the drugs to be very similar in their therapeutic effects (Sim *et al.*, 1975). Dothiepin showed markedly fewer unwanted effects and had an advantage in this respect. A study comparing two different dosage regimens for dothiepin showed once-daily dosage of the drug to be superior to thrice-daily dosage. In the first week placebo capsules were given, in the second week 75 mg dothiepin daily, in the third 150 mg daily and in the fourth week 225 mg daily. The patients were all suffering from depressive disorders and were treated as out-patients. The study showed once-daily dosage to be superior and attributed this effect to better compliance with the instructions given on the taking of medication (Pearce and Rees, 1974).

Opipramol

Although a tricyclic drug, opipramol, has a piperazine side-chain similar to that present in some phenothiazine drugs (*Figure 7.6*). In spite of this chemical similarity to some neuroleptic drugs opipramol resembles the tricyclic drugs in its pharmacological effects.

An early double-blind comparison of opipramol (average dosage 100 mg daily), phenobarbitone 50 mg daily, and placebo in depressed patients showed an improvement rate after three weeks' treatment of approximately 46 per cent, 20 per cent and 16 per cent respectively. The onset of improvement in patients on opipramol was general after 4–5 d of administration. Unwanted effects were similar in all treatment groups; opipramol showed evidence of sedative effects (Azima, Silver and Arthurs, 1962). These findings are supported by similar results from placebo controlled studies (Splitter, 1963; Shepherd, 1965; Carney, 1968).

In a comparative trial of opipramol 60 mg daily with imipramine 150 mg daily conducted in general practice very similar therapeutic results were observed over a four-week period. Unwanted effects were similar among patients receiving either drug as was the number of patients discontinuing the treatments (Murphy, 1975). A rather similar study also conducted in general practice compared the effects of opipramol 150 mg daily and desipramine 75 mg daily in the treatment of depressed patients. At two weeks desipramine showed greater effects but at four weeks the treatments were similar. Opipramol was more effective in controlling anxiety both after one and four weeks (Rogers, Davies and Galbraith, 1969). A double-blind comparison of the effects of opipramol with the combined effects of phenelzine and chlordiazepoxide in the treatment of depressed out-patients showed no advantage to either regimen at the end of six weeks. Opipramol was more effective in controlling tension, insomnia and bodily symptoms; the combined preparations more effective in the control of phobic and depressive symptoms. The patients favoured the combination; the doctors favoured opipramol (Capstick and Rooke, 1974).

A series of studies has been made of the effectiveness of opipramol in the treatment of anxiety. A sequentially analysed comparison with placebo showed differences between the treatments which were not statistically significant (Carney and Maxwell, 1967). Three studies comparing opipramol and chlordiazepoxide showed the treatments to be very similar (Grosser and Ryan, 1965; Murphy, Donald and Beaumont, 1971; Jepson and Beaumont, 1973). A comparison of the effects of opipramol 150 mg daily or more in the treatment of anxiety showed the drugs to be very similar with regard to both therapeutic and unwanted effects (Gringras and Beaumont, 1971). A study which involved comparison of opipramol 150–200 mg daily, dixyrazine 30–40 mg daily, diazepam 12–16 mg daily and placebo showed diazepam to give the best control of symptoms of anxiety and placebo the least, with the other substances giving an intermediate effect. Patient reports favoured diazepam. Unwanted effects were mild. The authors draw attention to the importance of adequate controls for trials of treatment of anxiety and to the relatively poor response even to the most effective treatment (Arfwidsson et al., 1971).

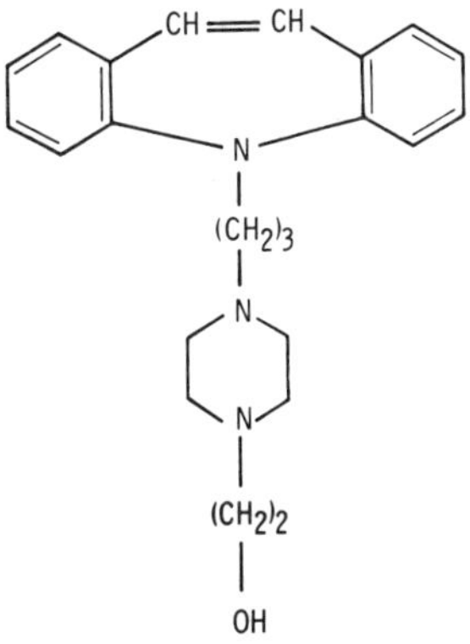

Figure 7.6 Opipramol

On this evidence opipramol would appear to have similar antidepressant properties to those of other tricyclic drugs and to have effects on anxiety which are similar to or somewhat less than those of benzodiazepines.

Butriptyline

Butriptyline is a tricyclic drug with an additional methyl group attached to its aliphatic side-chain; it is a tertiary amine (*Figure 7.7*). The drug has been shown to have less inhibitory effect on the uptake of noradrenaline and less anticholinergic effect than related drugs with an unbranched side-chain (Lippmann, 1971). Other animal experiments have shown the drug to have a similar potency to that of imipramine in a variety of pharmacological effects (Herr, Voith and Jaramillo, 1971).

A double-blind comparison of butriptyline and imipramine in the treatment of 28 depressed out-patients, using a flexible dosage schedule utilizing 25 mg tablets, showed butriptyline to be slightly superior in the relief of symptoms of depression and anxiety and to produce fewer unwanted effects (Levinson, 1974). A similar study compared the effects of butriptyline and amitriptyline, both given in a dosage of 225 mg daily in the treatment of out-patient depressives, and showed butriptyline to be slightly superior in the relief of depressive symptoms. Unwanted effects are similar in both groups of patients (Suy, 1976).

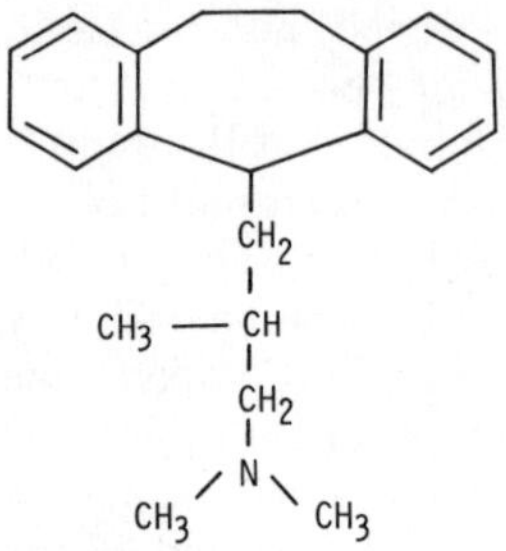

Figure 7.7 Butriptyline

Doxepin

Doxepin is a tricyclic drug with an oxygen atom in the middle ring and an aliphatic side-chain, resembling dothiepin in many respects (*Figure 7.5*). The drug has been shown to have pharmacological characteristics similar to other members of the tricyclic group (Hobbs, 1969). Open studies in a large number of patients showed the drug to have similar clinical characteristics to those of the group as a whole; to be less likely to produce hypotension and tachycardia; and to require administration in a dosage of about 150 mg daily (Pitts, 1969). In a sequentially analysed comparison of doxepin and placebo in 14 pairs of moderately depressed patients doxepin was shown to relieve symptoms of depression and anxiety during the course of three weeks' administration (Burrows, Mowbray and Davies, 1972).

Doxepin was compared with amitriptyline in a double-blind study of depressed out-patients who received the drugs for four weeks; amitriptyline 100–250 mg daily; doxepin 150–350 mg daily. The trial was stopped when 22 patients had been treated, when the treatments were found to have been equally effective. Amitriptyline was particularly effective in relieving agitation, insomnia and weight loss, doxepin in relieving anxiety, retardation and hypochondriacal symptoms, with both drugs showing effects in improving depressed mood, work performance and insight, and in relieving suicidal ideas (Grof *et al.*, 1974). A detailed study of the effects of overdosage of several tricyclic antidepressants on the heart were studied using the technique of Bundle of His electrocardiography: all the drugs, with the exception of doxepin, showed conduction abnormalities in a large proportion of the patients who had taken them (Burrows *et al.*, 1976). These findings suggest that doxepin may be safer in the treatment of patients with established heart disease.

Iprindole

Iprindole is a substance with an indole nucleus, a dimethyl-aminopropyl side-chain; and a cyclo-octane ring (*Figure 7.8*). The drug shows similar pharmacological effects to those shown by the tricyclic group but, unlike other tricyclics, does not inhibit the re-uptake of noradrenaline, has weak anticholinergic activity, weak antihistamine properties and does not block REM in sleep as seen in the EEG. Iprindole antagonizes the effects of reserpine in animals as does the tricyclic group of substances. No permanent toxic effects have been found in animals. These characteristics in animal experiments suggest that the substance has antidepressive properties with less anticholinergic activity than is seen with most of the tricyclic drugs.

Clinical trials of iprindole include several comparisons with placebo and many with imipramine and other tricyclic drugs. In a double-blind comparison with placebo in 33 depressed patients in a general practice, the drug being given in a dosage of 90 mg daily over a period of 10–62 d, the administration of the active drug was associated with a 93 per cent reduction of symptoms in the patients treated, as compared with 21 per cent in patients receiving placebo. No serious unwanted effects were reported (Hicks, 1965). In a similar general practice study 100 patients were treated for neurotic depressive disorders using a double-blind method of assessment. The dosage of iprindole used was 45–90 mg daily and was given for up to eight weeks. Eighty per cent of the patients receiving the active drug were considered to have shown an excellent response compared with 16 per cent on placebo (Daneman, 1967). Complaints of dryness of the mouth, constipation, and blurring of vision were reported by patients on either treatment.

A number of comparisons between iprindole and imipramine have been conducted and suggest that the drug in a dosage of 90 mg daily has similar effects to imipramine 150 mg daily but with fewer unwanted effects (El-Deiry, Forrest and Littman, 1967).

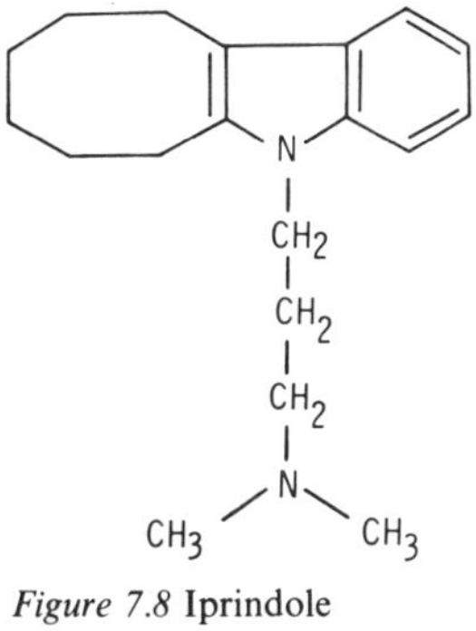

Figure 7.8 Iprindole

Iprindole has also been shown to be comparable in therapeutic effect with amitriptyline (Sterlin *et al.*, 1968).

Iprindole is generaly given in a dosage of 30–90 mg daily and in this dosage appears to have fewer unwanted effects than some other antidepressant drugs. The precautions to be observed in its administration are similar to those for tricyclic drugs.

Dibenzepin

Dibenzepin is a dibenzodiazepine derivative (*Figure 7.9*). Like imipramine it is a tertiary amine and has similar pharmacological effects. In animals dibenzepin antagonizes the effect of reserpine as do many substances showing antidepressive activity in man (Boissier *et al.*, 1966).

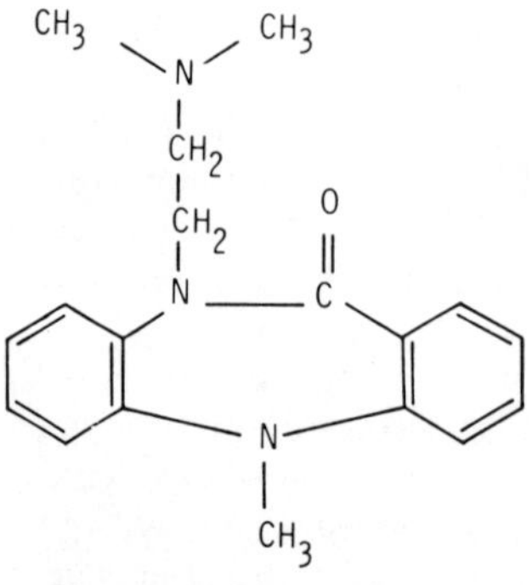

Figure 7.9 Dibenzepin

An early uncontrolled clinical assessment suggested that the drug had an effect comparable with, but slightly inferior to that of imipramine and that it was most helpful to the retarded depressed patient, as in the case of imipramine. It was found to exhibit less unwanted effects than imipramine and to be better tolerated (Angst and Kind, 1964).

Subsequent double-blind trials tend to confirm the early reports. A double-blind comparison of the effects of dibenzepin, 480 mg daily, and of imipramine, 150 mg daily, in 22 moderately severely depressed in-patients and day-patients showed the regimens to be equally effective. The speed of action was shown to be similar at all stages of the study. The type, severity and frequency of unwanted effects was similar among patients on both treatments. In both groups the frequency of unwanted effects decreased with time (Fielding, 1969). In a similar study dibenzepin was compared with imipramine in 71 depressed in-patients (Sim *et al.*, 1971). In this case a flexible drug dosage regimen was used; patients receiving imipramine 85 mg daily or dibenzepin, 240 mg daily at first, rising as necessary to a maximum of 150 mg daily or 48 mg daily, respectively. Treatment continued for six weeks in most of the patients studied. The drugs were found to have a similar effect although it was noted that imipramine had a slight advantage in the treatment of the most severely affected patients. Dibenzepin showed more unwanted effects than imipramine but had a slightly quicker action.

In a comparison of the effects of dibenzepin with amitriptyline in 79 depressed in-patients the drugs were shown to be equally effective (Ekdawi, 1971). The drugs were administered in a low dosage at first but this was raised to 150 mg of amitriptyline daily or 48 mg of dibenzepin daily by the end of the fourth day; after 14 d on the full dosage the dose could be raised to 225 mg daily or 560 mg daily respectively at the psychiatrist's discretion. Similar proportions of patients complained of unwanted effects on each drug but the author felt that the effects produced by dibenzepin were less severe than those produced by amitriptyline.

The reports available suggest that dibenzepin is similar in most respects to other tricyclic antidepressants. There appear to be no special indications for its use nor particular dangers from its administration. A daily dosage of 480 mg appears to give similar clinical effects to those of imipramine and amitriptyline given in a dosage of 150 mg daily.

Maintenance therapy

From their follow-up study of patients who had recovered from depressive illness following treatment with imipramine Kiloh and Ball (1961) were unable to give precise advice on the length of the period for which medication should be continued. They gained the impression that relapse was most likely within two months of recovery but the intervals observed varied widely. The mean duration of treatment with drugs in their study was six months with a range of 1–14 months. In general a lower dosage of imipramine (75–100 mg daily) was adequate in the follow-up period compared with a treatment level of 150–200 mg daily with a maximum of 250 mg daily, but a few patients seemed to require more.

A number of studies have attempted to discover whether the continued adminis-tration of tricyclic antidepressants to patients after they have recovered from a depressive illness which has responded to treatment, is associated with a lower rate of recurrence than giving no treatment in the follow-up period (Seager and Bird, 1962; Imlah, Ryan and Harrington, 1964; Hordern et al., 1964; Kay, Fahy and Garside, 1970). These studies, in which initial treatment was with ECT, suggest that patients do gain an advantage from continued medication with antidepressants as compared with those given placebo, no drugs, or other preparations such as sedatives.

More recently two studies of continuation therapy have been conducted in which depressed patients were first treated with amitriptyline or imipramine. In a study conducted under the aegis of the Medical Research Council of Great Britain patients suffering from moderately severe depressive illness were initially treated with amitriptyline or imipramine and then, after full clinical recovery, were randomly allocated to six months' further treatment with the drug to which they had recently responded or to placebo. When continuation therapy was started all the patients were well but as the study progressed patients relapsed. The relative benefit to the patients was shown by the difference between the relapse rate among the patients who received the active drugs and that among those who received placebo. At the end of the six-month period of continuation therapy 22 per cent of those on the active drugs had relapsed compared with 50 per cent of those on placebo (*Figure 7.10*). The only clinical factor which was associated with benefit from active treatment was the presence of minor symptoms at the time at which continuation therapy was commenced (Mindham et al., 1973).

A rather similar study was conducted at Yale at about the same time as the study just described. In this study all the patients received amitriptyline initially and were then divided into three groups to receive amitriptyline, placebo or no medication for six months. These groups were further subdivided into those groups who received supportive psychotherapy from a social worker in addition to other measures, and those who were followed by a psychiatrist routinely. Thus there were six treatment cells

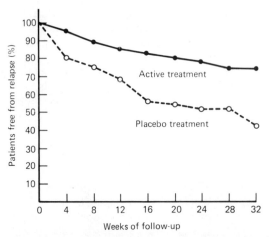

Figure 7.10 Effects of maintenance antidepressant therapy compared with placebo in two trial groups compared at 4-weekly intervals (the active treatment group were taking imipramine or amitriptyline)

in all. The trial showed an advantage, as far as relapse was concerned, to the patients who received amitriptyline, irrespective of other measures (Paykel *et al.*, 1975).

These studies appear to demonstrate conclusively that some patients benefit from continued medication for a six-month period after recovery from a depressive illness which has responded to the same drug. In some ways both of the trials described above concern the management of patients during the later stages of treatment rather than prophylaxis proper. The results now seem rather obvious but an enquiry before the first study was completed shows that the psychiatrists participating were unable to foresee the outcome (Mindham, 1981). The authors of both studies draw attention to the finding that not all patients require continued medication as many of those allocated to placebo did not relapse.

The introduction and widespread use of lithium salts in the prophylaxis of affective disorders raises the question of the relative effectiveness of lithium and tricyclic drugs (Mindham, 1978). A study conducted over a two-year period examined this issue. The findings showed that in both unipolar and bipolar manic depressive illness, lithium carbonate reduces the risk of relapse into mania or depressive states; whereas imipramine protected only against relapse into depression and might have increased the risk of mania (Prien, Caffey and Klett, 1972). Thus tricyclic drugs can only be recommended in patients who suffer from recurrent depressive episodes; the choice between lithium salts and tricyclic drugs being mainly one of convenience and preference. In patients subject to both episodes of depression and mania lithium salts are to be preferred.

Comparisons between tricyclic drugs and other antidepressive treatments

Imipramine compared with electroconvulsive therapy (ECT)

A number of studies have compared the effects of imipramine with those of electroconvulsive therapy in the treatment of depressive illness. In an early study 50 patients suffering from depressive illness were randomly allocated to receive either

ECT or imipramine 150–255 mg daily for four weeks. Of 22 patients given ECT 21 were much better after four weeks' treatment, as were 16 out of the 19 patients treated with imipramine. The results were marginally in favour of ECT although there were some patients who did not respond to either treatment (Bruce *et al.*, 1960). In another study patients suffering from depressive illnesses considered to require ECT were randomly allocated to receive ECT or imipramine. The patients on imipramine had anaesthesia without ECT, and those receiving ECT had placebo tablets resembling imipramine. Progress was assessed using the Hamilton rating scale and behavioural ratings performed by nursing staff. ECT was clearly superior in bringing about a greater general improvement and in reducing the severity of individual symptoms (Robin and Harris, 1962).

The medical research council study of treatments for depression

An important study of the effects of imipramine on depressive illness was that organized under the auspices of the Medical Research Council of Great Britain (MRC, 1965). In this study a comparison was made between the effects of imipramine, phenelzine, ECT and placebo in the treatment of a group of 250 moderately severely depressed patients of both sexes. ECT was the most effective treatment in the short term (four weeks) but over a longer period (12 weeks) both ECT and imipramine brought improvement to about two-thirds of the patients who received these treatments. Phenelzine and placebo were associated with improvement in about one-third of the patients who received them.

Comparisons between tricyclic drugs and monoamine oxidase inhibiting drugs

The Medical Research Council study showed that imipramine is superior to phenelzine in the treatment of depressed in-patients. Although it is likely that these findings can be generalized to reflect differences between the tricyclic drugs and the monoamine oxidase inhibiting drugs as groups, this cannot be assumed. This issue has been examined in a number of trials and some of these will be outlined here and also in Chapter 9.

An early study concerned a comparison of the effects of imipramine 50–200 mg daily and phenelzine 45–60 mg daily in 96 patients suffering from depressive disorders. Of these 79 were in-patients and 17 out-patients; 95 were diagnosed as suffering from endogenous depression and one from reactive depression. After four weeks' therapy 76 per cent of the patients on imipramine had responded compared with 57 per cent of responders on phenelzine. At four months after continued medication the figures were 67 per cent and 49 per cent respectively (Martin, 1963). The findings of this study are rather similar to those of the MRC study and suggest that imipramine is superior to phenelzine in the more severe forms of depressive illness. As no placebo treatment group was used it is impossible to say whether phenelzine is an effective treatment.

A comparison of imipramine, amitriptyline, isocarboxazid and tranylcypromine in depressed out-patients over a three-week period showed more of the drugs to be associated with much symptomatic improvement. The authors conclude that all of these drugs are ineffective in an out-patient population (Richmond and Roberts, 1964). This conclusion should be qualified as the drugs were given for only three weeks. In a population of this kind spontaneous recovery would be expected in a proportion of patients, and one suspects that the method of rating symptoms used was too crude for the purpose for which it was employed or, alternatively, that it was not properly administered.

The relative merit of tricyclic drugs and monoamine oxidase inhibiting drugs has been studied in two recent trials. In the first 135 mildly or moderately severely depressed out-patients were randomly allocated to one of five treatment regimens for six weeks of treatment: namely trimipramine, phenelzine, isocarboxazid, trimipramine plus phenelzine, trimipramine plus isocarboxazid. Symptomatology was assessed using various scales after one, three and six weeks of treatment. Trimipramine was found to be superior to phenelzine and to isocarboxazid and to the combined treatments. Flexible dosage schedules were used throughout, and it is interesting to note that the same average dosage of the drugs was used whether they were administered singly or in combination (Young, Lader and Hughes, 1979). In the second study 30 depressed subjects newly admitted to hospital were randomly allocated to receive amitriptyline up to 300 mg daily; tranylcypromine up to 40 mg daily; or a combination of amitriptyline up to 150 mg daily and tranylcypromine up to 20 mg daily. Treatment was continued for four weeks. Patients in all three groups showed a similar degree of improvement (White, Pistole and Boyd, 1980). Unwanted effects were slightly more troublesome among the patients on the combined treatment but this was not statistically significantly different from unwanted effects in the other two groups. No patients dropped out of the study on account of unwanted effects.

The studies described suggest that tricyclic drugs are more effective than the monoamine oxidase drugs in the treatment of both in-patients and out-patients suffering from depressive illness. The issue is clouded by difficulties in diagnosing depressive illness, including depressive–anxiety states, and the concept of atypical depression. This important issue is dealt with in Chapter 9.

Although lithium salts are not generally considered to possess antidepressive properties comparable with the tricyclic drugs and electroconvulsive therapy there is some evidence that they have some beneficial effects in mild depressive states (Fieve, Platman and Plutchik, 1968; Goodwin, Murphy and Bunney, 1969; Greenspan et al., 1970; Mendels, Secunda and Dyson, 1972) but not in severe depressive illness (Fieve, Platman and Plutchik, 1968). A study is reported from Japan in which the effects of imipramine and lithium carbonate were compared in a mixed group of depressed in-patients and out-patients. Patients on either drug showed marked improvement, and after three and five weeks of treatment the degree of improvement seen was similar in both treatment groups (Watanabe, Ishino and Otsuki, 1975). The implication of this study is that lithium carbonate has antidepressive properties comparable with those of imipramine and that this is seen in a variety of depressive states. This finding requires confirmation from other centres.

Combinations of tricyclic antidepressants with other drugs

Although it is widely held that tricyclic drugs should not be given with drugs which inhibit monoamine oxidase, a number of psychiatrists have consistently advocated such combinations in the treatment of refractory cases (Gander, 1965; Sargant, 1971; Schuckit, Robins and Feighner, 1971; Sethna, 1974). A serious interaction between the two types of drugs can certainly occur (see below). Because of the possible dangers the use of combinations of tricyclic drugs and monoamine oxidase inhibitors has been largely confined to the treatment of refractory cases and until quite recently no attempts had been made to compare the effects of combined drugs with the drugs individually or with placebo.

Two of the studies described above (Young, Lader and Hughes, 1979; White, Pistole and Boyd, 1980) also examined the benefits of combining tricyclic drugs with monoamine oxidase inhibitors in the treatment of depressive states. In the first study there was no advantage gained from the combination of trimipramine with either phenelzine or isocarboxazid; in fact, trimipramine alone was superior even though it was given in no greater dosage than in the combination. In the second study the combination of amitriptyline with tranylcypromine was as effective as either of the two drugs given alone but in a higher average dosage. Again interpretation of the findings, especially of the second study, is made more difficult by our limited knowledge of the efficacy of monoamine oxidase inhibitors in depressive states. A number of studies show tranylcypromine to be the most effective antidepressant of the monamine oxidase inhibiting drugs (Tyrer, 1979) and this may explain the rather different findings of the two studies.

The authors of these studies report few unwanted effects, a low level of drop-outs from drug effects and no serious complications of treatment. They claim to have demonstrated the feasibility and safety of combining the drugs in the treatment of depressed subjects other than those who have failed to respond to all other methods of treatment. Earlier experience suggests that tricyclic drugs should not be added to the treatment of patients already stabilized on a monoamine oxidase inhibitor; rather, the two drugs should be prescribed together (Pare, 1965; Sethna, 1974). In general the sedative tricyclics are safer than the stimulant members of the group and similarly stimulant monoamine oxidase inhibitors (e.g. tranylcypromine) should be avoided in combination. Dietary restrictions naturally apply to patients taking monoamine oxidase inhibiting drugs in combination as well as in other circumstances.

Tricyclic antidepressants and amine precursors

See p. 274.

Tricyclic drugs compared or combined with psychotherapy in depressive illness

Although studies have occasionally been made of the relative place of drugs and psychotherapy in the treatment of various psychiatric disorders (Uhlenhuth, Lipman and Covi, 1969) few attempts have been made to compare the efficacy of the tricyclic antidepressant drugs with that of psychotherapy in the management of depressive illness (Luborsky *et al.*, 1971).

A study primarily concerned with the evaluation of continuation therapy with drugs after recovery from depressive illness was used in the evaluation of psychotherapy both in the prevention of depressive relapse and in promoting social adjustment (Weissman *et al.*, 1974). This study is described more fully in the section on continuation therapy (Paykel *et al.*, 1975). One hundred and fifty female patients who were suffering from 'neurotic depression' as defined in DSMII were initially treated with amitriptyline. The patients were then randomly allocated to receive amitriptyline, placebo or no medication for a further period of six months. The groups were further subdivided to receive either psychotherapy from a social worker or to have normal out-patient follow-up by a psychiatrist. The psychotherapy consisted of 1 or 2 h per week; one hour was spent in individual psychotherapy and the second hour was devoted to family or group treatment with the same therapist. The therapy was mainly concerned with current problems and difficulties in interpersonal relationships. Patients were helped to identify recurring maladaptive patterns in their behaviour and assisted to adopt more favourable patterns of response especially in interpersonal and family matters. No attempt was made to establish 'regressive transference' or to deal with unconscious material or infantile drives. Five therapists were concerned; the process of psycho-therapy was studied during the main investigation, and this served to keep some similarity of goals and methods between the therapists.

Social adjustment was assessed using a number of established rating scales which were at the same time assessed for reliability and validity. Performance in work, in social and leisure activities, in family relationships, in the marriage and as parents, was assessed. These factors were examined afer two and six months of continuation therapy. At two months there were no differences between the groups with regard to social adjustment but the patients on active medication showed less impairment on other variables. At six months, however, patients receiving psychotherapy showed evidence of better social adjustment than those experiencing low-contact with the follow-up team. The differences between the findings of two months and at six months suggests that short-term psychotherapy has no value in these particular circumstances. No evidence of interaction between maintenance therapy with drugs and psycho-therapy was demonstrated. The design of this particular study was such that those entering the phase of continuation therapy had responded to drug therapy already and, furthermore, patients were not included in the analysis of the effects of psychotherapy unless they completed the six-month follow-up period; that is they remained psychiatrically well for six months. The authors conclude that an extended period of psychotherapy is desirable after recovery from a depressive illness, for the best results to be obtained. This area clearly merits further research.

Tricyclic drugs in the treatment of enuresis

The effectiveness of imipramine in the treatment of nocturnal enuresis was first reported by MacLean (1960) in an uncontrolled study. Since then many reports have appeared and, although the majority of them are not methodologically satisfactory, there appears to be good evidence to support the claim that the tricyclic drugs as a group are helpful in some cases of nocturnal enuresis. Two of the more useful studies will be described in detail.

In a study of the effects of amitriptyline in nocturnal enuresis 60 children who wet themselves frequently were studied in a double-blind, cross-over comparison with placebo (Poussaint, Ditman and Greenfield, 1966). The children were aged 5–15 years and included about 35 per cent of girls. Physical investigations were normal. Allocation to the treatment was at random and medication was continued for four weeks before changing to the other regimen with the majority; there was a smaller group of patients who continued the initial treatment uninterrupted for eight weeks. Amitriptyline was given in a dosage of 25 mg at night to the under-12s and 50 mg at night to the over-12s. Among those patients who changed medication amitriptyline was the better treatment in 60 per cent, placebo better in 9 per cent and there was no difference between the regimens in 31 per cent. In all groups there was a reduction in the reported incidence of enuresis. The main unwanted effects reported were drowsiness, fatigue, headache, loss of appetite, irritability and waking at night.

After eight weeks' treatment all the children were given amitriptyline and the dosage manipulated in the 25–75 mg range and continued for varying periods. Ten per cent of children continued to be dry after the gradual withdrawal of amitriptyline, 62 per cent showed varying degrees of improvement which in the majority continued after drug withdrawal; 28 per cent failed to benefit from treatment.

The authors suggest that the observed therapeutic effects may be attributed to:

(1) an antidepressant effect leading to improvement in mood;
(2) an anticholinergic effect leading to relaxation of the detrusor muscle of the bladder and contraction of the sphincter muscle;
(3) an awakening effect allowing the child to respond to a full bladder by wakening;
(4) a combination of these effects.

A slightly later study of the effects of imipramine in childhood enuresis is worth describing in some detail as it was exceptionally well-designed and conducted (Shaffer, Costello and Hill, 1968). After initial screening 62 children entered a double-blind placebo controlled trial of imipramine at two levels of dosage; and 59 completed the three months of the trial. Dosage of imipramine was calculated according to surface area, and the schedules were arranged to give a maximum of 75 mg in the high dosage group and 50 mg in the low dosage group. In practice the low dosage group was given approximately 25 mg for ages 4–7 years, 35 mg for 8–11 years and 50 mg over 11 years. Treatments were given in all possible orders and patients were stratified for age, sex, previous psychiatric treatment and evidence of current emotional disturbance.

The results showed imipramine to be markedly superior to placebo, but no difference between the high and low dosage levels was found. Drug withdrawal was almost always followed by relapse but, unlike Poussaint and colleagues, these workers did not show the effect to be modified by sudden or gradual drug withdrawal. Unwanted effects were very infrequent, restlessness, irritability, tearfulness, difficulty in concentration, deterioration of school work, nightmares and difficulty in getting off to sleep being the worst. Follow-up periods of 3–14 months showed variable results. The majority have shown benefit from imipramine but most had relapsed when the drug was withdrawn.

The authors conclude that imipramine is effective in controlling enuresis in a high proportion of children but that it cannot be regarded as a pharmacological cure for the disorder.

A study of the use of imipramine in enuresis showed that optimum effects were obtained when plasma steady-state levels of imipramine plus desipramine reached a level of 60 μg. ℓ^{-1}; above that level no further benefit was obtained (Jorgensen *et al.*, 1980). Below this level there was a correlation between steady-state plasma levels of imipramine and frequency of enuresis.

There is good evidence that the tricyclic drugs can control the symptoms of enuresis in a high proportion of physically normal subjects. Relapse following the withdrawal of drugs is common but some subjects do enjoy long-term improvement. The drugs are particularly useful for achieving short-term control of symptoms where the use of bell and pad is impracticable such as during holidays and short absences from home.

General topics concerning the tricyclic drugs

Since the discovery and development of the tricyclic antidepressants a number of important issues have arisen concerning the validity of the findings of studies of their clinical effects, suggestions as to the mechanisms by which their effects are mediated, possible advantages of newer preparations, and studies of plasma levels of the drugs and their relationship with clinical effects. Some of these topics will be briefly reviewed.

Validity of trials

Following the introduction and acceptance of imipramine and amitriptyline as effective antidepressant substances, they have been widely used clinically and have, moreover, become the standards against which new preparations have been clinically tested. This development has placed great reliance upon the findings of the earlier studies of imipramine and amitriptyline, and has made the trials in which they were compared with placebo particularly important. In the case of imipramine there were relatively few studies in which a satisfactory clinical comparison with placebo was made, and even by the time amitriptyline was introduced some authors felt that comparison with placebo was either unnecessary or unethical. Questions which have been frequently asked are whether these early studies gave valid results and whether we can continue to assume that the antidepressive activity of these drugs has been conclusively demonstrated (Leyburn, 1967).

An important consideration is whether it is possible to conduct a double-blind study comparing a drug with strong anticholinergic effects with a placebo, without breaking the code and allowing observer biases to affect the results of assessment. Reservations of this kind have led to the use of atropine as a control treatment in a very few studies. The weight of evidence is that the tricyclics are superior to placebo in the treatment of depressed patients. Reviews of large numbers of studies of the clinical effects of tricyclic antidepressant drugs (Wechsler, Grosser and Greenblatt, 1965; Bennett, 1966; Klein and Davis, 1969; Angst, 1970; Morris and Beck, 1974) show that most controlled studies support the claim that drugs are antidepressive substances although there is considerable variability in the findings of the reported studies, and some show negative results.

The more recent studies of continuation therapy also give support to the claim that the tricyclic drugs have antidepressive effects. Two of the studies described above (Mindham, Howland and Shepherd, 1973; Paykel et al., 1975) concerned the later stages of treatment; in both the withdrawal of the drug used increased the risk of relapse. The pattern of relapse extending as it does over several months is not compatible with the suggestion that relapse was simply due to drug withdrawal. The design of both studies shows the effect to be due to pharmacological effects rather than to other attendant factors.

Studies of the unwanted effects of medication show that they are greatly diminished after the first few days of treatment and that after a further period are not prominent in the majority of patients (Åsberg et al., 1970). This phenomenon would tend to reduce the risk of breaking the code as long as assessment was carried out some days after treatment was initiated. Furthermore, it is clear that unwanted effects may also be experienced by patients receiving placebo. In the study of continuation therapy already quoted (Mindham, Howland and Shepherd, 1973) there was a high incidence of unwanted effects among patients on placebo, and on all criteria but one it was impossible to distinguish between those patients receiving the active drug and those receiving the placebo. In the case of dryness of the mouth the symptom was twice as common in those receiving active drug as among those on placebo, but the symptom nevertheless occurred in one-third of those receiving placebo and, had its presence been used as a criterion for separating the groups, there would have been many errors.

Clinical effects of tricyclic antidepressants

There has been speculation as to how antidepressants might affect the course of depressive disorders. There are two main clinical hypotheses as to how they might act;

one is that the drugs reverse the disorder underlying the symptoms so that medication might rationally be stopped once the symptoms are controlled; the other is that the drugs simply suppress the symptoms without altering an underlying disorder, the implication being that drugs should be continued until the underlying disorder has run its natural course. Clinical observation and the results of trials of continuation therapy tend to support the second hypothesis.

An important question is whether the tricyclic antidepressants should properly be regarded as antidepressive substances at all. It has been suggested that their advantage over placebo in the treatment of depressed patients is a non-specific one, possibly due to a sedative effect (Hollister *et al.*, 1967; Paykel *et al.*, 1968).

A particularly instructive study of the effects of various treatments in depressive disorder was conducted in a general practice in Australia (Blashki, Mowbray and Davies, 1971). Depressed female patients were randomly allocated to receive amitriptyline 75 mg daily; amitriptyline 150 mg daily; amylobarbitone 150 mg daily; or placebo for a period of four weeks. During the course of the trial patients receiving each of the treatments showed improvement. At the assessment after 7 d of treatment there was a reduction in the severity and prevalence of depressive symptoms. The decline in symptoms as measured by the Zung scale was similar in all groups. At 28 d the patients receiving amitriptyline in the higher dosage showed greater improvement than those on the other treatments. There was some variation between the changes in the severity of symptoms shown by different rating scales. Overall the findings of the study suggest that the superior effects of amitriptyline were due to more than a simple sedative effect.

The apparently well-established observation that the tricyclic drugs vary in their sedative effects has recently been questioned (Beaini, Hindmarch and Snaith, 1980). A double-blind comparison of the effects of amitriptyline and imipramine in similar dosage in the treatment of depressive illness showed them to have very similar therapeutic effects. In addition to rating scales for depression and anxiety, tests of critical flinker fusion and of sensorimotor coordination were used to measure sedative effects of the drugs. The drugs were not significantly different in the degree of sedation they produced, and moreover this was not related to their efficacy in controlling symptoms of anxiety or depression; somewhat paradoxically, some patients who were sedated by medication suffered continuing anxiety. The findings of the study demand further investigation in studies examining drug effects in larger groups of patients. The markedly different effects of drugs on different subjects is notable and has been observed by large numbers of investigators.

A consistent clinical finding is that there is a delay of two to three weeks following initiation of treatment before a therapeutic effect is seen. This is a much longer period than is required by most drugs: why should this be so? It is suggested that the onset of depressive disorder is associated with a change in the synthesis of amine transmitter substances in the nerve cell. This qualitative change may be corrected by the administration of antidepressive drugs. Once the drug is given the process of amine synthesis is corrected, but it takes two to three weeks for the normal transmitter amines to migrate down the nerve axon to the nerve endings where they become active. This time interval is in keeping with the migration of other substances in nerve cells (Dunleavy *et al.*, 1972).

The pharmacological effects of this group of drugs are attributed to their effect on the re-uptake of amine neurotransmitter substances after their release from the nerve endings. This effect is mediated by a change in permeability of the cell membrane. Different drugs selectively influence different series of amines; tertiary amines principally decrease the re-uptake of indole amines, whereas secondary amines reduce the re-uptake of noradrenaline. A number of drugs inhibit the re-uptake of both series of amines, and this may be because tertiary amines, such as amitriptyline and imipramine, are demethylated to secondary amines, i.e. nortriptyline and desipramine, in the body. Several drugs have been developed which predominantly affect the re-uptake of particular amines, e.g. clomipramine is a potent inhibitor of re-uptake of indole amines; the clinical relevance of this information is as yet uncertain.

A full review of the pharmacology of these drugs is beyond the scope of this chapter, and the reader is referred to recent reviews of the topic (Iversen and Mackay, 1979; Peet and Coppen, 1979; Green and Costain, 1979).

Speed of action of drugs

As new tricyclic drugs have appeared they have been found to share many characteristics but to vary in certain respects; some, such as amitriptyline and trimipramine, are markedly sedative; others, such as imipramine and desipramine, much less so. There is also variation in the intensity of anticholinergic effects and in effects on transmitter amines in the nerve cells.

Claims of rapid action have been made for many of the drugs, e.g. desipramine. The notion was that desipramine, not imipramine, was the therapeutically active substance in the body and that by giving desipramine the time required for imipramine to be demethylated to the active substance could be saved. In the clinical situation no difference was shown between the speeds of action of the two substances (Edwards, 1965).

A study in which the clinical effects of amitriptyline 150 mg daily and protriptyline 45 mg daily were compared in depressed patients showed protriptyline to have given greater relief of symptoms after 5 d of treatment but that by 17 d the treatments were equally effective (Lewis and Silverstone, 1970). Protriptyline gave better control of symptoms of anxiety, and this may have contributed to its apparent advantage in giving more general early relief of symptoms. Anticholinergic effects were more severe with protriptyline, and this raises the possibility that equivalent dosages of the two drugs were not used leading to an early therapeutic advantage to patients on protriptyline. It is questionable whether such a transient advantage is of significant benefit to depressed patients.

A greater speed of action has occasionally been attributed to amitriptyline and other sedative tricyclic antidepressant drugs; this claim is probably more appropriately attributed to the benefits of their sedative effects than to their antidepressant effects as demonstrated in the study by Blashki, Mowbray and Davies (1971). At present there appears to be no tricyclic antidepressant drug which has an advantage over other members of the group by virtue of a more rapid antidepressant effect. It should be recognized, however, that there are great methodological difficulties in demonstrating such an effect.

Unwanted effects

All the tricyclic drugs have similar unwanted effects but these vary in severity in the different preparations. The most frequently reported unwanted effects are due to the anticholinergic properties of the drugs. It has been demonstrated that the severity of the unwanted effects of nortriptyline are directly related to plasma levels of the drug

(Åsberg *et al.*, 1970). Dryness of the mouth, difficulty with visual accommodation, difficulty in initiating micturition, constipation, palpitations and postural hypotension are often seen. Retention of urine, paralytic ileus, heart failure, and the precipitation of glaucoma are possible, but uncommon, sequelae of these anticholinergic effects. Electrocardiographic changes resembling those due to quinidine are also occasionally seen. Cases of sudden death in patients receiving amitriptyline have been reported (Coull *et al.*, 1970; Boston Collaborative Drug Surveillance Program, 1972).

Amitriptyline and trimipramine often cause drowsiness but this usually passes off after the first few days of administration. Imipramine and closely related drugs cause less drowsiness.

The tricyclic antidepressant drugs may precipitate excitement or even hypomania sometimes on drug withdrawal but these are rare (Leyberg and Denmark, 1959; Mirin, Schatzberg and Creasey, 1981). Severe attacks of anxiety may also be precipitated by drug withdrawal (Gawin and Markoff, 1981). Visual hallucinations can occur, probably as the first symptoms of a toxic state. Other effects seen include excessive sweating, dizziness, tremor, ataxia, parkinsonism, lactation and oedema. Skin rashes occur occasionally but agranulocytosis rarely. Tricyclic antidepressants may be taken in attempts at suicide, and these patients present great problems in management.

Interactions between tricyclic antidepressants and other drugs

Interaction between tricyclic drugs and monoamine oxidase inhibitors is well documented (Hamilton and Mahapatra, 1972; Hollister, 1975; Blackwell, 1977). The typical clinical picture seen is of excitement, restlessness, dilatation of the pupils, flushing, sweating, muscular twitching and rigidity, hyperpyrexia and loss of consciousness. This syndrome is rare and tends to occur after overdosage (*see* Chapter 9) but it can occur in normal dosage if a tricyclic drug is given to patients already taking a monoamine oxidase inhibiting drug (Beaumont, 1973).

SYMPATHOMIMETIC AMINES

The tricyclic antidepressant drugs potentiate the pressor effects of the sympathomimetic amines and may produce attacks of severe hypertension. Dental patients receiving local anaesthetic preparations containing noradrenaline are in particular danger. A number of reports of severe headaches precipitated by the combination of noradrenaline with tricyclic drugs, leading to death, have appeared occasionally (Boakes *et al.*, 1972, 1973; Hollister, 1975).

AMPHETAMINES

The effects of amphetamines are potentiated by tricyclic antidepressants (Beaumont, 1973). This action may lead to clinical effects from very small doses of amphetamines. When amphetamine is given in therapeutic dosage its actions may be enhanced and prolonged.

HYPOTENSIVE DRUGS

Tricyclic drugs antagonize the hypotensive effects of a number of substances including guanidines, guanethidine, bethanidine, debrisoquine and bretylium (Stockley, 1972; Hollister, 1975). Centrally acting hypotensive agents such as clonidine are also antagonized by tricyclic drugs. The importance of this effect in the management of depressed hypertensive patients is clear.

PHENOTHIAZINE DRUGS AND ANALOGUES

Phenothiazine drugs and their analogues inhibit the metabolism of the tricyclic antidepressants (Gram and Overø, 1972). This is thought to be due to a blocking of hydroxylation which in turn leads to high levels of excretion of unchanged tricyclic drugs and other metabolites (Crammer and Rolfe, 1972).

ANTICOAGULANTS

Nortriptyline increases the half-life of coumarin anticoagulants and prolongs and intensifies the anticoagulant effect (Loeliger, 1972; Stockley, 1973).

OTHER INTERACTIONS

Administration of barbiturates leads to an increased rate of metabolism of tricyclic drugs. The concurrent administration of other drugs is one of the many factors which may affect the levels which a tricyclic drug achieves in the plasma (Luscombe, 1977). Benzodiazepines do not appear to influence plasma levels of tricyclic drugs (Silverman and Braithwaite, 1973). The action of imipramine is potentiated by L-triiodothyronine (Whybrow et al., 1972).

Many further interactions between tricyclic antidepressants and other drugs will undoubtedly be reported in due course. The possibility of a dangerous interaction should always be kept in mind when drugs are given together.

Choice of tricyclic antidepressant

The choice of an antidepressant drug involves three separate judgements: first, is there a superior antidepressant; secondly, are there particular features of depressive states, be they clinical, genetic, historical, psychological or biochemical, which are related to a good response to drugs; and finally, are there drugs which are especially suited to the treatment of particular depressive syndromes?

The criteria for choosing an antidepressive drug have occasionally been reviewed (Bennett, 1966; *British Medical Journal*, 1978; Herrington, 1978; *Drug and Therapeutics Bulletin*, 1980). The best *evidence for efficacy* favours the earlier drugs which have been thoroughly investigated and tested against placebo controls. Newer preparations may have advantages in producing fewer unwanted effects in therapeutic dosage. In purely therapeutic terms there does not appear to be a tricyclic antidepressant which, given in appropriate dosage, is superior to the others as regards final outcome of treatment.

Features of depressive illness which may be predictors of the outcome of treatment by drug therapy have been studied in a large number of trials, most of them primarily concerned with drug effects but others specifically designed to discover predictors of outcome (Paykel, 1972; Paykel, 1979; Stern, Rush and Mendels, 1980).

A personal or family history of response to a particular tricyclic drug increases the chance of a good response in a further episode in the individual or in a relative (Pare and Mack, 1971). A history of *neurotic pre-morbid traits* has generally been held to suggest a poor response to tricyclic drugs. This is difficult to interpret, however, on account of the difficulty in separating neurotic disorders from anxious depression of other types, and from personality disorders. One study showed a good response to tricyclics in anxious depressives although more generally neurotic patients showed poor progress on treatment. (Paykel, 1972). An *insidious onset* of depression suggests a good response to tricyclic drugs but the absence of a recognizable precipitant does not (Bielski and Friedel, 1976).

In general, *psychotically depressed* patients do well on tricyclic drugs especially where there are many 'vegetative' or 'vital' symptoms. The presence of delusions or hypochondriasis, possibly indications of severe disorder, are bad features of depressive illness as regards outcome of drug treatment (Ball and Kiloh, 1959; Kiloh, Ball and Garside, 1962; Raskin and Crook, 1976; Paykel, 1979).

Biological predictors of antidepressant response include tests of urinary metabolites, cerebrospinal fluid amine concentrations, the response to amphetamines, erythrocyte catechol-*o*-methyl transferase concentrations, and of the electroencephalographic characteristics of sleep (Stern, Rush and Mendels, 1980). None of these approaches is yet at the stage of clinical application but they are of great theoretical interest.

The *choice of a tricyclic antidepressant* drug is still largely a matter of clinical judgement and individual preference. The tricyclic antidepressant drugs are said to be divisible into three groups according to the degree of sedation produced: for example, amitriptyline and trimipramine have marked sedative effects; others have a stimulant effect and this group includes nortriptyline, desipramine and protriptyline; and, finally there are those drugs which are neither sedative nor stimulant, such as imipramine. Sedative properties might make the drugs suitable for the treatment of agitated patients, and stimulant properties might be expected to make the drugs more suitable for the treatment of retarded patients. This kind of classification may be an oversimplification, as the drugs appear to show a great variety of effects in different patients.

The relationship between the sedative and antidepressive effects of tricyclic drugs has been examined recently and shown not to conform with longstanding beliefs (Beaini, Hindmarsh and Snaith, 1980). A problem in evaluation is that symptomatic relief from sedative effects of a drug early in treatment may not be closely related to the more delayed antidepressive effect (Bielski and Friedel, 1976).

Considerable stress has been laid on the pharmacological differences between drugs in influencing the metabolism of different brain amines: as yet the relevance of these differences for the treatment of patients is uncertain.

Thus, little firm advice can be given on the choice of a tricyclic antidepressant drug and, in practice, this is very much a matter of personal preference based on experience of the use of particular drugs.

Prescription of tricyclic drugs

Our knowledge of the properties of the tricyclic drugs indicates that they should be given in optimal dosage for a period of four to six weeks initially (*Drug and Therapeutics Bulletin*, 1980). During this time most of those patients who will eventually respond will have begun to do so. If clinical improvement occurs the drugs should be continued for a total of 8–10 weeks during which time improvement will progress and be consolidated. Where a patient fails to respond to a drug given for 4–6 weeks the choice lies between giving electroconvulsive therapy (ECT), a quite different antidepressive drug, or changing to another tricyclic drug. Where the clinical condition of the patient does not require administration of ECT and the illness is of a type which might be expected to respond to a tricyclic drug, a change to another tricyclic drug may well be the best course to take. When this is done it is best to choose a tricyclic of a different type rather than to change to one which is closely related both chemically and pharmacologically to the drug of first choice. Beyond this little advice can be given. During the initial treatment of patients who do not respond promptly to the first drug used it should be remembered that the careful evaluation of the effects of a drug in a particular patient can be of great value in the treatment of subsequent episodes. Conversely, the half-hearted use of antidepressive drugs, in inadequate dosage for insufficient periods of time, makes the rational use of drug treatment in depressive states impossible. A recent study of the use of tricyclic drugs in general practice showed a high rate of 'non-compliance' among doctors in that drugs were not administered in a way appropriate to their pharmacological effects (Johnson, 1981).

After initial treatment it is less clear what should be done for the patient's good. Studies of continuation therapy have shown that some patients benefit from continued therapy but by no means all. One study suggests that patients who make an incomplete recovery, even when this is shown only by the remnant of a single symptom, are likely to benefit from continued administration of the drug (Mindham, Howland and Shepherd, 1973). Where recovery is complete there appears to be much less advantage to be gained from continued administration. The studies so far completed are of relatively short periods of continuation therapy, and the advantages and possible dangers of giving tricyclic drugs for longer periods are uncertain.

The tricyclic drugs are generally given orally, and the soundness of this procedure is supported by the knowledge of their absorption and metabolism. The drugs may also be given by intramuscular injection but on the evidence of current knowledge this method is unlikely to be of any advantage unless there is a defect of absorption from the gut.

References

AGUIRRE, E. A. One experience in the treatment of depressive states with 3-chloro-5-(3-dimethylamino propyl-)10, 11-dihydro-5,4-dibenzodiazepine hydrochloride, preparation G34586, *Revista Folia Neuropsiquiatrica del Sur de Espana* **3**, 1–8 (1968)

ALEXANDERSON, B., EVANS, D. A. P. and SJÖQVIST, F. Steady state plasma levels of nortriptyline in twins. Influence of genetic factors and drug therapy, *British Medical Journal* **4**, 764 (1969)

AMSTERDAM, J., BRUNSWICK, D. and MENDELS, J. The clinical application of tricyclic antidepressant pharmacokinetics and plasma levels, *American Journal of Psychiatry* **137**, 653–662 (1980)

ANGST, J. Clinical aspects of imipramine. In *Tofranil (imipramine)* (Eds. J. ANGST and W. THEOBALD), Verlag Stampfli & Cie AG, Berne (1970)

ANGST, J. and KIND, H. Clinical experience with W91/HF1927 in the in- and out-patient treatment of depressive states, *Schweizerische Medizinische Wochenschrift* **94**, 759–764 (1964)

ARFWIDSSON, L., ARN, L., BESKOW, J., OTTOSSON, J-O. and PERSSON, G. A comparison between diazepam, dixyrazine, opipramol and placebo in anxiety states, *Acta Psychiatrica Scandinavica* **221**, Suppl., 19–32 (1971)

ÅSBERG, M. On the clinical importance of plasma concentrations of tricyclic antidepressant drugs—a review of the evidence. In *Clinical Pharmacology in Psychiatry* (Ed. E. USDIN), Wiley, Chichester (1980)

ÅSBERG, M., CRONHOLM, B., SJÖQVIST, F. and TUCK, D. Correlation of subjective side effects with plasma concentrations of nortriptyline, *British Medical Journal* **4**, 18–21 (1970)

ÅSBERG, M., CRONHOLM, B., SJÖQVIST, F. and TUCK, D. Relationship between plasma level and therapeutic effect of nortriptyline, *British Medical Journal* **3**, 331–334 (1971)

ÅSBERG, M. and SJÖQVIST, F. On the role of plasma level monitoring of tricyclic antidepressants in clinical practice, *Communications in Psychopharmacology* **2**, 381–391 (1978)

AZIMA, H., SILVER, A. and ARTHURS, D. The effects of G-33040 in depressive states: a multi-blind study, *American Journal of Psychiatry* **119**, 465–466 (1962)

BALL, J. R. B. and KILOH, L. G. A controlled trial of imipramine in treatment of depressive states, *British Medical Journal* **2**, 1052–1055 (1959)

BAN, T. A. and LEHMANN, H. E. Clinical trial with desmethyl imipramine (G35020), a new antidepressive compound, *Canadian Medical Association Journal* **86**, 1030–1031 (1962)

BEAINI, A. Y., HINDMARCH, I. and SNAITH, R. P. A re-examination of the clinical effects of imipramine and amitriptyline in depressive illness, *Journal of Affective Disorders* **2**, 89–94 (1980)

BEAUMONT, G. Drug interaction with clomipramine (Anafranil), *Journal of International Medical Research* **1**, 480–483 (1973)

BENNETT, I. F. Is there a superior antidepressant?, *Proceedings of First International Symposium, Milan*, Institutio di Recherche Farmacologiche Mario Negri (1966)

BIELSKI, R. J. and FRIEDEL, R. O. Prediction of tricyclic antidepressant response: a critical review, *Archives of General Psychiatry* **33**, 1479–1489 (1976)

BLACKWELL, B. Drugs used in depression and mania. In *Side Effects of Drugs Annual* **I** (Ed. M. N. G. DUKES), Excerpta Medica, Amsterdam (1977)

BLASHKI, T. G., MOWBRAY, R. and DAVIES, B. Controlled trial of amitriptyline in general practice, *British Medical Journal* **1**, 133–138 (1971)

BOAKES, A. J., LAURENCE, D. R., LOVEL, K. W., O'NEIL, R. and VERRILL, P. J. Adverse reactions to local anaesthetic/vasoconstrictor preparations, *British Dental Journal* **133**, 137–140 (1972)

BOAKES, A. J., LAURENCE, D. R., TEOH, P. C., BARAR, F. S. K., BENEDIKTER, L. T. and PRICHARD, B. N. C. Interactions between sympathomimetic amines and antidepressant agents in man, *British Medical Journal* **1**, 311–315 (1973)

BOISSIER, J-R., SIMON, P., FICHELLE-PAGNY, J. and LWOFF, J-M. La dibenzepine (Noveril); quelques aspects de pharmacologie prévisionelle, *Thérapie* **21**, 773–780 (1966)

BORGÅ, O., AZARNOFF, D. L., FORSHELL, G. P. and SJÖQVIST, F. Plasma protein binding of tricyclic anti-depressants in man, *Biochemical Pharmacology* **18**, 2135–2143 (1969)

BORGÅ, O., HAMBERGER, B., MALMFORS, T. and SJÖQVIST, F. The role of plasma protein binding in the inhibitory effect of nortriptyline on the neuronal uptake of norepinephrine, *Clinical Pharmacology and Therapeutics* **11**, 581–588 (1970)

BOSTON COLLABORATIVE DRUG SURVEILLANCE PROGRAM. Adverse reactions to the tricyclic-antidepressant drugs, *Lancet* **1**, 529–531 (1972)

BRAITHWAITE, R. A., GOULDING, R., THEANO, G., BAILEY, J. and COPPEN, A. Plasma concentration of amitriptyline and clinical response, *Lancet* **1**, 1297–1300 (1972)

BRAITHWAITE, R. A., NARRA, B. R. S. and GAIND, R. Steady-state plasma concentrations during single and multiple dosage schedules of amitriptyline, *Psychological Medicine* **4**, 338–341 (1974)

BRAITHWAITE, R. A. and WIDDOP, B. A specific gas-chromatographic method for the measurement of steady-state plasma levels of amitriptyline and nortriptyline in patients, *Clinica Chimica Acta* **35**, 461–472 (1971)

BRITISH MEDICAL JOURNAL. Choosing an antidepressant, *British Medical Journal* **1**, 128 (1978)

BRITISH MEDICAL JOURNAL. Tricyclic antidepressant concentrations and clinical response, *British Medical Journal* **2**, 783–784 (1978)

BROADHURST, A. D., JAMES, H. D. and CORTE, L. D. Clomipramine plasma level and clinical response, *Postgraduate Medical Journal* **4**, Suppl., 139–145 (1977)

BRODIE, B. B., BICKEL, M. H. and SULSER, F. Desmethylimipramine, a new type of antidepressant drug, *Excerpta Medica* **5**, 454–458 (1962)

BRODIE, B., DICK, P., KIELHOLZ, P., POELDINGER, W. and THEOBALD, W. Preliminary pharmacological and clinical results with demethylimipramine (DMI) G35020, a metabolite of imipramine, *Psychopharmacologia* **2**, 467–474 (1961)

BRUCE, E. M., CRONE, N., FITZPATRICK, G., FREWIN, S. J., GILLIS, A., LASCELLES, C. F., LEVENNE, L. J. and MERSKEY, H. A comparative trial of ECT and Tofranil, *American Journal of Psychiatry* **117**, 76 (1960)

BURCH, J. and HULLIN, R. P. The absorption rate and bioavailability of amitriptyline in the form of Lentizol, *Neuropharmacology* **17**, 1069–1071 (1978)

BURKE, B. V., SAINSBURY, M. J. and MEZO, B. A. A comparative trial of amitriptyline and trimipramine in the treatment of depression, *Medical Journal of Australia* **1**, 1216–1218 (1967)

BURNS, B. H. Preliminary evaluation of a new antidepressant, trimipramine, by a sequential method, *British Journal of Psychiatry* **111**, 1155–1157 (1965)

BURROWS, G. D., MOWBRAY, R. M. and DAVIES, B. A sequential comparison of doxepin (Sinequan) and placebo in depressed patients, *Medical Journal of Australia* **1**, 364–366 (1972)

BURROWS, G. D., NORMAN, T. R., MAGUIRE, K. P., RUBENSTEIN, G., SCOGGINS, B. A. and DAVIES, B. A new antidepressant butriptyline: plasma levels and clinical response, *Medical Journal of Australia* **2**, 604–606 (1977)

BURROWS, G. D., VOHRA, J., HUNT, D., SLOMAN, J. G., SCOGGINS, B. A. and DAVIES, B. Cardiac effects of different tricyclic antidepressant drugs, *British Journal of Psychiatry* **129**, 335–341 (1976)

BURT, C. G., GORDON, W. F., HOLT, N. F. and HORDERN, A. Amitriptyline in depressive states: a controlled trial, *Journal of Mental Science* **108**, 711–730 (1962)

CAPSTICK, N. and ROOKE, K. C. A comparative trial of opipramol with phenelzine and chlordiazepoxide in the treatment of depression, *Journal of International Medical Research* **2**, 293–297 (1974)

CARLSSON, A. Modification of sympathetic function, *Pharmacological Reviews* **18**, 541–549 (1966)

CARNEY, M. W. P. Investigations of the clinical effects of opipramol, *Proceedings of the Fourth World Congress of Psychiatry* **3**, 1904–1908 (1968)

CARNEY, M. W. P. and MAXWELL, C. Sequential double-blind controlled trial of opipramol in anxiety neurosis, *International Journal of Neuropsychiatry* **3**, 491–493 (1967)

COPPEN, A., MONTGOMERY, S., GHOSE, K., RAO, V. A. R., BAILEY, J., CHRISTIANSEN, J., MIKKLESON, P. L., VANPRAAG, H. M., VAN DE POEL, F., MINSKER, E. J., KOZULJA, V. G., MATUSSEK, N., KUNGKUNZ, G. and JØRGENSEN, A. Amitriptyline plasma-concentration and clinical effect. A World Health Organisation collaborative study, *Lancet* **1**, 63–66 (1978)

COULL, D. C., CROOKS, J., DINGWALL-FORDYCE, I., SCOTT, A. M. and WEIR, R. D. Amitriptyline and cardiac disease, *Lancet* **2**, 590–591 (1970)

CRAMMER, J. L. and ROLFE, B. Interaction of imipramine and chlorpromazine in man. VIII C.I.N.P. Congress, Copenhagen (1972)

DANEMAN, E. A. Imipramine in office management of depressive reactions (a double blind clinical study), *Diseases of the Nervous System* **22**, 213–217 (1961)

DANEMAN, E. A. Treatment of depressed patients with iprindole, *Psychosomatics* **8**, 216–221 (1967)

DENCKER, H., DENCKER, S. J., GREEN, A. and NAGY, A. Intestinal absorption, demethylation and enterohepatic circulation of imipramine, *Clinical Pharmacology and Therapeutics* **19**, 584–586 (1976)

DRUG AND THERAPEUTICS BULLETIN. How to use antidepressant drugs more effectively, *Drug and Therapeutics Bulletin* **18**, 73–74 (1980)

DUNLEAVY, D. L. F., BREZINOVA, V., OSWALD, I., MACLEAN, A. W. and TINKER, M. Changes during weeks in effects of tricyclic drugs on the human sleeping brain, *British Journal of Psychiatry* **120**, 663–672 (1972)

EDWARDS, G. Comparison of the effect of imipramine and desipramine on some symptoms of depressive illness, *British Journal of Psychiatry* **111**, 889–897 (1965)

EKDAWI, M. Y. Dibenzepin and amitriptyline in the treatment of depression, *British Journal of Psychiatry* **118**, 523–524 (1971)

EL-DEIRY, N. K., FORREST, A. D. and LITTMANN, S. K. Clinical trial of a new antidepressant (WY 3263), *British Journal of Psychiatry* **113**, 999–1004 (1967)

FIELDING, J. M. A double-blind comparative trial of dibenzepin and imipramine, *Medical Journal of Australia* **1**, 614–616 (1969)

FIEVE, R. R., PLATMAN, S. R. and PLUTCHIK, R. R. The use of lithium in affective disorders: I Acute endogenous depression, *American Journal of Psychiatry* **125**, 487–491 (1968)

FRIEDMAN, C., DE MOWBRAY, M. S. and HAMILTON, V. Imipramine (Tofranil) in depressive states: a controlled trial with in-patients, *Journal of Mental Sciences* **107**, 948–953 (1961)

GANDER, D. R. Treatment of depressive illnesses with combined antidepressants, *Lancet* **2**, 107–109 (1965)

GARRY, J. W. and LEONARD, T. J. Trial of amitriptyline in chronic depression, *British Journal of Psychiatry* **109**, 54–55 (1963)

GAWIN, F. H. and MARKOFF, R. A. Panic anxiety after abrupt discontinuation of amitriptyline, *American Journal of Psychiatry* **138**, 117–118 (1981)

GENERAL PRACTITIONER RESEARCH GROUP. Two new psychotropic drugs: (1) A new antidepressant, *Practitioner* **198**, 135–141 (1967)

GENERAL PRACTITIONER RESEARCH GROUP. Protriptyline in depression, *Practitioner* **201**, 506–509 (1968)

GLASSMAN, A. H., PEREL, J. M., SHOSTAK, M., KANTOR, S. J. and FLEISS, J. L. Clinical implications of imipramine plasma levels for depressive illness, *Archives of General Psychiatry* **34**, 197–204 (1977)

GLOWINSKI, J. and AXELROD, J. Inhibition of uptake of tritiated-noradrenaline in the intact rat brain by imipramine and structurally related compounds, *Nature (London)* **204**, 1318–1319 (1964)

GOODWIN, F. K., MURPHY, D. L. and BUNNEY, W. E. Jr. Lithium carbonate treatment in depression and mania, *Archives of General Psychiatry* **21**, 486–496 (1969)

GORE, C. P. Clomipramine (Anafranil), Tofranil (imipramine) and placebo: a comparative study in relation to electroconvulsive therapy, *Journal of International Medical Research* **1**, 347–351 (1973)

GRAM, L. F., ANDREASEN, P. B., FREDRICSON-OVERØ, K. and CHRISTIANSEN, J. Comparison of single-dose kinetics of imipramine, nortriptyline and antipyrine in man, *Psychopharmacology* **50**, 21 (1976)

GRAM, L. F. and OVERØ, K. F. Drug interaction—inhibitory effect of neuroleptics on metabolism of tricyclic antidepressants in man, *British Medical Journal* **1**, 463–465 (1972)

GREEN, A. R. and COSTAIN, D. W. The biochemistry of depression. In *The Psychopharmacology of Affective Disorders* (Eds. E. S. PAYKEL and A. COPPEN), Oxford University Press, Oxford (1979)

GREENSPAN, K., SCHILDKRAUT, J. J., GORDON, E. K., BAER, L., ARONOFF, M. S. and DURELL, J. Catecholamine metabolism in affective disorders—III. MHPG and other catecholamine metabolites in patients treated with lithium carbonate, *Journal of Psychiatric Research* **7**, 171–183 (1970)

GRINGRAS, M. and BEAUMONT, G. A double-blind comparison of opipramol and diazepam in the treatment of anxiety in general practice, *British Journal of Clinical Practice* **25**, 455–458 (1971)

GROF, P., SAXENA, B., CANTOR, R., DAIGLE, L., HETHERINGTON, D. and HAINES, T. Doxepin versus amitriptyline in depression: a sequential double-blind study, *Current Therapeutic Research* **16**, 470–476 (1974)

GROSSER, H. H. and RYAN, E. Drug treatment of anxiety: a controlled study of opipramol and chlordiazepoxide, *British Journal of Psychiatry* **111**, 134–141 (1965)

HAEFLIGER, F. Chemistry of Tofranil, *Canadian Psychiatric Association Journal* **4**, Suppl., 69–74 (1959)

HAIDER, I. A comparative investigation of desipramine and nortriptyline in the treatment of depression, *British Journal of Psychiatry* **114**, 1293–1294 (1968)

HAMILTON, M. and MAHAPATRA, S. B. Antidepressive drugs. In *Side Effects of Drugs, Chapter 2* (Eds. L. MEYLER and A. HERXHEIMER), Excerpta Medica, Amsterdam (1972)

HAMMER, W. and SJÖQVIST, F. Plasma levels of monomethylated tricyclic antidepressants during treatment with imipramine-like compounds, *Life Sciences* **6**, 1895–1903 (1967)

HARDING, T. A comparative clinical trial of oral clomipramine (Anafranil) against amitriptyline, *Journal of International Medical Research* **1**, 343–346 (1973)

HARGREAVES, M. A. and MAXWELL, C. The speed of action of desipramine: a controlled trial, *International Journal of Neuropsychiatry* **3**, 140–141 (1967)

HAYDU, G. G., DHRYMIOTIS, A. and QUINN, G. P. Plasma imipramine level in syndromes of depression, *American Journal of Psychiatry* **119**, 574–575 (1962)

HAYS, P. and STEINART, J. A blind comparative trial of nortriptyline and isocarboxazid in depressed out-patients, *Canadian Psychiatric Association Journal* **14**, 307–308 (1969)

HERR, F., VOITH, K. and JARAMILLO, J. The pharmacology of butriptyline, *Journal of Medicine* **2**, 258–270 (1971)

HERRINGTON, R. N. The new antidepressants: how much of an improvement are they?, *Modern Medicine* **June**, 73–77 (1978)

HICKS, J. T. Iprindole, a new antidepressant for use in general office practice, *Illinois Medical Journal* **128**, 622–626 (1965)

HOBBS, D. C. Distribution and metabolism of doxepin, *Biochemical Pharmacology* **18**, 1941–1954 (1969)

HOLLISTER, L. E. Antidepressant drugs. In *Side Effects of Drugs* (Ed. M. N. G. DUKES), Excerpta Medica, Amsterdam (1975)

HOLLISTER, L. E. Tricyclic antidepressants, *New England Journal of Medicine* **299**, 1106–1109 (1978)

HOLLISTER, L. E., OVERALL, J. E., JOHNSON, M., KATZ, G., KIMBELL, I. Jr and HONIGFELD, G. Evaluation of desipramine in depressive states, *Journal of New Drugs* **3**, 161–166 (1963)

HOLLISTER, L. E., OVERALL, J. E., JOHNSON, M., PENNINGTON, V., KATZ, G. and SHELTON, J. Controlled comparison of amitriptyline, imipramine and placebo in hospitalised depressed patients, *Journal of Nervous and Mental Diseases* **139**, 370–375 (1964)

HOLLISTER, L. E., OVERALL, J. E., SHELTON, J., PENNINGTON, V., KIMBELL, I. and JOHNSON, M. Drug therapy of depression. Amitriptyline, perphenazine and their combination in different syndromes, *Archives of General Psychiatry* **17**, 486–493 (1967)

HORDERN, A., BURT, C. G., GORDON, W. F. and HOLT, N. F. Amitriptyline in depressive states: six-month treatment results, *British Journal of Psychiatry* **110**, 641–647 (164)

HYNES, M. V. A comparative clinical trial of oral clomipramine (Anafranil) against amitriptyline, *Journal of International Medical Research* **1**, 338–342 (1973)

IMLAH, N. W., RYAN, E. and HARRINGTON, J. A. The influence of antidepressant drugs on the response to electroconvulsive therapy and on subsequent relapse rates, *Proceedings IV International Congress of Neuropharmacology Birmingham 1964*, 438–442, Elsevier, Amsterdam (1964)

IVERSEN, L. L. and MACKAY, A. V. P. Pharmacodynamics of antidepressants and antimanic drugs. In *Psychopharmacology of Affective Disorders* (Eds. E. S. PAYKEL and A. COPPEN), Oxford University Press, Oxford (1979)

JEPSON, K. and BEAUMONT, G. A comparative trial of opipramol and chlordiazepoxide in the treatment of anxiety, *Journal International Medical Research* 1, 145–150 (1973)

JOHNSON, D. A. W. Depression: treatment compliance in general practice, *Acta Psychiatrica Scandinavica* 63, Suppl. 290, 447–453 (1981)

JOHNSON, F., SACCO, F. A. and YELLOWLEY, T. W. Chlordiazepoxide and dothiepin compared in anxiety/depression in general practice, *Practitioner* 211, 362–364 (1973)

JORGENSEN, O. S., LOBER, M., CHRISTIANSEN, J. and GRAM, L. F. Plasma concentration and clinical effect in imipramine treatment of childhood enuresis, *Clinical Pharmacokinetics* 5, 386–393 (1980)

JUNGKUNZ, G. and KUSS, H. J. Amitriptyline and its demethylation rate, *Lancet* 2, 1263–1264 (1978)

KAY, D. W. K., FAHY, T. and GARSIDE, R. F. A seven-month double-blind trial of amitriptyline and diazepam in ECT-treated depressed patients, *British Journal of Psychiatry* 117, 667–671 (1970)

KENNING, I. S., RICHARDSON, N. L. and TUCKER, F. G. The treatment of depressive states with imipramine hydrochloride, *Canadian Psychiatric Association Journal* 5, 60–64 (1960)

KILOH, L. G. and BALL, J. R. B. Depression treated with imipramine: a follow-up study, *British Medical Journal* 1, 168–171 (1961)

KILOH, L. G., BALL, J. R. B. and GARSIDE, R. F. Prognostic factors in treatment of depressive states with imipramine, *British Medical Journal* 1, 1225–1227 (1962)

KLEIN, D. F. and DAVIS, J. M. *Diagnosis and Drug Treatment of Psychiatric Disorders*, Williams & Wilkins Co., Baltimore (1969)

KRAGH-SØRENSEN, P., ÅSBERG, M. and EGGERT-HANSEN, C. Plasma nortriptyline levels in endogenous depression, *Lancet* i, 113–115 (1973)

KRAGH-SØRENSEN, P., HANSEN, C. E. and BAASTRUP, P. C. Self-inhibiting action of nortriptyline's antidepressive effect at high plasma levels, *Psychopharmacologia* 45, 305–316 (1976)

KRAKOWSKI, A. J. Protriptyline in treatment of severe depressions: a long-range pilot study, *American Journal of Psychiatry* 121, 807–809 (1965)

KUHN, R. Uber die Behaudlung depressiver Zustände mit einen Iminodibenzylderivat (G22355), *Schweizerische medizinische Wochenschrift* 87, 1135–1140 (1957)

KUHN, R. The treatment of depressive states with G-22355 (imipramine hydrochloride), *American Journal of Psychiatry* 115, 459–464 (1958)

KUPFER, D. J., HANIN, I., SPIKER, D. G., GRAU, T. and COBLE, P. Amitriptyline plasma levels and clinical response in primary depression, *Clinical Pharmacology and Therapeutics* 22, 904–911 (1977)

LAFAVE, H. G., MARCH, B. W., KARGAS, A. K. and SHUFFLER, S. Y. Desipramine and imipramine in an out-patient setting: a comparative study, *American Journal of Psychiatry* 122, 698–701 (1965)

LEAHY, M. R. and MARTIN, I. C. A. Double-blind comparison of nortriptyline and amitriptyline in depressive illness, *British Journal of Psychiatry* 113, 1433–1434 (1967)

LEAN, T. H. and SIDHU, M. S. Comparative study of imipramine (Tofranil) and trimipramine (Surmontil) in depression associated with gynaecological conditions, *Proceedings of Obstetrical and Gynaecological Society* 3, 222–228 (1972)

LEVINSON, B. Butriptyline hydrochloride and imipramine hydrochloride in the treatment of non-psychotic depression, *South African Medical Journal* 48, 873–875 (1974)

LEWIS, A. G. and SILVERSTONE, J. T. The speed of action of protriptyline. A double-blind controlled trial, *Clinical Trials Journal* 7, 423–430 (1970)

LEYBERG, J. T. and DENMARK, J. C. The treatment of depressive states with imipramine hydrochloride (Tofranil), *Journal of Mental Science* 105, 1123–1126 (1959)

LEYBURN, P. A critical look at antidepressant during trials, *Lancet* ii, 1135–1138 (1967)

LIPPMANN, W. Effects of butriptyline and structurally-related drugs on norepinephrine uptake and gastric acid secretion in rodents, *Journal of Medicine* 2, 250–257 (1971)

LIPSEDGE, M. S., REES, W. L. and PIKE, D. J. A double-blind comparison of dothiepin and amitriptyline for the treatment of depression with anxiety, *Psychopharmacologia* 19, 153–162 (1971)

LOELIGER, E. A. Drugs affecting blood clotting and fibrinolysis. In *Side Effects of Drugs* (Eds. L. MEYLER and A. HERXHEIMER), Excerpta Medica, Amsterdam (1972)

LUBORSKY, L., AUERBACH, A. H., CHANDLER, M., COHEN, J. and BACHRACH, H. M. Factors influencing outcome of psychotherapy, *Psychological Bulletin* 75, 145–185 (1971)

LUSCOMBE, D. K. Factors influencing plasma drug concentrations, *Journal of International Medical Research* 5, Suppl., 82–97 (1977)

LYLE, W. H., BROOKS, P., EARLY, D. F., LEGGETT, W. P., SILVERMAN, G., BRAITHWAITE, R. A., GUTHILL, J. M., GOULDING, R., PEARSON, I. B., SNAITH, R. P. and STRANG, G. E. Plasma concentration of nortriptyline as a guide to therapy, *Postgraduate Medical Journal* 50, 282–287 (1974)

McCONAGHY, N., JOFFE, A. D., KINGSTON, W. R., STEVENSON, H. G., ATKINSON, I., COLE, E. and FENNESSY, L. A. Correlation of clinical features of depressed out-patients with response to amitriptyline and protriptyline, *British Journal of Psychiatry* 114, 103–106 (1968)

MacLEAN, R. E. G. Imipramine hydrochloride (Tofranil) and enuresis, *American Journal of Psychiatry* **117**, p. 551 (1960)

MacCLEAN, R. and REES, W. L. A controlled trial of nortriptyline (Aventyl) in the treatment of depressive illness, *Clinical Trials Journal* **3**, 567–570 (1966)

MANN, A. M. and HESELTINE, G. F. D. The desmethyl metabolite if imipramine (G-35020) in the treatment of depression: further clinical experience, *Canadian Medical Association Journal* **88**, 1102–1107 (1963)

MARKS, I. M., STERN, R. S., MAWSON, D., COBB, J. and McDONALD, R. Clomipramine and exposure for obsessive-compulsive rituals, *British Journal of Psychiatry* **136**, 1–25 (1980)

MARSHALL, W. K. and MICEV, V. Clomipramine (Anafranil) in the treatment of obsessional illnesses and phobic anxiety states, *Journal of International Medical Research* **1**, 403–412 (1973)

MARTIN, M. E. A comparative trial of imipramine and phenelzine in the treatment of depression, *British Journal of Psychiatry* **109**, 279–285 (1963)

MEDICAL RESEARCH COUNCIL. Clinical trial of the treatment of depressive illness, *British Medical Journal* **1**, 881–886 (1965)

MENDELS, J. Comparative trial of nortriptyline and amitriptyline in 100 depressed patients, *American Journal of Psychiatry* **124**, Suppl., 59–62 (1968)

MENDELS, J., SECUNDA, S. K. and DYSON, W. L. A controlled study of the antidepressant effects of lithium carbonate, *Archives of General Psychiatry* **26**, 154–157 (1972)

MINDHAM, R. H. S. The use of drugs in the prevention of relapse in affective disorders, *International Journal of Mental Health* **6**, 88–103 (1978)

MINDHAM, R. H. S. Continuation therapy with tricyclic antidepressants in relapsing depressive illness, *Bibliotheca Psychiatrica* **160**, 49–55 (1981)

MINDHAM, R. H. S., HOWLAND, C. and SHEPHERD, M. An evaluation of continuation therapy with tricyclic antidepressants in depressive illness, *Psychological Medicine* **3**, 5–17 (1973)

MIRIN, S. M., SCHATZBERG, A. F. and CREASEY, D. E. Hypomania and mania after withdrawal of tricyclic antidepressants, *American Journal of Psychiatry* **138**, 87–89 (1981)

MONTGOMERY, S. and BRAITHWAITE, R. The relationship between plasma concentration of amitriptyline and therapeutic response. Paper presented at a Meeting of the British Association for Psychopharmacology, London (1975)

MONTGOMERY, S., BRAITHWAITE, R., DAWLING, S. and McAULEY, R. High plasma nortriptyline levels in the treatment of depression, *Clinical Pharmacology and Therapeutics* **23**, 309–314 (1978)

MOODY, J. P., WHYTE, S. F., McDONALD, A. J. and NAYLOR, G. J. Pharmacokinetic aspects of protriptyline plasma levels, *European Journal of Clinical Pharmacology* **11**, 51–56 (1977)

MORRIS, J. B. and BECK, A. T. The efficacy of antidepressant drugs. A review of research (1958–1972), *Archives of General Psychiatry* **30**, 667–674 (1974)

MURPHY, J. E. A comparative clinical trial of Org GB94 and imipramine in the treatment of depression in general practice, *Journal of International Medical Research* **3**, 251–260 (1975)

MURPHY, J. E., DONALD, J. E. and BEAUMONT, G. A comparative clinical trial of opipramol and chlordiazepoxide employing a method of patient self-assessment, *Clinical Trials Jou. nal* **8** No. 2, 28–32 (1971)

MUSCETTOLA, G., GOODWIN, F. K., POTTER, W. Z., CLAEYS, M. M. and MARKEY, S. P. Imipramine and desipramine in plasma and spinal fluid. Relationship to clinical response and serotonin metabolism, *Archives of General Psychiatry* **35**, 621–625 (1978)

NAGY, A. On the kinetics of imipramine and related antidepressants, *Acta Psychiatrica Scandinavica* **61**, Suppl. 280, 147–156 (1980)

NAGY, A. and HANSEN, T. The kinetics of imipramine-N-oxide in man, *Acta Pharmacology and Toxicology* **42**, 58–67 (1978)

NAGY, A. and JOHANSSON, R. The demethylation of imipramine and clomipramine as apparent from their plasma kinetics, *Psychopharmacology* **54**, 125–131 (1977)

NIES, A., ROBINSON, D. S., FRIEDMAN, M. J., GREEN, R., COOPER, T. B., RAVARIS, C. L. and IVES, J. O. Relationship between age and tricyclic antidepressant plasma levels, *American Journal of Psychiatry* **134**, 790–793 (1977)

OLIVIER-MARTIN, R., MARZIN, D., BUSCHENSCHULTZ, E., PICHOT, P. and BOISSIER, J. Concentrations plasmatiques de l'imipramine et de la desmethylimipramine et effet antidepresseur au couis d'un traitment controle, *Psychopharmacologia (Berlin)* **41**, 187–195 (1975)

PARE, C. M. B. Combining the antidepressant drugs, *British Medical Journal* **1**, 384 (1965)

PARE, C. M. B. and MACK, J. W. Differentiation of two genetically specific types of depression by the response to antidepressant drugs, *Journal of Medical Genetics* **8**, 306–309 (1971)

PAYKEL, E. S. Depressive typologies and response to amitriptyline, *British Journal of Psychiatry* **120**, 147–156 (1972)

PAYKEL, E. S. Predictors of treatment response. In *Psychopharmacology of Affective Disorders* (Eds. E. S. PAYKEL and A. COPPEN), 193–220, Oxford University Press, Oxford (1979)

PAYKEL, E. S., DIMASCIO, A., HASKELL, D. and PRUSOFF, B. A. Effects of maintenance amitriptyline and psychotherapy on symptoms of depression, *Psychological Medicine* 5, 67–77 (1975)

PAYKEL, E. S., PRICE, J. S., GILLAN, R. U., PALMAI, G. and CHESSER, E. S. A comparative trial of imipramine and chlorpromazine in depressed patients, *British Journal of Psychiatry* 114, 1281–1287 (1968)

PEARCE, J. B. and REES, W. L. A double-blind comparison of three times daily and single night dosage of the tricyclic antidepressant dothiepin, *Journal of International Medical Research* 2, 12–19 (1974)

PEET, M. and COPPEN, A. The pharmacokinetics of antidepressant drugs: relevance to their therapeutic effect. In *Psychopharmacology of Affective Disorders* (Eds. E. S. PAYKEL and A. COPPEN), Oxford University Press, Oxford (1979)

PITTS, N. E. The clinical evaluation of doxepin—a new psychotherapeutic agent, *Psychosomatics* X, 164–171 (1969)

POUSSAINT, A. F., DITMAN, K. S. and GREENFIELD, R. Amitriptyline in childhood enuresis, *Clinical Pharmacology and Therapeutics* 7, 21–25 (1966)

PRIEN, R. F., CAFFEY, E. M. and KLETT, C. J. Comparison of lithium carbonate and chlorpromazine in the treatment of mania, *Archives of General Psychiatry* 26, 146–153 (1972)

PRIEST, R. G. A comparative trial of protriptyline and nortriptyline, *Current Medical Research and Opinion* 3, 710–715 (1976)

RACK, P. H. A comparative clinical trial of oral clomipramine (Anafranil) against imipramine, *Journal of International Medical Research* 1, 332–337 (1973)

RASKIN, A. and CROOK, T. H. The endogenous-neurotic distinction as a predictor of response to antidepressant drugs, *Psychological Medicine* 6, 59–70 (1976)

REES, L., BROWN, A. C. and BENAIM, S. A controlled trial of imipramine (Tofronil) in the treatment of severe depressive states, *Journal of Mental Science* 107, 552–559 (1961)

REISBY, N., GRAM, L. F., BECK, P., NAGY, A., PETERSEN, G. O., ORTMANN, J., IBSEN, I., DENKER, S. J., JACOBSEN, O., KRAUTWALD, O., SONDERGAARD, I. and CHRISTIANSEN, J. Imipramine: clinical effects and pharmacokinetic variability, *Psychopharmacology* 54, 263–272 (1977)

RICHMOND, P. W. and ROBERTS, A. H. A comparative trial of imipramine, amitriptyline, isocarboxazid and tranylcypromine in out-patient depressive illness, *British Journal of Psychiatry* 110, 846–850 (1964)

RICKELS, K., GORDON, P. E., WEISE, C. C., BRAZILIAN, S. E., FELDMAN, H. S. and WILSON, D. A. Amitriptyline and trimipramine in neurotic depressed out-patients: a collaborative study, *American Journal of Psychiatry* 127, 208–218 (1970)

RISCH, S. C., HUEY, L. Y. and JANOWSKY, D. S. Plasma levels of tricyclic antidepressants and clinical efficacy: review of the literature—Part II, *Journal of Clinical Psychiatry* 40, 58–69 (1979)

ROBIN, A. A. and HARRIS, J. A. A controlled comparison of imipramine and electroplexy, *Journal of Mental Science* 108, 217–219 (1962)

ROBIN, A. A. and LANGLEY, G. E. A controlled trial of imipramine, *British Journal of Psychiatry* 110, 419–422 (1964)

ROGERS, S. C. and CLAY, P. M. A statistical review of controlled trials of imipramine and placebo in the treatment of depressive illnesses, *British Journal of Psychiatry* 127, 599–603 (1975)

ROGERS, S. C., DAVIES, F. J. and GALBRAITH, A. W. A study of depression in two general practices. A double-blind comparison of desipramine and opipramol, *Clinical Trials Journal* 6, 5–11 (1969)

ROSE, J. T. and WESTHEAD, T. T. Comparison of desipramine and imipramine in depression, *American Journal of Psychiatry* 121, 496–498 (1964)

ROULET, N., ALVAREZ, R. R., DUFFY, J. P., LENKOSKI, L. D. and BIDDER, T. G. Imipramine in depression: a controlled study, *American Journal of Psychiatry* 119, 427–431 (1962)

SARGANT, W. Safety of combined antidepressant drugs, *British Medical Journal* 1, 555–556 (1971)

SATIJA, D. C., ADVANI, G. B. and BANSAL, A. K. A double-blind clinical trial of a new antidepressant 'Surmontil', *Indian Journal of Psychiatry* 15, 341–346 (1973)

SCHILDKRAUT, J. J. Neuropsychopharmacology and the affective disorders, *New England Journal of Medicine* 281, 197–201, 248–255, 302–308 (1969)

SCHUCKIT, M., ROBINS, E. and FEIGHNER, J. Tricyclic antidepressants and monoamine oxidase inhibitors. Combination therapy in the treatment of depression, *Archives of General Psychiatry* 24, 509–514 (1971)

SEAGER, C. P. and BIRD, R. L. Imipramine with electrical treatment in depression—controlled trial, *Journal of Mental Science* 108, 704–707 (1962)

SETHNA, E. R. A study of refractory cases of depressive illnesses and their response to combined antidepressant treatment, *British Journal of Psychiatry* 124, 265–272 (1974)

SHAFFER, D., COSTELLO, A. J. and HILL, I. D. Control of enuresis with imipramine, *Archives of Diseases in Childhood* **43**, 665–671 (1968)

SHEPHERD, F. S. A study of opipramol in general practice, *Practitioner* **195**, 92–95 (1965)

SILVERMAN, G. and BRAITHWAITE, R. A. Benzodiazepines and tricyclic antidepressant plasma levels, *British Medical Journal* **3**, 18–20 (1973)

SIM, M., ARMITAGE, G. H., DAVIES, W. H. and GORDON, E. B. The treatment of depressive states. A comparative trial of dibenzepin (Novenil) with imipramine (Tofranil), *Clinical Trials Journal* **8**, No. 2, 29–34 (1971)

SIM, M., REID, D., PALLETT, J. and GORDON, E. The Hamilton rating scale and the Sim record card: a comparative assessment based on a dothiepin (Prothiaden) v. imipramine (Tofranil) clinical trial, *Journal of Pharmacology Clinics II* **1**, 52–59 (1975)

SKARBEK, A. and SMEDBERG, D. Amitriptyline: a controlled trial in chronic depressive states, *Journal of Mental Science* **108**, 859–861 (1962)

SPLITTER, S. R. Comprehensive treatment of office patients with the aid of a new psychophysiologic agent, opipramol (Insidon), *Psychosomatics* **4**, 283–289 (1963)

STERLIN, C., LEHMANN, H. E., OLIVEROS, R. F., BAN, T. A. and SAXENA, B. M. A preliminary investigation of WY3263 v. amitriptyline in depressions, *Current Therapeutic Research* **10**, 576–582 (1968)

STERN, S. L., RUSH, A. J. and MENDELS, J. Toward a rational pharmacotherapy of depression, *American Journal of Psychiatry* **137**, 545–552 (1980)

STEWART, J. A. and MITCHELL, P. H. A comparative trial of desipramine and nortriptyline in depression, *British Journal of Psychiatry* **114**, 469–471 (1968)

STOCKLEY, I. H. Interactions with anti-hypertensive agents, *Pharmaceutical Journal* **209**, 445–452 (1972)

STOCKLEY, I. H. Interactions with oral anticoagulants, *Pharmaceutical Journal* **210**, 339–000 (1973)

SULZER, F. and BRODIE, B. B. On mechanisms of the antidepressant action of imipramine, *Biochemical Pharmacology* **8**, 16 (Abstract) (1961)

SUTHERLAND, M. S., SUTHERLAND, S. S. and PHILLIP, A. E. Depressive illness. Comparison of effects of iprindole WY3263 and imipramine, *Clinical Trials Journal* **7**, 857–860 (1970)

SUY, E. Comparison of butriptyline hydrochloride and amitriptyline hydrochloride in the therapeutic management of non-psychotic depression, *Acta Therapeutica* **2**, 245–352 (1976)

SYMES, M. H. Monochlorimipramine: a controlled trial of a new antidepressant, *International Journal of Neuropsychiatry* **3**, 60–65 (1967)

THIELE, J. and HOZINGER, O. Über o-diamidodibenzyl, *Justus Liebigs Annual of Chemistry* **305**, 96 (1899)

TYRER, P. Clinical use of monoamine oxidase inhibitors. In *Psychopharmacology of Affective Disorders* (Eds. E. S. PAYKEL and A. COPPEN), Oxford University Press, Oxford (1979)

UHLENHUTH, E. H., LIPMAN, R. S. and COVI, L. Combined pharmacotherapy and psychotherapy, *Journal of Nervous and Mental Disease* **148**, 52–64 (1969)

UHLENHUTH, E. H. and PARK, L. C. The influence of medication (imipramine) and doctor in relieving depressed psychoneurotic out-patients, *Journal of Psychiatric Research* **2**, 101–122 (1964)

VESTRE, N. D., JANECEK, J. and ZIMMERMANN, R. A controlled study of desipramine in the treatment of hospitalized depressive disorders, *Journal of Neuropsychiatry* **3**, 354–359 (1967)

WALDMEIER, P. C., BAUMANN, P., GREENGRASS, P. M. and MAÎTRE, L. Effects of clomipramine and other tricyclic antidepressants on biogenic amine uptake and turnover, *Postgraduate Medical Journal* **52**, Suppl. 3, 33–39 (1976)

WALDRON, J. and BATES, T. J. N. The management of depression in hospital: a comparative trial of desipramine and imipramine, *British Journal of Psychiatry* **111**, 511–516 (1965)

WALTER, C. J. S. Drug plasma levels and clinical effect, *Proceedings of Royal Society of Medicine* **64**, 282–285 (1970)

WALTER, C. J. S. Clinical impressions on treatment of obsessional states with intravenous clomipramine (Anafranil), *Journal of International Medical Research* **1**, 413–420 (1973)

WATANABE, S., ISHINO, H. and OTSUKI, S. Double-blind comparison of lithium carbonate and imipramine in treatment of depression, *Archives of General Psychiatry* **32**, 659–668 (1975)

WATT, D. C., CRAMMER, J. L. and ELKES, A. Metabolism, anticholinergic effects and therapeutic outcome of desmethylimipramine in depressive illness, *Psychological Medicine* **2**, 397–405 (1972)

WECHSLER, H., GROSSER, G. H. and GREENBLATT, M. Research evaluating antidepressant medications on hospitalised mental patients: a survey of published reports during a five year period, *Journal of Nervous and Mental Diseases* **141**, 231–239 (1965)

WEISSMAN, M. M., KLERMAN, G. L., PAYKEL, E. S., PRUSOFF, B. and HANSON, B. Treatment effects on the social adjustment of depressed patients, *Archives of General Psychiatry* **30**, 771–778 (1974)

WHITE, K., PISTOLE, T. and BOYD, J. L. Combined monoamine oxidase inhibitor-tricyclic antidepressant treatment: a pilot study, *American Journal of Psychiatry* **137**, 1422–1425 (1980)

WHYBROW, P. C., COPPEN, A., PRANGE, A. J., NOQUERA, R. and BAILEY, J. E. Thyroid function and the response to liothyronine in depression, *Archives of General Psychiatry* **26**, 242–245 (1972)

WILSON, I. C., VERNON, J. T., GUIN, T. and SANDIFER, M. G. JR. A controlled study of treatments of depression, *Journal of Neuropsychiatry* **4**, 331–337 (1963)

YOUNG, J. P. R., LADER, M. H. and HUGHES, W. C. Controlled trial of trimipramine, monoamine oxidase inhibitors and combined treatment in depressed out-patients, *British Medical Journal* **2**, 1315–1317 (1979)

ZIEGLER, V. E., CO, B. T. and BIGGS, J. T. Plasma nortriptyline levels and ECG findings, *American Journal of Psychiatry* **134**, 441–443 (1977)

ZIEGLER, V. E., CLAYTON, P. J., TAYLOR, J. R., CO, B. T. and BIGGS, J. T. Nortriptyline plasma levels and therapeutic response, *Clinical Pharmacology and Therapeutics* **20**, 458–463 (1976)

Chapter 8

New generation of antidepressants

T. R. E. Barnes and P. K. Bridges

In the 1950s were laid the foundations of modern psychiatry with its emphasis on relatively specific psychotropic medication which has proved to be highly effective in treating the functional psychoses, illnesses that can be seriously incapacitating and potentially fatal. These include schizophrenia, mania and endogenous depression. The drugs that became available fall into three groups—antianxiety, antidepressant and antipsychotic. Their prime importance is that, not only were they new drugs, serendipitously discovered, but they were found to have psychotropic activities which were unknown before. For example, for the treatment of depression amphetamines were previously available but these compounds, unlike the antidepressants, lack specificity and produce effects in both the psychiatric patient and the normal subject. Specific antidepressant activity was a new property for a drug.

It is also surprising that two chemically dissimilar compounds, which became available within a few years of each other, were both found to have antidepressant effects. The monoamine oxidase inhibitors derived from the original preparation, iproniazid, which was developed from isoniazid. Tricyclic antidepressants were a development from the aliphatic phenothiazines which have a somewhat similar three-ring structure, although the tricyclic antidepressants are not usually of value in schizophrenic illnesses.

Not only are the antidepressants clinically effective but their pharmacological activity, when the effects on animals are studied, offer the possibility of improving knowledge of the metabolic associations of depressive illnesses, an essential step towards the elucidation of their aetiology and their biochemical detection. As a result of these scientific investigations we can now define an antidepressant in relatively precise biological terms rather than relying on vague, clinical descriptions. Thus, an antidepressant is a substance administered to a patient that increases the availability of certain monoamine neurotransmitters in the brain, the more important of which are 5-hydroxytryptamine (5-HT), noradrenaline (NA) and dopamine (DA). The specificity of the antidepressants should be stressed because they do not modify mood in healthy subjects and their activity is thus different from the amphetamines which are better classed as psychostimulants.

This summary of antidepressant medication remained valid until a few years ago but since then a number of compounds, chemically different from both the monoamine inhibitors and the tricyclics, have been introduced. Obviously there is a need to be sure that new compounds actually have antidepressant activity and this is best assessed against a placebo in a double-blind investigation. These studies have been carried out with all the new drugs but there are methodological difficulties. For one thing, the response to antidepressants tends to be delayed even after the optimum dose has been reached. This introduces problems as to the amount of the optimum dose, which will vary from subject to subject, and there will be difficulty in assessing the period of time required on the drug to be sure of absence of response. Another very important aspect is the ethical one. Many clinicians feel that the older antidepressants are now established as being effective. Therefore a patient with a suitable type of depression should not be denied effective medication by being given a placebo for a period, especially because of the risks, sometimes considerable, of suicidal behaviour encountered in those with affective disorders. Hence, most trials have necessarily compared the new preparations with established antidepressant medication, usually imipramine or amitriptyline, despite the real need for decisive information concerning the effects of the new drugs. This latter approach is scientifically unsound but perhaps clinically unavoidable. Investigations with a reference drug are unable to take into account the possibility of placebo responses and finding that a new preparation seems to produce a therapeutic response similar to that of an established tricyclic, does not necessarily mean that both substances have similar antidepressant activity. Furthermore, there may be different side effects which cause problems of interpretation as to the effect of the drug on a patient.

However, pharmacological findings with animals may help. There is no useful animal model for human affective illnesses but antidepressants can be recognized, using animal studies, by a profile of biochemical effects which do not themselves produce antidepressant activity. For example, maprotiline was found to produce dose-dependent protective effects against ptosis in rats given reserpine and against catalepsy due to tetrabenazine. It potently inhibits the uptake of noradrenaline in a number of organs of the rat, cat and chick, the effects being dose-dependent. This gives a spectrum of metabolic activity which can be expected of an antidepressant drug. There are other means of recognition, for example, the 'thymoleptic' electroencephalogram (EEG) (Itil, Polvan and Hsu, 1972). It appears that mianserin was discovered to have antidepressant activity because general screening included EEG investigations on volunteers receiving the drug.

When a preparation has been shown to have the necessary metabolic spectrum for an antidepressant and has been compared with an established antidepressant in a clinical trial, it has to be assessed in a more general way in relation to the antidepressant medication already available. It could be that some newly-introduced antidepressant compounds might be found to be clinically effective but have no advantages compared with the established tricyclic group and monoamine oxidase inhibitors, or it may have more disadvantages. Hence new compounds need to be considered in relation to clinical experience with the established drugs.

Tricyclic antidepressants

Advantages

(1) Can be highly effective.
(2) Their use is now familiar to clinicians as they have been available for 20 or more years.

(3) Generally safe in normal use. With some patients, the sedative effects, especially of amitriptyline and trimipramine can be exploited by giving the total dose at night to help insomnia.
(4) They tend to be cheap in price.

Disadvantages

(1) With a number of patients the side effects can be troublesome—these include excessive sedation (especially amitriptyline and trimipramine), dry mouth, blurring of vision, excessive sweating and micturition difficulties.
(2) Contraindicated with acute closed-angle glaucoma.
(3) Hypotension may occur.
(4) The activity of some antihypertensive drugs are reversed.
(5) Epileptic fits may be precipitated.
(6) Dangerous in overdose.
(7) Can be cardiotoxic.
(8) Antidepressant activity is usually delayed for about two weeks on optimum dosage, and it may also take time to reach optimum dosage. In this period the depression can worsen and suicidal behaviour may result.

MAO inhibitors

Advantages

(1) May be effective with some depressive illnesses when the tricyclics have not produced improvement. It is uncertain whether they act more specifically with certain types of depression.
(2) Do not cause fits.

Disadvantages

(1) Hypotension.
(2) Diet with a low tyramine content is necessary. Tyramine-containing foods may cause hypertensive crises and even cerebral haemorrhages.
(3) Potentially dangerous interaction with anaesthetics, barbiturates, with pethidine and its derivatives, and with ephedrine, to be found widely in cough 'cures', nasal sprays, etc.
(4) Therapeutic response may be delayed for two weeks or more on optimum dosage.
(5) MAO inhibition is produced irreversibly, therefore on stopping the drug the effects will remain for about two weeks until adequate new MAO is formed.
(6) Dangerous in overdose.

Hence the ideal antidepressant would have characteristics such as these:

(1) Minimal side effects; no anticholinergic activity, no interaction with other drugs or particular foods.
(2) No effects on blood pressure.
(3) No tendency to produce fits.
(4) Not cardiotoxic.

(5) There is a shorter period before a therapeutic response is apparent.
(6) Relatively safe in overdose.

An attempt can now be made to relate the effects of the new antidepressants against these practical clinical considerations.

Maprotiline (Ludiomil)

Rather ingeniously, maprotiline (Ludiomil) was introduced as a 'tetracyclic' antidepressant. This tends to suggest that it is a new type of antidepressant without indicating whether the implied four-ring structure makes a significant difference in the psychopharmacological properties of the compound. Maprotiline is an anthracene with a formula that is similar to that of nortriptyline except for an ethylene link across the central ring of the basic tricyclic structure (*Figure 8.1a* and *b*). However, this bridge imposes a rigid flexure on the molecular skeleton which could have pharmacokinetic implications (Wilhelm, 1972). It also has considerable structural similarity to the anxiolytic drug benzoctamine (Tacitin) (*see* p. 159). The main difference between them is in the length of the side chain, although this comparatively minor modification gives rise to considerable differences in the pharmacological and therapeutic effects of the two drugs.

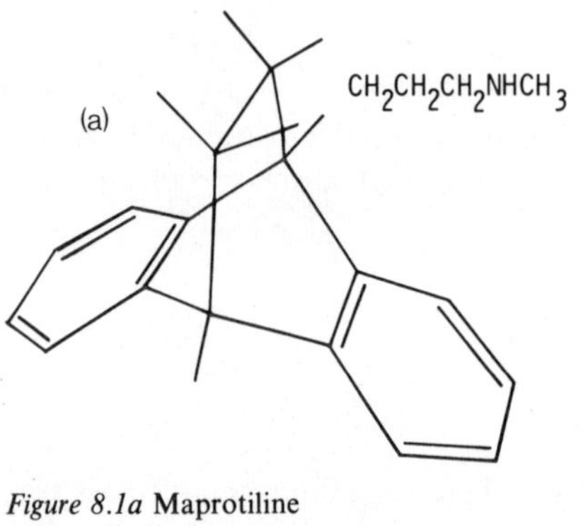

Figure 8.1a Maprotiline 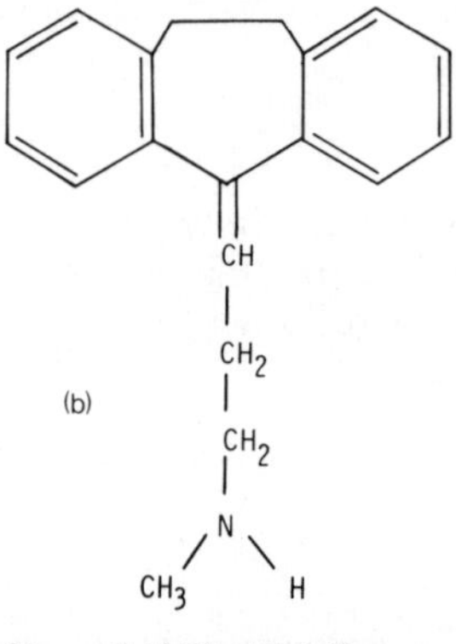   Figure 8.1b Nortriptyline

Maprotiline resembles the tricyclic antidepressants in many of its pharmacological properties but there are some differences. For example, while imipramine tends to produce excitatory effects in animals, maprotiline has marked sedative and anti-aggressive properties, but it differs from the benzodiazepines in that it does not protect against induced seizures nor impair spinal reflex transmission (Delini-Stula, 1972). Maprotiline suppresses excitation induced in mice by giving them a combination of pargyline and reserpine, but this effect is not produced by imipramine or amitriptyline. Maprotiline differs from imipramine in having fewer cardiovascular effects in animals (Brunner *et al.*, 1971). It seems to be less likely to induce seizures than the tricyclics (Trimble, 1978), it is reported to have weak anticholinergic activity and less alpha-adrenoceptor blocking effects than amitriptyline. However, like the tricyclic compounds, it must be regarded as dangerous in overdose (Park and Proudfoot, 1977).

Mode of action

Like the tricyclics, maprotiline blocks the membrane pump re-uptake of transmitter in the synapse. But the effect is specifically on NA and there is no appreciable action on 5-HT re-uptake, even with high doses (Maitre *et al.*, 1975). It is presumably this activity that is associated with the antidepressant properties, although the clinical significance of the NA-uptake blocking drugs as opposed to those mainly blocking 5-HT uptake is uncertain (Ridges, 1975).

Pharmacokinetics

Maprotiline, when taken orally, is slowly and completely absorbed. Its half-life, following rapid intravenous administration, is 40 ± 15 h (Maguire *et al.*, 1980) and it is bound to plasma protein. As with many psychopharmacological preparations, considerable variation is found in blood levels following standard doses and this may relate to body weight. Coppen *et al.*, (1976) found a significant negative correlation between body weight and maprotiline plasma levels. The compound is eliminated almost completely as metabolites, mainly the desmethyl derivative. Chronic effects in animals have been studied by Delini-Stula, Radeke and Vassout (1978).

In a study of plasma levels it was found that a steady state was achieved in one week but the values showed much variation and there was no correlation between plasma or blood levels with side effects and clinical response (Miller *et al.*, 1977).

Therapeutic trials

In a large number of trials carried out internationally no significant differences have been found between the antidepressant activity of maprotiline when compared with amitriptyline, imipramine and clomipramine (Pinto *et al.*, 1972). A study by Balestrieri *et al.* (1971) tended to show that the drug was more effective in patients diagnosed as having neurotic depression than in patients with endogenous depression, and a report by Kessell and Holt (1975) suggested that maprotiline might be more effective than imipramine for patients with neurotic depression. Placebo controlled trials have been carried out by Jukes (1975) and by McCallum and Meares (1975). In the first study the two groups of patients were not well matched and in the second study amitriptyline seemed more effective. On the other hand, Kay and Davies (1974) found no significant difference between the effects of the drug and amitriptyline, using a biochemical marker with each tablet for detection in the urine. Forrest (1975), studying elderly patients, found amitriptyline to be less effective and maprotiline seemed to have more rapid action. Forrest (1977) also carried out an open multicentre trial into which 2270 patients were entered, with most taking maprotiline 75 mg at night. Using an extract from the Hamilton Depression Scale, the mean score fell from an initial 9.5 to 2.5 on day 28. In another large multicentre trial involving 1440 hospital outpatients, maprotiline given in two doses was compared with doxepin and no differences in clinical effects were found except that more patients with reactive depression responded to maprotiline and it has been suggested that maprotiline might be used as a substitute for monoamine oxidase inhibitors in patients with neurotic depression (Bartholini and Pinto, 1973), although there is some controversy as to whether the MAO inhibitors have specificity for neurotic depression. With regard to speed of therapeutic effect, Sims (1980) found both maprotiline and sustained-release ami-triptyline to have similar effectiveness and there was a similar period before the therapeutic response was seen.

Adverse effects

In general maprotiline produces side effects similar to those of the tricyclic antidepressants and there does not seem to be a clear relationship to dose. The side effects include hypotension, palpitations, sweating, tremor, constipation and visual disturbances. Also, as with the tricyclic drugs, grand mal seizures may occur occasionally (Shepherd and Kerr, 1978; Marks *et al.*, 1979) but the incidence is less with maprotiline (Trimble, 1978). There have been several reports of hallucinations, usually in elderly people although the symptoms settled rapidly on stopping the medication. In the multicentre trial described above (Bartholini and Pinto, 1973) side effects occurred in about 25 per cent, mainly dry mouth. The incidence of vertigo and dizziness was more common with the patients on maprotiline. In the other large trial (Forrest, 1977) the commonest side effects were drowsiness and dry mouth.

Maprotiline has some effects on the cardiovascular system, said to be less than with the tricyclic compounds. The drug interacts with adrenergic blockers but this has also been said to be less than with tricyclics. The evidence for cardiotoxicity is not strong and the compound has been shown to differ from imipramine in the cardiovascular effects produced in animals (Brunner *et al.*, 1971). Khan (1980) reviewed the cardiac conduction effects of maprotiline and mianserin and concluded that no conduction abnormality or evidence of myocardial lesion was found in patients on either preparation.

DOSE

As for most of the tricyclics, from 75 mg daily usually up to 150 mg daily, probably best given in one dose at night.

Mianserin (Bolvidon, Norval)

Both mianserin and maprotiline were introduced as tetracyclic antidepressants. Mianserin, with its piperazine–dibenzapine structure, has a three-ring molecular configuration similar to that of the tricyclic group but differs from these drugs by the addition of a fourth ring instead of a side chain (*Figure 8.2*).

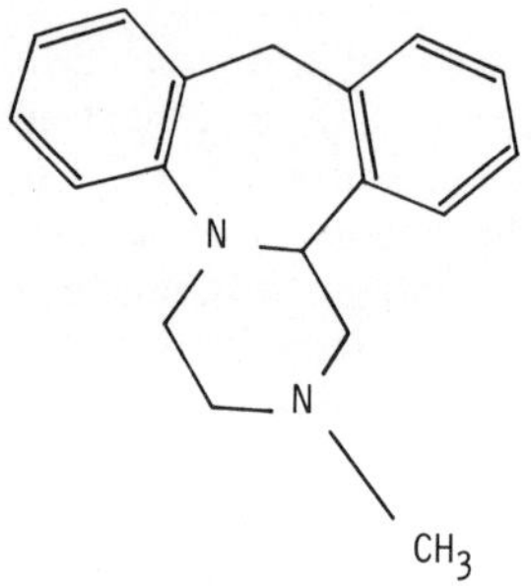

Figure 8.2 Mianserin

Mianserin was developed by transformation of the structure of an antihistamine, phenbenzamine, with the aim of synthesizing an anti-asthma, anti-migraine compound, but the possibility of other therapeutic effects was investigated. Mianserin was developed as a potential antidepressant on the basis of the 'thymoleptic EEG' mentioned above, even though it failed to exhibit the full pharmacological profile in animals characteristic of the tricyclics.

Mode of action

Mianserin is a potent histamine antagonist, a property it shares with iprindole and the tricyclic antidepressants (Green and Maayani, 1977; Kanof and Greengard, 1978) but this is unlikely to be related to its antidepressant effects (Black, 1978). Mianserin does not seem to affect catecholamine re-uptake (Leonard, 1974; Kafoe, de Ridder and Leonard, 1976) but it apparently increases the synaptic availability of noradrenaline by blocking pre-synaptic alpha$_2$-adrenoceptors.

These auto-receptors regulate pre-synaptic release of noradrenaline and operate through a negative feedback system (Baumann and Maître, 1977; Langer, 1978). Some other antidepressants, including amitriptyline, nortriptyline and trazodone, also appear to block these negative (α)-receptors while others, such as desipramine and viloxazine are inactive. Many antidepressants after chronic treatment 'down regulate' positive(β) receptors, adding to their antidepressant efficacy. This may explain why tolerance does not develop to their antidepressant effects after prolonged dosage. Collis and Shepherd (1980) consider the modulation of noradrenaline release via pre-synaptic receptors to be a more efficient mechanism for increasing synaptic noradrenaline levels than re-uptake inhibition.

Mianserin also blocks post-synaptic 5-HT receptors (Maj et al., 1977). The combination of noradrenaline potentiation and 5-HT antagonism would seem to put mianserin in a unique position to test the concept of two possible subtypes of depression, one involving a functional deficiency of NA and the other of 5-HT (Maas, Fawcett and Dekirmenjian, 1972; Garver and Davies, 1979). However, mianserin shows no marked treatment selectivity, producing benefit in patients classified as having either neurotic or endogenous depression (Coppen et al., 1976; Murphy, Donald and Molla, 1976; Okamoto, Nakano and Inanaga, 1978; Daly, Browne and Morgan, 1979; Mehta, Spear and Whittington, 1980). The results from a few studies suggest that the drug is particularly effective in agitated depression (Kretschmer, 1980; Saletu and Grünberger, 1980) but this may merely reflect its anxiolytic effects (Murphy, 1978; Conti and Pinder, 1979).

Pharmacokinetics

Mianserin is rapidly absorbed following oral administration, with a peak plasma level of 30–150 ng. ml^{-1} occurring 2–3 h after ingestion. The elimination half-life is estimated at 10–17 h (Fink, Irwin and Gastpar, 1977; Van der Veen et al., 1980). No relationship between mean, steady state, plasma levels and clinical response was found by Coppen et al. (1976), whereas the results of Montgomery, McAuley and Montgomery (1978) suggested a curvilinear relationship, patients with plasma mianserin concentrations above 70 μg. ml^{-1} or below 15 μg. ml^{-1} showing a poorer clinical response. Thus mianserin may share with nortriptyline a plasma level range for optimum therapeutic response, the so-called 'therapeutic window' effect (Åsberg et al., 1971; Kragh-Sørensen, Åsberg and Eggert-Hansen, 1973; Gram, 1977).

Therapeutic trials

Brogden *et al.* (1978) surveyed seven double-blind trials comparing mianserin and amitriptyline, and four similar trials of mianserin versus imipramine. These authors had reservations regarding the methodology of these studies, commenting that, in general, the patient numbers were relatively small, the trials were of short duration and the treatment groups of dubious comparability.

Since the review by these authors there have been three further double-blind studies comparing mianserin and amitriptyline in depressed patients (Daly, Browne and Morgan, 1979; Kretschmar, 1980; Mehta, Spear and Whittington, 1980), all of which failed to detect any difference between the drugs in terms of antidepressant effect. In addition there have been three similar studies comparing mianserin with imipramine. Two of these (Pull *et al.*, 1980; Montgomery *et al.*, 1980) found no differences in responses between mianserin- and imipramine-treated patients, but in the third (Svestka *et al.*, 1979) imipramine proved to be superior, producing a greater percentage of 'full remissions'. Mianserin has also been compared with clomipramine (De Buck, 1980; Blaha, Pinder and Stulemeijer, 1980; Pinder *et al.*, 1980), and maprotiline (Khan and Moslehuddin, 1980), in double-blind trials that did not reveal any significant differences in therapeutic response.

The antidepressant effect of mianserin has been tested against placebo in four studies. Murphy, Donald and Molla (1976), Magnus (1979) and Smith, Naylor and Moody (1978) found mianserin superior to placebo while Perry *et al.* (1978) found no significant differences between mianserin, imipramine and placebo. In the latter study, real differences between the treatments may have been obscured by the non-specific effects of hospital admission and concurrent psychotherapy. Mianserin has also been tested against a benzodiazepine, as an 'ethical placebo' in two studies with depressed patients (Russell *et al.*, 1978; Hamouz, Pinder and Stulemeijer, 1980). Mianserin was found to be significantly superior as an antidepressant in both trials.

Adverse effects

Most comparative drug studies involving mianserin and a tricyclic antidepressant have noted fewer side effects with mianserin. Drowsiness during the first few weeks of treatment seems to be the most common problem with mianserin therapy. The compound is said to be virtually devoid of anticholinergic activity. For example, it does not decrease salivary flow and may even cause a limited increase (Ghose, Coppen and Turner, 1976; Kopera, 1978; Wilson, Petrie and Ban, 1980). Nevertheless, dry mouth as well as blurred vision, constipation and urinary retention have occasionally been reported in association with mianserin administration (Pinder *et al.*, 1980; Blaha, Pinder and Stulemeijer, 1980; Hamouz, Pinder and Stulemeijer, 1980; Khan and Moslehuddin, 1980), although to a far lesser extent than with the tricyclic antidepressants. Whether these symptoms reflect anticholinergic effects has been doubted. Mehta, Spear and Whittington (1980) found such symptoms present prior to antidepressant treatment in a depressed population and subsequent mianserin treatment produced little change in side effects except that the number of patients complaining of drowsiness and headache was significantly reduced.

A few cases of epileptic fits, apparently induced by mianserin have been described (Tyrer, Steinberg and Watson, 1979; Mikhail, 1979; Evans and Lander, 1980). In one case the possibility of lorazepam withdrawal as a cause of the convulsions was suggested (Einarson, 1980). By November 1979, 30 such cases had been reported to the Committee on Safety of Medicines (Edwards, 1979). However, Edwards claimed that these CSM data might be unreliable. He had investigated many cases of alleged mianserin-induced seizures and the cause was usually uncertain. Patients were often receiving other potentially epileptogenic drugs concurrently or being withdrawn from benzodiazepines. According to Crome, and Chand (unpublished material quoted by Shaw, 1980), who collected information on 84 mianserin overdoses, only one patient had experienced convulsions. Trimble (1980a) considered that mianserin was probably less convulsant than the tricyclics although there was insufficient information to be certain. Nevertheless, it seems as if mianserin must join the list of antidepressants, headed by the tricyclics, that should be used with caution or avoided in patients where there is the suspicion of a reduced seizure threshold.

Unlike the tricyclics, mianserin appears to be free of any significant cardiotoxic effects, producing no significant ECG changes in therapeutic doses (Burrows et al., 1979; Kopera, Klein and Schenk, 1980; Montgomery, 1980). First degree heart-block has occurred in one patient following an overdose of 580 mg of mianserin (Green and Kendall-Taylor, 1977) but the ECG recordings returned to normal 16 h after ingestion. Wester and Siegers (1980) compared the effects of amitriptyline and mianserin on cardiac function using non-invasive techniques. They found a loss of myocardial contractility with the tricyclic-treated patients but not the mianserin patients. Burgess et al. (1979) measured systolic time intervals in depressed patients receiving mianserin and found evidence of both increased and decreased contractility, although these authors considered these changes related to drug effects on the peripheral circulation rather than a direct action on the myocardium. In overdose, serious cardiotoxic effects are rare (Newman and Crome, 1980; Shaw, 1980).

Anorexia is a common depressive symptom and appetite might be expected to improve with antidepressant therapy. Mianserin, however, has apparently been associated with excessive weight gain, appetite increase and changes in food preference (Harris and Harper, 1980). Hopman (1980) reported 'remarkable' increases in body weight in 10 per cent of his patients receiving mianserin and felt that the associated increase in appetite might be partly due to a direct pharmacological action of the drug.

Agranulocytosis is a rare complication of treatment with tricyclic antidepressants (Albertini and Penders, 1978) which usually recovers if the drug is discontinued early. A case of leucopenia (McHarg and McHarg, 1979) and a case of agranulocytosis (Curson and Hale, 1979) with mianserin therapy have been described, both of which recovered spontaneously after the drug was stopped. The second report mentioned that four cases of blood dyscrasias associated with mianserin treatment had been reported to the Committee on Safety of Medicines, with only nine cases where mianserin was 'probably responsible' reported up to 1982.

In overdose, mianserin does not cause the serious complications of respiratory depression, convulsions and cardiac arrythmias associated with the tricyclics. Shaw (1980, quoting Crome and Chand, unpublished material) reported on 84 mianserin overdose cases, half of whom took a combination of drugs. All 42 patients who took mianserin alone apparently 'recovered promptly'. There were no reports of deep coma, seizures, serious cardiotoxicity or respiratory depression; the most common problem being drowsiness in 16 cases. For the 42 patients who ingested mianserin with other drugs serious complications were relatively frequent and two patients died.

DOSE

From 30 mg daily to 200 mg daily or more if necessary. Probably best given in one dose at night.

Viloxazine (Vivalan)

Viloxazine is structurally distinct from the tricyclic and tetracyclic antidepressants (*Figure 8.3*). It is a bicyclic tetrahydroxazine and was introduced as a potential psychotropic agent in 1972 (Mallion *et al.*, 1972). Early animal research revealed a

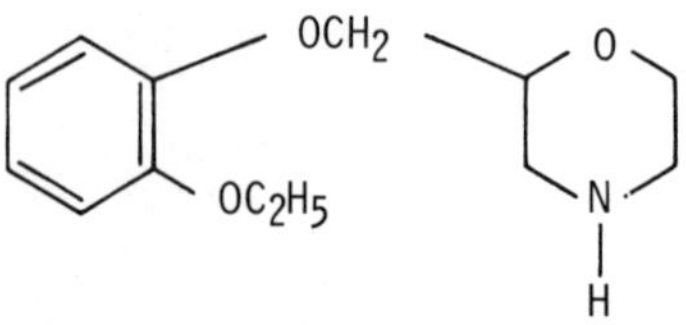

Figure 8.3 Viloxazine

pharmacological profile similar, in some aspects, to that of the tricyclic anti-depressants. But viloxazine differs from the tricyclics in certain properties. For example, it fails to inhibit both 5-HT uptake into human blood platelets and noradrenaline uptake in rat medulla and hypothalamus (Mallion *et al.*, 1972).

Mode of action

In terms of brain amines, viloxazine inhibits noradrenaline re-uptake in both the central and peripheral nervous systems, and generally potentiates noradrenergic phenomena (Greenwood, 1975; Lippman and Pugsley, 1976; Blackburn *et al.*, 1978), properties it shares with some tricyclic antidepressants. Viloxazine also potentiates 5-HT activity, probably via a pre-synaptic mechanism (Martin, Baker and Mitchell, 1978; Pawlowski, Ruczynska and Wojtasik, 1979). The drug has minimal effects on DA re-uptake or release and is virtually devoid of peripheral anticholinergic activity although the possibility of central activity remains (Weinstock and Cohen, 1976).

   Following the monoamine hypothesis of affective disorder, the potentiation of either noradrenergic or serotonergic activity, or both, is likely to be the mode of action, with an associated mood-elevating effect in depressed patients. However, alternative although less likely theories exist. For example, Vogel (1975) believes that the antidepressant effects of a drug relate to its ability to suppress rapid eye movement (REM) sleep with an associated build up of REM 'pressure', i.e. following withdrawal of the drug there will be a rebound increase in REM sleep. Viloxazine fulfils these criteria, markedly reducing REM sleep and producing a withdrawal rebound (Brezinova *et al.*, 1977).

Pharmacokinetics

Viloxazine is rapidly and almost completely absorbed, with peak blood concentrations occurring approximately 2 h after oral administration. There are no active metabolites, the ingested drug being responsible for the pharmacological effects. In depressed patients the inter-individual plasma level variation is only two-fold, in contrast to the tricyclic antidepressants where a ten-fold range is seen, and the elimination half-life is just under 5 h (Adams, Barnes and Gaind, unpublished material; Müller-Oerlinghausen and Rüther, 1979; Elwan and Adam, 1980).

Therapeutic trials

Pinder *et al.* (1977) reviewed nine double-blind studies comparing viloxazine with imipramine or amitriptyline in in-patients and out-patients with depression. These authors considered that the trials did not show a difference between the antidepressant efficacy of viloxazine and the tricyclics. Similar recent studies have produced equivalent findings (Nugent, 1979; Botter, 1979; Floru and Tegeler, 1979). Pinder *et al.* (1977) also reviewed two placebo-controlled trials. Mahapatra (1975) found no difference between viloxazine and placebo in the overall reduction of Hamilton rating scores although viloxazine produced a significant reduction in scores for certain specific items such as 'depressed mood', 'suicidal tendencies' and 'guilt', within the first few days of treatment. In the second study by Magnus (1975) viloxazine had significantly superior antidepressant effects compared to placebo.

In the same year as the review by Pinder *et al.* (1977), Edwards (1977a) assessing the potential for an early antidepressant effect, reported that viloxazine produced fewer beneficial results than placebo in the first week of treatment. Von Knorring (1980), in a placebo-controlled trial in elderly depressed patients, failed to find a difference between viloxazine and placebo after 7 d but by the end of the third week there was a statistically significant difference in depression scores between the two treatment groups, favouring the patients on viloxazine. McEvoy *et al.* (1980) found no differences between viloxazine, doxepin or placebo in a four-week double-blind clinical trial involving patients with depressive neurosis. The disparity between the findings in these studies may be partly explained by the wide dose range prescribed for the patients (150–400 mg daily) and also perhaps by the diagnostically diverse patient populations included.

Adverse effects

In most comparative studies viloxazine has been found to have a lower incidence of side effects, especially those due to anticholinergic activity. However, nausea and vomiting have been common complaints, particularly in UK studies and often necessitating drug withdrawal (Peet, 1973; Wheatley, 1974; Edwards, 1977a; Nugent, 1979; Botter, 1979; Von Knorring, 1980; McEvoy *et al.*, 1980). Headache is another symptom frequently associated with viloxazine administration (Wheatley, 1974; Mukherjee and Holland, 1979; McEvoy *et al.*, 1980). In the context of an open study of viloxazine in 30 patients Barnes, Kidger and Greenwood (1979) reported classic migraine symptoms in three patients and severe one-sided headache in two further patients, none of whom had a history of migraine. Although nausea and vomiting are usually ascribed to a local gastrointestinal action of viloxazine, its association with headache suggests a possible cerebrovascular or central mechanism. Viloxazine may precipitate migraine by virtue of its 5-HT potentiating properties.

Edwards (1977b) drew attention to the possibility of epileptogenic properties in man despite evidence that viloxazine protects rodents from fits induced electrically or by drugs (Mallion *et al.*, 1972). He reported that, in a double-blind placebo-controlled trial, one patient on 300 mg viloxazine daily, experienced three convulsive seizures. Previously Magnus (1975) had recorded an increase in the frequency of fits in one epileptic patient receiving viloxazine and a convulsion in another patient not previously known to be an epileptic. However, both Brion (1975) and Kress *et al.* (1978) have used the drug in the treatment of depression in epileptic patients without provoking seizures. Five patients taking viloxazine overdoses have had convulsions but two had also taken other centrally-acting compounds (Holland and Brosnon, 1979). The evidence for viloxazine-induced fits remains largely circumstantial and the phenomenon is clearly rare. Up to November 1979 a total of six cases of fits associated with viloxazine were reported to the Committee on Safety of Medicines, one of which apparently proved fatal (Edwards, 1979). Based on the data from animal experiments and clinical reports, Trimble (1980a) concludes that tricyclic antidepressants are more inclined to induce fits rather than the non-tricyclic antidepressants and, of the latter, considers viloxazine as one of the least likely.

There is little evidence of cardiotoxicity with viloxazine. Serious dysrhythmias have not been reported even with overdose (Holland and Brosnan, 1979). ECG changes in patients receiving the drug have occasionally been reported but viloxazine has been well tolerated in a few studies including patients with concurrent cardiac disease (Bayle, 1979; Von Knorring, 1980; Samat, Grazzini and Duvic, 1980).

The risks associated with self poisoning would appear to be less than those with tricyclic antidepressant overdose. Brewer (1975) described an overdose of 6.5 g of viloxazine which was followed by an uneventful recovery. Holland and Brosnan (1979) reported on 64 overdoses of which only four were fatal. Of the four who died, one had been taking a variety of psychotropic preparations and the other three had probably taken at least 5 g of viloxazine. In general, the most common central nervous system effect was drowsiness or clouding of consciousness, with transient coma in a quarter of the cases.

DOSE

From 150 mg daily up to 400 mg daily. Probably best given in divided doses.

Flupenthixol (Fluanxol)

The thioxanthine derivative, flupenthixol, is an effective antipsychotic drug which is available as an intramuscular depot injection of flupenthixol decanoate (Depixol). Flupenthixol is also available in tablet form as the dihydrochloride (Fluanxol) which, it is claimed, has specific antidepressant effects, being also non-sedative and anxiolytic. Flupenthixol is not the first antipsychotic drug to be investigated for antidepressant properties. There is evidence that thioridazine is similar to impramine in this respect (Overall et al., 1964; General Practice Clinical Trials, 1972). Chlorpromazine has also been compared with imipramine, an equivalent antidepressant effect being found (Fink, Klein and Kramer, 1965; Paykel et al., 1968). Raskin et al. (1970) confirmed this result although they reported that imipramine was significantly better than chlorpromazine in relieving motor retardation.

Pharmacokinetics

The active isomer, alpha-(cis) flupenthixol, taken orally, is relatively slowly absorbed with a peak serum concentration at 3–6 h, and with an elimination half-life of 19–39 h (Jørgensen, 1980). Flupenthixol is generally stated to be antidepressant only in small doses (1–4 mg daily), much larger doses being required in the treatment of schizophrenia, 20–100 mg depot intramuscularly every 2–4 weeks, or more (Crammer, Barraclough and Heine, 1978; Trimble, 1980b). How far this therapeutic distinction between low antidepressant doses and high antipsychotic doses is clinically valid, is unclear.

Jørgensen (1980) measured alpha-flupenthixol serum levels in normal healthy volunteers receiving both oral and depot preparations of the drug. Based on the results, Jørgensen considered 10 mg of oral flupenthixol daily to be pharmacokinetically equivalent to 25 mg of the depot injection each week. He pointed out that the fluctuations in serum level between maximum and minimum occur within 24 h after tablet administration but over 2–4 weeks following depot injection, so this pharmacokinetic equivalence does not necessarily correspond to clinical efficacy. However, if this equivalence ratio holds true as a 'useful guideline', through the dose range, 4 mg daily orally is equivalent to 10 mg depot every week and thus the antidepressant and the antipsychotic dose ranges appear to overlap.

Therapeutic trials

There were early reports that flupenthixol was beneficial with depressed patients (Holst, 1965; Sonne, 1966). Reiter (1969) treated 130 depressed out-patients and noted that the drug possessed 'interesting normalizing properties', with few adverse effects and an onset of therapeutic effect within a few days. The remission rate was about 60 per cent, similar to the generally accepted level for tricyclic antidepressants. However, two further studies, by Sonne (1971) and Frølund (1974) with out-patients and general practice patients respectively, led both workers to conclude that if improvement had not occurred within one week there was little to be gained from further treatment with flupenthixol, and alternative medication was indicated.

In a double-blind controlled study undertaken by Young, Hughes and Lader (1976), 60 depressed out-patients were treated with either amitriptyline or flupenthixol for six weeks, using flexible dosage regimens. The authors concluded that flupenthixol was 'at least as effective as amitriptyline as both an antidepressant and an anxiolytic'. They found no difference between the two drugs in speed of onset of action, both treatment groups showing a marked improvement within the first week. This result was interpreted by Kellett (1976) as reflecting the sedative properties of the drugs and placebo responses, rather than specific antidepressant action. The anxiolytic action claimed is also difficult to interpret since the majority of patients also received a benzodiazepine.

Robertson and Trimble (1981) in an open study of flupenthixol found 1 mg daily to be an adequate antidepressant dose. However, they also allowed benzodiazepines to be prescribed. The effects of this additional medication on outcome may not be limited to anxiety reduction. Johnson (1979) found no significant difference between the antidepressant effects of flupenthixol, nortriptyline and diazepam in patients with neurotic depression. Comparisons between the antidepressant effects of flupenthixol and placebo have not demonstrated impressive differences (Predescu et al., 1973; Frølund, 1974; Ovhed, 1976). The largest study was a double-blind general practice trial on 231 patients (Frølund, 1974). Improvement was obtained in 65 per cent of the flupenthixol treated patients and 50 per cent of the placebo patients. Frølund considered the difference between the two groups 'slight'.

Adverse effects

Side effects with flupenthixol are generally reported as minimal with only occasional drowsiness, agitation and mild parkinsonism (Johnson, 1979). However, Robertson and Trimble (1981) reported akathisia in five out of 16 patients, four of whom were receiving only 2 mg flupenthixol daily. Three normal male subjects, receiving relatively low doses of flupenthixol as part of a pharmacokinetic investigation experienced 'restlessness' (Jørgensen, 1980). Parkinsonism and akathisia are both dose-dependent side effects that reflect the central dopamine antagonist properties of the drug. The possibility of tardive dyskinesia developing with chronic treatment must be considered.

DOSE

1 mg twice daily up to 1 mg three times daily.

Nomifensine (Merital)

Nomifensine is a tetrahydroisoquinoline compound which has a three-ring structure, but of different configuration from that of the tricyclic group (*Figure 8.4*). This tends to show that classifying antidepressants by the number of ring components in the formula seems to be of little clinical value. Nomifensine has no chemical relationship with any other antidepressant. However, it resembles imipramine and other antidepressants in the usual animal screening tests for antidepressant substances. It has antagonizing activity on reserpine-induced hypothermia in mice, it reverses catalepsy produced by tetrabenzine and reserpine in mice and rats, and in some of these effects it is more potent than imipramine (Hoffman, 1977).

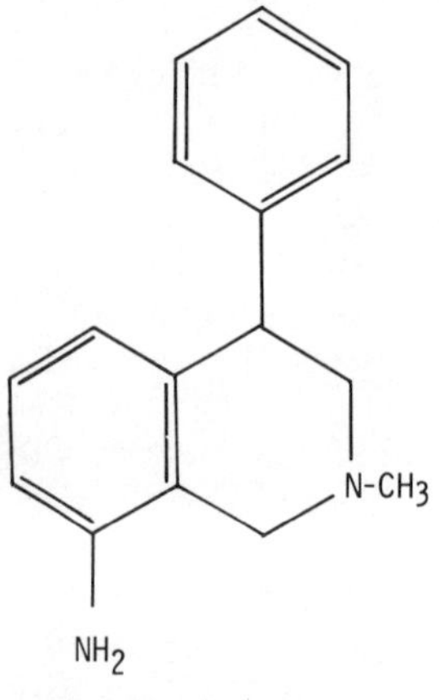

Figure 8.4 Nomifensine

Like some of the tricyclic preparations, nomifensine produced marked inhibition of NA re-uptake but there is little effect on 5-HT re-uptake. However, so far uniquely among the antidepressants, it has a potent inhibitory effect on DA re-uptake (Horn, Coyle and Snyder, 1971). The most active inhibitors of DA re-uptake so far reported have been the amphetamines and the antiparkinsonian drug benztropine (Cogentin). Nomifensine has been found to be twice as active in this respect as benztropine in animal experiments, and amphetamine was the least active (Hunt, Kannengiessen and Raynaud, 1974). Considering the close relationship between DA transmission and blood prolactin levels it has been suggested (Müller, Genazzani and Murru, 1978) that a single oral dose of nomifensine might be a test for differentiating between patients with hyperprolactinaemia who have pituitary tumours and those who have not. However, Dunne *et al.* (1979) found no differences in the prolactin response of those taking nomifensine and the effects with those taking a placebo.

Mode of action

The antidepressant activity of nomifensine could be associated with the increased availability of NA resulting from inhibition of NA re-uptake, as with some of the tricyclics. Other tricyclic compounds, clomipramine for example, almost exclusively block 5-HT re-uptake, a property possessed only weakly by nomifensine (Tuomisto, 1977) although the active metabolite is more potent in this respect. The compound is characterized by its powerful inhibition effect on DA re-uptake and so there is the possibility that dopaminergic systems should now be reconsidered in relation to the biochemical concomitants of affective disorders.

The agonist effect on DA is shared with the amphetamines and apomorphine. However, it seems clear that the actions of the three substances on DA transmission are different and so account for the intense addictive properties of amphetamine but not of nomifensine. Amphetamine acts by releasing DA and blocking its re-uptake (Beall *et al.*, 1976). Apomorphine, another DA agonist, has a direct stimulatory effect on the DA receptor while the action of nomifensine appears to be similar to that of many antidepressants, that is inhibition of the membrane pump re-uptake mechanism into the pre-synaptic neuron (Gerhards, 1978). According to some authors nomifensine does not stimulate release of NA and DA from synaptosomes and stimulated brain slices (Schacht and Leven, 1978), and does not seem to alter endogenous brain concentrations of NA and DA. These properties suggest the action of nomifensine is quite unlike that of the amphetamines, but there is some controversy over the issue as others have found that DA release is stimulated by nomifensine (Braestrup and Scheel-Krüger, 1976).

Pharmacokinetics

Nomifensine is readily absorbed after oral administration in man and there is a steady state peak blood concentration within 5 d of repeated ingestion. Nearly all excretion is via the kidney and the half-life is short, about 2–4 h, although this may be prolonged in renal failure. All of an ingested dose is excreted in 2 d. The peak blood concentration occurs about 1–4 h after a single dose. There are three main metabolites, of which only one appears to be consistently pharmacologically active both *in vitro* and *in vivo*.

Therapeutic trials

As with other new antidepressants there have been many therapeutic trials using nomifensine. The trials vary widely as to the research design and the reliability of the results. With all investigations into antidepressant medication, there is the ever present problem concerning the definition of depression, which will be crucial for the reliable inclusion of patients with appropriate illnesses.

On the one hand there was a study carried out in France which involved 958 patients and 135 psychiatrists. On the other hand Forrest, Hewett and Nicholson (1977) carefully compared the effects of nomifensine with those of imipramine in 34 out-patients. There was a good response with both drugs and the ratings of depression for all the patients fell significantly within one week. An antianxiety effect was noted, which confirms other reports. Nomifensine has been compared in double-blind studies with imipramine, desipramine, nortriptyline, clomipramine, amitriptyline and doxepin (Brogden et al., 1979).

In another ambitious trial involving 47 general practitioners in 43 centres, nomifensine was compared to maprotiline and imipramine over six weeks using a double-blind method (Bogie, Hewett and Baird, 1980). Montgomery et al. (1980) studied 42 patients, all older than 50 years, with a primary affective disorder. All subjects were given a placebo for the first week and thereafter three groups were prescribed imipramine, mianserin or nomifensine. While there were no differences in the therapeutic responses produced by imipramine and mianserin, nomifensine was significantly less effective than both imipramine and mianserin on some measures of response at the third and fourth weekly assessments. A longer-term study over six months using imipramine and nomifensine has been reported by Storer, Eastwood and Bailey (1980). The two drugs were found to be equally effective and there was a reduced incidence of side effects in the nomifensine-treated group.

Adverse effects

Most studies suggest that there are fewer side effects with nomifensine than with reference drugs of the tricyclic group in particular. Taeuber (1974) reported the side effects observed with 1369 depressed patients taking nomifensine. The most common complaint was of sleep disturbance and this was found in about 6 per cent of the cases. The next most common side effect was restlessness which occurred in about 3 per cent. Trimble, Meldrum and Anlezark (1977) reported that nomifensine showed less epileptic activity in animals than did imipramine or clomipramine. It seems not to be epileptogenic in man, unlike maprotiline and mianserin (Edwards, 1979), and convulsions do not occur when the drug is taken in an overdose (Dawling, Braithwaite and Crome, 1979; Montgomery, Crome and Braithwaite, 1978). Nomifensine seems relatively safe in overdose (Dawling, Braithwaite and Crome, 1979; Montgomery, Crome and Braithwaite, 1978) with drowsiness, tremor, transient hypertension, sinus tachycardia and coma described in a few patients. However, there has been a report of renal failure after an overdose of nomifensine, possibly taken with chlordiazepoxide and nitrazepam (Prescott et al., 1980).

It has less anticholinergic activity than the tricyclic compounds and it is not sedative (Chan et al., 1980). Detailed cardiological testing, including Bundle of His cardio-graphy (Vohra et al., 1978; Burrows et al., 1978) showed no abnormality with patients on nomifensine. In particular, the quinidine-like cardiac effects of many tricyclics, including prolongation of the QRS interval and of distal conduction, were not observed. A study by Burgess et al. (1979) compared the electrocardiographic effects of amitriptyline, mianserin, zimelidine and nomifensine in depressed patients, and nomifensine was reported only as decreasing T-wave height while amitriptyline, in particular produced a considerable number of significant changes.

DOSE

From 75 mg daily to 200 mg daily, or more if necessary, in divided doses.

Trazodone (Molipaxin)

This is a triazolopiridine derivative which is not chemically related to any other antidepressant or group of antidepressants (*Figure 8.5*). It was first synthesized in Italy and described by Palazzo and Baiocchi (1966). Trazodone has been reported to produce therapeutic effects within a few days (Ban *et al.*, 1973; Agnoli *et al.*, 1974; Kellams, Klapper and Small, 1979).

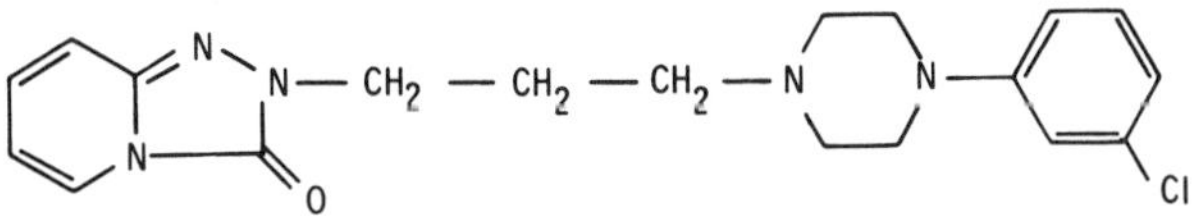

Figure 8.5 Trazodone

Some aspects of the pharmacological profile of trazodone indicate that it has central nervous system effects, but it lacks many of the effects considered characteristic of antidepressants (Silvestrini *et al.*, 1968). Like mianserin it does not reverse reserpine-induced hypothermia in mice, it does not antagonize reserpine and is inactive in other tests of potentiation of central monoaminergic functions. It does not potentiate responses to levodopa, it lacks significant cataleptic properties and has only weak hypothermic activity (Boissier *et al.*, 1974; Silvestrini *et al.*, 1968; Longo and De Carolis, 1974). Baran *et al.* (1979) reported central antagonism of 5-HT and Maj, Palider and Rawlow (1979) considered that there is central antagonism at low doses but 5-HT potentiation at high doses and this may account for the clinical observation that trazodone is anxiolytic at lower doses and sedative at higher doses (Muratorio *et al.*, 1974; Karniol, Dalton and Lader, 1976). It resembles the phenothiazines in reducing self-stimulation behaviour, antagonizing the effects of amphetamine and producing peripheral alpha-adrenergic blockade (Silvestrini *et al.*, 1968; Taylor, Hyslop and Riblet, 1980). Also, like many neuroleptics trazodone reduces spontaneous motor activity and aggressiveness. The compound blocks the responses to painful stimuli and conditioned avoidance reflexes (Loizzo and Massotti, 1973; Silvestrini *et al.*, 1968). Acute and chronic toxicity studies have been reported by Rivett and Barcellona (1974).

Mode of action

Like some of the tricyclic preparations, trazodone blocks 5-HT uptake by brain synaptosomes. In this, trazodone has weak, but selective activity as there are negligible effects on NA re-uptake (Boissier *et al.*, 1974; Allori, Cioli and Silvestrini, 1975; Riblet, Gatewood and Mayol, 1979; Stefanini *et al.*, 1976). The central 5-HT antagonism has been mentioned and this is considered to be a property associated with the anxiolytic effects of some antidepressant preparations (Clements-Jewery and Robson, 1980; Clements-Jewery, Robson and Chidley, 1980). If the 5-HT antagonism is also associated with the antidepressant effect, then this would accord with a suggestion implicating post-synaptic super-sensitivity as a cause of affective disorders (Shaw, Riley and Michalakeas, 1977).

Trazodone does not affect the cerebral concentrations of NA, DA and 3-methoxy-4-hydroxyphenylglycol but increases in the concentrations of homovanillic acid and dihydroxyphenylacetic acid have been reported after high doses (Angellucci and Bolle, 1974; Stefanini *et al.*, 1976). It has been noted that mianserin has an affinity for both alpha$_1$- and alpha$_2$-receptor sites. While mianserin binds to both, trazodone has six times the affinity for the alpha$_2$-receptor. Evidence for this comes from the report of increased turnover of NA in the rat brain (Garattini, 1974) and the reversal of the central cardiovascular effects of clonidine (Van Zwieten, 1977).

In reviewing the effects of trazodone, Clements-Jewery, Robson and Chidley (1980) came to the conclusion that the 5-HT membrane pump re-uptake blockade produced by trazodone may not have functional significance because of the associated more potent 5-HT receptor antagonism. It was suggested that the anxiolytic and anti-depressant properties of trazadone are pharmacologically separate and the former is a result of blockade of central 5-HT receptors while the antidepressant effect is produced by a combination of alpha$_2$-receptor antagonism and NA releasing effects (Peroutka and Snyder, 1979). The possibility of complex interactions of this type, with one drug having different and even opposite effects on various neuron systems, themselves interacting, suggests that the simplistic hypotheses that depression is associated with reduced availability of monoamine neurotransmitters, or post-synaptic receptor supersensitivity, may have to be reconsidered.

Therapeutic trials

There have been a large number of open trials, reviewed by Brogden *et al.* (1981). Gershon and Newton (1980) studied 262 patients in a multicentre trial who were divided into three groups, the patients in each of which had trazodone, imipramine or placebo over a 28-d period. Similar therapeutic results were found for both trazodone and imipramine, both of which were significantly more effective than the placebo. Gerner *et al.* (1980) investigated the effect of trazodone on 60 elderly patients with depression, comparing therapeutic effectiveness against that found for patients receiving imipramine or placebo. Trazodone was as effective as imipramine but there was a high drop-out rate from those taking imipramine because of side effects.

Rickels *et al.* (1980) compared the efficacy of trazodone with that of amitriptyline and a placebo in 202 depressed patients and found trazodone to be as effective as amitriptyline and significantly more so than placebo. De Gregorio and Dionisio (1969) studied 281 depressed patients with seven investigators, and trazodone was found to be as effective as amitriptyline. Another study comparing trazodone with amitriptyline was carried out by Lapierre, Sussman and Ghadirian (1980). The group of patients was divided into 20 who were retarded and 20 who were agitated. Trazodone gave better results with the retarded patients but was less effective than amitriptyline with agitated patients.

Pierce (1980) used a non-cross-over single-blind design to compare the comparative effects of trazodone and dothiepin in a group of patients, some with neurotic depression and some with endogenous depression, over a period of at least four weeks. The therapeutic effect was measured by several rating scales and it was found that with both compounds there was a significant improvement in depressive symptoms but there were no apparent differences in efficacy between the group of patients with neurotic depression as opposed to those with endogenous depression.

There have been studies with trazodone given as an intravenous infusion to patients with endogenous depression. Pariante (1974) and Roccatagliata *et al.* (1977) reported studies of this type and the former found marked sedative effects but also specific improvement with certain symptoms including depressed mood, guilt, suicidal ideas and anxiety.

Deutsch, Ban and Lehmann (1977) gave trazodone to unselected patients with schizophrenia and it was found to be less effective than chlorpromazine, although in those cases with depression as well as with schizophrenic symptoms, it was helpful. Singh, Saxena and Helson (1978) compared the effect of trazodone with that of a placebo in 60 chronic schizophrenic patients who were all receiving phenothiazine therapy. The trial lasted for six weeks and adverse effects were rare. Headache was the commonest complaint, but it was reported by only three patients. It was concluded that trazodone was pharmacologically compatible with phenothiazine medication and was superior to placebo in antidepressant efficacy in patients with chronic schizophrenia. It has been suggested that trazodone might be preferable to the tricyclic compounds in cases of schizophrenia because of the weak inhibitory effect trazodone has on DA uptake.

Loeb and Roccatagliata (1980) used intravenous trazodone given twice daily for a small number of patients with tardive dyskinesia and parkinsonism and the symptoms were almost eliminated in three patients of eight. The decrease in tremor was accompanied by reduction in anxiety, which may be the mechanism of action in these circumstances. Roccatagliata *et al.* (1980) gave trazodone to patients with chronic alcoholism who were also suffering from depression and anxiety. There was considerable improvement in the anxiety rating scales and tremor disappeared after a few days.

Pharmacokinetics

This compound is usually taken orally but its clinical effects have been evaluated with the drug given intramuscularly and intravenously. Oral trazodone is rapidly absorbed with peak plasma levels reached in 0.5–2 h but usually within 1 h. Maximum blood levels are several times higher in fasted than in non-fasted animals, and enhancement of absorption in fasting volunteers has been observed (Catanese and Lisciani, 1970). The drug, following oral administration, seems to be almost completely absorbed as shown by the almost identical urinary excretion pattern following oral, intravenous or intramuscular administration (Koss and Busch, 1978).

Trazodone is extensively metabolized and less than 1 per cent is recovered in the urine unchanged. The elimination half-life is about 4 h and it is cleared almost entirely by urinary and biliary excretion of free and conjugated metabolites. Clearance of the unchanged drug from plasma is complete within 24 h. Trazodone is metabolized by hydroxylation, splitting at the piridine ring and oxidation, and by N-oxidation (Koss and Busch, 1978).

Adverse effects

In general, side effects do not appear to be a major problem with trazodone and the incidence is dose-related. Furthermore, a trend has been noticed towards reduced frequency with time (Rickels *et al.*, 1980). Pohlmeier, De Gregorio and Sieroslawski (1980) found that with 1621 patients treated with trazodone, drowsiness was the most frequent complaint, reported by 8.7 per cent. Gastrointestinal disorders, dizziness and dry mouth were complained of by about 3 per cent of the patients, while insomnia, headache and agitation occurred in about 1 per cent. Other reported side effects included weakness, insomnia, hypotension and tremor.

Cardiovascular side effects, such as hypotension, tachycardia and palpitations have been infrequently reported with trazodone even when given to patients with pre-existing cardiovascular disorders (Bufalari, 1972). Gershon and Newton (1980) studied the incidence of the four main anticholinergic effects, namely, dry mouth, blurred vision, bowel movement disturbance and delayed urine flow among 379 patients from 15 centres treated either with trazadone, imipramine or a placebo. When compared statistically there were no differences in the side effects for the groups on trazodone and on placebo, but comparison between trazodone and imipramine showed that trazodone was associated with significantly fewer of these side-effects. Gomoll, Byrne and Deitchman (1979) carried out cardiovascular studies on anaesthe-tized dogs given trazodone or imipramine. With trazodone there was alpha-adrenergic blockade and slowing of heart rate only, whereas imipramine caused more disturb-ances. It was concluded that imipramine compromises the pump function of the heart in a way that trazodone does not. Gomoll and Byrne (1979) carried out conduction studies on dogs and found that trazodone produced no effects whereas imipramine significantly slowed impulse conduction as well as atrial transmission. These results suggest that trazodone is not cardiotoxic in the way that the tricyclics are.

Daniele and Fiore (1972) found that trazodone, given to healthy subjects and to patients with open-angle glaucoma, tended to lower intra-ocular pressure and thus did not adversely effect glaucoma.

Trazodone potentiates the effects of barbiturates and is likely to increase sedation with sedative antidepressants, with hypnotics and alcohol. As with other drugs with alpha-adrenergic blocking activity, inhibition of the antihypertensive effect of clonidine may be caused. It is possible that trazodone may also inhibit the antihypertensive effect of guanethidine and other neuron blocking drugs.

DOSE

From 100 mg daily to 600 mg daily, usually given in one dose at night.

Zimelidine

Zimelidine is a new antidepressant drug that has only just been introduced to clinical practice (*Figure 8.6*). It is the first 'pure' 5-HT selective re-uptake inhibitor to be used in psychiatry, although its purity is relative, for it does have a small inhibitory effect on the

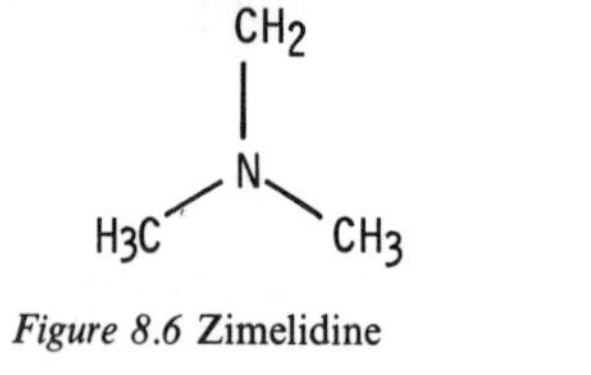

Figure 8.6 Zimelidine

re-uptake of noradrenaline (Ögren *et al.*, 1981). In clinical studies its relative purity is confirmed by the absence of cholinergic unwanted effects such as dry mouth, constipation and blurred vision (Coppen, Swade and Wood, 1981). Comparison with amitriptyline, desipramine and maprotiline in clinical trials suggests that zimelidine is better tolerated, has greater antianxiety effects in depressed patients than tricyclic antidepressants, but shows no superiority in antidepressant efficacy (Montgomery *et al.*, 1981; d'Elia *et al.*, 1981; Åberg, 1981). In one recent study zimelidine was significantly more effective than placebo in the treatment of depression (Georgotas, Krakowski and Gershon, 1982).

Comments

It is probably too early to make a satisfactory assessment of the place of the new antidepressants in the pharmacological treatment of psychiatric illnesses. But at least some of them appear to constitute an advance, especially with regard to reduced side effects. To make some very general points; maprotiline has a number of pharmacological properties which are different from those of tricyclic antidepressants, but whether the drug is clinically different to a significant extent is uncertain. Mianserin, nomifensine and trazodone seem on present evidence to be effective antidepressants and to show considerably fewer side effects, with reduced anticholinergic activity and cardiotoxicity, compared to the tricyclic group. Mianserin and trazodone are sedative and perhaps useful especially in cases of agitated depression. Zimelidine may also have anxiety reducing properties in depressed patients, but further studies are required.

Nomifensine is not sedative and may worsen agitated states, so it should be considered especially with patients with retarded depression. Mianserin and trazodone in lower doses seem to be indicated with the elderly or the infirm; drowsiness is the most likely side effect. Maprotiline and mianserin occasionally produce fits, and perhaps viloxazine. Nomifensine and trazodone, on present evidence, do not cause convulsions. Viloxazine seems to be associated with some troublesome side effects. One very noteworthy advance is that on current information mianserin, nomifensine and trazodone appear to be relatively safe in overdose.

Not all new preparations live up to their expectations; sometimes it may be some years during which a drug is used before a particular side effect becomes apparent. The headache following cheese ingestion with monoamine oxidase inhibitors and the cardiotoxic effects of the tricyclic antidepressants are examples. Clinical acceptance in the long term may be based more on personal and collective clinical experience, than on molecular structure, animal studies and clinical trials. Especially is this true of clinical trials, which come in for much criticism because the design is unconvincing, there are insufficient patients or the diagnostic selection is unacceptable, among many other possible defects. It must be admitted that a great deal of scientific and clinical work has been carried out on these new drugs, not of uniformly high standard it is true, and large numbers of trials have been undertaken. It seems that trials are going to become even more difficult with the recent evidence that fewer patients are becoming available for possible inclusion in trials, and the cry has gone up 'Where are the untreated depressives?' (Little, Kerr and McLelland, 1978).

Summary

(1) While the evidence is not always convincing, in general the new drugs seem to have definite antidepressant activity. However, there is no claim for greater efficacy of

antidepressant effect for any of the new drugs compared with the tricyclic group and the MAO inhibitors.

(2) A number of the new compounds seem to have significantly fewer side effects and therefore better compliance can be expected.

(3) Some of the newer drugs would appear to be more suitable for older and frailer patients.

(4) Some of the new compounds seem very safe in overdose but clinical experience is relatively limited at present.

(5) They have quite different formulae from the previously available antidepressants and this could contribute to the development of research into the biochemistry of depression, at present necessarily largely dependent on the known actions of the tricyclics and MAO inhibitors.

(6) The different formulae may become associated with different antidepressive drug effects. An example has been given above with regard to the sedative effects of mianserin and trazodone in cases of agitated depression, but no more definite special indications are apparent at the moment.

(7) The new drugs tend to be considerably more expensive than the older antidepressants and, as the new compounds are not necessarily more effective, this is an aspect which should be borne in mind, although no doubt with increasing use the prices will fall.

References

ÅBERG, A. Controlled cross-over study of a 5-HT uptake inhibiting and an NA uptake inhibiting antidepressant, *Acta Psychiatrica Scandinavica* **63**, Suppl. **290**, 244–255 (1981)

AGNOLI, A., PICCIONE, M., CASACCHIA, M. and FAZIO, C. Trazodone versus despiramine. A double-blind study on the rapidity of the antidepressive effect. In *Trazodone. Proceedings of the First International Symposium*, Montreal, Quebec, October 1973 **9** (Eds. T. A. BAN and B. SILVESTRINI). Modern Problems of Pharmacopsychiatry, p. 190, Karger, Basel (1974)

ALBERTINI, R. S. and PENDERS, T. M. Agranulocytosis associated with tricyclics, *Journal of Clinical Psychiatry* **39**, 483–485 (1978)

ALLORI, L., CIOLI, V. and SILVESTRINI, B. Experimental and clinical data indicating a potential use of trazodone in acute stroke, *Current Therapeutic Research* **18**, (3) 410–416 (1975)

ANGELLUCCI, L. and BOLLE, P. Considerations on biochemical studies with trazodone, *Proceedings of the First International Symposium*, Montreal, Quebec, October 1973 **9**. Modern Problems of Pharmacopsychiatry 29–46, Karger, Basel (1974)

ÅSBERG, M., CRÖNHOLM, B., SJÖQVIST, F. and TUCK, D. Relationship between plasma level and therapeutic effect of nortriptyline, *British Medical Journal* **3**, 331–334 (1971)

BALESTRIERI, A., BENASSI, P., CASSANO, G. P., CATROGIOVANNI, P., CATALANO, A., COLOMBI, A., CONFORTO, C., DEL SOLDATO, G., GILBERTI, F., LUCCHELLI, P. E., MURATORIO, A., NISTRI, M. and SARTESCHI, P. Clinical comparative evaluation of maprotiline, a new antidepressant drug. A multicentre study, *International Pharmacopsychiatry* **6**, p. 236 (1971)

BAN, T. A., LEHMAN, H. E., AMIN, M., GALVAN, L., NAIR, N. P. V., VERGARA, L. and ZOCH, G. Comprehensive clinical studies with trazodone, *Current Therapeutic Research* **15**, 540–551 (1973)

BARAN, L., MAJ, J., ROGOZ, Z. and SKUZA, G. On the central anti-serotonin action of trazodone, *Polish Journal of Pharmacology* **31**, 25–33 (1979)

BARNES, T. R. E., KIDGER, T. and GREENWOOD, D. T. Viloxazine and migraine, *Lancet* **2**, 1368 (1979)

BARTHOLINI, E. and PINTO, O. DE S. A comparison of two different Ludiomil dose levels. In *Masked Depression* (Ed. KIELHOLZ), p. 256, Hans Huber, Berne (1973)

BAUMANN, P. A. and MAITRE, L. Blockade of presynaptic α-receptors and of amine uptake in the rat brain by the antidepressant mianserin, *Naunyn-Schmiedeberg's Archives of Pharmacology* **300**, 31–37 (1977)

BAUMANN, P. A. and MAITRE, L. Neurobiochemical aspects of maprotiline (Ludiomil) action, *Journal of International Medical Research* **7**, 391–400 (1979)

BAYLE, B. J. Clinical trial of a new antidepressive: viloxazine, *Psychologie Medicale* **11**, 2241–2249 (1979)

BEALL, J. E., MARTIN, R. F., APPLEBAUM, A. E. and WILLIS, W. D. Inhibition of primate spinothalamic tract neurons by stimulation in the region of the nucleus raphe magnus, *Brain Research* **114**, 328–333 (1976)

BLACK, J. W. Antidepressants and histamine, *Lancet* **2**, 53–54 (1978)

BLACKBURN, T. P., FOSTER, G. A., GREENWOOD, D. T. and HOWE, R. Effects of viloxazine, its optical isomers and its major metabolites on biogenic amine uptake mechanisms *in vitro* and *in vivo*, *European Journal of Pharmacology* **52**, 367–374 (1978)

BLAHA, L., PINDER, R. M. and STULEMEIJER, S. M. Double-blind comparative trial of mianserin versus clomipramine, *Current Medical Research Opinion* **6**, Suppl. 7, 99–106 (1980)

BOGIE, W., HEWETT, A. J. and BAIRD, C. M. Multi-centre clinical comparison of nomifensine, maprotiline and imipramine in depressed patients in general practice, *Royal Society of Medicine International Congress Symposium Series* No. 25, 95–101 (1980)

BOISSIER, J. R., PORTMANN-CRISTESCO, E., SOUBRIE, P. and FICHELLE, J. Pharmacological and biochemical features of trazodone. In *Trazodone. Modern Problems of Pharmacopsychiatry* (Eds. BAN, T. A. and SILVESTRINI, B.), **9**, 18–28, Karger, Basel (1974)

BOTTER, P. A. A double-blind comparison of viloxazine and amitriptyline in involutional and endogenous depression, *Acta Psychiatrica Belgique* **79**, 198–209 (1979)

BRAESTRUP, C. and SCHEEL-KRÜGER, J. Methylphenidate-like effects of the new antidepressant drug, nomifensine, *European Journal of Pharmacology* **38**, 305–312 (1976)

BREWER, C. A safer antidepressant?, *British Medical Journal* **4**, 409 (1975)

BREZINOVA, V., ADAM, K., CHAPMAN, K., OSWALD, I. and THOMSON, J. Viloxazine, sleep and subjective feelings, *Psychopharmacology* **55**, 121–128 (1977)

BRION, S. Open studies with viloxazine (Vivalan), *Journal of International Medical Research* **3**, Suppl. 3, 87–91 (1975)

BROGDEN, R. N., HEEL, R. C., SPEIGHT, T. M. and AVERY, G. S. Mianserin: a review of its pharmacological properties and therapeutic efficacy in depressive illness, *Drugs* **16**, 273–301 (1978)

BROGDEN, R. N., HEEL, R. C., SPEIGHT, T. M. and AVERY, G. S. Nomifensine: a review of its pharmacological properties and therapeutic efficacy in depressive illness, *Drugs* **18**, 1–24 (1979)

BROGDEN, R. N., HEEL, R. C., SPEIGHT, T. M. and AVERY, G. S. Trazodone: a review of its pharmacological properties and therapeutic use in depression and anxiety, *Drugs* **21**, 401–429 (1981)

BRUNNER, H., HEDWALL, P. R., MEIER, M. and BEIN, H. J. Cardiovascular effects of preparation CIBA 34, 276-Ba and imipramine, *Agents and Actions* **2**, 69 (1971)

BUFALARI, A. The use of trazadone in internal medicine, *Clinica Europea* **11**, 1–11 (1972)

BURGESS, C. D., MONTGOMERY, S., WADSWORTH, J. and TURNER, P. Cardiovascular effects of amitriptyline, mianserin, zimelidine and nomifensine in depressed patients, *Postgraduate Medical Journal* **55**, 704–708 (1979)

BURROWS, G. D., DAVIES, B., HAMER, A. and VOHRA, J. Effect of mianserin on cardiac conduction, *Medical Journal of Australia* **2**, 97–98 (1979)

BURROWS, G. D., VOHRA, J., DUMOVIC, P., SCOGGINS, B. A. and DAVIES, B. Cardiological effects of nomifensine, a new antidepressant, *Medical Journal of Australia* **1**, 341–343 (1978)

CATANESE, B. and LISCIANI, R. Investigations on the absorption and distribution of trazodone or AF 1161 in rats, dogs and humans, *Bolletino Chimico Farmaceutico* **109**, 369–373 (1970)

CHAN, M-Y., EHSANUCCAH, R., WADSWORTH, J. and McEWEN, J. A comparison of the pharmacodynamic profiles of nomifensine and amitriptyline in normal subjects, *British Journal of Clinical Pharmacology* **9**, 247–253 (1980)

CLEMENTS-JEWERY, S. and ROBSON, P. A. The *in vivo* and *in vitro* occupation of (3H)-spiperone binding sites in the frontal cortex and striatum by putative 5-hydroxytryptamine antagonists, *Neuropharmacology* **19**, 657–661 (1980)

CLEMENTS-JEWERY, S., ROBSON, P. A. and CHIDLEY, L. J. Biochemical investigations into the mode of action of trazodone, *Neuropharmacology* **19**, 1165–1174 (1980)

COLLIS, M. G. and SHEPHERD, J. T. Antidepressant drug action and presynaptic α-receptors, *Mayo Clinic Proceedings* **55**, 567–572 (1980)

CONTI, L. and PINDER, R. M. A controlled comparative trial of mianserin and diazepam in the treatment of anxiety states in psychiatric outpatients, *Journal of International Medical Research* **7**, 285–289 (1979)

COPPEN, A., GUPTA, R., MONTGOMERY, S., GHOSE, K., BAILEY, J., BURNS, B. and DE RIDDER, J. J. Mianserin hydrochloride: a novel antidepressant, *British Journal of Psychiatry* **129**, 342–345 (1976a)

COPPEN, A., MONTGOMERY, S. A., GUPTA, R. K. and BAILEY, J. E. A double-blind comparison of lithium carbonate and maprotiline in the prophylaxis of the affective disorders, *British Journal of Psychiatry* **128**, 479–486 (1976b)

COPPEN, A., SWADE, C. and WOOD, K. The action of antidepressant drugs on 5-hydroxytryptamine uptake by platelets—relationship to therapeutic effect, *Acta Psychiatrica Scandinavica* **63**, 236–243 (1981)

CRAMMER, J., BARRACLOUGH, B. and HEINE, B. *The use of drugs in psychiatry*, Gaskell, London (1978)

CURSON, D. A. and HALE, A. S. Mianserin and agranulocytosis, *British Medical Journal* **1**, 378–379 (1979)

DALY, R. J., BROWNE, P. J. and MORGAN, E. Mianserin in the treatment of depressive illness: a comparison with amitriptyline, *Irish Journal of Medical Science* **148**, 145–148 (1979)

DANIELE, S. and FIORE, C. Hypotensive effect on intraocular tension by AF-1161 (Trazodone), *Annales di Ottalmologia et Clinica Oculistica (Pharma)* **98**, 1–6 (1972)

DAWLING, S., BRAITHWAITE, R. and CROME, P. Nomifensine overdose and plasma drug concentration, *Lancet* **1**, 56 (1979)

DE BUCK, R. A comparison of the efficacy and side-effects of mianserin and clomipramine in primary depression: a double-blind randomized trial, *Current Medical Research Opinion* **6**, Suppl. 7, 88–97 (1980)

DE GREGORIO, M. and DIONISIO, A. Ricerche cliniche su un nuovo psicofarmaco (AF-1161). Valutazione preliminare, *Medicina Psicosomatica* **14**, 477–493 (1969)

D'ELIA, G., HÄLLSTRÖM, T., NYSTRÖM, C. and OTTOSON, J-O. Zimelidine versus maprotiline in depressed out-patients: a preliminary report, *Acta Psychiatrica Scandinavica* **63**, Suppl. 290, 225–235 (1981)

DELINI-STULA, A. The pharmacology of Ludiomil. In *Depressive Illness, Diagnosis, Assessment, Treatment* (Ed. KEILHOLZ), 113–124, Hans Huber, Berne (1972)

DELINI-STULA, A., RADEKE, E. and VASSOUT, A. Some aspects of the psychopharmacological activity in maprotiline (Ludiomil): Effects of single and repeated treatments, *Journal of International Medical Research* **6**, 421–429 (1978)

DEUTSCH, M., BAN, T. A. and LEHMANN, H. E. A standard controlled clinical study with trazodone in schizophrenic patients, *Psychopharmacology Bulletin* **13**, 13–14 (1977)

DUNNE, M. J., WALKER, J., COWDEN, E. A. and RATCLIFFE, J. G. Nomifensine test for investigation of hyperprolactinaemia, *Lancet* **2**, 1243 (1979)

EDWARDS, J. G. Viloxazine: assessment of potential rapid antidepressant action, *British Medical Journal* **2**, 1327 (1977a)

EDWARDS, J. G. Convulsive seizures and viloxazine, *British Medical Journal* **2**, 96–97 (1977b)

EDWARDS, J. G. Antidepressants and convulsions, *Lancet* **2**, 1368–1369 (1979)

EINARSON, T. R. Lorazepam withdrawal seizures, *Lancet* **1**, 151 (1980)

ELWAN, O. and ADAM, H. K. Relationship between blood and cerebrospinal levels of the antidepressant agent viloxazine, *European Journal of Clinical Pharmacology* **17**, 179–182 (1980)

EVANS, L. and LANDER, C. M. Mianserin and epilepsy, *Medical Journal of Australia* **2**, 462–463 (1980)

FINK, M., IRWIN, P., GASTPAR, M. and DE RIDDER, J. J. EEG, blood level and behavioural effects of the antidepressants mianserin (Org. GB94), *Psychopharmacology* **54**, 249–254 (1977)

FINK, M., KLEIN, D. F. and KRAMER, J. C. Clinical efficacy of chlorpromazine-procyclidine combination, imipramine and placebo in depressive disorders, *Psychopharmacologia (Berlin)* **7**, 27–36 (1965)

FLORU, L. and TEGELER, J. Eine vergleichende Untersuchung der beiden Antidepressiva Viloxazin und Imipramin, *Pharmakopsychiatrie Neuropsychopharmakologie* **12**, 313–320 (1979)

FORREST, W. A. A comparison between daily and nightly dose regimen of amitriptyline and maprotiline (Ludiomil) in the treatment of reactive depression in general practice, *Journal of International Medical Research* **3**, Suppl. 2, 120–125 (1975)

FORREST, W. A. Maprotiline (Ludiomil) in depression. A report of a monitored release study in general practice, *Journal of International Medical Research* **5**, Suppl. 4, 112–115 (1977)

FORREST, A., HEWETT, A. and NICHOLSON, P. Controlled randomized group comparison of nomifensine and imipramine in depressive illness, *British Journal of Clinical Pharmacology* **4**, Suppl. 2, 215s–220s (1977)

FRØLUND, F. Treatment of depression in general practice: a controlled trial of flupenthixol (Fluanxol), *Current Medical Research Opinion* **2**, 78–89 (1974)

GARATTINI, S. Biochemical studies with trazodone: a new psychoactive drug. *Trazodone. Proceedings of the First International Symposium* (Eds. T. A. BAN and B. SILVESTRINI), Montreal, Quebec, October 1973. Modern Problems of Pharmacopsychiatry 29–46, Karger, Basel (1974)

GARVER, D. L. and DAVIS, J. M. Biogenic amine hypotheses of affective disorders, *Life Sciences* **24**, 383–394 (1979)

GENERAL PRACTICE CLINICAL TRIALS. Thioridazine as an antidepressant, *Practitioner* **209**, 95–98 (1972)

GEORGOTSA, A., KRAKOWSKI, M. and GERSHON, S. Treatment of depression with 5-HT re-uptake inhibitors, *American Journal of Psychiatry*, (to be published)

GERHARDS, H. J. Effects of antidepressants on peripheral and central metabolism of catecholamines. In *Depressive Disorders* (Ed. GARATTINI, S.), 37–47, Schattauer, Stuttgart (1978)

GERNER, R., ESTABROOK, W., STEUER, J. and JARVIK, L. Treatment of geriatric depression with trazodone, imipramine and placebo. A double-blind study, *Journal of Clinical Psychiatry* **41**, (6), 216–220 (1980)

GERSHON, S. and NEWTON, R A multicentred controlled evaluation of trazodone in endogenous depression. In *Trazodone: a new broad-spectrum antidepressant* (Eds. S. GERSHON, K. RICKELS and B. SILVESTRINI). Proceedings of the 11th Congress of the Collegium Internationale Neuro-Psycho pharmacologicum July 9–14, 1978, 42–53, Excerpta Medica, Amsterdam (1980)

GHOSE, K., COPPEN, A. and TURNER, P. Autonomic actions and interactions of mianserin hydrochloride (Org. GB94) and amitriptyline in patients with depressive illness, *Psychopharmacology* **49**, 201–204 (1976)

GOMOLL, A. W. and BYRNE, J. E. Trazodone and imipramine. Comparative effects of canine cardiac conduction, *European Journal of Pharmacology* **57**, 335–342 (1979)

GOMOLL, A. W., BYRNE, J. E. and DEITCHMAN, D. Hemodynamic and cardiac actions of trazodone and imipramine in the anaesthetized dog, *Life Sciences* **24**, 1841–1848 (1979)

GRAM, L. F. Plasma level monitoring of tricyclic antidepressant therapy, *Clinical Pharmacokinetics* **2**, 237–251 (1977)

GREEN, J. P. and MAAYANI, S. Tricyclic antidepressant drugs block histamine H_2 receptor in brain, *Nature* **269**, 163–165 (1977)

GREEN, S. D. R. and KENDALL-TAYLOR, P. Heart block in mianserin hydrochloride overdose, *British Medical Journal* **2**, 1190 (1977)

GREENWOOD, D. T. Animal pharmacology of viloxazine (Vivalan), *Journal of International Medical Research* **3**, Suppl. 3, 18–28 (1975)

HAMOUZ, W., PINDER, R. M. and STULEMEIJER, S. M. A double-blind group comparative trial of mianserin and diazepam in depressed out-patients, *Current Medical Research Opinion* **6**, Suppl. 7, 72–79 (1980)

HARRIS, B. and HARPER, M. Unusual appetites in patients on mianserin, *Lancet* **1**, 590 (1980)

HOFFMANN, I. A comparative review of the pharmacology of nomifensine, *British Journal of Clinical Pharmacology* **4**, Suppl. 2, 69s–75s (1977)

HOLLAND, R. P. C. and BROSNAN, R. D. Overdosage with viloxazine. Paper presented at 15th International Congress of Therapeutics, Brussels, September 5–9 (1979)

HOLST, B. N7009 ved behandling af angsttilstande, *Nordisk Psykiatrisk Tidsskrrift* **19**, 59–66 (1965)

HOPMAN, H. Mianserin in outpatients with depressive illness, in dosage up to 130 mg daily, *Current Medical Research Opinion* **6**, Suppl. 7, 107–112 (1980)

HORN, A. S., COYLE, J. T. and SNYDER, S. H. Catecholamine uptake by synaptosomes from rat brain. Structure-activity relationships of drugs with differential effects on dopamine and norepinephrine neurons, *Molecular Pharmacology* **7**, 66–80 (1971)

HUNT, P., KANNENGIESSER, M-H. and RAYNAUD, J-P. Nomifensine a new potent inhibitor of dopamine uptake into synaptosomes from rat brain corpus striatum, *Journal of Pharmacy and Pharmacology* **26**, 370–371 (1974)

ITIL, T. M., POLVAN, N. and HSU, W. Clinical and EEG effects of GB-94, a 'tetracyclic' antidepressant (EEG model in discovery of a new psychotropic drug), *Current Therapeutic Research* **14**, 395–413 (1972)

JOHNSON, D. A. W. A double-blind comparison of flupenthixol, nortriptyline and diazepam in neurotic depression, *Acta Psychiatrica Scandinavica* **59**, 1–8 (1979)

JØRGENSEN, A. Pharmacokinetic studies in volunteers of intravenous and oral cis (z)-flupenthixol and intramuscular cis (z)-flupenthixol decanoate in Viscoleo, *European Journal of Clinical Pharmacology* **18**, 356–360 (1980)

JUKES, A. M. A comparison of maprotiline (Ludiomil) and placebo in the treatment of depression, *Journal of International Medical Research* **3**, Suppl. 2, 84–88 (1975)

KAFOE, W. F., DE RIDDER, J. J. and LEONARD, B. E. The effect of a tetracyclic antidepressant compound, Org GB94, on the turnover of biogenic amines in rat brain, *Biochemical Pharmacology* **25**, 2455–2460 (1976)

KANOF, P. D. and GREENGARD, P. Brain histamine receptors as targets for antidepressant drugs, *Nature* **272**, 329–333 (1978)

KARNIOL, I. G., DALTON, J. and LADER, M. Comparative psychotropic effects of trazodone, imipramine and diazepam in normal subjects, *Current Therapeutic Research* **20** (3), 337–348 (1976)

KAY, N. E. and DAVIES, B. A controlled trial of maprotiline (Ludiomil) and amitryptiline in general practice, *Medical Journal of Australia* **1**, 704–705 (1974)

KELLAMS, J. J., KLAPPER, M. H. and SMALL, J. G. Trazodone. A new antidepressant: efficacy and safety in endogenous depression, *Journal of Clinical Psychiatry* **40**, 390–395 (1979)

KELLET, J. M. Flupenthixol for depression, *British Medical Journal* **1**, 1405 (1976)

KESSELL, A. and HOLT, N. F. A controlled study of a tetracyclic antidepressant—maprotiline (Ludiomil), *Medical Journal of Australia* **1**, 773–776 (1975)

KHAN, M. C. A review of cardiac conduction effects of maprotiline and mianserin, *British Journal of Clinical Practice* Suppl. 7, 96–99 (1980)

KHAN, M. C. and MOSLEHUDDIN, K. A double-blind comparative trial of mianserin and maprotiline in the treatment of depression, *Current Medical Research Opinion* **6**, Suppl. 7, 63–70 (1980)

KOPERA, H. Anticholinergic and blood pressure effects of mianserin, amitriptyline and placebo, *British Journal of Clinical Pharmacology* **5** Suppl. 1, 29s–34s (1978)

KOPERA, H., KLEIN, W. and SCHENK, H. Psychotropic drugs and the heart: clinical implications, *Progress in Neuro-psychopharmacology* **4**, 527–535 (1980)

KOSS, F. W. and BUSCH, U. Pharmacokinetics and metabolism of trazodone in different species. In *Depression and the Role of Trazodone in Antidepressant Therapy*. Proceedings of the USSR The Serbsky Central Research Institute of Forensic Psychiatry and the F. Angelini Research Institute. Rome Italy. Moscow. June 28–30 1977 (Eds. G. MOROZOV, J. SAARMA and B. SILVESTRINI), Rome: Edizioni Luigi Pozzi S.p.A. (1978)

KRAGH-SØRENSEN, P., ÅSBERG, M. and EGGERT-HANSEN, C. Plasma-nortriptyline levels in endogenous depression, *Lancet* **1**, 113–115 (1973)

KRESS, J. J., CLEDES, A., HILLION, C. and GENTIL, G. The treatment of depression using viloxazine—A trial in twenty cases, *Psychologie Medicale* **10**, 1777–1785 (1978)

KRETSCHMAR, J. H. Mianserin and amitriptyline in elderly hospitalized patients with depressive illness: a double-blind trial, *Current Medical Research Opinion* **6**, Suppl. 7, 144–150 (1980)

LANGER, G. Neuroendokrinologie der Depression und der Schizophrenie, *Arzneimittel-Forschung* **28**, 1280–1281 (1978)

LAPIERRE, Y. D., SUSSMAN, P. and GHADIRIAN, A. Differential antidepressant properties of trazodone and amitriptyline in agitated and retarded depression, *Current Therapeutic Research* **28**, 845–856 (1980)

LEONARD, B. E. Some effects of a new tetracyclic antidepressant compound, Org GB94, on the metabolism of monoamines in the rat brain, *Psychopharmacologia (Berlin)* **36**, 221–236 (1974)

LITTLE, J. C., KERR, T. A. and McCLELLAND, H. A. Where are the untreated depressives? *British Medical Journal* **1**, 1593–1594 (1978)

LIPPMANN, W. and PUGSLEY, T. A. Effects of viloxazine, an antidepressant agent on biogenic-amine uptake mechanisms and related activities, *Canadian Journal of Physiology and Pharmacology* **54**, 494–509 (1976)

LOEB, C. and ROCCATAGLIATA, G. Trazodone therapy in depressed patients. In *Trazodone—A New Broad Spectrum Antidepressant*. Proceedings of the 11th Congress of the Collegium Internationale Neuropsychopharmacologicum July 10–14, 1978 (Eds. S. GERSHON, K. RICKELS and B. SILVESTRINI), 60–63, Amsterdam: Excerpta Medica (1980)

LOIZZO, A. and MASSOTTI, M. Taming effect of non-narcotic analgesics on the septal syndrome in rats, *Pharmacology, Biochemistry and Behavior* **1**, 367–370 (1973)

LONGO, V. G. and DE CAROLIS, A. S. Pharmacological features of trazodone. In *Trazodone. Proceedings of the First International Symposium*. Montreal Quebec. October 1973, **9** Modern Problems of Pharmacopsychiatry (Eds. T. A. BAN and B. SILVESTRINI), 4–10, Basel: Karger (1974)

MAAS, J. W., FAWCETT, J. A. and DEKIRMENJIAN, H. Catecholamine metabolism, depressive illness and drug response, *Archives of General Psychiatry* **26**, 252–262 (1972)

McCALLUM, P. and MEARES, R. A controlled trial of maprotiline (Ludiomil) in depressed outpatients, *Medical Journal of Australia* **2**, 392–393 (1975)

McEVOY, J. P., SHERIDAN, W. F., STEWART, W. R. C., BAN, T. A., WILSON, W. H., GUY, W. and SCHAFFER, J. D. Viloxazine in the treatment of depressive neurosis: a controlled clinical study with doxepin and placebo, *British Journal of Psychiatry* **137**, 440–443 (1980)

McHARG, A. M. and McHARG, J. F. Leucopenia in association with mianserin treatment, *British Medical Journal* **1**, 623–624 (1979)

MAGNUS, R. V. A placebo-controlled trial of viloxazine with and without tranquillisers in depressive illness, *Journal of International Medical Research* **3**, 207–213 (1975)

MAGNUS, R. V. Mianserin—a study of different dosage regimes in psychiatric outpatients, *British Journal of Clinical Practice* **33**, 251–258 (1979)

MAGUIRE, K. P., NORMAN, T. R., BURROWS, G. D. and SCOGGINS, B. A. An evaluation of maprotiline—intravenous kinetics and comparison of two oral doses, *European Journal of Clinical Pharmacology* **18**, 249–254 (1980)

MAHAPATRA, S. B. Short-term effects of viloxazine (vivalan) compared with placebo in depression: A double-blind study, *Journal of International Medical Research* **3**, Suppl. 3, 70–74 (1975)

MAITRE, L., WALDMEIER, P. C., GREENGRASS, P. M., JAEKEL, J., SEDLACEK, S. and DELINI-STULA, A. Maprotiline—its position as an antidepressant in the light of recent neuropharmacological and neurochemical findings, *Journal of International Medical Research* **3**, 1–15 (1975)

MAJ, J., BARAN, L., RAWLÓW, A. and SOWINSKA, H. Central effects of mianserin and danitracen—new antidepressants of unknown mechanism of action, *Polish Journal of Pharmacology and Pharmacy* **29**, 213–214 (1977)

MAJ, J., PALIDER, W. and RAWLÓW, A. Trazodone, a central serotonin antagonist and agonist, *Journal of Neural Transmission* **44**, 237–248 (1979)

MALLION, K. B., TODD, A. H., TURNER, R. W., BAINBRIDGE, J. G., GREENWOOD, D. T., MADINAVEITIA, J., SOMERVILLE, A. R. and WHITTLE, B. A. 2- (2-Ethoxyphenoxy-methyl) tetrahydro-1, 4-oxazine hydrochloride, a potential psychotropic agent, *Nature* **238**, 157–158 (1972)

MARKS, P., ANDERSON, J., VINCENT, R., HUTCHINSON, J. T. and REES, H. M. Epileptiform seizures with maprotiline hydrochloride, *Postgraduate Medical Journal* **55**, 742 (1979)

MARTIN, I. L., BAKER, G. B. and MITCHELL, P. R. The effect of viloxazine hydrochloride on the transport of noradrenaline, dopamine, 5-hydroxytryptamine and gamma-amino-butyric acid in rat brain tissue, *Neuropharmacology* **17**, 421–423 (1978)

MEHTA, B. M., SPEAR, F. G. and WHITTINGTON, J. R. A double-blind controlled trial of mianserin and amitriptyline in depression, *Current Medical Research Opinion* **7**, 14–22 (1980)

MIKHAIL, W. I. Epileptogenic effect of mianserin, *Lancet* **2**, 969 (1979)

MILLER, P. I., BEAUMONT, G., SELDRUP, J., JOHN, V., LUSCOMBE, D. K. and JONES, R. Efficacy, side-effects, plasma and blood levels of maprotiline (Ludiomil), *Journal of International Medical Research* **5**, Suppl. 4, 101–111 (1977)

MONTGOMERY, S. The effect of mianserin on sleep and cardiac function, *Current Medical Research Opinion* **6**, Suppl. 7, 23–28 (1980)

MONTGOMERY, S., CROME, P. and BRAITHWAITE, R. Nomifensine overdose, *Lancet* **1**, 828–829 (1978)

MONTGOMERY, S., McAULEY, R. and MONTGOMERY, D. B. Relationship between mianserin plasma levels and antidepressant effect in a double-blind trial comparing a single night-time and divided daily dose regimens, *British Journal of Clinical Pharmacology* **5**, Suppl. 1, 71s–76s (1978)

MONTGOMERY, S. A., RANI, S. J., McAULEY, R., ROY, D. and MONTGOMERY, D. A. The antidepressant efficacy of zimelidine and maprotiline, *Acta Psychiatrica Scandinavica* **63**, Suppl. 290, 219–224 (1981)

MONTGOMERY, S. A., ROY, D., RANI, J. S., McAULEY, R. and MONTGOMERY, D. B. A comparative clinical study of nomifensine, mianserin and imipramine. In *Nomifensine*. Royal Society of Medicine International Congress and Symposium Series No. 25 (Eds. P. D. STONIER and F. A. JENNER). Published jointly by Academic Press London and The Royal Society of Medicine, New York, Grune and Stratton (1980)

MUKHERJEE, P. K. and HOLLAND, R. P. C. Study of 'Vivalan' in geriatric patients suffering from depression, *Journal of International Medical Research* **7**, 588–591 (1979)

MÜLLER, E. E., GENAZZANI, A. R. and MURRU, S. Nomifensine: diagnostic test in hyper-prolactinemic states, *Journal of Clinical Endocrinology and Metabolism* **47**, 1352–1357 (1978)

MÜLLER-OERLINGHAUSEN, B. and RÜTHER, E. Clinical profile and serum concentration of viloxazine as compared to amitriptyline, *Pharmakopsychiatrie Neuro-Psychopharmakologie* **12**, 321–337 (1979)

MURATORIO, A., MAGGINI, C., COCCAGNA, G. and GUAZZELLI, M. Polygraphic study of the all-night sleep pattern in neurotic and depressed patients treated with trazodone. In *Trazodone*, Proceedings of the First International Symposium. Montreal, Quebec. October 1973, **9**, Modern Problems of Pharmacopsychiatry, 182–189 (Eds. T. A. BAN and B. SILVESTRINI), Basel: Karger (1974)

MURPHY, J. E. Mianserin in the treatment of depressive illness and anxiety states in general practice, *British Journal of Clinical Pharmacology* **5**, Suppl., 81s–85s (1978)

MURPHY, J. E., DONALD, J. F. and MOLLA, A. L. Mianserin in the treatment of depression in general practice, *Practitioner* **217**, 135–138 (1976)

NEWMAN, B. and CROME, P. The clinical toxicology of mianserin hydrochloride, *Veterinary and Human Toxicology* **21** Suppl., 60–63 (1980)

NUGENT, D. A double-blind study of viloxazine (vivalan) and amitriptyline in depressed geriatric patients, *Clinical Trials Journal* **16**, 13–17 (1979)

ÖGREN, S. O., ROSS, S. B., HALL, H., HOLM, A. C. and RENYL, A. L. The pharmacology of zimelidine: a 5-HT selective reuptake inhibitor, *Acta Psychiatrica Scandinavica* **63**, Suppl. 290, 127–151 (1981)

OKAMOTO, K., NAKANO, T. and INANAGA, K. Clinical experience with Org GB94 (mianserin hydrochloride), a new tetracyclic antidepressant, *Folia Psychiatrica et neurologica Japonica* **32**, 171–183 (1978)

OVERALL, J. E., HOLLISTER, L. E., MEYER, F., KIMBELL, I. and SHELTON, J. Imipramine and thioridazine in depressed and schizophrenic patients, *Journal of the American Medical Association* **189**, 605–608 (1964)

OVHED, I. A double-blind study of flupenthixol (Fluanxol) in general practice, *Current Medical Research Opinion* **4**, 144–150 (1976)

PALAZZO, G. and BAIOCCHI, L. Derivati mesoinici con un anello piridico condensato, *Annali de chimica* **56**, 190–206 (1966)

PARIANTE, F. Clinical effect of intravenous trazodone administration in severe depression. In *Trazodone*. Proceedings of the First International Symposium. Montreal, Quebec. October 1973, **9**, Modern Problems of Pharmacopsychiatry, 176–181 (Eds. T. A. BAN and B. SILVESTRINI), Karger, Basel (1974)

PARK, J. and PROUDFOOT, A. T. Acute poisoning with maprotiline hydrochloride, *British Medical Journal* **1**, 1573 (1977)

PAWLOWSKI, L., RUCZYŃSKA, J. and WOJTASIK, E. An evidence for the central serotoninergic activity of viloxazine, *Polish Journal of Pharmacology and Pharmacy* **31**, 261–269 (1979)

PAYKEL, E. S., PRICE, J. S., GILLAN, R. U., PALMAI, G. and CHESSER, E. S. A comparative trial of imipramine and chlorpromazine in depressed patients, *British Journal of Psychiatry* **114**, 1281–1287 (1968)

PEET, M. A clinical trial of ICI 58,834—a potential antidepressant, *Journal of International Medical Research* **1**, 624–626 (1973)

PEROUTKA, S. J. and SNYDER, S. H. Multiple serotonin receptors: differential binding of (3H) 5-hydroxytryptamine, (3H) lysergic acid diethylamide and (3H) spiroperidol, *Molecular Pharmacology* **16**, 687–699 (1979)

PERRY, G. F., FITZSIMMONS, B., SHAPIRO, L. and IRWIN, P. Clinical study of mianserin, imipramine and placebo in depression: blood level and MHPG correlations, *British Journal of Clinical Pharmacology* **5**, Suppl. 1, 35s–41s (1978)

PINDER, R. M., BLUM, A., STULEMEIJER, S. M., BARRES, M., MOLCZADZKI, M., RIGAUD, A., CHARBAUT, J., ISRAEL, L. and KAMMERER, T. A double-blind, multi-centre trial comparing the efficacy and side-effects of mianserin and clomipramine in depressed inpatients and outpatients, *Current Medical Research Opinion* **6**, Suppl. 7, 115–125 (1980)

PINDER, R. M., BROGDEN, R. N., SPEIGHT, T. M. and AVERY, G. S. Viloxazine: A review of its pharmacological properties and therapeutic efficacy in depressive illness, *Drugs* **13**, 401–421 (1977)

PIERCE, D. A comparison of trazodone and dothiepin in depression, *Neuropharmacology* **19**, 1219–1220 (1980)

PINTO, O. DE S., AFEICHE, S. P., BARTHOLINI, E. and LOUSTALOT, P. International experience with Ludiomil. In *Depressive Illness, Diagnosis, Assessment, Treatment* (Ed. KIELHOLZ), 253–266, Hans Huber, Berne (1972)

POHLMEIER, H., DE GREGORIO, M. and SIEROSLAWSKI, H. Clinical data on trazodone: A review of the literature. In *Trazodone—A New Broad-Spectrum Antidepressant*. Proceedings of the 11th Congress of the Collegium Internationale Neuro-Psychopharmacologicum July 9–14 (Eds. S. GERSHON, K. RICKELS and B. SILVESTRINI), pp. 8–26, Amsterdam, Excerpta Medica (1980)

PREDESCU, V., CIUREZU, T., TIMTOFTE, G. and ROMAN, I. Symptomatic relief with flupenthixol (Fluanxol) of the anxious-algetic-depressive syndrome complex in neurotic states, *Acta Psychiatrica Scandinavica* **49**, 15–27 (1973)

PRESCOTT, L. F., ILLINGWORTH, R. N., CRITCHLEY, J. A. J. H., FRAZER, I. and STIRLING, M. L. Acute haemolysis and renal failure after nomifensine overdosage, *British Medical Journal* **281**, 1392–1393 (1980)

PULL, C. B., PICHOT, P., PULL, M. C. and DREYFUS, J. F. A double-blind controlled multi-centre study comparing mianserin and imipramine, *Current Medical Research Opinion* **6**, Suppl. 7, 81–87 (1980)

RASKIN, A., SCHULTERBRANDT, J. G., REATIG, N., CHASE, C. and McKEON, J. J. Differential response to chlorpromazine, imipramine and placebo. A study of subgroups of hospitalized depressed patients, *Archives of General Psychiatry* 23, 164–173 (1970)

REITER, P. J. On flupenthixol, an antidepressant of a new chemical group, *British Journal of Psychiatry* 115, 1399–1402 (1969)

RIBLET, L. A., GATEWOOD, C. F. and MAYOL, R. F. Comparative effects of trazodone and tricyclic antidepressants on uptake of selected neurotransmitters by isolated rat brain synaptosomes, *Psychopharmacology* 63, 99–101 (1979)

RICKELS, K., CSANALOSI, H., NEWMAN, A., HUROWITZ, J., WERBLOWSKY, J. and WHITE, N. Trazodone and amitriptyline in depressed outpatients—a controlled study. In *Trazodone—A New Broad-Spectrum Antidepressant.* Proceedings of the 11th Congress of the Collegium Internationale Neuro-Psycho pharmacologicum July 9–14 1978 (Eds. S. GERSHON, K. RICKELS and B. SILVESTRINI), 86–101, Excerpta Medica, Amsterdam (1980)

RIDGES, A. P. Biochemistry of depression: a review, *Journal of International Medical Research* 3, Suppl. 2, 42–54 (1975)

RIVETT, K. F. and BARCELLONA, P. S. Toxicology of trazodone. In *Trazodone.* Proceedings of the First International Symposium. Montreal, 9. Modern Problems of Pharmacopsychiatry (Eds. T. A. BAN and B. SILVESTRINI), 76–86, Karger, Basel (1974)

ROBERTSON, M. M. and TRIMBLE, M. R. The antidepressant action of flupenthixol, *Practitioner* 225, 761–763 (1981)

ROCCATAGLIATA, G., ABBRUZZESE, G., ALBANO, C. and GANDALFO, C. Trazodone intravenously administered in depressive syndromes, *Drugs in Experimental and Clinical Research* 1, 389–395 (1977)

ROCCATAGLIATA, G., ALBANO, C., MAFFINI, M. and FARELLI, S. Alcohol withdrawal syndrome. Treatment with trazodone, *International Pharmacopsychiatry* 15, 105–110 (1980)

RUSSELL, G. F. M., NIAZ, U., WAKELING, A. and SLADE, P. D. Comparative double-blind trial of mianserin hydrochloride (Organon GB94) and diazepam in patients with depressive illness, *British Journal of Clinical Pharmacology* 5, Suppl. 1, 57s–65s (1978)

SALETU, B. and GRÜNBERGER, J. Changes in clinical symptomatology and psychometric assessments in depressed patients during mianserin and combined amitriptyline/chloridazepoxide therapy: a double-blind comparison, *Current Medical Research Opinion* 6, Suppl. 7, 52–61 (1980)

SAMAT, J., GRAZZINI, J. P. and DUVIC, C. Viloxazine in depressive states encountered in general medical practice, *Lyon Mediteranee Medical* 16, 2905–2909 (1980)

SCHACHT, U. and LEVEN, M. Synaptosomes and brain slices as *in vitro* models for the characterisation of antidepressant drugs. In *Depressive Disorders* (Ed. S. GARATTINI), 17–35, Schattauer, Stuttgart (1978)

SHAW, W. L. The comparative safety of mianserin in overdose, *Current Medical Research Opinion* 6, Suppl. 7, 44–50 (1980)

SHAW, D. M., RILEY, G., MICHALAKEAS, A. C., TIDMARSH, S. F., BLAZEK, R. and JOHNSON, A. L. New direction to the amine hypothesis. A cause of affective disorders, *Lancet* 1, 1259–1260 (1977)

SHEPHERD, G. A. A. and KERR, F. Maprotiline hydrochloride and grand-mal seizures, *British Medical Journal* 1, 1523 (1978)

SILVESTRINI, B., CIOLI, V., BURBERI, S. and CATANESE, B. Pharmacological properties of AF 1161, a new psychotropic drug, *International Journal of Neuropharmacology* 7, 587–599 (1968)

SIMS, A. C. P. Comparison of the efficacy of sustained-release amitriptyline with maprotriline in the treatment of depressive illness, *Current Medical Research and Opinion* 6, 534–539 (1980)

SINGH, A. N., SAXENA, B. and HELSON, H. L. A controlled clinical study of trazodone in chronic schizophrenic patients with pronounced depressive symptomatology, *Current Therapeutic Research* 23 (4), 485–501 (1978)

SMITH, A. H. W., NAYLOR, G. S. and MOODY, J. P. Placebo-controlled double-blind trial of mianserin hydrochloride, *British Journal of Clinical Pharmacology* 5, Suppl. 1, 67s–70s (1978)

SONNE, L. M. Behandlung af depressive tilstande med flupenthixol, *Nordisk Psykiatrisk Tidsskrift* 20, 322–324 (1966)

SONNE, L. M. Behandlung af depressive tilstande med flupenthixol, *Nordisk Psykiatrisk Tidsskrift* 25, 454–463 (1971)

STEPHANINI, E., FADDA, F., MEDDA, L. and GESSA, G. L. Selective inhibition of serotonin uptake by trazodone. A new antidepressant agent, *Life Sciences* 18, 1459–1466 (1976a)

STEPHANINI, E., FADDA, F., PORCEDDU, M. L. and GESSA, G. L. Effect of trazodone on brain dopamine metabolism, *Journal of Pharmacy and Pharmacology* 28, 925–927 (1976b)

STORER, D., EASTWOOD, P. and BAILEY, E. Long-term comparison of nomifensine and imipramine in the treatment of depression, *Royal Society of Medicine International Congress Symposium Series* 25, 109–115 (1980)

SVESTKA, J., NAHUNEK, K., CESKOVA, E., RYSANEK, R. and MISUREC, J. Controlled comparison of mianserin with imipramine in endogenous depressions, *Activitas nervosa superior (Praha)* **21**, 147–148 (1979)

TAEUBER, K. Relevance of screening tests in human psychopharmacology: the physiological point of view (Human screening tests for the clinical investigation of nomifensine), *Symposia Medica Hoechst* **10** (1), 51–60 (1974)

TAYLOR, D. P., HYSLOP, D. K. and RIBLET, L. A. Trazodone: a new non-tricyclic antidepressant without anticholinergic activity, *Biochemical Pharmacology* **29**, 2149–2150 (1980)

TRIMBLE, M. Non-monoamine oxidase inhibitor antidepressants and epilepsy: a review, *Epilepsia* **19**, 241–250 (1978)

TRIMBLE, M. R. Antidepressant drugs and convulsions, *Lancet* **1**, 307 (1980a)

TRIMBLE, M. R. Psychotropic drugs in epilepsy, *Journal of International Biomedical Information and Data* **1**, 37–44 (1980b)

TRIMBLE, M. R., MELDRUM, B. S. and ANLEZARK, G. Effect of nomifensive on brain amines and epilepsy in photosensitive baboons, *British Journal of Clinical Pharmacology* **4**, Suppl. 2, 101s–107s (1977)

TYRER, P., STEINBERG, B. and WATSON, B. Possible epileptogenic effect of mianserin, *Lancet* **2**, 798–799 (1979)

TUOMISTO, J. Nomifensine and its derivatives as possible tools for studying amine uptake, *European Journal of Pharmacology* **42**, 101–106 (1980)

VAN DER VEEN, F., DE RIDDER, J. J., VINK, J. and WIJNAND, H. P. Plasma levels of the antidepressant drug mianserin: relevance to clinical pharmacology and therapy, *Therapeutic Drug Monitoring* **2**, 95 (1980)

VAN ZWEITEN, P. A. Inhibition of the central hypotensive effect of clonidine by trazodone: a novel antidepressant, *Pharmacology* **15**, 331–336 (1977)

VOHRA, J. K., BURROWS, G. D., McINTYRE, I. and DAVIES, B. Cardiovascular effects of nomifensive, *Lancet* **2**, 902 (1978)

VOGEL, G. W. A review of REM sleep deprivation, *Archives of General Psychiatry* **32**, 749–761 (1975)

VON KNORRING, L. A double-blind trial: vivalan against placebo in depressed elderly patients, *Journal of International Medical Research* **8**, 18–21 (1980)

WEINSTOCK, M. and COHEN, D. Tricyclic antidepressant drugs as antagonists of muscarinic receptors in sympathetic ganglia, *European Journal of Pharmacology* **40**, 321–328 (1976)

WESTER, H. A. and SIEGERS, C-P. Cardiovascular effects of mianserin and amitriptyline in healthy volunteers, *International Journal of Clinical Pharmacology and Therapeutic Toxicology* **18**, 513–517 (1980)

WHEATLEY, D. *Psychopharmacology in Family Practice*, Heinemann Medical, London (1973)

WHEATLEY, D. Viloxazine—a new antidepressant, *Current Therapeutic Research* **16**, 821–828 (1974)

WILHELM, M. The chemistry of polycyclic psycho-active drugs—serendipity or systematic investigation? In *Depressive Illness. Diagnosis, Assessment, Treatment* (Ed. P. KIELHOLZ), 129–137, Hans Huber, Berne (1972)

WILSON, W. H., PETRIE, W. M. and BAN, T. A. Possible lack of anticholinergic effects with mianserin: a pilot study, *Journal of Clinical Psychiatry* **41**, 63–65 (1980)

YOUNG, J. P. R., HUGHES, W. C. and LADER, M. H. A controlled comparison of flupenthixol and amitriptyline in depressed outpatients, *British Medical Journal* **1**, 1116–1118 (1976)

Chapter 9

Monoamine oxidase inhibitors and amine precursors

P. J. Tyrer

Monoamine oxidase inhibitors were discovered in the search for more effective antituberculous agents. Iproniazid, the first drug to be clinically tested, is closely related to isoniazid, which is now well established as a highly effective antituberculous drug. Iproniazid was also used in the treatment of tuberculosis but was noted to produce euphoria in some patients. This probable antidepressant effect was one of the reasons why iproniazid was rejected as an antituberculous drug. Early in pharmacological evaluation iproniazid was noted to inhibit monoamine oxidase (Zeller *et al.*, 1952), but this was not felt to be of any clinical importance. Early studies suggested that iproniazid was of no value in treating depression but in 1957 encouraging results were reported in the treatment of chronic schizophrenics and depressed patients (Loomer, Saunders and Kline, 1957). These also suggested the therapeutic benefit of iproniazid was due to its inhibition of monoamine oxidase and that its main clinical effect was an improvement in energy and initiative. They coined the term 'psychic energizers' to describe the monoamine oxidase inhibitors and a search was started for more drugs in the same group.

Two main classes of MAOIs were subsequently discovered, one containing drugs structurally similar to iproniazid, including phenelzine, isocarboxazid, nialamide, pheniprazine and mebanazine. These are all hydrazine MAOIs. The second group are non-hydrazines and the only member in clinical use is tranylcypromine. tranylcypromine.

It is important to realize that the monoamine oxidase inhibitors were introduced before there were other antidepressant drugs available. The term 'psychic energizer' quickly became translated as 'antidepressants' and they were used initially for the treatment of the large number of depressed hospital in-patients for whom there were no effective treatments available apart from electroconvulsive therapy. Many clinical trials were carried out. These showed that there was little difference in efficacy between the MAOIs (Bates and Douglas, 1961) and that in many groups of depressed patients the drugs were relatively ineffective (Harris and Robin, 1960; Greenblatt, Grosser and Wechsler, 1964; Hare, Dominian and Sharpe, 1962). Soon after these reports the tricyclic antidepressants were introduced to clinical practice and proved to be more effective as antidepressants. This was followed by a series of adverse reports with MAOIs, particularly in combination with other drugs and certain foodstuffs. The well known 'cheese reaction' was first described by Blackwell in 1963 and was followed by reports of serious adverse reactions, particularly fatal hepatocellular jaundice (Pare,

1964; Cole, 1964). The further evidence that MAOIs could also interact fatally with other drugs (Sjöqvist, 1965) almost spelt the deathknell for this class of agents in psychiatry. In the last 15 years it has been recognized that the drugs are safe if used appropriately and are of specific benefit in some psychiatric disorders not helped by other drug treatment. Their use is, however, a great deal less than that of the tricyclic antidepressants and associated compounds.

Pharmacology

The class of monoamine oxidase inhibitors indicates a common property of these drugs. Monoamine oxidase inactivates catecholamines, including dopamine, noradrenaline and 5-hydroxytriptamine, and its inhibition thereby leads to a rise in central and peripheral catecholamine levels. This may be particularly relevant in the synaptic clefts where the fundamentals of neurotransmission take place. By preventing the breakdown of catecholamines the levels of amines rise in the synaptic cleft and in neurons (Spector, Hirsh and Brodie, 1963). This demonstration of a rise in central catecholamine levels with compounds that appeared to be antidepressant was the impetus for the catecholamine hypothesis of depression. In its simplest form this states that depression is caused by a relative deficit of monoamine neurotransmitters and that in mania there is a relative abundance of the neurotransmitters (Schildkraut, 1965). It is supported by the additional evidence that tricyclic antidepressants inhibit re-uptake of monoamines from the synaptic cleft. The hypothesis was disarmingly simple; tricyclic antidepressants increase functional monoamines by preventing their re-uptake into neurons, and MAOIs have the same effect by preventing the amines from being broken down (*Figure 9.1*). Further support came from animal pharmacological studies with reserpine. Reserpine is the hypotensive drug that is most at risk in inducing depressive illness (Tyrer, 1981) and in animals it produces an immobile state similar to that of psychomotor retardation (Brodie, Pletscher and Shore, 1956). Monoamine oxidase inhibitors counteract this effect of reserpine in animals and it was reasonable to suppose that they did so by preventing central monoamine depletion.

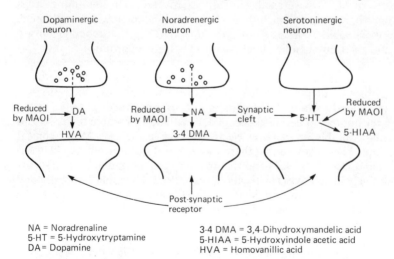

NA = Noradrenaline
5-HT = 5-Hydroxytryptamine
DA = Dopamine

3-4 DMA = 3,4-Dihydroxymandelic acid
5-HIAA = 5-Hydroxyindole acetic acid
HVA = Homovanillic acid

Figure 9.1 Mechanism of action of monoamine oxidase inhibitors

Although the cathecholamine hypothesis of depression has been of tremendous value in stimulating research it is clear that, as originally formulated, it is no longer tenable. No convincing evidence has been given that an increase in functional neurotransmitter monoamines result from MAO inhibition although there is a general rise in brain monoamine levels. There is also evidence that MAOIs have many other pharmacological actions apart from inhibition of monoamine oxidase, including the inhibition of re-uptake of noradrenaline and other monoamines from the synaptic cleft (Hendley and Snyder, 1968). Some MAOIs such as pargyline (not commercially marketed) are hypotensive and this is impossible to reconcile with the catecholaminc hypothesis as originally formulated; all MAOIs should have the potential for increasing blood pressure but not reducing it.

In the last decade the inhibition of monoamine oxidase has been shown to be more complex than first thought. It exists in two functional forms, A and B (Johnston, 1968) and also shows great substrate specificity (i.e. its effects vary in different parts of the brain (Youdim *et al.*, 1972). This may be relevant to clinical response. Although all marketed MAOIs inhibit both MAO-A and MAO-B clinical studies with a selective MAO-A inhibitor, clorgyline, suggest that clinical antidepressant effects follow from inhibition of MAO-A as they are not shown with the partially selective MAO-B inhibitor, pargyline (Murphy *et al.*, 1981). Deprenyl, a selective MAO-B inhibitor, has been used in the treatment of parkinsonism in combination with levodopa (Birkmayer *et al.*, 1977) and is discussed fully in Chapter 5. Unlike other monoamine oxidase inhibitors it does not give rise to the 'cheese reaction' with foodstuffs containing tyramine. Unfortunately it probably does not have the mood enhancing properties of other MAOIs and is unlikely to be used in psychiatry. The implications are that inhibitors of MAO-A are both clinically effective in altering mood and carry risks of dangerous drug and food interactions whereas inhibitors of MAO-B have neither of these properties. Thus although there appears to be great scope for advances with MAOIs in the near future it seems unlikely that newer agents will be produced which are safer but which retain the same clinical efficacy.

Hydrazine monoamine oxidase inhibitors differ from non-hydrazine ones in that they produce irreversible inhibition of monoamine oxidase. With non-hydrazine MAOIs the inhibition is slowly reversible. There are important clinical implications of this property. When treatment with a MAOI is stopped the drug may be completely eliminated from the body within a few days but monoamine oxidase levels remain low. It takes many days to synthesize new monoamine oxidase, and during this time the subject will still be liable to dangerous reactions if he consumes food with a high tyramine or dopamine content. Tranylcypromine, the only non-hydrazine MAOI in clinical use, differs from the other agents in releasing dopamine as well as blocking its uptake. This probably explains its more rapid clinical action and its amphetamine-like stimulant properties.

Although MAO inhibition is achieved rapidly after administration of a MAOI the clinical effects take much longer to become manifest (*see* p. 259). No satisfactory explanation for this delay has been put forward. Inhibition of monoamine oxidase takes place in all parts of the body and the measurement of platelet MAO inhibition has been used in several clinical studies. Platelets contain MAO-B only (Donnelly and Murphy, 1977) but there is good evidence that to achieve clinical response at least 80 per cent inhibition of platelet MAO is necessary (Robinson *et al.*, 1973; Robinson *et al.*, 1978; Davidson, McLeod and Blum, 1978).

Taking all the evidence into consideration the working hypothesis that monoamine oxidase inhibitors exert their clinical action by inhibition of monoamine oxidase still seems the most plausible. It nonetheless has to explain why these drugs are not particularly effective in severe depression, why clinical effects are delayed so markedly, and why some MAOIs such as nialamide inhibit MAO well but are relatively ineffective clinically. The fit between MAO inhibition and the clinical indications for the drug is not yet close enough to admire the final result as a feat of sartorial virtuosity.

When it comes to explaining the unwanted effects of MAOIs the fit is much more satisfactory. The interaction between MAOIs and high tyramine-containing foods such as Chianti wine, yeast extracts, cheese and pickled herrings, and food with a high dopamine content such as broad bean pods, is definitely a consequence of MAO inhibition. Indeed, it could have been predicted from pharmacological knowledge before the drugs were ever introduced to clinical psychiatry (Blackwell et al., 1967). Tyramine and dopamine are normally deaminated by MAO in the gut and liver but after prior treatment with a MAOI these protective mechanisms cease to work. Tyramine and dopamine are pressor amines which release noradrenaline at sympathetic nerve endings. Cardiac output and peripheral arterial resistance are raised and hypertension rapidly follows. This may lead to a cerebrovascular haemorrhage and sudden death. Severe headache may result without any arterial rupture.

Similarly, all drugs that can interact dangerously with MAOIs do so because of the consequence of MAO inhibition. These include the *indirectly acting* sympathomimetic amines such as phenylephrine and phenylpropanolamine which are also present in nasal decongestants sold without the need for a prescription. Predictably, levodopa also interacts with MAOIs to produce hypertensive reactions, but adrenaline and noradrenaline do not, as commonly believed, interact with MAOIs as they can be broken down by different metabolic pathways. The absence of interaction has been most clearly shown by Boakes and his colleagues (1973).

Monoamine oxidase inhibitors also inhibit other enzymes, particularly in the liver. These enzymes include those involved in the metabolism of barbiturates and opiates such as pethidine. Thus the clinical effects of both these classes of drugs tend to be more pronounced and prolonged when they are given to a patient already taking an MAOI. Inhibition of enzymes is also thought to be the reason why MAOIs also potentiate the effects of insulin and oral hypoglycaemic drugs.

Pharmacokinetics

The pharmacokinetics of monoamine oxidase inhibitors are poorly understood. This is surprising, as the compounds are relatively simple ones, but their metabolites have proved very difficult to isolate. The drugs are rapidly absorbed through the gut and are widely distributed through all parts of the body, including the brain. The metabolites of MAOIs are mainly inactive and play little part in their clinical effects. The metabolic pathways include acetylation (Tilstone, Margot and Johnstone, 1979) and possibly oxidation and oxidative deamination (Marshall, 1976). Tranylcypromine is metabolized rapidly to clinically inactive compounds.

The metabolic pathways may be of clinical importance if they alter the rate of metabolism of the parent drugs. If the drug is inactivated too rapidly it may never reach sufficiently high levels to produce clinical response, no matter what dosage is given. Acetylation is the pathway of metabolism that has aroused the most interest with the hydrazine MAOIs. This is because the population can be separated into slow or fast acetylators on the basis of a simple test. This involves taking a loading dose of a sulphonamide drug (which has shown to be metabolized by acetylation) and measuring the amount of free (i.e. non-metabolized) drug several hours later (Evans, 1969). Acetylator status describes whether an individual metabolizes a drug by acetylation slowly or rapidly, a phenomenon determined by a polygenic mode of inheritance. In most parts of the world there are roughly equal proportions of slow and fast acetylators, although there are important exceptions. Egyptians, for example, comprise only 18 per cent fast acetylators whereas Eskimos are almost all fast acetylators, making 95 per cent of the total (Whitford, 1978).

The clinical importance of this depends on whether the major metabolic pathway of MAOIs is through acetylation. If it is, slow acetylators might be expected to respond better than fast acetylators to hydrazine MAOIs, as the acetylator metabolite is clinically inactive. The first evidence that this might be the case came from Johnstone and Marsh (1973). Using a cross-over design in which phenelzine and placebo were taken for three weeks each they found that slow acetylators improved significantly more than fast acetylators when taking phenelzine. Side effects were also more marked in slow acetylators although not significantly so. A previous study (Evans, Davidson and Pratt, 1965) had also shown that side effects were more pronounced in slow acetylators but failed to show any difference between slow and fast acetylators in clinical response. Further investigators have produced the same pattern of conflicting results. Four studies have shown no difference in outcome between slow and fast acetylators (Davidson et al., 1978; Marshall et al., 1978; Tyrer et al., 1980; Nies and Robinson, 1981) and two (Johnstone, 1976; Rowan et al., 1981) have shown greater improvement in slow acetylators. The most comprehensive of these studies have been reported in more detail by Paykel and his colleagues (1982a). In this study the superiority of phenelzine over placebo was compared using double-blind procedure after two, four and six weeks in slow and fast acetylators. Slow acetylators showed significantly greater improvement than placebo after only two weeks but fast acetylators took six weeks to show a similar level of improvement. These results suggest that slow acetylators respond more rapidly than fast acetylators and, by inference, the fast acetylators should receive a higher dosage than slow acetylators. This in itself is not sufficient reason for estimating acetylator phenotype before treatment and the contradictory results from other studies make the value of these estimations even more dubious.

Clinical use

There is still controversy over the clinical indications for MAOIs. This is not surprising as the results of clinical trials have been conflicting and the list of adverse effects with these drugs is a formidable one. Before considering the place of any drug treatment in clinical use we first need evidence that it is superior to placebo or no treatment. Secondly, it needs to be compared with other accepted treatments for the condition. To be an established treatment in the clinician's armamentarium it needs to be at least of equivalent efficacy to these other treatments and preferably better. Because the response to monoamine oxidase inhibitors varies with diagnosis their use in different psychiatric disorders needs to be discussed separately.

Depressive psychosis

Following the results of the early studies it was to be expected that the MAOIs would receive the label of antidepressant drugs, and that depressive illnesses would be one of the main groups liable to be treated. The classification of depressive illness was still being agonized about during the course of these clinical trials so it is often difficult to decide which patients suffered from severe depressive illness (depressive psychosis) with characteristic pathophysiological features of loss of appetite and weight, sleep disturbance with early morning waking and delusions of guilt and unworthiness, and which had mild illnesses (depressive neurosis). In retrospect it is fairly clear that patients with severe depressive illness do not respond particularly well to MAOIs and certainly less well than other antidepressant treatments.

Many of the early studies were carried out with depressed in-patients and, although the type of depression was often unspecified, the fact that they were in-patients is suggestive that they were suffering from more severe forms of depression. Many studies in this group of patients showed little or no difference between the effects of MAOIs and placebo (Pare and Sandler, 1959; Harris and Robin, 1960; Greenblatt, Grosser and Wechsler, 1964; Medical Research Council, 1965). The last study was an influential multicentre trial that must have led to many clinicians abandoning MAOIs altogether from their psychiatric treatments. Electroconvulsive therapy (ECT), imipramine, phenelzine and placebo were all compared. ECT topped the list for efficacy, followed by imipramine, with phenelzine and placebo way behind. Indeed, in the depressed women treated phenelzine was marginly less effective than placebo.

Unfortunately as MAOIs were called antidepressants and as the catecholamine hypothesis of depression had such influence at this time the assumption was frequently made that these drugs were still only of value in severely depressed patients. Authoritative reviews recommended the MAOIs only for depressive illness non-responsive to tricyclic antidepressants (Atkinson and Ditman, 1965; Jarvik, 1970; Hollister, 1973). As tricyclic antidepressants are in the main given to patients with typical depressive illness it is hardly rational to recommend MAOIs for the hard core of resistant depressions who have failed to respond to the more effective drugs. It is as pointless as recommending that the only function of the horse is to shift heavy loads after mechanized vehicles have failed to move them.

It is a mistake to generalize from the findings in severe depression to psychiatric disorders as a whole. Statements such as 'in the absence of any clear-cut indications for specific response to a monoamine oxidase inhibitor, this (unpredictability) places these drugs clearly in the category of third-choice therapeutic agents behind the tricyclic antidepressant and newer second generation drugs' (Blackwell, 1981), imply that for all clinical indications MAOIs are inferior to tricyclics and tricyclic-like antide-pressants. The evidence shows that it is only true for severe depressive illness. Does this mean that MAOIs should only be used in severe depression after at least two other conventional antidepressant drugs have been tried and found wanting? This is arguable. Shaw (1977) suggests using a MAOI immediately after a tricyclic antide-pressant has failed to produce improvement and the amphetamine-like stimulant properties of tranylcypromine make it the most suitable MAOI for severe depressive illness. Two other factors, one pharmacogenetic, the other pharmacokinetic, may also influence response. Pare and his colleagues (Pare, Rees and Sainsbury, 1962; Pare and Mack, 1971) have found familial evidence of clinical response to both tricyclic antidepressants and MAOIs. Thus if a first degree relative of the patient has responded to a MAOI in the past it is more likely that the patient will respond to the same drug even if the clinical presentation may suggest otherwise. Obviously this only covers a very small proportion of patients and there is often difficulty in separating placebo responders from pharmacological ones on the basis of a retrospective account by a relative.

The second factor is dosage. This is described later in more detail but there is evidence from a review of published controlled trials that patients with depressive illnesses are more likely to respond to a monoamine oxidase inhibitor if it is given in a higher dose than those normally recommended (i.e. the upper limit of the dosages given in *Table 9.1* p. 258) (Tyrer, 1979a). As most published comparisons of MAOIs with other drugs have used much lower dosage they may have placed the MAOIs at a disadvantage.

Depressive neurosis (including atypical depression)

Depressive neurosis is an unsatisfactory diagnostic label that includes a heterogeneous group of disorders. There are those who sometimes argue that classification is a sterile and therapeutically unproductive exercise but its value is well illustrated by the confusion thrown up by studies with the MAOIs. The first study to suggest that these drugs were effective in other depressed patients apart from 'endogenous' ones was by West and Dally in 1959. They found that patients responding to iproniazid had few typical depressive symptoms but had a mixture of hysterical, phobic and anxiety symptoms together with lack of energy and diurnal mood swing. They were among the first to use the term 'atypical depression' to describe these patients, and further studies, mainly from St Thomas's Hospital in London, developed this theme (Sargant, 1961; Sargant and Dally, 1962; Lascelles, 1966). Lascelles described the beneficial effects of MAOIs in atypical facial pain, in which overt depression was conspiciously absent, illustrating how little connection these disorders had with typical depressive illness.

Although the introduction of the term atypical depression emphasized that depression consisted of many disorders it did nothing to resolve the classification problems. Because it had no clear-cut identifying features it could easily be moulded to fit any neurotic disorder and the absence of depression allowed a range of other mood disturbance to be also included. In retrospect many conditions now described as personality disorders, anxiety neuroses, phobic state and hypochondriacal disorders were all included under the umbrella of 'atypical depression'. For this reason it is better not used without a clear definition.

As it is accepted that the differentiation of the neuroses is a difficult task it is often more fruitful to describe the main clinical features that are responsive to MAOIs. From the evidence of clinical trials in which separate analysis has been made of these features (Tyrer, 1976) it is possible to select patients with depressive illness that are more likely to respond to these drugs. Thus a strong anxiety component, rapid change in mood and other symptoms in response to circumstances, and somatization of symptoms tend to be associated with a good response, and insomnia, guilt feelings and weight loss with a poor one. Thus even within the confines of depressive neurosis as conventionally defined there is likely to be variation in response to MAOIs.

Pollitt and Young (1971) have pointed out that the clinical factors associated with response to MAOIs are more common in younger people and with increasing age the more typical symptoms of depressive illness become predominant. The significance of this is not clear and there is no good evidence that psychogeriatric patients as a whole are unresponsive to MAOIs (*see* p. 388).

Even if MAOIs are effective drugs in some patients with depressive neurosis the clinician needs evidence that they are superior to more conventional antidepressant drugs before they can be prescribed as first choice drug treatments. It has to be said that no such evidence exists. When patients with depressive neurosis have been carefully selected so that more severe (psychotic) depressive illness has been excluded and such patients treated with MAOIs or a tricyclic antidepressant no difference in overall efficacy has been shown, although patients with anxiety symptoms showed a trend for greater improvement than with the MAOI (phenelzine) (Rowan, Paykel and Parker, 1982; Nies and Robinson, 1981). In the first of these studies differential effects were also shown in patients. Those with depressive personality traits did significantly worse with phenelzine than those without these characteristics but no difference was shown in patients receiving amitriptyline (Paykel *et al.*, 1982b). In another study, two MAOIs, phenelzine and isocarboxazid, were compared with a tricyclic antidepressant, trimipramine, and combined therapy with both MAOIs and trimipramine (Young, Lader and Hughes, 1979). Trimipramine alone was superior to both MAOIs and the combination treatments. However, in the study no diagnostic separation of depression was made and all patients with moderate depression entered the study.

The finding that depressive neurosis associated with anxiety is a preferential indicator for MAOI therapy is also supported by studying the predictors of response to different drug treatments. Tricyclic-like and tricyclic antidepressants tend to lead to a poor clinical response when anxiety is a marked component of the depressive syndrome (Paykel, 1979). Investigators in the USA have studied this group, which they term depressive–anxiety states, in a number of clinical trials, confirming the superiority of one of the MAOIs, phenelzine, over a placebo control (Robinson *et al.*, 1973; Ravaris *et al.*, 1976; Nies and Robinson, 1981).

In summary, MAOIs are effective drugs in depressive neurosis but show little or no advantage over the tricyclic antidepressants unless there is a significant admixture of anxiety symptoms. The term 'atypical depression' describes a group of disorders which includes depression-cum-anxiety as well as others, but because it is so loosely defined it is better abandoned.

Anxiety neuroses

There are surprisingly few studies of monoamine oxidase inhibitors in the treatment of anxiety neuroses. This may be because anxiety neuroses are most commonly seen in primary care rather than in hospital practice and hospital referral is only made when depression or other symptoms supervene. There has only been one controlled study of the effectiveness of monoamine oxidase inhibitors in patients specifically diagnosed as having anxiety neurosis. This showed no difference between the MAOI, phenelzine, and placebo (Mountjoy *et al.*, 1977) but as all patients in the study were also taking an antianxiety drug, diazepam, significant differences between phenelzine and placebo were difficult to obtain. In another study, Sheehan, Ballenger and Jacobsen (1980) found phenelzine to be superior to imipramine in a group of patients who satisfy many of the diagnostic criteria for anxiety neurosis but also had additional phobic, hypochondriacal and hysterical symptoms. This is one of the few studies showing a MAOI to be superior to a tricyclic antidepressant and supports the other indicators that in pathological anxiety MAOIs have specific advantages.

Although convincing evidence is slim because of the relative absence of controlled studies anxiety neurosis is one of the clinical indications for treatment with monoamine oxidase inhibitors. Because there are a large number of other therapies available for anxiety states, both pharmacological and psychological (Tyrer, 1979b), MAOIs should be a relatively low choice on the list. It is probably best to reserve treatment for chronic anxiety states in which drugs such as benzodiazepines have not controlled the symptoms and psychological therapies such as biofeedback and relaxation training have either failed or been rejected.

Phobic anxiety states

Agoraphobia and social phobias constitute the main phobias suitable for treatment with monoamine oxidase inhibitors. Monosymptomatic (specific) phobias such as those of animals, thunder and heights are not, and have never been, recommended for treatment, although single phobias with a socially phobic content (e.g. that of vomiting in public) may occasionally be considered. Although some of the earlier published studies have suggested that phobic symptoms were specifically helped by MAOIs the first evidence that phobias as a diagnostic group might be a clinical indication for treatment came in an open retrospective study by Kelly and his colleagues (1970). Later prospective trials confirmed that iproniazid and phenelzine were significantly superior to placebo in the treatment of both agoraphobia and social phobias (Lipsedge *et al.*, 1973; Solyom *et al.*, 1973; Tyrer, Candy and Kelly, 1973), although in the study by Mountjoy and his colleagues (1977) already mentioned significant differences were not found between the phenelzine and placebo groups, both of which received diazepam as well as their trial drugs. No controlled comparisons have been made between MAOIs and tricyclic antidepressants in phobic states. This is hardly surprising as tricyclic antidepressants, with the exception of clomipramine, are not recommended for the treatment of phobias. However, in the study already mentioned by Sheehan, Ballenger and Jacobsen, (1980) many of the patients described included phobic patients with high levels of free-floating anxiety and in this group phenelzine was superior to imipramine.

The evidence from these studies indicates that MAOIs have marked antiphobic and anxiolytic activity and are generally superior to tricyclic antidepressants in these properties. At first sight this is difficult to reconcile with the known pharmacology of MAOIs. The catecholamine hypothesis and animal pharmacological studies suggested that these drugs were antidepressants with the same therapeutic profile as tricyclic antidepressants. Suggestions have been made that patients with phobic and anxiety symptoms who respond to MAOIs have 'masked depression' (Pollitt and Young, 1971) but this is difficult to prove unless in all other respects such patients are indistinguishable from depressed patients. It is also possible that antianxiety activity is achieved by the side effect of sedation, a well-established phenomenon with tricyclic antidepressants that is quite unrelated to antidepressant activity. This is more difficult to argue with MAOIs as there have only been a few reports of sedation with them (Hare, Dominian and Sharpe, 1962) and the opposite unwanted effect of stimulation and consequent insomnia is more common (Sargant and Slater, 1962; Tyrer, 1976). In phobic and anxious patients who respond to MAOIs clinical improvement is more consistent with a stimulant action; there is improved confidence, energy and self-esteem rather than drowsiness and torpor. This recalls the MAOIs' original label of 'psychic energizers' and has led to their description as 'delayed psychostimulants' (Tyrer, 1976) which accounts for their therapeutic activity in phobic and anxiety disorders as well as mild depressives ones.

Obsessional neurosis

Although there have been no systematic studies of the value of MAOIs in obsessional neurosis there are some clinicians who recommend their use for this therapeutically resistant group. Short-term improvement in obsessional neurosis occurring as a consequence of non-specific or placebo factors is rare, and so more credence can be attached to the results of single case studies.

Annesley (1969) reported a gradual but steady improvement over six months in an obsessional man treated with phenelzine 60 mg daily. The patient had not previously responded to a range of other therapies, including tricyclic antidepressants, ECT and phenothiazines. In a similar case of chronic obsessional ruminations resistant to therapy a dramatic response to treatment with phenelzine was noted after two weeks (Jain, Swinson and Thomas, 1970). Phenelzine (75 mg daily) also produced dramatic improvement in a woman with an 18 year history of compulsions and rituals who had failed to respond to imipramine (Isberg, 1981). Treatment with tranylcypromine (20–30 mg daily) has also been associated with consistent improvement in two severely obsessional patients, the improvement occurring after only a few days of treatment (Jenike, 1981).

One consistent feature of these reports is the presence of phobic and anxiety symptoms in the patients who responded. It is therefore difficult to know if it is obsessions-with-anxiety that are responsive to MAOIs or obsessional symptoms alone. In most of the reports relapse has been noted if the MAOI has been withdrawn after recovery although the maintenance dose is lower than that required to achieve response.

Dosage and clinical response

There is a greater range of dosage with MAOIs than with tricyclic antidepressants. This may be conveniently divided into low and high dose regimens (*Table 9.1*). The most employed dose of each drug is usually at the boundary between the two ranges and few clinicians use the whole range of dosage shown in the table.

TABLE 9.1 Dosage range of monoamine oxidase inhibitors

Monoamine oxidase inhibitor	Low dose (mg) (daily)	High dose (mg) (daily)
Tranylcypromine	10–30	40–60
Iproniazid	25–75	100–150
Phenelzine	15–45	60–90
Isocarboxazid	10–30	40–60

Qualitative differences between low and high dosage

There is little point in separating dosage unless there are important qualitative differences between them. The most clear-cut evidence of such differences comes from Ravaris and his colleagues (1976). They showed that depressive–anxiety states treated with phenelzine in two dosage strengths or with placebo, showed differential response. Patients treated with 60 mg daily showed significantly greater improvement than the other group and patients treated with 30 mg daily showed no superiority over placebo treatment.

There is another hypothesis that received some support from published evidence; that clinical response in severe depressive illness (depressive psychosis) only occurs when high dosage is used. In clinical trials showing significant benefit from MAOIs in severe depressive illness (Rees and Davies, 1961; Hutchinson and Smedberg, 1963) high dosage has always been used. Although this hypothesis is far from proved, it is reasonable to consider dosage in the higher range when more severe depressive illness is treated with MAOIs. The same may also apply in the treatment of obsessional neurosis.

Quantitative differences between low and high dosage

There is now good evidence that patients treated with higher dosage of MAOIs respond more rapidly than those on low dosage. Reviews of clinical trials (Tyrer, 1976, 1979a; Paykel, 1979) suggests that when lower dosage is used clinical response is delayed. In a prospection study, using phenelzine in two daily dosages of 45 mg and 90 mg, significantly greater improvement was found in the higher dosage group after four weeks (Tyrer et al., 1980). The results of self-ratings suggested that these differences begin after only one week on higher dosage.

These differences are clinically important, because the latent period between starting treatment and the onset of subjective improvement can vary from a few days to eight weeks. The non-hydrazine MAOI, tranylcypromine, has a more rapid effect than hydrazines with clinical response occurring within two weeks, and with this drug the different rates of improvement with high and low dosage are less important.

In phobic and obsessional illnesses the delay in response to drug treatment can be many weeks (Tyrer, Candy and Kelly, 1973), possibly because the pharmacological effects only facilitate changes in phobic and obsessional behaviour rather than act directly on them. The speed of response will therefore be more important with these disorders. Compliance is very difficult to achieve unless the patient can be assured that improvement is likely to start within four weeks of treatment. In these circumstances an increase in dosage is often advisable.

Not surprisingly, unwanted effects are more common with higher dosage. Unsteadiness or dizziness, probably due to postural hypotension, is a common symptom (Tyrer et al., 1980), and dry mouth, constipation and feelings of general weakness are also frequently noticed. As with other psychotropic drugs, the unwanted effects are more marked early in treatment and tolerance to them develops over time. It is therefore preferable to build up to high dosage slowly over 1–2 weeks and to reassure patients that any unpleasant effects are likely to be temporary.

Dosage recommendation and prescribing practice

All patients starting treatment with a MAOI should receive dosage in the lower range (*Table 9.1*). If the patient has severe depressive illness the dose should be increased to the higher range after 1–2 weeks. The same procedure may be necessary in other patients, particularly those with obsessional and phobic disorders, unless the patient has a chronic illness and is prepared to tolerate a long delay before clinical response is achieved. If a rapid response is considered necessary tranylcypromine is preferable to hydrazine MAOIs although other factors will also dictate the final choice. There is no evidence of differences in the speed of response between individual hydrazine MAOIs.

Another aspect of response also deserves emphasis. In clinical trials groups of patients are treated and the mean speed of response recorded. This gives the mistaken impression of *gradual* improvement in clinical symptoms. Response to a monoamine oxidase inhibitor is rarely like this; a sudden and dramatic change in mood and other symptoms takes place within 24 h. The reasons for this are not known and are certainly not related to parameters such as extent of MAO inhibition in platelets or other structures, which are maximal long before clinical response occurs. It seems that a 'switch mechanism' in the brain must be operating to produce such a qualitative change in such a short time. This view is favoured by the similar dramatic onset of suppression of rapid eye movement (REM) sleep in patients treated with MAOIs. The change from about 20 per cent to 100 per cent suppression occurs within 24 h and coincides with the dramatic change in mood (Dunleavy and Oswald, 1973).

In practical terms this means that the clinician and patient should not despair if after 2–3 weeks of treatment there is no vestige of improvement. The patient should be reassured that this is a common occurrence and that they should continue in the same dosage to ensure that later response is not jeopardized. Poor compliance with tricyclic depressants in general practice has been highlighted by Johnson (1981) and is likely to be even lower in patients taking MAOIs as the delay in response may be longer than with tricyclic antidepressants. The doctor is the best guardian against poor compliance but may sometimes falter when there is delay in response. In my clinical practice I treat patients with tranylcypromine for up to three weeks and up to seven weeks with hydrazine MAOIs before abandoning them as ineffective. In short, the advice is 'do not give up too soon'.

Maintenance therapy

It is very satisfying for patient and clinician to see a marked therapeutic response with any treatment, but it is perhaps even greater with MAOIs as the response is often so unexpected. When it has been achieved one is very reluctant to do anything which might reverse it. Unfortunately, there is no published evidence to indicate either the duration of maintenance therapy or the appropriate dose. In the absence of data many extrapolate from the evidence at least six months' maintenance therapy with tricyclic antidepressants after relief of depressive symptoms (Mindham, Howland and Shepherd, 1973), although this is not really justified.

Nevertheless there is considerable anecdotal evidence that relapse is frequent if an MAOI is stopped within a few weeks of response being achieved (Sargant and Slater, 1962; Lipsedge et al., 1973; Solyom et al., 1973) and even when withdrawal takes place after several months relapse is not uncommon (Tyrer and Steinberg, 1975). In a recent (non-blind) study of the incidence of relapse and withdrawal phenomena after chronic consumption of MAOI, phenelzine and tricyclic antidepressants, the patients on phenelzine had a significantly greater incidence of symptoms on withdrawal than those taking tricyclic antidepressants (Tyrer, 1982).

This suggests that MAOIs may produce a form of mild dependence similar to that occurring with benzodiazepines. Tolerance and an increase in dosage to maintain pharmacological effects is rare but patients have difficulty in stopping their medication because of withdrawal symptoms. There is an alternative explanation; that the conditions that are treated with MAOIs tend to be chronic neurotic disorders so that relapse occurs on drug withdrawal because of a return of symptoms. Whatever the explanation the possibility of dependence must be taken into account before prescribing a MAOI.

When clinical response has occurred it is common to reduce the dose of the MAOI by about one-third at some point in the next three months. This could be regarded as the start of maintenance therapy. It is good policy to attempt a prediction of the duration of maintenance treatment and to try and keep to it. The psychiatrist's work is far from done at this stage even though the patient may have no symptoms. I usually fix on a time between 6 and 12 months of treatment but this depends on many other factors, including the progress of behaviour therapy in phobic disorders and the duration of illness before treatment with the MAOI. Because there have been more

instances of true pharmacological dependence with tranylcypromine than with hydrazine MAOIs it is advisable to keep the duration of tranylcypromine treatment as short
as possible. Clearly there will be instances in which the possibilities of dependence
will be considered acceptable and long-term therapy becomes the lesser of two evils.

After maintenance therapy is completed it is probably preferable to reduce MAOIs
gradually, even though abrupt cessation of treatment does not lead to any sudden
pharmacological changes. Because all the marketed hydrazine MAOIs are 'suicide
inhibitors' (i.e. they irreversibly inhibit monoamine oxidase) normal levels of
monoamine oxidase take several weeks to be regained as they are dependent on the
synthesis of new enzyme. Tranylcypromine, a non-hydrazine drug, produces partially
reversible MAO inhibition and levels of enzyme return to normal more rapidly.
Dietary restrictions need to be continued for at least four weeks after stopping long-
term treatment with a hydrazine MAOI and at least two weeks after stopping
tranylcypromine. Just as patients may dramatically improve after a latent period of
2–6 weeks when starting therapy, they may relapse just as dramatically several weeks
after stopping the drug. In an individual subject the timing of response may predict the
time of relapse (*Figure 9.2*). Reducing the drugs gradually should help to avoid such
dramatic changes. Occasionally patients may only remain well when taking a small
dose of the drug, often so low that MAO inhibition may be negligible. Some patients I
have treated have reduced their dosage to as little as 10 mg of isocarboxazid on
alternate days but cannot reduce further without a return of symptoms. Although this
may only reflect psychological dependence it could be a manifestation of pharmacodynamic effects unrelated to monoamine oxidase inhibition .

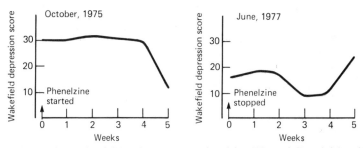

Figure 9.2 Example of delayed response to phenelzine (45 mg·d^{-1}) and delayed relapse on withdrawal
in the same patient

Unwanted effects

MAOIs are probably better known for their unwanted effects than their therapeutic
ones. This is because their unwanted effects are somewhat unusual and, in the
phraseology of journalism, 'make good copy' because they illustrate

(1) that a little learning is a dangerous thing in psychopharmacology,
(2) that knowledge of pharmacology can often predict unwanted effects before they
    happen, and
(3) doctors should always be receptive to the unusual when detecting unwanted effects
    of a drug.

Unwanted effects of MAOIs are best separated into those that are due to interaction
with foodstuffs and those that are due to the drugs alone.

Interaction with foodstuffs

Monoamine oxidase inhibitors were in clinical use for five years before it was recognized that they could produce hypertensive crises when taken with certain foods (Blackwell, 1963). The offending substance in the foods was the pressor amine, tyramine, which enters the systemic circulation if not inactivated by endogenous MAO, leading to a sudden rise in blood pressure. The first symptom is headache, usually sudden and localized to the temporal or occipital regions. Sweating, pallor, stiff neck, chest pains and palpitations may follow, and in a small proportion of patients there are cerebral haemorrhages that may be fatal.

Although this pharmacological interaction was predictable from the knowledge available at the time monoamine oxidase inhibitors were introduced to clinical practice (Blackwell *et al.*, 1967) it was not anticipated. Even in the early testing of iproniazid in the treatment of tuberculosis it was realized that hypertensive crises could occur (Ogilvie, 1955) although the association with food was first made by a pharmacist, Rowe, and followed up by a pharmaceutical representative and a psychiatrist (Samuel and Blackwell, 1968). Since the interaction was discovered all patients taking MAOIs are issued with a card giving a list of foods (and drugs) that should not be consumed while they are taking MAOIs (*Figure 9.3*). Over the years the number of prohibited foods has oscillated greatly, largely related to the level of acceptance of MAOIs as therapeutic agents rather than to any advance in pharmacological knowledge. It is now known that dopamine and tyramine are the important pressor amines that must be avoided by patients taking MAOIs and whether foodstuffs are acceptable is dependent on dopamine and tyramine content (*Table 9.2*).

Only foods containing high concentrations of tyramine and dopamine are absolutely contraindicated with MAOIs. Thus, in general, the smellier a cheese the higher its tyramine content and the more potent its interaction, although some cheeses,

TREATMENT CARD

Carry this card with you at all times. Show it to any doctor who may treat you other than the doctor who prescribed this medicine, and to your dentist if you require dental treatment.

INSTRUCTIONS TO PATIENTS

Please read carefully

While taking this medicine and for 10 days after your treatment finishes you must observe the following simple instructions:–

1 Do not eat CHEESE, PICKLED HERRING OR BROAD BEAN PODS.

2 Do not eat or drink BOVRIL, OXO, MARMITE or ANY SIMILAR MEAT OR YEAST EXTRACT.

3 Do not take any other MEDICINES (including tablets, capsules, nose drops, inhalations or suppositories) whether purchased by you or previously prescribed by your doctor, without first consulting him.

   NB   *Cough and cold cures, pain relievers and tonics are medicines.*

4 Drink ALCOHOL only in moderation and avoid CHIANTI WINE completely.

Report any severe symptoms to your doctor and follow any other advice given by him.

Prepared by The Pharmaceutical Society and the British Medical Association on behalf of the Health Departments of the United Kingdom.

11530/1963 R16S 558905 250m 11/77 AG 3640/4

Figure 9.3 Diet and drug warning card issued to patients taking MAOIs

TABLE 9.2 Tyramine and dopamine content of foods and recommendation concerning consumption in patients taking monoamine oxidase inhibitors

Foodstuff	Tyramine content	Dopamine content	Avoidance in patients on MAOIs
Cheese			
Stilton	High	—	Absolute
Emmenthal	Moderate	—	Absolute
Camembert	Low	—	Recommended
Cheddar	Low–high	—	Absolute
Cottage	Very low	—	Nil
Pickled herring	Very high	—	Absolute
Caviar	Moderate	—	Recommended
Chianti wine	Moderate	—	Recommended
Port	Very low	—	Nil
Seasoned game	Moderate	—	Recommended
Chicken and beef liver	Low	—	Quantities not important unless large
Bovril, Oxo	Moderate	—	Absolute
Marmite	Low	—	Recommended
Broad beans	—	Low	Recommended
Broad bean pods	—	High	Absolute

such as Cheddar, show tremendous variation in tyramine content depending on maturity. Similar variation is shown with yeast and meat extracts (Blackwell, Marley and Taylor, 1965). Broad bean pods have a very high dopamine content and are also contraindicated with MAOIs. With other foodstuffs the dangers are much less and some clinicians may allow patients the option of taking them in small amounts. These now include Marmite (which has had its tyramine content reduced by the manufacturers in recent years), Chianti and other fortified wines, caviar and seasoned game. In fact, the foods that should be completely avoided are very few. In the UK the forbidden foods seldom constitute more than a small fraction of the total diet but in some countries, such as Norway and Sweden, they are more important. (It may be no coincidence that in Norway and Sweden MAOIs are rarely prescribed.)

Some other foods have crept on to the forbidden list in recent years because of adverse clinical reports. Without exception they have very low tyramine and dopamine content and are highly unlikely to be associated with untoward reactions. They include bananas, red wine, port, sherry and beer, yoghurt, chocolate and avocado pears. Commercial brands of these products are safe, but occasionally home-made wines, beers and yoghurt may achieve a higher tyramine content and should be avoided.

It is interesting that before the adverse interactions with foodstuffs were recognized many patients took them together with MAOIs with no ill effects (Blackwell, Marley and Taylor, 1965). One possible reason for this was that tyramine (and dopamine) might be metabolized by other pathways, particularly sulphate conjugation. Investigation of patients who have had no reactions despite taking high tyramine foods and those who have experienced reactions has showed no difference between their tyramine-conjugating abilities (Bonham Carter, 1974). It is therefore unlikely that conjugation of tyramine is an important metabolic pathway and so yet another attempt to separate the adverse effects of MAOIs from their clinical ones has failed. Indeed, the latest view is that a potential 'cheese-reaction' is not only a necessary accompaniment to MAOI therapy but may be the important pharmacological factor associated with response (Sandler, 1981).

Unwanted effects due to drugs alone

MOOD DISORDER

MAOIs have frequently been implicated as a cause of iatrogenic mania and in this respect are similar to the tricyclic antidepressants. This is a difficult subject to investigate as mood swings are part of the natural history of most depressive disorders and can occur independently of drug treatment. Nevertheless, the known energizing properties of MAOIs make them highly suspect and when patients on them become overactive and show elevated mood it is wise to stop the MAOIs immediately. It is difficult to assess the incidence of mania but in 168 patients with depressive, phobic or anxiety neuroses treated with phenelzine in personal practice manic disturbance has only occurred in three (1.8 per cent). If more severely depressed patients are treated, or if tranylcypromine is used, this figure is likely to be higher.

HEPATOTOXICITY

The first MAOI to be used in clinical practice, iproniazid, was reported to produce hepatocellular jaundice, sometimes fatally, soon after its introduction (Pare, 1964). Other hydrazine MAOIs may also produce hepatocellular jaundice, and one, pheniprazine, was withdrawn from clinical use because of this danger. Non-hydrazine MAOIs do not carry this risk. Because the hepatocellular jaundice produced by drugs is histologically and clinically similar to that of infectious hepatitis there have been suggestions that the MAOIs have been unfairly blamed for causing jaundice of viral origin (Sargant, 1963a).

Certainly the incidence of jaundice with phenelzine and isocarboxazid is extremely low and even laboratory evidence of hepatic toxicity from raised liver enzymes is uncommon. Nevertheless it is wise to avoid treatments with MAOIs in patients with known liver disease and to check liver enzyme levels at regular intervals in patients who have either had liver disease in the past or are currently at risk (e.g. those with drinking problems).

OTHER UNWANTED EFFECTS

Insomnia is a frequent complaint in patients taking MAOIs. This is to be expected with drugs that have energizing properties and the problems can be partially compensated by taking the drug in twice daily dosage in the morning and at noon. Curiously, a small percentage of patients develop the opposite problem of drowsiness when on MAOIs and prefer to take their drugs in a single night time dose. Ten (6 per cent) of the 168 patients treated with phenelzine in my practice came into this group and rapidly lost their drowsiness when phenelzine was withdrawn.

Hypertensive crises may sometimes develop in the absence of drug or food interactions. They are more common with tranylcypromine but in recent years have been reported much less frequently than during the decade of alarm between 1960 and 1970. Skin rashes are sometimes found and a lupus-like eruption has been reported (Swartz, 1978). Dizziness is also a fairly common symptom, probably due in most cases to postural hypotension, and the largely anticholinergic side effects of dry mouth, constipation, delay in micturition and ejaculation are not uncommon. Indeed, MAOIs have sometimes been suggested as a treatment for premature ejaculation because of this property. Oedema is an unusual unwanted effect (Dunleavy, 1977) which may misleadingly be diagnosed as cardiac in origin. It affects the arms and legs mainly and, less commonly, the face. Although it can be compensated by the administration of a diuretic it is better to stop the MAOI. The incidence of oedema with phenelzine was 2.4 per cent in the 168 patients personally studied.

Frank addiction has occasionally been reported with the MAOIs. Patients exceed the recommended dose several fold in order to get the stimulant action of the drug, tolerance develops and on stopping the drug there are severe withdrawal symptoms (Le Gassicke, 1963; Pitt, 1974; Ben-Arie and George, 1979). Addiction has been reported more frequently with tranylcypromine than with hydrazine MAOIs. In view of the amphetamine-like properties of tranylcypromine this is not unexpected and in some respects it is surprising that addiction is not more common. The relatively long delay between ingestion of the drug and therapeutic response may be an important preventative factor (Tyrer, 1976).

Drug interactions

SYMPATHOMIMETIC AMINES

There has been some confusion over the interactions between the sympathomimetic amines and MAOIs. Early reports suggested that all amines were dangerous when combined with MAOIs and in 1966 the Committee on Safety of Drugs produced a warning list that included adrenaline and noradrenaline. This was a mistake; it has been shown clearly that adrenaline and noradrenaline do not interact with MAOIs (Elis et al., 1967; Boakes et al., 1973), although their pressor effects are potentiated by tricyclic antidepressants. Indirectly acting sympathomimetics are all dangerous when given to patients treated with MAOIs as their metabolism is inhibited, so prolonging their elimination half-life, and as MAOIs also increase the amount of noradrenaline at peripheral nerve endings the administration of sympathomimetic amines leads to a sudden increase in blood pressure by two independent mechanisms (Stockley, 1973). These hypertensive reactions are even more serious than the interactions between MAOIs and foodstuffs and fatalities are not uncommon. The main amines implicated are those in nasal decongestants and bronchial dilators such as pseudoephedrine, phenylephrine, phenylpropanolamine and ephedrine. The appetite suppressants, fenfluramine and phentermine should also be included in this group. Some of these drugs may be dispensed as nasal or eye drops and in this form are still potentially dangerous. Many of these drugs may be present in preparations that can be bought over the counter at any chemists without a prescription and so it is worth stressing to all patients on MAOIs that drugs are still drugs no matter how they are obtained. Amphetamine and methylamphetamine are also potentially fatal in combination with MAOIs (Lloyd and Walker, 1965) and any patient suspected of illegal drug use should not be prescribed MAOIs. Predictably, levodopa is also liable to produce hypertensive reactions when given with MAOIs (Hunter et al., 1970) and should be avoided.

TREATMENT OF HYPERTENSIVE REACTIONS

The specific antidote to hypertensive crises due to drug and food interactions with MAOIs is an alpha-adrenergic blocking drug such as phentolamine mesylate. This has little use in the routine treatment of hypertension but when given intravenously reverses the increase in peripheral resistance that is mainly responsible for the rise in blood pressure. Between 5 and 10 mg given by intravenous injection reverses the rise in blood pressure within minutes, although further injections may be necessary later. If phentolamine (or the other potent alpha-adrenergic blocking drug, phenoxyben-zamine) is not available a phenothiazine such as chlorpromazine, which also has alpha-adrenergic blocking properties, may be given intramuscularly in a dose of 50 to 150 mg.

OPIATES

The effects of opiate analgesics (methadone, morphine and particularly pethidine) may be greatly potentiated in patients on MAOIs. As mentioned earlier this is likely to be a pharmacokinetic effect through the inhibition of liver enzymes responsible for the metabolism of the opiates. Only a small proportion of patients show marked potentiation of drug effects. By giving a test dose of one-tenth or one-twentieth of the intended therapeutic dose of the opiate these susceptible patients can be identified (Churchill-Davidson, 1965; Evans-Prosser, 1968), and compensated by gradual increase of dosage to therapeutic levels.

The effects of barbiturates and oral hypoglycaemic drugs may also be potentiated in patients on MAOIs but not to the same extent as with opiates. In most instances a small revision in dosage will be the only action necessary. The effects of chloral hydrate and local anaesthetic agents may also be marginally increased in patients taking MAOIs by a similar mechanism but with these drugs it is of doubtful clinical significance. Patients can be reassured that conventional analgesics (e.g. aspirin, paracetamol) are safe provided they are not taken in combination with an opiate. It is usually advisable to avoid analgesic preparations containing codeine although many patients I have treated report they have taken codeine with complete impunity.

COMBINED ANTIDEPRESSANT THERAPY

During the 1960s, when the hazardous interactions of MAOIs were first reported, a combination of MAOIs and tricyclic antidepressants came in for critical scrutiny. Nine deaths had been reported from the combination (Ananth and Luchins, 1977) but none had definite evidence of hypertensive crises, and at least five followed overdoses. This and other evidence suggests that the combination is much safer than at first thought (Schuckit, Robins and Feighner, 1971) and vindicates those who defended the combination as safe from the beginning (Sargant, 1963a; Davies, 1963). Nevertheless, there are still dangers in the combination. If a tricyclic antidepressant is added to the drug regimen of a patient already taking a MAOI there is likely to be an increased incidence of unwanted effects, particularly postural hypotension and confusion, and wherever possible the combined drugs should be started simultaneously or the MAOI given after the patient has become stabilized on the tricyclic drug. In clinical practice it is more common to consider combined antidepressant therapy when a tricyclic drug has been relatively ineffective in the treatment of depression and so this order of prescription seldom poses problems. Some combinations of MAOIs and tricyclic antidepressants should be avoided. Because tranylcypromine is more prone to unwanted affects it is best to avoid it in combination with other antidepressants, particularly imipramine and clomipramine, and no account should parenteral antidepressants be given with MAOIs. Phenelzine is best combined with one of the amitriptyline group but can be given safely with the newer antidepressants, mianserin, maprotiline and nomifensine.

The list of potential drug interactions between MAOIs and other drugs is given in *Table 9.3* and represents an amplified form of the restrictions given to patients in the warning cards issued on the first occasion an MAOI is given. It is better to have a supply of these cards available to give to the patient rather than relying on the chemist or the pharmacy to give the warning card with the first prescription. This enables the doctor to go over the list with the patient before prescription so that any misconceptions can be sorted out. Some patients, for example, are initially reluctant to eat any form of meat when taking MAOIs or they think that even the natural gravy from cooked meat is a 'meat extract' and potentially dangerous.

TABLE 9.3 Drug interactions with monoamine oxidase inhibitors

Drug class	Comments
Indirectly acting sympathomimetic amines (e.g. phenylephrine, amphetamines, phenylpropanolamine)	Absolutely contraindicated
Directly acting sympathomimetic amines (e.g. adrenaline, noradrenaline)	Safe to use with MAOIs
Opiates (e.g. pethidine)	Usually contraindicated, but potentiation can be compensated by initial test doses (Evans-Prosser, 1968)
Levodopa	Absolutely contraindicated
Tricyclic antidepressants Newer antidepressants	May be used together provided that MAOI is not given first
Barbiturates Oral hypoglycaemic drugs (e.g. chlorpropamide, tolbutamide)	Care needed when given with MAOIs because of potentiation of drug effects

Individual monoamine oxidase inhibitors

Hydrazine MAOIs

IPRONIAZID

Iproniazid was the first MAOI to be introduced to psychiatry and was responsible for the early reports of antidepressant efficacy (*Figure 9.4*) (Crane, 1957; Loomer, Saunders and Kline, 1957). Its hepatotoxic effects (Pare, 1964) led to its gradual loss of popularity and it is now rarely prescribed. It has been shown to be effective in the treatment of phobias (Lipsedge *et al.*, 1973) and there is no doubt that it is an effective

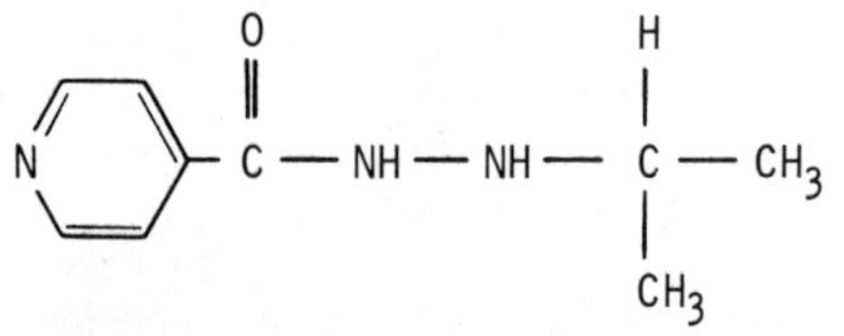

Figure 9.4 Iproniazid

antidepressant, probably the most powerful of the MAOI series. Its risks, unfortunately, are also considerable and its use is likely to remain very limited.

PHENELZINE

Phenelzine is now the most commonly used hydrazine MAOI and is the source of most recent clinical studies (Figure 9.5). It is a relatively simple molecule and pharmacodynamically lies in the middle range of both efficacy and dangers (Table 9.4). It therefore tends to be the preferred MAOI of those who want an effective drug that is not associated with any unpredictable dangers. It has been reported to produce hypertensive reactions with foodstuffs but no fatalities have occurred when the food and the drug have been taken in normal dosage and reactions are much less common than with tranylcypromine. In the original series described by Blackwell (1963), out of 12 hypertensive reactions 11 occurred with tranylcypromine and only one with phenelzine, despite very similar prescribing figures for each drug in the hospitals concerned. The effectiveness of phenelzine in depressive, phobic and anxiety disorders has already been mentioned. Because phenelzine is the best documented MAOI one frequently has to generalize from its studies to MAOIs as a group. It seems reasonable to do this for other hydrazine MAOIs but not for tranylcypromine.

The effects of differential dosage have also been described. In most instances it is reasonable to start at a dosage of 15 mg morning and noon, increasing to 60–75 mg daily over the next few weeks with the understanding that clinical response is likely to be more rapid on the higher dosage. In the few patients who complain of drowsiness the total dose may be given at night. If there has been no improvement after six or eight weeks it is probably better to stop treatment rather than change to another MAOI or to add another antidepressant because of the likelihood of unwanted effects. It is

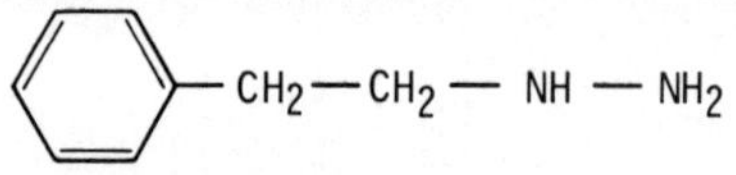

Figure 9.5 Phenelzine

TABLE 9.4 Summary of differences between MAOIs

Drug	Efficacy	Interaction risk	Unwanted effects
Iproniazid	High	High	Very serious
Tranylcypromine	High	High	Serious
Phenelzine	Moderate	Moderate	Moderate
Isocarboxazid	Fair	Low	Low

important to realize that even if phenelzine is stopped the effects of MAO inhibition persists for several weeks and care must be taken not to give another drug known to produce dangerous interactions with MAOIs for up to four weeks afterwards.

ISOCARBOXAZID

Isocarboxazid is in many respects a weaker form of phenelzine, although its relative freedom from unwanted effects and dangerous interactions makes it a preferable alternative in some patients (*Figure 9.6*). It should be prescribed in a similar way to phenelzine, beginning with a dose of 10 mg twice daily and increasing to 40–60 mg daily if necessary over the ensuing four weeks. Because it has lower energizing properties than phenelzine it has less impact on sleep and it is not too important to prescribe the last dose early in the day.

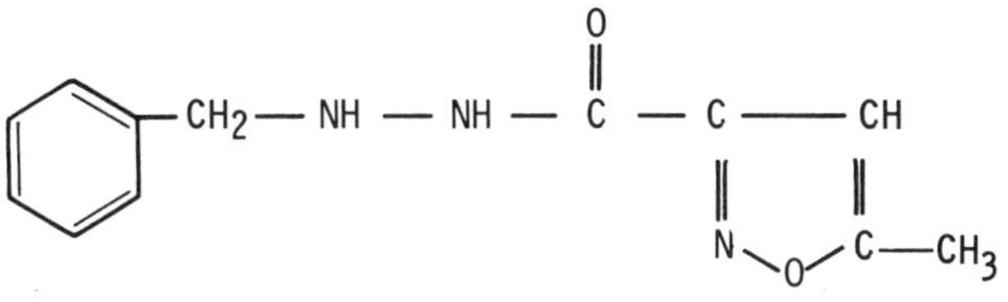

Figure 9.6 Isocarboxazid

Because isocarboxazid has a lower incidence of unwanted effects than other MAOIs it may sometimes be appropriate to change from another MAOI to isocarboxazid during maintenance therapy if side effects are particularly troublesome. I have found this helpful in cases of iatrogenic hypomania, oedema, insomnia and constipation with phenelzine or tranylcypromine.

TRANYLCYPROMINE

Tranylcypromine is the only non-hydrazine MAOI currently marketed in psychiatry (*Figure 9.7*), although pargyline (Eutonyl) is another non-hydrazine MAOI used for the treatment of resistant hypertension. Tranylcypromine also has a similar molecule that is structurally similar to amphetamines (p. 314). This appears to confirm greater stimulant properties to the drug and it is the MAOI that is most like amphetamine in its pharmacological effects. It therefore has greater euphoriant and antidepressant effects than phenelzine and isocarboxazid and is more prone to dependence. Initial dosage is 10 mg once or twice daily, increasing up to 60 mg daily with the last dose of the day taken no later than 4 pm. Tranylcypromine has been compared with tricyclic antidepressants and found to be similar in efficacy (Hutchinson and Smedberg, 1963; Spear, Hall and Stirland, 1964) although there are no comparative studies of MAOIs suggesting that tranylcypromine is superior to the others in antidepressant effects.

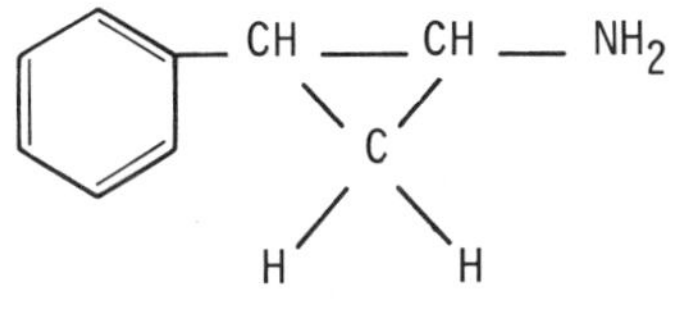

Figure 9.7 Tranylcypromine

Tranylcypromine has not been specifically tested for benefit in phobic and anxiety states although from personal experience it appears to have similar actions to the hydrazine MAOIs. Its speed of action is more rapid than the hydrazines and it is seldom worthwhile persisting with treatment if improvement has not occurred after 3–4 weeks. Because of the dangers of dependence it is best to limit prescription to a few months wherever possible.

Other MAOIs

Mebanazine and nialamide were marketed until recently in the UK. They have similar actions to other MAOIs but are less effective and have gradually become redundant. The selective monoamine oxidase inhibitors have already been mentioned. Clorgyline preferentially inhibits MAO-A and deprenyl only inhibits MAO-B. Neither is marketed for clinical use in psychiatry although they are interesting and important drugs in research studies.

Main clinical indications for MAOIs

It is not easy to summarize the clinical indications for MAOIs because they are far from agreed. They have a spectrum of pharmacodynamic activity that is unique and which has potential application in anxiety states, phobic disorders, hypochondriacal and depressive neurosis, obsessional neurosis and, possibly, more severe depressive illness. Klein (1976, 1981) also claims that MAOIs (and tricyclic antidepressants) specifically block panic attacks and so have a definite place in disorders characterized by recurrent panic. There are many other treatments available for these disorders and it is not easy to place the MAOIs in any order of preference. In general only the more resistant patients with severe symptoms should be considered for treatment, preferably after other approaches such as behaviour therapy have been tried. Because of their potential dangers and delay in clinical response MAOIs should seldom be given to patients who have a disorder which has lasted less than a month. Where their use should be considered more often is when patients have had a range of other treatments without any response and the clinician then feels that, as he has tried everything, nothing further can be done. MAOIs often do not come into the 'everything' and may prove invaluable. Unfortunately there are relatively few comparisons between MAOIs and non-pharmacological treatments for these disorders with the one exception of behaviour therapy for phobias, in which MAOIs are of equivalent efficacy (Solyom *et al.*, 1973; Lipsedge *et al.*, 1973). Further comparisons are needed.

Combined therapy with MAOIs

COMBINED ANTIDEPRESSANTS

Although the combination of MAOIs and tricyclics (or newer) antidepressants may be safer than originally thought its use can only be justified if the combination is demonstrably better than MAOIs or tricyclic antidepressants alone. The evidence for this does not exist. Although there is a general impression from clinical studies that refractory cases of depressive illness are responsive to combined treatment after antidepressants alone have failed (Sethna, 1974) the only controlled trial of combined antidepressants against MAOIs and a tricyclic antidepressant (trimipramine) given separately showed that trimipramine alone was significantly superior to the other treatment (Young, Lader and Hughes, 1979). As the patients in the study had only 'moderate' depressive illness and would not have been considered appropriate for combined antidepressant therapy in ordinary clinical practice it may be unfair to generalize from this population to the chronic resistant group who have failed to respond to other treatments before starting combined therapy (Tyrer, 1980). The position remains open and at present there are no definite clinical indications for combined antidepressant therapy.

OTHER COMBINATIONS

Combined therapy with a MAOI and L-tryptophan is also recommended for depressive illness. L-Tryptophan is converted to 5-hydroxytryptamine (5-HT) after absorption and by combining it with a MAOI cerebral amine levels are boosted. There is good evidence that the MAOI-tryptophan combination is more effective (or at least exerts it effects more rapidly) than a MAOI alone (Pare, 1963; Coppen, Shaw and Farrell, 1963; Glassman and Platman, 1969) but the combination does not appear to be commonly used.

The most common drug combination with MAOIs is that with a benzodiazepine such as diazepam. This is rational, particularly for the disorders in which anxiety is prominent. It may also help to preserve compliance during the long latent period between initial prescription and response. When reducing the drugs after maintenance therapy I have found it preferable to reduce and stop the benzodiazepine under cover of the MAOI as this seems to prevent or attenuate any withdrawal symptoms. The MAOI is then reduced gradually as mentioned earlier. Other combinations that have no specific clinical indications but which may be used safely are with beta-blocking drugs such as propranolol in somatic anxiety and with lithium in recurrent affective disorders. As a general rule, however, polypharmacy should be avoided with the MAOIs in view of their potential drug interactions.

Amine precursors

Although amine precursors are in no way related to the MAOIs they are a group of drugs that may also raise cerebral monoamine levels, by increasing input rather than inhibiting their breakdown. They are L-tryptophan, 5-hydroxytryptophan and levodopa and are therefore discussed in this chapter.

Pharmacology

L-Tryptophan is a precursor of 5-hydroxytryptamine (5-HT) and levodopa one of dopamine (*Figure 9.8*). It is therefore natural that they would be tested for antidepressant efficacy when the catecholamine hypothesis of depression was formulated. By giving L-tryptophan or levodopa, which are both readily absorbed and penetrate the blood–brain barrier, it was postulated that central 5-HT and dopamine levels would rise and thereby relieve the depressive disorder. Improvement is therefore dependent on both a relative deficiency of dopamine or 5-HT in the brain and that this deficiency is directly related to the depressive disturbance.

The Dutch psychiatrist, van Praag, has long championed the hypothesis that a significant proportion of depressed patients have central 5-HT deficiency and that

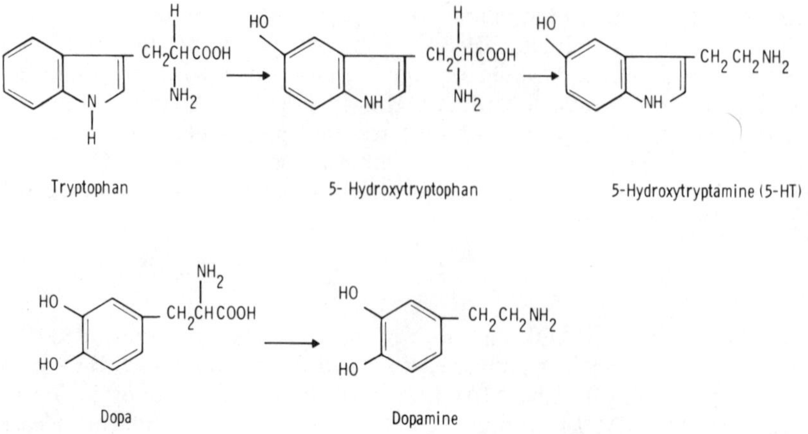

Figure 9.8

these patients will respond to treatment with amine precursors. He has identified these patients by the probenecid technique. This inhibits the transfer of the major metabolite of 5-HT, 5-hydroxyindole acetic acid (5-HIAA), and homovanillic acid, (HVA), the main metabolite of dopamine, from the brain to the bloodstream. 5-HIAA and HVA therefore accumulate in the brain and their levels can be used as a measure of their rate of synthesis. The probenecid test involves measurement of CSF 5-HIAA and HVA levels after a single dose of probenecid and clearly cannot be recommended as a routine clinical procedure. Nevertheless, in an important study, van Praag and his colleagues (1972) have shown that depressed patients with low rates of synthesis of 5-HIAA and HVA (i.e. with an inferred brain deficiency of 5-HT and dopamine) respond well to the precursor of 5-HT, 5-hydroxytryptophan (5-HTP), whereas those who have high rates of synthesis of 5-HIAA and HVA show little or no clinical response to 5-HTP.

This suggests that amine precursors will be valuable treatment in selected patients with depressive illness. It also suggests that other amine precursors as well as 5-HTP would be beneficial as antidepressants but there are no pharmacological studies with L-tryptophan or levodopa supporting this action in the same way as 5-HTP. Åsberg and her colleagues (1973) have found a bimodal distribution of 5-HIAA in the CSF of depressed patients, which supports van Praag's contention that a certain proportion of depressed patients have reduced central 5-HT levels.

The giving of L-tryptophan, 5-HTP or levodopa is dependent on their crossing the blood–brain barrier readily. There is reasonable evidence that 5-HTP does cross readily as an increase in 5-HIAA levels follows administration (van Praag and Korf, 1975) and the same probably occurs with L-tryptophan and levodopa but the evidence is not so clear.

Clinical use

L-TRYPTOPHAN

L-Tryptophan is the most frequently used amine precursor and is marketed as an antidepressant in a daily dose of 3–6 g. The tablets are large and some patients find difficulty in swallowing them; the drug may also be given in powdered form in a chocolate-flavoured drink. The evidence for the antidepressant efficacy of tryptophan is very confusing for reasons that are far from clear. An early study suggested that it was at least as good as ECT in its antidepressant effects (Coppen *et al.*, 1967) but the patients were not randomly allocated to treatment and part of the control group was retrospectively obtained. Later studies have shown ECT to be unequivocally superior (Carroll, Mowbray and Davies, 1970; Herrington *et al.*, 1974), although the difference in efficacy only becomes fully apparent after 2–3 weeks of treatment.

Later studies have compared L-tryptophan with placebo and tricyclic antidepressants under double-blind conditions. The results have been variable, with some showing no superiority over placebo (Murphy *et al.*, 1974; Mendels *et al.*, 1975) and others suggesting that L-tryptophan is at least at the same level of efficacy as the tricyclic antidepressants (Herrington *et al.*, 1976; Rao and Braodhurst, 1976; Thomson *et al.*, 1982). The variability in these results is difficult to explain. Tryptophan appears to have been given in adequate dosage for a reasonable length of time in each of the studies and no common feature separates the positive findings from the negative ones.

On present evidence tryptophan cannot be regarded as having an established place in the treatment of affective disorders. If, however, easier techniques (either clinical or biochemical) become available to identify these depressed patients with a functional deficiency of 5-HT, it may then have a recommended use. However, in combination with other drugs tryptophan appears to have definite merit (*see below*).

5-HYDROXYTRYPTOPHAN (5-HTP)

5-HTP has not been adequately evaluated as an antidepressant but there are some preliminary findings that are encouraging (Takahashi, Kondo and Kato, 1975; van Praag and Korf, 1975). From pharmacological evidence 5-HTP would appear to be the most promising of the amine precursors for treating depression but it is not commercially available.

LEVODOPA

Levodopa might be expected to have antidepressant efficacy following the hypothesis that some depressions are due to central dopamine deficiency. In fact levodopa is singularly ineffective as an antidepressant although it may occasionally induce mania in patients with bipolar affective psychosis (Murphy, 1971; Mendels *et al.*, 1975). These negative findings emphasize again that the catecholamine hypothesis of depression is inadequate in explaining much of the pharmacology of antidepressant drugs. The main clinical uses of levodopa are in the treatment of extrapyramidal disorders discussed in Chapter 5.

PYRIDOXINE

Pyridoxine (vitamin B6) is not an amine precursor but is involved in the metabolism of tryptophan. It has been postulated that the depressive symptoms occurring during therapy with oral contraceptives are due to 5-HT deficiency (Winston, 1969) and that this can be reversed by giving pyridoxine. One study supports this hypothesis (Adams *et al.*, 1973) but it stands alone. There is no other evidence that pyridoxine has antidepressant properties and at present it cannot be recommended.

Combined therapy with amine precursors and other drugs

TRICYCLIC ANTIDEPRESSANTS AND L-TRYPTOPHAN

L-Tryptophan, on theoretical grounds, might be expected to potentiate the effects of tricyclic antidepressants. The antidepressant effects of clomipramine have been reported to be enhanced by the addition of L-tryptophan (Wålinder *et al.*, 1976). Clomipramine is a potent 5-HT re-uptake inhibitor and it is pharmacologically plausible that L-tryptophan (and 5-HTP) would enhance its efficacy but the 'pure' 5-HT re-uptake inhibitor, zimelidine, does not appear to have its antidepressant effects potentiated by tryptophan in the same way (Wålinder, Carlsson and Persson, 1981). Tryptophan has also been used in combination with other tricyclic antidepressants. In one recent study L-tryptophan in a daily dose of 3 g was compared with L-tryptophan and amitriptyline (150 mg daily) and placebo in depressed patients in general practice (Thomson *et al.*, 1982). All the active treatments were significantly superior to placebo and the combination was slightly superior to the other active treatments alone, but the superiority only became manifest between the eighth and twelfth weeks of treatment.

COMBINATION THERAPY WITH 5-HYDROXYTRYPTOPHAN

5-HTP appears to potentiate the antidepressant effects of clomipramine (van Praag *et al.*, 1974). There is also some evidence that the selective monamine oxidase inhibitor, L-deprenyl, which has no antidepressant efficacy, may exert antidepressant effects when combined with 5-HTP (Mendelwicz and Youdim, 1980). If 5-HTP was accepted as having antidepressant effects through its conversion to 5-HT the inhibition of MAO-B by L-deprenyl would aid this by allowing 5-HT to accumulate. This work needs following up and at present neither drug is commercially available.

AMINE PRECURSORS AND MAOIS (*see* p. 271)

Unwanted effects
Tryptophan is a naturally occurring amino acid present in largest concentrations in high protein foods such as beef steak. It is therefore predictably free of adverse effects and even when given in doses as large as 8 g intravenously is free of untoward effects with the exception of mild drowsiness (Greenwood *et al.*, 1974). An increase in sexual arousal has been reported (Smith and Prockop, 1962); this has not been confirmed by others and, even if present, this effect may not always be unwanted. The unwanted effects of MAOIs may be potentiated by tryptophan and care should be taken not to start patients on full dosage immediately when using combined therapy.

Summary

Amine precursors are valuable drugs in psychopharmacological research and will continue to remain so. Their value as antidepressants remains to be established but there is reasonable evidence that L-tryptophan and 5-hydroxytryptophan have antidepressant activity although levodopa does not. On current evidence their most appropriate use is in combination with tricyclic antidepressants and monoamine oxidase inhibitors.

References

ADAMS, P. W., WYNN, Y., ROSE, D. P., SEED, M., FOLKARD, J. and STRONG, R. Effect of pyridoxine hydrochloride (Vitamin B6) upon depression associated with oral contraception, *Lancet* **1**, 897–904 (1973)

ANANTH, J. and LUCHINS, D. A review of combined tricyclic and MAOI therapy, *Comprehensive Psychiatry* **18**, 221–230 (1977)

ANNESLEY, P. T. Nardil response in a chronic obsessive compulsive, *British Journal of Psychiatry* **115**, 748 (1969)

ÅSBERG, M., BERTILSSON, L., TUCK, D., CRONHOLM, B. and SJÖQVIST, F. Indoleamine metabolites in the cerebrospinal fluid of depressed patients before and during treatment with nortriptyline, *Clinical Pharmacology and Therapeutics* **14**, 277–286 (1973)

ATKINSON, R. M. and DITMAN, K. S. Tranylcypromine: a review, *Clinical Pharmacology and Therapeutics* **6**, 631–655 (1965)

BATES, T. J. N. and DOUGLAS, A. D. M. A comparative trial of four monoamine oxidase inhibitors on chronic depressives, *Journal of Mental Sciences* **107**, 538–543 (1961)

BEN-ARIE, O. and GEORGE, G. C. W. A case of tranylcypromine (Parnate) addiction, *British Journal of Psychiatry* **135**, 273–274 (1979)

BIRKMAYER, W., RIEDERER, P., AMBROZI, L. and YOUDIM, M. B. H. Implications of combined treatment with Madopar and L-deprenil in Parkinson's disease, *Lancet* **1**, 439–443 (1977)

BLACKWELL, B. Hypertensive crisis due to monoamine oxidase inhibitors, *Lancet* **2**, 849–851 (1963)

BLACKWELL, B. Adverse effects of antidepressant drugs. Part 1, monoamine oxidase inhibitors and tricyclics, *Drugs* **21**, 201–219 (1981)

BLACKWELL, B., MARLEY, E. and RYLE, A. Hypertensive crisis associated with monoamine oxidase inhibitors, *Lancet* **1**, 722–723 (1964)

BLACKWELL, B., MARLEY, E. and TAYLOR, D. Effects of yeast extract after monoamine-oxidase inhibition, *Lancet* **1**, 1166 (1965)

BLACKWELL, B., MARLEY, E., PRICE, J. and TAYLOR, D. Hypertensive interactions between monoamine oxidase inhibitors and foodstuffs, *British Journal of Psychiatry* **113**, 349–365 (1967)

BONHAM CARTER, S. Tyramine conjugation defect and its identification. In *Colloquium on MAOI Therapy*, pp. 75–81, Dataspeed, London (1974)

BOAKES, A. J., LAURENCE, D. R., TEOH, P. C., BARAR, F. S. K., BENEDIKTER, L. T. and PRICHARD, B. N. C. Interactions between sympathomimetic amines and antidepressant agents in man, *British Medical Journal* **1**, 311–315 (1973)

BRODIE, B. B., PLETSCHER, A. and SHORE, P. A. Possible role of serotonin in brain function and in reserpine action, *Journal of Pharmacology* **116**, 9 (1956)

CARROLL, B. J., MOWBRAY, R. M. and DAVIES, B. M. Sequential comparison of L-tryptophan and ECT in severe depression, *Lancet* **1**, 967–969 (1970)

CHURCHILL-DAVIDSON, H. C. Anaesthesia and monoamine-oxidase inhibitors, *British Medical Journal* **1**, 520 (1965)

COLE, J. O. Therapeutic efficacy of antidepressant drugs, *Journal of the American Medical Association* **190**, 448–455 (1964)

COPPEN, A., SHAW, D. M. and FARRELL, J. P. Potentiation of the antidepressive effect of a monoamine oxidase inhibitor by tryptophan, *Lancet* **1**, 79–81 (1963)

COPPEN, A., SHAW, D. M., HERSBERG, B. and MAGGS, R. Tryptophan in the treatment of depression, *Lancet* **2**, 1178–1180 (1967)

CRANE, G. E. Iproniazid (Marsilid) phosphate, a therapeutic agent for mental disorders and debilitating diseases, *Psychiatric Research Reports* **8**, 142–152 (1957)

DAVIDSON, J., McLEOD, M. N. and BLUM, M. R. Acetylation phenotype, platelet monoamine oxidase inhibition and the effectiveness of phenelzine in depression, *American Journal of Psychiatry* **135**, 467–469 (1978)

DAVIES, E. B. Combining the antidepressant drugs, *Lancet* **2**, 781–782 (1963)

DONNELLY, C. H. and MURPHY, D. L. Substrate-related and inhibitor-related characteristics of human platelet monoamine oxidase, *Biochemical Pharmacology* **26**, 853–858 (1977)

DUNLEAVY, D. L. F. Phenelzine and oedema, *British Medical Journal* **1**, 1353 (1977)

DUNLEAVY, D. L. F. and OSWALD, I. Phenelzine, mood response and sleep, *Archives of General Psychiatry* **28**, 353–356 (1973)

ELIS, J., LAWRENCE, D. R., MATTIE, H. and PRICHARD, B. N. C. Modification by monoamine oxidase inhibitors of the effect of some sympathomimetics on blood pressure, *British Medical Journal* **2**, 75–78 (1967)

EVANS, D. A. P. An improved and simplified method of detecting the acetylator phenotype, *Journal of Medical Genetics* **6**, 405–407 (1969)

EVANS, D. A. P., DAVIDSON, K. and PRATT, R. T. C. The influence of acetylator phenotype on the effects of treating depression with phenelzine, *Clinical Pharmacology and Therapeutics* **6**, 430–435 (1965)

EVANS-PROSSER, C. D. G. The use of pethidine and morphine in the presence of monoamine oxidase inhibitor, *British Journal of Anaesthetics* **40**, 279–282 (1968)

GLASSMAN, A. H. and PLATMAN, S. R. Potentiation of a monoamine-oxidase inhibitor by tryptophan, *Journal of Psychiatric Research* 7, 83–88 (1969)

GREENBLATT, M., GROSSER, G. H. and WECHSLER, H. Differential response of hospitalized depressed patients to somatic therapy, *American Journal of Psychiatry* 120, 935–943 (1964)

GREENWOOD, M. H., FRIEDEL, J., BOND, A. J., CURZON, G. and LADER, M. H. The acute effects of intravenous infusion of L-tryptophan in normal subjects, *Clinical Pharmacology and Therapeutics* 16, 455–464 (1974)

HARE, E. H., DOMINIAN, J. and SHARPE, L. Phenelzine and dexamphetamine in depressive illness: a comparative trial, *British Medical Journal* 1, 9–12 (1962)

HARRIS, J. A. and ROBIN, A. A. A controlled trial of phenelzine in depressive reactions, *Journal of Mental Science* 106, 1432–1437 (1960)

HENDLEY, E. D. and SNYDER, S. H. Relationship between the action of monoamine oxidase inhibitors on the noradrenaline uptake system and their antidepressant efficacy, *Nature* 220, 1330–1331 (1968)

HERRINGTON, R. N., BRUCE, A., JOHNSTONE, E. C. and LADER, M. H. Comparative trial of L-tryptophan and ECT in severe depressive illness, *Lancet* 2, 731–734 (1974)

HERRINGTON, R., BRUCE, A., JOHNSTONE, E. and LADER, M. Comparative trial of L-tryptophan and amitriptyline in depressive illness, *Psychological Medicine* 6, 673–678 (1976)

HOLLISTER, L. E. *Clinical use of psychotherapeutic drugs*, Thomas, Springfield, Illinois (1973)

HORWITZ, D., LOVENBERG, W., ENGELMAN, K. and SJOERDSMA, A. Monoamine oxidase inhibitors, tyramine and cheese, *Journal of the American Medical Association* 188, 1108–1110 (1964)

HUNTER, K. R., BOAKES, A. J., LAURENCE, D. R. and STERN, G. M. Monoamine oxidase inhibitor and L-dopa, *British Medical Journal* 3, 388 (1970)

HUTCHINSON, J. T. and SMEDBERG, D. Treatment of depression: a comparative study of ECT and six drugs, *British Journal of Psychiatry* 109, 536–538 (1963)

ISBERG, R. S. A comparison of phenelzine and imipramine in an obsessive-compulsive patient, *American Journal of Psychiatry* 138, 1250–1251 (1981)

JAIN, V. K., SWINSON, R. P. and THOMAS, J. G. Phenelzine in obsessional neurosis, *British Journal of Psychiatry* 117, 237–238 (1970)

JARVIK, M. E. Drugs used in the treatment of psychiatric disorder. In *The Pharmacological Basis of Therapeutics* (Eds. L. S. GOODMAN and S. GILMAN), 4th edn, pp. 151–203, MacMillan, London (1970)

JENIKE, M. A. Rapid response of severe obsessive-compulsive disorder to tranylcypromine, *American Journal of Psychiatry* 138, 1249–1250 (1981)

JOHNSON, D. A. Depression: treatment compliance in general practice, *Acta Psychiatrica Scandinavica* 63, Suppl. 290, 447–453 (1981)

JOHNSTON, J. P. Some observations on a new inhibitor of monoamine oxidase in brain tissue, *Biochemical Pharmacology* 17, 1285–1297 (1968)

JOHNSTONE, E. C. The relationship between acetylator status and inhibition of monoamine oxidase excretion of free drug and antidepressant response in depressed patients on phenelzine, *Psychopharmacologia* 46, 289–294 (1976)

JOHNSTONE, E. C. and MARSH, W. Acetylator status and response to phenelzine in depressed patients, *Lancet* 1, 567–570 (1973)

KAUFMANN, J. S. Drug interaction involving psychotherapeutic agents. In *Drug Treatment of Mental Disorders* (Ed. L. L. SIMPSON), p. 302, Raven Press, New York (1976)

KELLY, D., GUIRGUIS, W., FROMMER, E., MITCHELL-HEGGS, N. and SARGANT, W. Treatment of phobic states with antidepressants: a retrospective study of 246 patients, *British Journal of Psychiatry* 116, 387–398 (1970)

KLEIN, D. F. Diagnosis of anxiety and differential use of antianxiety drugs. In *Drug Treatment of Mental Disorders* (Ed. L. L. SIMPSON), pp. 61–72, Raven Press, New York (1976)

KLEIN, D. F. Anxiety reconceptualized. In *Anxiety: New Research and Changing Concepts* (Eds. D. F. KLEIN and J. G. RABKIN), pp. 235–263, Raven Press, New York (1981)

LASCELLES, R. G. Atypical facial pain and depression, *British Journal of Psychiatry* 112, 651–659 (1966)

LE GASSICKE, J. Tranylcypromine, *Lancet* 1, 270 (1963)

LIPSEDGE, M. S., HAJIOFF, J., HUGGINS, P., NAPIER, L., PEARCE, J., PIKE, D. J. and RICH, M. The management of severe agoraphobia: a comparison of iproniazid and systematic desensitisation, *Psychopharmacologia* 32, 67–80 (1973)

LLOYD, J. T. and WALKER, D. R. H. Death after combined dexamphetamine and phenelzine, *British Medical Journal* 2, 168–169 (1965)

LOOMER, H. P., SAUNDERS, J. C. and KLINE, N. S. A clinical and pharmacodynamic evaluation of iproniazid as a psychic energiser, *Psychiatric Research Reports* 8, 129–141 (1957)

MARSHALL, E. F. The myth of phenelzine acetylation, *British Medical Journal* 2, 817 (1976)

MARSHALL, E. F., MOUNTJOY, C. Q., CAMPBELL, I. C., GARSIDE, R. F., LEITCH, I. M. and ROTH, M. The influence of acetylator phenotype on the outcome of treatment with phenelzine in a clinical trial, *British Journal of Clinical Pharmacology* **6**, 247–254 (1978)

MEDICAL RESEARCH COUNCIL. Report of Clinical Psychiatry Committee. Clinical trial of the treatment of depressive illness, *British Medical Journal* **1**, 881–886 (1965)

MENDELS, J., STINNETT, J. K., BURNS, D. and FRAZER, A. Amine precursors and depression, *Archives of General Psychiatry* **32**, 22–29 (1975)

MENDELWICZ, J. and YOUDIM, M. B. H. Antidepressant potentiation of 5-hydroxytryptophan by L-depronil in affective illness, *Journal of Affective Disorders* **2**, 137–146 (1980)

MINDHAM, R. H. S., HOWLAND, C. and SHEPHERD, M. An evaluation of continuation therapy with tricyclic antidepressants in depressive illness, *Psychological Medicine* **3**, 5–17 (1973)

MORGAN, M. H. and READ, A. E. Antidepressants and liver disease, *Gut* **13**, 697–701 (1972)

MOUNTJOY, C. Q., ROTH, M., GARSIDE, R. F. and LEITCH, I. M. A clinical trial of phenelzine in anxiety, depressive and phobic neuroses, *British Journal of Psychiatry* **131**, 486–492 (1977)

MURPHY, D. L. Regular induction of hypomania by L-dopa in bipolar manic-depressive patients, *Nature* **229**, 135–136 (1971)

MURPHY, D., BAKER, M. GOODWIN, F., MILLER, H., KOTIN, J. and BUNNEY, W. L-Tryptophan in affective disorders: indoleamine changes and differential clinical effects, *Psychopharmacologia* **34**, 11–20 (1974)

MURPHY, D. L., LIPPER, S., PICKAR, D., JIMERSON, D., COHEN, R. M., GARRICK, N. A., ALTERMAN, I. S. and CAMPBELL, I. C. Selective inhibition of monoamine oxidase Type A, clinical antidepressant and effects and metabolic changes in man. In *Monoamine Oxidase Inhibitors—The State of the Art* (Eds. M. B. H. YOUDIM and E. S. PAYKEL), pp. 189–205, John Wiley, Chichester (1981)

NIES, A. and ROBINSON, D. S. Comparison of clinical effects of amitriptyline and phenelzine treatment. In *Monoamine Oxidase Inhibitors. The State of the Art* (Eds. M. B. H. YOUDIM and E. S. PAYKEL), pp. 141–148, John Wiley, Chichester (1981)

OGILVIE, C. M. The treatment of pulmonary tuberculosis with iproniazid and isoniazid, *Quarterly Journal of Medicine* **24**, 175–189 (1955)

PARE, C. M. B. Potentiation of monoamine oxidase inhibitors by tryptophan, *Lancet* **2**, 527–528 (1963)

PARE, C. M. B. Toxicity of psychotropic drugs: Side-effects and toxic effects of antidepressants, *Proceedings of the Royal Society of Medicine* **57**, 757–778 (1964)

PARE, C. M. B. and SANDLER, M. A clinical and biochemical study of a trial of iproniazid in the treatment of depression, *Journal of Neurology, Neurosurgery and Psychiatry* **22**, 247–251 (1959)

PARE, C. M. B. and MACK, J. W. Differentiation of two genetically specific types of depression by the response to antidepressant drugs, *Journal of Medical Genetics* **8**, 306–309 (1971)

PARE, C. M. B., REES, L. and SAINSBURY, M. J. Differentiation of two genetically specific types of depression by the response to antidepressants, *Lancet* **2**, 1340–1343 (1962)

PAYKEL, E. S. Predictors of treatment response. In *Psychopharmacology of Affective Disorders* (Eds. E. S. PAYKEL and A. COPPEN), pp. 193–220, Oxford University Press, Oxford (1979)

PAYKEL, E. S., ROWAN, P. R., PARKER, R. R. and BHAT, A. V. Response to phenelzine and amitriptyline in sub-types of out-patient depression, *Archives of General Psychiatry* (in press) (1982b)

PAYKEL, E. S., WEST, P. S., ROWAN, P. R. and PARKER, R. R. Influence of acetylator phenotype on antidepressant effects of phenelzine, *British Journal of Psychiatry* **141**, 243–248 (1982a)

PITT, B. Withdrawal symptoms after stopping phenelzine? *British Medical Journal* **2**, 332 (1974)

POLLITT, J. and YOUNG, J. Anxiety states or masked depression? A study based on the action of monoamine oxidase inhibitors, *British Journal of Psychiatry* **119**, 143–149 (1971)

RAO, B. and BROADHURST, A. D. Tryptophan in depression, *British Medical Journal* **1**, 460 (1976)

RASKIN, A. Adverse reactions to phenelzine: result of a nine-hospital depression study, *Journal of Clinical Pharmacology* **12**, 22–25 (1972)

RAVARIS, C. L., NIES, A., ROBINSON, D. S., IVES, J. O., LAMBORN, K. R. and KORSON, L. A multiple dose, controlled study of phenelzine in depression-anxiety states, *Archives of General Psychiatry* **33**, 347–350 (1976)

REES, L. and DAVIES, B. A controlled trial of phenelzine (Nardil) in the treatment of severe depressive illness, *Journal of Mental Science* **107**, 560–566 (1961)

ROBINSON, D. S., NIES, A., RAVARIS, C. L. and LAMBORN, K. R. The monoamine oxidase inhibitor phenelzine, in the treatment of depressive-anxiety states: a controlled clinical trial, *Archives of General Psychiatry* **29**, 407–413 (1973)

ROBINSON, D. S., NIES, A., RAVARIS, C. L., IVES, J. O. and BARTLETT, D. Clinical pharmacology of phenelzine, *Archives of General Psychiatry* **35**, 629–635 (1978)

ROWAN, P. R., PAYKEL, E. S. and PARKER, R. R. Phenelzine and amitriptyline: effects on symptoms of neurotic depression, *British Journal of Psychiatry* (In press) (1982)

ROWAN, P. R., PAYKEL, E. S., WEST, P. S., RAO, B. M. and TAYLOR, C. N. Effects of phenelzine and acetylator phenotype, *Neuropharmacology* **20**, 1353–1354 (1981)

SAMUEL, G. and BLACKWELL, B. Monoamine oxidase inhibitor and cheese: a process of discovery, *Hospital Medicine*, 942–943 (1968)

SANDLER, M. Monoamine oxidase inhibitor efficacy in depression and the 'cheese effect', *Psychological Medicine* **11**, 455–458 (1981)

SARGANT, W. Drugs in the treatment of depression, *British Medical Journal* **1**, 225–227 (1961)

SARGANT, W. Antidepressant drug and liver damage, *British Medical Journal* **2**, 806 (1963a)

SARGANT, W. Combining the antidepressant drugs, *Lancet* ii, 634–635 (1963b)

SARGANT, W. and SLATER, E. *Introduction to physical methods of treatment in psychiatry*, 5th edn, Churchill Livingstone, Edinburgh (1962)

SARGANT, W. and DALLY, P. Treatment of anxiety states by antidepressant drugs, *British Medical Journal* **1**, 6–9 (1962)

SCHILDKRAUT, J. J. The catecholamine hypothesis of affective disorders: a review of supporting evidence, *American Journal of Psychiatry* **122**, 509–522 (1965)

SCHUCKIT, M., ROBINS, E. and FEIGHNER, J. Tricyclic antidepressants and monoamine oxidase inhibitors, *Archives of General Psychiatry* **24**, 509–514 (1971)

SETHNA, E. R. A study of refractory cases in depressive illnesses and their response to combined antidepressant treatment, *British Journal of Psychiatry* **124**, 265–272 (1974)

SHAW, D. The practical management of affective disorders, *British Journal of Psychiatry* **130**, 432–451 (1977)

SHEEHAN, D. V., BALLENGER, J. and JACOBSEN, G. Treatment of endogenous anxiety with phobic, hysterical and hypochondriacal symptoms, *Archives of General Psychiatry* **37**, 51–59 (1980)

SJÖQVIST, F. Psychotropic drugs (2): interaction between monoamine oxidase (MAO) inhibitors and other substances, *Proceedings of the Royal Society of Medicine* **58**, 967–978 (1965)

SMITH, B. and PROCKOP, D. J. CNS effects of ingestion of L-tryptophan by normal subjects, *New England Journal of Medicine* **267**, 1338–1341 (1962)

SOLYOM, L., HESELTINE, G. F. D., McCLURE, D. J., SOLYOM, C., LEDWIDGE, B. and STEINBERG, G. Behaviour therapy versus drug therapy in the treatment of phobic neurosis, *Canadian Psychiatrical Association Journal* **18**, 25–32 (1973)

SPEAR, F. G., HALL, P. and STIRLAND, J. D. A comparison of subjective responses to imipramine and tranylcypromine, *British Journal of Psychiatry* **110**, 53–55 (1964)

SPECTOR, S., HIRSH, C. W. and BRODIE, B. B. Association of behavioural effects of pargyline, a non-hydrazine MAO inhibitor with increase in brain norepinephrine, *International Journal of Neuropharmacology* **2**, 81–93 (1963)

STOCKLEY, I. H. Monoamine oxidase inhibitors. 1. Interactions with sympathomimetic amines, *Pharmaceutical Journal* **210**, 590–594 (1973)

SWARTZ, C. Lupus-like reaction to phenelzine, *Journal of the American Medical Association* **239**, 2693 (1978)

TAKAHASHI, S., KONDO, H. and KATO, M. Effect of L-5-hydroxytryptophan on brain monoamine metabolism and evaluation of its clinical effect in depressed patients, *Journal of Psychiatric Research* **12**, 177–187 (1975)

THOMSON, J., RANKIN, H., ASHCROFT, G. W., YATES, C. M., McQUEEN, J. K. and CUMMINGS, S. W. The treatment of depression in general practice: a comparison of L-tryptophan, amitriptyline and a combination of L-tryptophan and amitriptyline with placebo. *Psychological Medicine* (In press) (1982)

TILSTONE, W. J., MARGOT, P. and JOHNSTONE, E. C. Acetylation of phenelzine, *Psychopharmacology* **60**, 261–263 (1979)

TYRER, P. Towards rational therapy with mono-amine oxidase inhibitors, *British Journal of Psychiatry* **128**, 354–360 (1976)

TYRER, P. Clinical use of monoamine oxidase inhibitors. In *Psychopharmacology of Affective Disorders* (Eds. E. S. PAYKEL and A. COPPEN), pp. 159–178, Oxford University Press, Oxford (1979a)

TYRER, P. Anxiety States. In *Recent Advances in Clinical Psychiatry* (Ed. K. L. GRANVILLE-GROSSMAN) **3**, 161–183, Churchill Livingstone, Edinburgh (1979b)

TYRER, P. J. Combined antidepressant treatment, *British Medical Journal* **280**, 183 (1980)

TYRER, P., CANDY, J. and KELLY, D. A study of the clinical effects of phenelzine and placebo in the treatment of phobic anxiety, *Psychopharmacologia* **32**, 237–254 (1973)

TYRER, P. Drug-induced depression, *Prescribers Journal* **21**, 237–242 (1981)

TYRER, P. Consequences of stopping tricyclic antidepressants and monoamine oxidase inhibitors after chronic therapy (to be published) (1982)

TYRER, P. and STEINBERG, D. Symptomatic treatment of agoraphobia and social phobias: a follow-up study, *British Journal of Psychiatry* **127**, 163–168 (1975)

TYRER, P., GARDNER, M., LAMBOURN, J. and WHITFORD, M. Clinical and pharmacokinetic factors affecting response to phenelzine, *British Journal of Psychiatry* **136**, 359–365 (1980)

VAN PRAAG, H. M. Indoleamines in depression. In *Neuroregulators and Psychiatric Disorders* (Eds. E. USDIN, D. HAMBURG and J. BARCHAS), pp. 163–176, Oxford University Press, London (1977)

VAN PRAAG, H. and KORF, D. Central monoamine deficiency in depression, *Pharmacopsychotherapy* **8**, 322–326 (1975)

VAN PRAAG, H. M., KORF, J., DOLS, L. C. W. and SCHUT, T. A pilot study of the predicted value of the probenecid test in the application of 5-hydroxytryptophan as an antidepressant, *Psychopharmacologia* **25**, 14 (1972)

VAN PRAAG, H. M., VAN DEN BURG, W., BOS, E. R. H. and DOLS, N. C. W 5-hydroxytryptophan in combination with clomipramine in therapy resistant depression, *Psychopharmacologia* **38**, 267–269 (1974)

WÅLINDER, J., CARLSSON, A. and PERSSON, R. 5-HT reuptake inhibitors plus tryptophan in endogenous depression, *Acta Psychiatrica Scandinavica* **63**, Suppl. 290, 179–190 (1981)

WÅLINDER, J., SKOTT, A., CARLSSON, A., NAGY, A. and ROOS, B. E. Potentiation of the antidepressant action of clomipramine by tryptophan, *Archives of General Psychiatry* **33**, 1384–1389 (1976)

WEST, E. D. and DALLY, P. J. Effects of iproniazid in depressive syndromes, *British Medical Journal* **1**, 1491–1494 (1959)

WHITFORD, G. M. Acetylator phenotype in relation to monoamine oxidase inhibitor antidepressant drug therapy, *International Pharmacology and Psychiatry* **13**, 126–132 (1978)

WINSTON, F. Oral contraceptives and depression, *Lancet* **1**, 1209 (1969)

YOUDIM, M. D. H., COLLINS, G. G. S., SANDLER, M., BEVAN JONES, A. B., PARE, C. M. B. and NICHOLSON, W. J. Human brain monoamine oxidase, multiple forms and selective inhibitors, *Nature* **236**, 225–228 (1972)

YOUNG, J. P. R., LADER, M. H. and HUGHES, W. C. Controlled trial of imipramine, monoamine oxidase inhibitors, and combined treatment in depressed outpatients, *British Medical Journal* **2**, 1315–1317 (1979)

ZELLER, E. A., BARSKY, J., BERMAN, E. R. and FOUTS, J. R. Action of isonicotinic acid hyrdazide and related compounds on enzymes involved in the autonomic nervous system, *Journal of Pharmacology* **106**, 427–428 (1952)

Chapter 10

Lithium carbonate

S. Tyrer and D. M. Shaw

Introduction and historical aspects

The use of lithium in medicine dates back to the fourth century AD when the waters of Ephesus were recommended for the treatment of those with ill humour. It has been found since that these natural springs contain appreciable lithium salts. However, lithium was not discovered until 1817 and its first recorded use was by Ure, who used lithium carbonate as a solvent for bladder calculi (1843). However, the drug was hardly used in practice until Garrod (1859) showed that pieces of cartilage coated with urate deposits were more readily dissolved in a solution of lithium carbonate than in equimolar solutions of sodium or potassium carbonate. On this basis Garrod recommended lithium for the treatment of gout and the 'uric acid diathesis', the inherited predisposition to develop excess uric acid in the blood. Lithium is not actually a uricosuric agent when given in subtoxic doses, but the use of lithium compounds increased in conditions associated with uric acidaemia, including hypertension, diabetes, rheumatism and chronic nephritis. It was thought that these illnesses were caused by periodic surges of uric acid in the blood, of which gout was one manifestation. Lithium was employed to wash out these periodic deposits of uric acid (Mendelsohn, 1893).

It was also suggested that periodic depression was a manifestation of the uric acid diathesis and lithium salts were proposed for this condition. Their first recorded use was 20 years after Garrod by the Danish neurologist, Carl Lange (1896). Independently Alexander Haig (1892) in London used lithium in the treatment of depression on the same premise that there was increased excretion of uric acid in this illness. The dosage of lithium used by these authors, 8 mmol of lithium daily is 20–30 per cent of the dosage of lithium at present used in the prophylaxis of affective disorder.

Lithium was available in over-the-counter remedies from as far back as 1867. More preparations became available following these publications and there was increasing recognition of the side effects following 'the excessive consumption of lithia tablets' (*Practitioner*, 1907). Their use fell into decline and reached their apogee in 1949 when deaths occurred in patients with cardiac failure receiving lithium as a salt substitute (Corcoran, Taylor and Page, 1949). 'Stop using this dangerous poison at once', thundered *Time* (1949).

As it happened, this same year marked the publication of a report that led to the revival of lithium in psychiatry (Cade, 1949). Working on the hypothesis that mania

280

was due to intoxication by a normal metabolite of the body circulating in excess, Cade investigated the toxicity of urine from manic patients. High urine urea content was associated with toxicity but was not sufficient in itself to account for the more toxic properties of urine from manic patients. Other metabolites might be enhancing the toxicity of urea. Uric acid was a possible candidate for this purpose but is difficult to administer experimentally as it is insoluble in water. The most soluble urate, the lithium salt, was consequently used instead. Contrary to expectations, the urea/lithium urate solution reduced toxic manifestations in guinea pigs when compared with the same concentration of urea administered alone, making them placid and lethargic. After confirmation of the calming properties of lithium alone in guinea pigs, the next logical step was the administration of lithium to manic patients, with gratifying results.

Although these findings were confirmed by other Australian investigators (Noack and Trautner, 1951; Glesinger, 1954), the earlier American reports on the dangers of lithium discouraged clinical research in Europe and the New World. It was the patient investigative work of Schou and his colleagues in Denmark that established the value of lithium in manic-depressive disorder. After determining the limits of toxicity of lithium in the body (Schou, 1958), the effectiveness of lithium in preventing both manic and depressive episodes in recurrent affective illness was shown conclusively (Baastrup and Schou, 1967; Baastrup et al., 1970).

Pharmacology

Lithium is the third element in the periodic table, a monovalent alkaline metal in the same group as sodium, potassium, caesium and rubidium. It is widespread in nature and occurs in material of igneous origin, in greater abundance than tin, lead or silver. Lithium occurs mainly in the form of silicate in rocks such as spodumene, petalite and lepidolite. It is from these sources that the lithium carbonate used in medicine is derived. The earliest proprietary preparations of lithium included the citrate, hippurate, acetate, aspartate, sulphate, carbonate and tartrate. Lithium carbonate is now the most commonly prescribed lithium salt as it contains weight for weight more lithium than most lithium products and has a longer shelf-life than other lithium salts.

Although we know that lithium affects a number of cellular processes it is not known which of these is responsible for its action in the treatment of mania and the prophylaxis of manic-depressive psychosis. This is not too surprising as the primary cause of affective illness is itself unknown.

Considerable attention has been paid to the theory that there is an alteration of monoamine availability or metabolism in affective illness. Lithium has varying effects on monoamine activity depending on whether it is given for short or long periods. With acute administration lithium increases the retention and turnover of noradrenaline (Corrodi et al., 1967) but has inconsistent effects on 5-hydroxytryptamine (5-HT) (Knapp and Mandell, 1973). When given for longer periods lithium stimulates turnover of 5-HT (Perez-Cruet et al., 1970), possibly by inducing tryptophan hydroxylase activity (Mandell and Knapp, 1979). Chronic lithium administration also increases noradrenaline transport across synaptosomal membranes (Colburn et al., 1967). Lithium decreases acetylcholine synthesis (Dawes and Vizi, 1973) and affects the metabolism of γ-aminobutyric acid (GABA) (Gottesfeld, Ebstein and Samuel, 1971).

There are inconsistent reports of the effect of lithium on dopaminergic systems. Friedman and Gershon (1973) demonstrated that dopamine synthesis was inhibited in rats treated with lithium for two weeks. Pre-treatment with lithium prevents the dopamine receptor supersensitivity induced by chronic treatment with haloperidol (Klawans, Weiner and Nausieda, 1977). Furthermore, lithium prevents striatal dopamine receptor binding when administered in this way (Pert *et al.*, 1978). In contrast, pre-treatment with lithium enhanced receptor sensitivity induced by reserpine (Friedman, Dallob and Levine, 1979). Lithium only inhibits dopamine-sensitive adenylate cyclase when administered in clinically toxic concentrations (Stefanini *et al.*, 1978).

These findings seem contradictory and more work is required to determine how lithium affects dopaminergic pathways. Clinically, parkinsonian side effects certainly occur in patients maintained on lithium (Shopsin and Gershon, 1975; Tyrer, Lee and Trotter, 1981), but the mechanism of this needs to be elucidated.

The clinical relevance of these observations of the effects of lithium on aminergic function is difficult to determine. They do suggest that lithium may be exerting different effects when given acutely to control mania than when administered chronically in the prophylaxis of manic-depressive illness. However, the effect of lithium on monoamine activity does not seem sufficient alone to account for its profound clinical actions.

Lithium inhibits the hormone-induced formation of adenosine 3′,5′-monophosphate (cyclic AMP) in the brain, kidney and thyroid. Cyclic AMP is formed from adenosine triphosphate (ATP), the reaction catalysed by adenylate cyclase and a divalent cation, usually magnesium. Lithium inhibits adenylate cyclase activity and consequent cyclic AMP production in the organs concerned. Cyclic AMP is required for many hormones to exert their action on their target cells so lithium indirectly reduces the responsiveness of these cells. This explains why lithium reduces release of thyroxine from the thyroid gland and inhibits the effect of antidiuretic hormone (ADH) upon the distal tubule of the kidney. Cyclic AMP is the so-called second messenger required for the hormones to exercise their full activity.

The effects of lithium on adenylate cyclase are most clinically relevant in explaining the side effects of lithium. Reduced thyroid activity and polyuria are direct consequences. However, cyclic AMP is involved in the physiology of synaptic transmission in the CNS, and the therapeutic effects of lithium may be related to the inhibition of some but not all adenylate cyclases (Ebstein and Belmaker, 1979).

Lithium affects a number of other enzymes when given in therapeutic doses, including pyruvate kinase and some functions of $Na^+ - K^+$ adenosine triphosphatase. The reader is referred to pharmacological journals for a consideration of these and other effects, which are beyond the scope of this chapter.

Pharmacokinetics

Lithium carbonate is only administered orally in man. When given in standard form it is rapidly absorbed from the gastrointestinal tract. Most absorption takes place in the small intestine with much smaller amounts taken up in the large intestine and stomach (Amdisen and Sjögren, 1968). The nature of the attached anion has little effect on the rate and extent of lithium absorption.

Lithium is absorbed more rapidly than it can be distributed to the tissues. Following administration of a single dose of a standard lithium carbonate preparation, two phases of the plasma concentration-time curve can be detected (*Figure 10.1*)

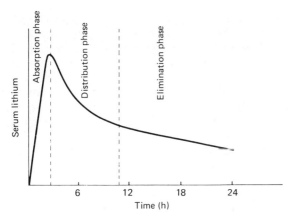

Figure 10.1 Diagrammatic representation of the course of the serum lithium level following a single dose of a standard lithium preparation

The elimination half-life for this second phase varies considerably, from 5 to 42 h with a mean of 13 h (Amdisen, 1977).

The lithium ion, as befits its elemental nature, passes readily into every compartment of the body. It is not bound to plasma or tissue proteins and there are consequently no profound differences in the lithium content of most organs, although high concentrations of lithium can occur in the brain (Amdisen *et al.*, 1974). The concentration of lithium in the cerebrospinal fluid (CSF) is about one-third that of the lithium concentration in the serum (Platman, Rohrlich, and Fieve, 1968). Steady-state CSF levels are reached somewhat later than in the serum. Elimination of lithium from the CSF is also slower than from the serum and this fact should be taken into account in patients recovering from lithium toxicity.

About 90 per cent of the ingested lithium dose is excreted through the kidneys (Kent and McCance, 1941). Five per cent of the lithium dose is lost in the faeces (Tyrer *et al.*, 1976), probably representing unabsorbed drug. A small amount of lithium is found in the sweat and saliva but no more than 1 per cent of the dose under normal conditions. Although lithium is filtered freely through the basement membrane of the glomerulus, 80 per cent of the filtered fraction is reabsorbed. Virtually all this exchange takes place in the proximal tubules (Thomsen and Schou, 1968). The renal clearance of lithium, i.e. the amount of plasma totally cleared of lithium in a defined period of time, varies from $8-45\ ml \cdot min^{-1}$. The variation is considerable and is only partly accounted for by the progressive reduction of lithium clearance with age (Hewick *et al.*, 1977).

Clinical relevance of lithium pharmacokinetics

Lithium is a hazardous drug to use unless a number of precautions are taken. The problem arises because the therapeutic ratio, i.e. the ratio of the effective therapeutic concentration of the drug to the toxic concentration is low, of the order of $1:2.5$. In many cases, therefore, doubling of the necessary lithium dose to achieve optimal treatment will cause the patient to become toxic. Lithium toxicity is highly dangerous. Some patients die and others are left with irreversible neurological sequelae. It is for this reason that it is important to obtain an indication of the patient's therapeutic requirements for lithium and to monitor serum lithium concentrations during treatment with the drug.

The usual method for determining the most appropriate dose for a patient is to administer a small dose of lithium and take blood samples at weekly intervals, increasing the dose if necessary once the weekly serum lithium values are known, until the desired serum lithium concentration is reached. There is a direct proportional relationship between lithium dosage and subsequent serum lithium levels (Amdisen, 1977). This is an accurate way of determining the lithium requirements for the patient as long as the patient is compliant with his medication. However, it necessitates the patient making weekly visits to the clinic and depends upon the patient following the prescribed regimen of tablets.

Alternative methods exist for the determination of lithium dose requirements before starting treatment. Schou (1968) originally recommended creatinine and lithium clearance determinations in patients about to receive lithium if there was any doubt about the integrity of renal function. The dosage of any drug eliminated entirely by renal routes required to maintain a desired drug concentration is indicated by the following formula:

$$D = C \times LiCl \times 1.44$$

where   D = dosage of drug over 24 h (mmol)
         C = average serum drug concentration (mmol $\cdot \ell^{-1}$)
         LiCl = lithium clearance (ml $\cdot$ min^{-1}).

Baastrup showed that the lithium clearance prior to lithium treatment correlated well with subsequent steady-state serum lithium levels (1971).

Lithium clearance estimation involves collection of urine from the patient for a period of some hours. At the beginning and end of this period blood is taken for measurement of serum lithium (Srinivasan and Hullin, 1980). This test is inconvenient and time-consuming for the patient as well as being subject to error because of faulty urine collection. Pharmacokinetic analysis of subjects starting on lithium suggested an easier test (Bergner et al., 1973). The serum lithium level taken 24 h after a loading dose of 600 mg of lithium carbonate was found to correlate very highly with subsequent steady-state serum lithium levels (Cooper and Simpson, 1976; Cooper, Bergner and Simpson, 1973).

TABLE 10.1 Table to determine dosage of lithium required to maintain serum lithium level of 0.6–1.2 mmol.ℓ^{-1}

24-h serum lithium level after single loading dose of 500 mg of standard lithium carbonate (mmol $\cdot \ell^{-1}$)	Daily lithium dosage required (mg)
<0.05	3000
0.05–0.09	2250
0.10–0.14	1500
0.15–0.19	1000
0.20–0.23	750
0.24/0.30	500
>0.30	400

(Derived from work by Cooper, Bergner and Simpson, 1973)
See p. 289 for dose schedules

TABLE 10.2 Determination of lithium dosage from lithium clearance

Lithium clearance (ml.min^{-1})	Recommended dose of standard lithium carbonate to maintain serum lithium level of 0.8 mmol.ℓ^{-1} (mg)
< 10	$\leq$ 600
10	800
15	1050
20	1300
25	1550
30	1800
35	2100
> 35	$\geq$ 2300

(Derived from Tyrer *et al.* 1980)
See p. 289 for dose schedules

Prediction tables have been compiled for the use of this test so that the lithium dose required to attain a desired lithium level can be calculated from the 24-h lithium level (Cooper, Bergner and Simpson, 1973). A recent comparison of a modification of this loading dose test and lithium clearance showed that both tests were of comparable accuracy (Tyrer *et al.*, 1981) (*Tables 10.1* and *10.2*).

In most clinics the 24-h loading dose test should be preferred. It is much simpler to carry out with less likelihood of fault but cannot be repeated in identical form once lithium treatment has started. The lithium clearance test is liable to error because of faulty urine collection in unsupervised hands, but has the advantage of providing a baseline measure of renal function with regard to lithium which can be repeated once the patient is stabilized on the drug.

The serum level of lithium following a single dose varies appreciably during the course of 24 h (*see Figure 10.1*). For this reason it is essential to standardize the interval of time between the last dose of lithium tablets and withdrawal of blood for serum lithium estimation. The time taken for absorption and distributio˙ of lithium following a dose of the drug varies from individual to individual but is not normally more than 8 h. For this reason it is recommended that blood should be withdrawn for serum lithium estimation at least 8 h after the last intake of tablets. Largely owing to the efforts of Amdisen (1975), it has now been generally accepted that when blood is withdrawn for lithium estimation in a patient maintained on lithium, the interval of time between the last lithium tablet and the blood sample should be 12 h. This is known as the standardized 12-h serum lithium concentration. Unless otherwise stated, when referring to serum lithium levels in patients receiving lithium, a serum lithium value is normally assumed to be a standardized one. Although Amdisen recommends that blood should be withdrawn for the standardized serum lithium concentration 30 min each side of the 12-h period, samples taken 10–14 h after the last tablet are suitable in practice.

What is the optimal serum lithium concentration? The therapeutic range at steady state is normally considered to be 0.6–1.2 mmol$\cdot\ell^{-1}$. However, these values were derived empirically and were largely concerned with the treatment of manic subjects. A number of studies show that manic patients require more lithium when elated than when normothymic (Greenspan *et al.*, 1968; Almy and Taylor, 1973). Recent work has suggested that lithium is effective in prophylaxis when the steady-state serum lithium level is maintained as low as $0.4 \, \text{mmol} \cdot \ell^{-1}$ (Hullin, 1980). Patients from clinics where low maintenance doses of lithium are administered have less renal functional impairment (Tyrer, 1979; Hullin *et al.*, 1979). Our recommendation for patients receiving prophylactic lithium is that the serum lithium level should be maintained between 0.6 and $0.8 \, \text{mmol} \cdot \ell^{-1}$ in most cases. Individual patients may require to be maintained at higher or lower lithium levels depending upon response and side effects. In general, manic patients require higher lithium levels. In one retrospective study, serum lithium levels above $0.9 \, \text{mmol} \cdot \ell^{-1}$ were required for therapeutic response (Prien, Caffey and Klett, 1972a).

Lithium can also be clinically monitored by measuring the concentration of the drug in red blood cells (RBCs) or saliva. Lithium exerts its effects intracellularly and it would seem more appropriate to look at the concentration of the drug in readily available cells. RBC lithium concentration is normally represented in relation to the serum lithium level, usually as the ratio between the concentration of lithium in the red cell and its concentration in the serum. There is some evidence that if this ratio becomes progressively greater during the course of lithium treatment that toxicity is more likely to occur (Dunner, Meltzer and Fieve, 1978). It has also been shown that patients with higher ratios have a better response than those with consistently low ones (Johnston *et al.*, 1980). However, the main value of RBC lithium estimation may be in determining compliance. The RBC/serum lithium ratio is normally stable over time for any one individual once steady state has been reduced. Patients maintained on lithium who have a fluctuating ratio are often found to be poorly compliant with their medication (Carroll and Feinberg, 1977). Entry of lithium into the RBC is slower than into the serum, so patients who take their tablets intermittently will have low ratios. This may explain, in part at least, the results from Dundee referred to earlier (Johnston *et al.*, 1980).

Earlier work suggested that patients with a high RBC/serum lithium ratio were more likely to respond to lithium when depressed (Mendels and Frazer, 1973). This work has not been replicated, even by the same authors (Frazer *et al.*, 1978).

The concentration of lithium in saliva has been used to monitor lithium levels, particularly in children (Lena and Bastable, 1978). The ratio between serum and saliva lithium varies from individual to individual but is relatively constant within each subject (Neu, DiMascio and Williams, 1975), although it is affected by activity in some individuals (Shimizu and Smith, 1977). Lithium is present in higher concentration in the saliva than in the serum; the ratio varies from 1:2 to 1:3.4 (Sims, 1980). Considerable variation in the ratio occurs depending on the time of saliva and serum samples in relationship to drug intake (Evrard *et al.*, 1978). Unless there are particular reasons why blood cannot be regularly withdrawn from a patient, we do not recommend estimation of saliva lithium as a guide to monitoring lithium concentrations in the body. The relationship between saliva and serum lithium varies too much from centre to centre for confidence in relying on these determinations.

Determination of lithium concentration

Lithium is measured in the laboratory by means of two techniques, flame emission and atomic absorption. These tests are based upon the same principle. When lithium salts are introduced into a flame part of the element dissociates into free atoms. A small proportion of these free atoms will absorb energy from the flame and will become excited. The emission of energy of these excited atoms in the form of light is the basis for flame emission spectrophotometry. The absorption of energy from the flame by the excited atoms is the foundation of atomic absorption spectrometry. It is generally agreed that flame emission is more sensitive than atomic absorption but at the concentrations of lithium measured in the blood these differences are unimportant. Flame photometry is the simpler and cheaper method.

Lithium preparations

There are over 50 different lithium preparations available throughout the world. Eighty per cent of these consist of lithium carbonate, the remainder include the citrate, sulphate, aspartate, glutamate and gluconate. Sustained and slow release lithium preparations have been produced although the nature and extent of the slow release properties of these preparations differ considerably.

In Britain, four lithium preparations are produced: Camcolit (Norgine Ltd), Priadel (Delandale Laboratories), Phasal (Pharmax Ltd) and Liskonum (Smith, Kline and French Ltd). All of these consist of lithium carbonate but they are marketed with different designations according to their degree of dissolution *in vitro*. Camcolit is provided in 250 mg and 400 mg tablets as a standard product. Priadel and Liskonum are termed controlled-release preparations and the manufacturers of Phasal specify their product a prolonged release preparation. The differences in terminology are accurate in terms of their dissolution. Under identical conditions, the percentage of lithium released from three of the products was 85 per cent for Camcolit, 33 per cent for Priadel and 12 per cent for Phasal (Tyrer *et al.*, 1976). However, in the same study, no difference was found in the rate of absorption and excretion of Camcolit and Priadel *in vivo*, although Phasal was poorly absorbed by half the subjects taking this product. This investigation was carried out on different subjects and the design did not allow for direct comparison of the pharmacokinetics of the two products.

These results differed from the findings of earlier studies. Coppen, Bailey and White (1969) found that a single dose of Priadel maintained remarkably steady serum lithium levels over the subsequent 24 h, although between-patient variation was considerable. These findings could not be replicated by Crammer, Rosser and Crane (1974), and it was later found that the formulation of Priadel had been changed in the intervening period (Amdisen, 1977). Shaw *et al.* (1974) found that Priadel and Phasal had similar kinetics in schizophrenic patients maintained on the drug. Bennie *et al.* (1977) in a complex but obscure design, discovered that Priadel, administered in a single daily dose to certain patients was able to maintain lithium levels within the therapeutic range during 24 h, whereas Camcolit was only able to maintain lithium levels within this range if administered on a thrice daily schedule. It is difficult to interpret these findings because no indication is given of the renal handling of lithium for each patient.

In order to overcome the considerable interindividual variability in the handling of lithium it is essential to employ a cross-over design in any comparison of different lithium preparations. Such comparisons can be made in single dose investigations or ideally, in volunteers or patients maintained on the drug for a sufficient period of time for steady state to be achieved. Results from single-dose studies are not necessarily directly applicable to the situation when steady state has been reached. However, lithium is readily distributed to all compartments of the body and single-dose investigations have been shown to relate accurately to subsequent steady-state kinetics

(Bergner *et al.*, 1973). Indeed, the correlation between single-dose studies and subsequent steady-state levels was as high as 0.97 in a well-planned investigation (Cooper, Bergner and Simpson, 1973). It is apparent, with regard to lithium, that single-dose kinetic information is very closely related to the kinetics of maintenance lithium treatment.

A single-dose cross-over trial of Camcolit and Priadel in six medical student volunteers showed differences between the two preparations that were not detected in the earlier work (Tyrer, 1978). The two products had equivalent bioavailability but there were differences in the rate of release of lithium (*Figure 10.2*). Priadel is released more slowly than Camcolit, reaching maximum concentration significantly later, although the height of peak serum lithium does not differ for the two products. These results are in accord with those of previous investigators. Grof *et al.* (1976) found no significant differences between Priadel and two standard Canadian lithium preparations in a six-week cross-over maintenance study in 12 volunteers. Van Kempen and Fabius (1978) in Holland found higher peak lithium values 2 h after administration of Priadel than with a slow release preparation, Litarex, in patients maintained on lithium. Johnson *et al.* (1979) have recently shown very similar results to those of Tyrer in an identical investigation. Their conclusion, as has been previously reported (Tyrer, 1978), is that Priadel is delayed-release rather than a true slow-release preparation. This is underlined by a comparison of Priadel and Litarex, a controlled-release lithium citrate product recently marketed. This preparation, Litarex (Dumex Ltd), has more of the characteristics of the ideal slow-release product. There is no initial serum lithium peak, there is less variation in serum lithium levels between individuals yet the drug has similar bioavailability to standard preparations (Amdisen, 1975, 1977 (*Figure 10.3*).

Similar properties have been shown by a new American slow-release preparation, Lithobid (Rowell Laboratories) (Cooper *et al.*, 1978).

What are the advantages of sustained-release preparations and why should there be concern to establish that such products fulfil the claims of the manufacturers? Slow-release preparations give rise to fewer side effects, they assist compliance and they are probably safer if swallowed as an overdose. It has been postulated that high peak serum lithium values may be associated with greater likelihood of renal impairment because of the large doses of lithium appearing in the renal collecting duct (Amdisen, 1979). However, no conclusive evidence has been produced to show that high peak

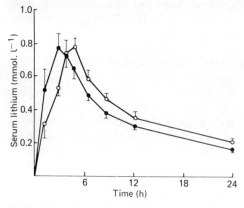

Figure 10.2 Mean serum lithium levels ± SD following administration of 1000 mg of Camcolit (●) and Priadel (○)

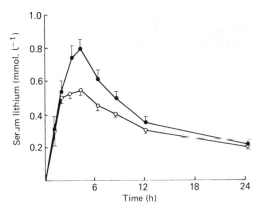

Figure 10.3 Mean serum lithium levels ±SD following administration of 27 mmol of lithium in the form of Priadel (●) and Litarex (○) (Tyrer *et al.*, 1982)

serum lithium levels (as opposed to high maintenance steady-state lithium levels) are associated with increased pathology, although they are clearly associated with more side effects (Persson, 1977). Indeed, it has been suggested that it is the change in serum lithium concentration in the body that is responsible for its metabolic effects (Plenge, 1978).

The evidence suggests that it does not greatly matter in what schedule lithium is administered or in what form, as long as toxicity is avoided. Nevertheless, it is necessary for us to be cautious with any drug that is administered for long periods for maintenance purposes and it would seem wise to administer most lithium preparations, whatever their designation, in a twice-daily dose at present (*Drug and Therapeutics Bulletin*, 1981). Litarex and Lithobid can be given once daily in many cases, but a divided dose schedule may be required in patients who excrete lithium rapidly.

Clinical use

The many assessments of the therapeutic effects of lithium have been fraught with methodological problems, some of which have complicated the interpretation of the results of an otherwise excellent study. The problems come both from the nature of the condition and from characteristics of the drug.

The first hurdle is that to the best of our knowledge, affective illness is peculiar to humans, so that all therapeutic trials must be on patients and/or on normal volunteers. Most of the studies have been done by psychiatrists on their in-patients. This imposes a bias in sampling. The in-patients may have an over-representation of the more severely ill, the more compliant, or those who have either secondary difficulties or complications unrelated to their psychiatric illness.

Even within this selected sample there is further bias particularly in mania in the assessment of the effect of lithium on the episode. Very disturbed patients cannot take part in a 'wash-out' period, or if they take part in the trial to this point, may be too uncontrolled to stay to the end of the period of assessment. Similarly, most studies of the effects of lithium on the depressive phase will tend to exclude the severely suicidal, very agitated or deluded individuals.

Investigation of prophylactic therapy is a source of its own biases. Such trials by their very nature have to be prolonged so that an appreciable number of patients 'fall-out *en route*'. Some investigations have used the discontinuation technique where patients already on lithium are assigned to lithium, placebo or some other treatment. Taking this group ('responders' and people who tolerate lithium well) as the individuals under investigation, ignoring those who find lithium difficult to take for one reason or another, or who have failed to respond in an earlier attempt at treatment, biases the sample.

On the whole 'end points' have been fairly straightforward—admission to hospital with an episode, and the need for additional treatment were the usual markers for the end of a cycle, but again how can the researchers cope adequately with the problem of the high proportion of their sample lasting to the end of a reasonable period of study and remaining well? This has complicated the analysis and has limited conclusions, particularly if the placebo group had relapsed quickly in comparison to the treated group. The treated group were then at risk for relapse for a longer period than were the placebo group.

In earlier studies (not just of lithium), where antimanic or antidepressant drugs were being used, many designs required administering treatment soon after admission. This means that those patients, perhaps 17–30 per cent or more (depending on the series), who are going to respond rapidly without drug treatment to admission to hospital 'dilute' the treated sample who are not 'placebo responders' and increase the variance.

Classification has been more than a minor stumbling block and continues to be so. So long as psychiatrists are unable to agree on whether there should not be any subdivision of depressed patients, or which of the classificatory systems should be used, there will be confusion.

In this chapter the simplest assumptions have been made, i.e. that affective illness includes manic-depressive psychosis; this has bipolar and unipolar forms which are distinct from neurotic/reactive illnesses, but that these latter forms of depression can and do co-exist with affective illness and may be secondary to it. It is also assumed that there is an entity which does not fit into either affective or schizophrenic groups—the schizo-affective illnesses, which show distinct features of both kinds of functional psychoses.

When it comes to running trials, on acute illness or on prophylactic therapy, the side effects of lithium make it difficult to keep a study double blind, and this was found by Platman (1970) in a comparison of lithium and chlorpromazine.

Whereas unipolar illness is a fairly common condition, in most centres manic individuals, or rather manic individuals fulfilling all the research trial criteria and lasting the course, tend to be few and far between. Running a trial on mania becomes a triumph of hope over experience and of patience over the natural urge to complete the trial. The researcher may be tempted to include patients with fewer and fewer of the selection criteria.

One of the stumbling blocks in any trial is detection of those who are non-compliers, but who for their own reasons continue to attend taking enough lithium before their visit to give just the 'right' plasma level. This 'game' is one detected usually only by chance, natural suspicion or with the help of the spouse.

While the above gives some idea of some of the complications and difficulties facing the researcher running a trial of lithium, the main controversy of the past lay in the initial studies of lithium as a prophylactic therapy. One of the objections raised was that the design used the patient as his or her own retrospective control by taking the past history of recurrences when the patient was not on lithium, and compared this with the prospective pattern of recurrences while on lithium. Separate controls were not employed. It was assumed that the incidence of illness in the prospective and retrospective periods would be similar. The study could not be double blind because both rater and patient were well aware of what was happening.

Use of lithium in the prophylaxis of affective illness

The term prophylaxis has had its critics, but has become accepted for want of a more accurately descriptive term to describe a treatment which, when given to a patient long term abolishes, attenuates or makes less frequent attacks of affective illness. It is a form, therefore, of preventative or 'protective' treatment.

As partly described above, most trials have been of one of several types:

(1) comparison of frequency/severity of recorded episodes before treatment with that after establishing lithium therapy;
(2) allocating patients randomly to lithium and placebo double blind either starting from the patient's first exposure to the drug, or taking patients, who were already established on the therapy and giving them 'active' or placebo treatments.

There have been many trials of lithium, and a proportion of them will be discussed here.

The history of prophylactic therapy began with the independent observations of Hartigan (1963) and Baastrup (1964) that the antimanic effect of lithium might apply also to recurrences of illness and that therefore the drug might have potential as a prophylactic agent. Baastrup and Schou (1967) then published data which claimed that patients with these frequent recurrences of affective illness if put on to continuous treatment with lithium experienced a reduction in illness—either abolition, attenuation or reduced frequency of episodes. It was this trial which raised the argument mentioned above.

Further studies arose, some of which were directed at criticism of this paper. Schou, Thomsen and Baastrup (1970) were not able to find any difference in the rate of relapse between patients discontinued blind or double blind, and Laurell and Ottosson (1968), Isaksson, Ottoson and Perris (1969) and Angst, Grof and Schou (1969) all found that the incidence of retrospective recurrences was not significantly different from the prospective incidence following an admission to hospital for an episode, the explanation therefore being that previous relapses predicted similar future episodes.

Similarly, when Schou, Thomsen and Baastrup (1970) took patients in whom lithium had been discontinued for a period, they showed that the rate of relapse was high before lithium had been started in the first place, low when the individual was on lithium and rose to its earlier level on discontinuation of treatment. The vulnerability to suffer relapse did not appear with a period of treatment with lithium.

In examining the actions of lithium in bipolar, unipolar and schizoaffective patients Angst et al., (1970) found shortened episodes in bipolar patients, but episodes of unchanged length in individuals with unipolar schizoaffective illness. However, the interval between episodes of illness was prolonged by 61 and 76 per cent in bipolar and unipolar patients, but by only 30 per cent in schizoaffective patients. Better results would have been obtained if the cycles, which had not come to an end at the end of the study, had not been counted as a relapse.

Since the original publication of Baastrup and Schou (1967) a large number of open trials have been done, most of which have supported the finding of a prophylactic effect of lithium in both unipolar and bipolar illness (e.g. Angst *et al.*, 1970). Not all have found lithium to be unfavourable in schizoaffective illness (e.g. Egli, 1971).

Trials using two groups and a double-blind design began appearing with that of Melia (1970). He took patients whose maximum remissions had been nine months or less in the preceding two years, the length of the trial was fixed to a maximum period of two years or to an episode, and the patients receiving lithium were allocated to either lithium or placebo randomly (discontinuation design). The patient groups were mixed unipolar and bipolar, nine lithium and nine placebo and the results of the two therapies were not significantly different.

Baastrup *et al.* (1970) had a similar format but used a sequential design; and a larger sample (50 bipolar, 34 unipolar). The results were highly significant at the 0.1 per cent level of probability in favour of lithium.

Coppen *et al.* (1971) took 38 bipolar and 25 unipolar patients who were starting lithium therapy on the criterion of two or more episodes in two years. The trial period was five months and gave differences favouring lithium at the $P < 0.001$ and $P \leq 0.01$ levels respectively. This paper produced important data giving some measure of the severe level of morbidity and disruption produced by affective illness.

Hullin, McDonald and Allsopp (1972) with a criterion of three episodes or more in three years, had a trial period of 14 months, a discontinuation design, and had a mixed group of 32 mixed unipolar and bipolar patients. Lithium was superior to placebo at the $P = 0.05$ level.

Of four other double-blind trials (Cundall, Brooks and Murray, 1972; Stallone *et al.*, 1973; Prien, Caffey and Klett, 1973; Prien, Klett and Caffey, 1973) all were on a discontinuation or mixed start and discontinuation design (Stallone *et al.*, 1973). Most produced statistically significant results with the exception of Cundall, Brooks and Murray (1972) in a very small sample of unipolar patients (four active, four placebo treated), and Prien's study showed only possible attenuation in depressives. In addition, in the trial of Cundall, Brooks and Murray (1972) and that of Hullin, McDonald and Allsopp (1972) some patients were included who were found to have lithium levels below the agreed minimum level, which might have reduced the significance of levels.

In general the trials of lithium have produced a large body of evidence establishing the efficacy of lithium as a prophylactic agent in bipolar illness. Although many reviews have stated that lithium is less effective in the prophylaxis of unipolar patients, and lithium is not an approved treatment for this purpose in the USA, many of the studies do not show lack of preventative activity in this disorder. Indeed the recent investigation by the MRC Drug Trials Committee (1981) found lithium and amitriptyline to be equally effective prophylactive agents (and superior to placebo).

Establishing and continuing prophylactic therapy with lithium

Lithium is a useful drug, but as the section on side and toxic effects shows, is not the ideal.

Some patients experience side effects which they cannot tolerate, the therapeutic index (ratio between toxic and therapeutic levels) is low and there is a risk of thyroid and kidney damage. It behoves the clinician therefore to be quite clear about the criteria for starting lithium. If these criteria are unclear or insufficient, then the motivation on the part of doctor and patient will be inadequate to carry both through a long-term treatment programme. Having said this there are no absolute indications.

The usually accepted criterion is two or more attacks in two years of a severity to warrant antidepressant or antimanic therapy. This is with the proviso that the second attack of only two should not be so close to the first that it may have been just a recrudescence of the first episode. In addition, however, there are some less clear indications which may apply to a minority of individuals.

Occasionally, patients have recurrences fairly regularly but at less frequent intervals, but the episodes are both severe and intractable to therapy, or are accompanied by an active drive towards suicide, etc. The same might apply to more widely spaced manic attacks if these are extreme, and the patient's behaviour is particularly destructive at these times.

Such instances are uncommon; for the great majority of patients the criterion stated above is sufficient guide. There is ample evidence to show that when there is yearly or more frequent illness further recurrences can be anticipated.

When deciding whether or not to give lithium it would be helpful if there were adequate guides as to the likelihood of success of the treatment. According to Coryell and Winokur (1980) a family history in which there is bipolar illness extending to second degree relatives is a favourable factor. Kukopulos et al., (1975) claimed that only 60 per cent of unipolar patients achieved prophylaxis quickly; and trials report failure rates varying from 20–50 per cent.

The only generally accepted and reasonably well established indicant of likely failure in prophylaxis with lithium is where the patient has rapidly recurring illness to the point of four or more illnesses per year. At this stage of the illness it appears to become refractory to lithium at least as a 'solo' therapy.

Lithium in the treatment of mania

Some of the pitfalls in trials of lithium were discussed in the previous section. With studies of lithium in mania the main difficulties have been in sampling (because of the management of severely ill patients), and the maintenance of the double blind.

As mentioned earlier the modern history of lithium in psychiatry began when Cade (1949) gave lithium salts to a group of patients suffering from mania, depression or schizophrenia. The drug seemed beneficial to the former as an acute treatment and his findings were replicated by Noack and Trautner (1951) and others. There have been many uncontrolled and single-blind trials which overall have supported Cade's original findings, and some of the major double-blind trials will be discussed here.

The first of these was by Schou et al., (1954) who gave lithium or placebo to 38 manic patients, 30 of which were classified as typical and eight as atypical. The periods of treatment varied, and prevention was included as one criterion of improvement, so assessment of the results was difficult. However, 12 and 15 of the typical cases out of the 30 were considered to have responded or possibly responded respectively.

In the double-blind study by Maggs (1963) a pilot study showed that one-third of patients were too severely ill to cooperate sufficiently to take drugs orally and such individuals were excluded. His criteria for selection were no treatment for the current episode and remaining in the trial for a six-week period. Treatments were randomly given in two-week 'blocks' of lithium, rest period and placebo, or placebo, rest period and lithium. A fixed dose of 1.5 g lithium carbonate was given during active treatment daily for 6 d per week. Five patients were withdrawn because of severity of illness, two for toxicity and three for other reasons. Of the remaining, 18 who completed the trial showed significant superiority of lithium over placebo. These effects were greater in the second week of treatment than the first.

Goodwin, Murphy and Bunney (1969a) gave lithium carbonate to 12 manic patients and blindly interposed periods of placebo. All patients had lithium first. Eight patients recovered completely during two weeks of treatment with lithium, one improved and three deteriorated. Of the eight who recovered, four relapsed on placebo.

Stokes *et al.* (1971) compared lithium and placebo double blind using a design in which there were four alternate periods of 7–10 d of active or placebo treatment, active therapy being the starting therapy in alternate patients. (34 patients had 98 periods of treatment—56 of lithium, 42 of placebo). There was a mean plasma level of $0.91 \, \text{mmol} \cdot \ell^{-1}$ but this covered a wide range with some at inadequate concentrations. The difference between lithium and placebo was statistically significant (in 75 per cent on active therapy as compared to 40.5 per cent of placebo). In this trial atypical patients fared as well as those with typical symptoms.

The overall results of these trials point to an expectation of improvement in 75–80 per cent of mild to moderately severe manic patients given two weeks of treatment of lithium, a number which might be greater with closer control of plasma levels. The situation with severely ill manic patients was not established by the studies.

Information in this area came from comparisons of the effects of lithium and chlorpromazine by Prien, Caffey and Klett (1972b). This was a large multicentre trial in which 255 manic patients were subdivided into 'highly active' and 'mildly active' groups. In the 'highly active' group 38 per cent of those given lithium dropped out of the trial, but only 8 per cent on chlorpromazine. Of the 21 lithium treated patients who dropped out, ten were for lack of response, six for 'uncooperative behaviour' and five for toxicity. Both treatments given over the three weeks of the trial were successful in ameliorating manic symptoms but the neuroleptic was the superior therapy. It brought symptoms under control within days whereas there was a delay with lithium until the second week. On the basis of this study, lithium would not be the treatment of choice in the severe manic patient.

On the debit side also there were severe side effects in 31 per cent of the lithium group, but in only 18 per cent of those taking chlorpromazine. The lesser side effects of somnolence, dry mouth, sluggishness, fatigue, constipation and slurred speech with chlorpromazine however, were probably more troublesome than the transient gastric discomfort and tremor produced by lithium.

In summary, for the mild to moderate manic patient lithium can be a useful treatment with the proviso that there is significant delay in the appearance of remission. Because of this slowness of response to lithium, it is unsuitable for the severely ill patient.

Combining lithium with neuroleptics in mania

This problem is discussed below (p. 301). Briefly, it comes from the doubts raised about potentiation of parkinsonian side effects, acute brain syndrome and possible permanent effects of two types of neuroleptics (butyrophenones and phenothiazines) when given with lithium.

Treatment of depression with lithium

Despite a number of investigations, the effectiveness of lithium as an antidepressant for use in the management of the acute episode remains uncertain. Whether or not further studies will appear in significant number is doubtful when so many new antidepressants are awaiting evaluation.

Many of the authors have claimed that there is a subgroup of patients who are 'lithium responsive' and have attempted to categorize these individuals.

Controlled studies of the antidepressant effect of lithium

Fieve, Platman and Plutchik (1968) did a trial of lithium versus imipramine in 29 patients and concluded that the tricyclic drug was clearly the more effective drug. Stokes *et al.* (1971) used lithium and placebo in 38 patients with depression (lithium 17, placebo 21), and found a trend towards some improvement with the active drug in that depressive symptoms were reduced by the periods of lithium compared with ratings on the day preceding the start of lithium, but this was not significantly different from the improvement with placebo. The periods of treatment may have been too short (10 d) to have given lithium an adequate trial.

Goodwin, Murphy and Bunney (1969b) and Goodwin *et al.* (1972) also used lithium and placebo, giving them alternately. Of 52 patients there was complete remission in only 15 but partial recovery in 21, especially in bipolar patients, and their criteria for improvement included the stipulation of recurrence of illness during placebo.

Mendels, Secunda and Dyson (1972) found lithium as effective as desimipramine in a 'mixed' group of 24 depressed patients and Noyes *et al.* (1974) in similarly heterogeneous patients got 13 responses out of 22 with nine relapses on withdrawal and replacement by placebo. Their group had six bipolar patients (all responders) and 16 unipolar individuals (seven responders).

On the other hand, as mentioned above, Fieve, Platman and Plutchik (1968) found imipramine better than lithium, and Stokes *et al.* (1971) could not detect any antidepressant response. The study of Lingjaerde *et al.* (1974) was unable to support the idea that lithium and tricyclics might be more efficacious than tricyclics alone. However, in a randomized double-blind trial in 63 unipolar and bipolar depressed females lithium was superior in efficacy to imipramine. Lithium's antidepressant response did not appear until the second or third week (Worrall *et al.*, 1979).

In all, the claimed antidepressant response to lithium requires some further study, although Worrall and colleagues' investigation was very supportive of a positive role. It may be that as suggested by some of the supporters of this action for lithium that certain subgroups as yet unidentified (despite effects to delineate them) may be lithium responders. What few indications there are in the trials point to a greater likelihood of lithium being of use in bipolar than unipolar depressive patients.

Lithium and schizoaffective disorders

Of all the types of illness related to affective illness, the diagnosis of schizoaffective illness is the most difficult. It presents as an apparent mixture of the acute active symptoms of schizophrenia and of affective illness, is phasic, and is not followed by the defect state of chronic schizophrenia. In addition, with one exception, the samples in the studies of lithium treatment of this condition have been small.

Johnson *et al.* (1971) gave lithium to seven and chlorpromazine to six such patients and found the phenothiazine to be the better drug. However, the dose of lithium used was high (plasma levels of 1.16–1.97 mmol · ℓ^{-1}) and nearly all (six out of the seven) were in a state of lithium intoxication.

Shopsin, Kim and Gershon (1971) included only four patients with schizoaffective illness in their trial of lithium versus chlorpromazine so that their data on this group was too meagre to be useful.

Brockington *et al.* (1978) also compared lithium and chlorpromazine in 19 selected patients. Of the eight on lithium two were lost from the trial, five made a complete or partial recovery and one was unchanged. Of 11 patients given chlorpromazine, three were lost from the trial, three were withdrawn and of the remaining five, four made a complete or partial recovery.

The most informative trial is that of Prien, Caffey and Klett (1972c) in whose multicentre trial lithium and chlorpromazine were compared in 83 schizoaffective patients, 42 classified as highly active (25 chlorpromazine; 17 lithium) and 41 as mildly active (21 chlorpromazine; 20 lithium). The mean lithium levels were 1.3 and 1.0 mmol $\cdot \ell^{-1}$ in the highly active and mildly active group respectively with a range of 0.65–1.28 mmol $\cdot \ell^{-1}$.

In the highly active group 41 per cent on lithium dropped out because of inadequate response or toxicity as compared to none on chlorpromazine, and in the mildly active group there was a higher incidence of withdrawal on chlorpromazine, but this was not statistically significant.

The authors' assessment was that chlorpromazine was the better therapy for the highly active group, but that for the mildly active there was little to choose between them. There was the possibility that schizoaffective patients were relatively sensitive to lithium, certainly were less tolerant than manic patients, and that therefore doses and levels should be monitored carefully.

Lithium and other conditions

Aggression

A number of authors including Sheard *et al.* (1976), Tupin and Smith (1972), Sheard (1971), Worrall, Moody and Naylor (1975), Sheard (1970), Tupin *et al.* (1973), and Sheard (1975) have discussed the effect of lithium on aggression in animals and man.

Sheard *et al.* (1976) described a double-blind placebo controlled trial of the effect of lithium on chronically impulsively aggressive behaviour of male prisoners aged 16–24. The participants had lithium or placebo for up to three months, preceded and followed by one drug-free month. Of the 66, 34 received lithium (20 for three months, eight for two months and six for one month), 32 had placebo (21 for three months, nine for two months and two for one month). Lithium had a significant antiaggressive effect compared with placebo, and there was a tendency towards return of previous aggressive behaviour in the month (drug free) after stopping the drug.

There was an equivocal effect on aggression in epileptic subjects (Marini and Sheard, 1977), but Worrall, Moody and Naylor (1975) demonstrated some antiaggressive action of lithium on mentally subnormal individuals in a double-blind trial, and this was supported by Dale (1980).

Other uses of lithium

Other applications of lithium require further exploration but the following are areas of promise:

(1) neutropenia (e.g. after anti-cancer drugs),
(2) inappropriate secretion of ADH,
(3) alcoholism (mainly associated with mood swings (Merry *et al.* (1976)),
(4) cluster headaches (Mathew, 1977),
(5) Kleine–Levin syndrome (Jeffries and Lefevre, 1973; Ogura *et al.*, 1976; Abe, 1977),
(6) cancer of thyroid (Turner, Brownlie and Rogers, 1976),
(7) as an immunological adjuvant.

Unwanted effects

Contraindications

The effect of lithium on the kidneys is discussed below, and at our present stage of knowledge consists of some impairment of concentrating ability with relatively little glomerular or other damage in long-term treated patients. In addition, lithium is excreted by the kidney where it is reabsorbed by the proximal tubules in competition with sodium. At times of sodium depletion or reduced glomerular filtration rate, lithium may accumulate in the body. As lithium levels rise, lithium, though not itself reabsorbed by the distal tubules, may decrease distal sodium uptake leading to a self-perpetuating situation (sodium depletion—lithium accumulation—increasing toxicity—sodium depletion, etc.).

It follows that using lithium in patients with sodium depletion or who have severely reduced glomerular function may be too hazardous. If thiazide diuretics have to be used then lithium dosage must be reduced and levels must be watched carefully and regularly (*see* p. 299).

Sodium depletion is not in itself a contraindication to treatment with lithium if it is a brief phenomenon such as due to sweating in hot weather or an acute attack of diarrhoea. However, when it is likely to be a continuing feature of the patient's life—in chronic diarrhoea as with ulcerative colitis, Crohn's disease or the use of diuretics—special care and regular monitoring of levels are needed. The precipitation of acute toxicity in such patients is a real hazard.

A decision by the patient to go on a diet may reduce his sodium excretion over a prolonged period and lead to lithium accumulation, and patients stabilized in hospital on a diet relatively rich in sodium may similarly suffer at home if their mode of preparation of food contains less salt (sometimes seen in the elderly).

Cardiac disease

Use of lithium in cardiac disease requires particularly careful consideration, especially in those bipolar patients where lithium may be particularly needed. Unfortunately, some data suggest that lithium has an effect on cardiac functioning, and has been associated with failure, arrhythmias, sinoatrial and atrioventricular block and ventricular ectopic beats (Swedberg and Winblad, 1974; Demers and Heninger, 1970; Wilson *et al.*, 1976; Eliasen and Andersen, 1975; Wellens, Cats and Duren, 1975; Tangedahl and Gau, 1972; Jaffe, 1977). These changes may be exacerbated by anaesthesia (Azar and Turndorf, 1977).

Lithium slows cardiac conduction in some patients, leading to reversible sinoatrial block (Roose *et al.*, 1979), and to a reduction of atrial arrhythmias (Tilkian *et al.*, 1976).

At toxic doses lithium can cause cardiac failure and ventricular arrhythmias (Swedberg and Winblad, 1974). It may be, however, that the dangers of cardiac effects in the non-toxic state have been overemphasized (Tyrer, 1981).

Clearly, caution is needed after coronary thrombosis, especially as the period after the infarct may require the use of digoxin and antidiuretics, and reduction of salt intake. Thus apart from its effects at toxic levels, care is needed with lithium in patients with a vulnerability to develop ventricular arrhythmias with this drug, and lithium should be withdrawn for two weeks after a myocardial infarct.

At usual dose ranges in normal individuals lithium may cause flattening of the T-wave in the ECG.

Epilepsy

There are no conclusive data on the results of giving lithium to patients with existing epilepsy. There are a few reports which include fits as a result of lithium therapy, including increased temporal lobe epilepsy and epilepsy during toxicity, but often there has been a reduction in frequency of fits (Schou, Amdisen and Trap-Jensen, 1968; Erwin et al., 1973; James and Reilly, 1971; Gershon and Yuwiler, 1960; Jus et al., 1973; Glesinger, 1954; Gershon and Trautner, 1956).

Lithium should be tried cautiously at low dosage in epileptics and any deterioration in frequency or worsening of the EEG pattern should be the signal to discontinue the drug and seek other methods of control. This does not apply to the established association of seizures and toxic states.

Parkinsonism

Lithium has a complex and as yet incompletely understood relationship to Parkinson's disease. Parkinsonism can be made worse, or can appear as a toxic phenomenon (Shopshin, Johnson and Gershon, 1971). This is despite the fact that many patients have had lithium and antiparkinsonian drugs with no ill effects (see below). At the time of writing, the safest course is to try to avoid giving lithium to patients with parkinsonism with affective illness whenever possible.

Cerebellar disease

Lithium in toxic dosage gives rise to symptoms of cerebellar disease—ataxia and intention tremor. Whether it should or should not be given to patients with pre-existing cerebellar disease is not known, but toxicity might give especially severe side effects.

Thyroid disease

There are ample data now on the effect of lithium in blocking the production of thyroid hormone and giving rise to a reversible hypothyroidism (Schou et al., 1968). This is usually no problem in that replacement with thyroxine will allow therapy to be continued so thyroid disease is not considered a contraindication to lithium.

Psoriasis

Rashes have been reported following treatment with lithium, but of more importance is the possibility that lithium may precipitate or aggravate psoriasis (Carter, 1972;

Skoven and Thorman, 1979). In the authors' limited experience of such cases, some can be managed on lithium despite this tendency, whilst for others the lithium has to be stopped.

Pregnancy, labour and breast feeding

Because of sampling problems the question of the teratogenicity of lithium and its degree has not been resolved with accuracy, mainly because normal births of mothers on lithium tend not to be recorded. Nevertheless, the data available from the collaborative study of Schou, Villeneuve, Goldfield and Weinstein (Weinstein, 1980) suggested an excess of Ebstein's anomaly and other cardiovascular malformations. These were associated with lithium, or lithium and other drugs in the first trimester of pregnancy. Given this tendency, it has been proposed that lithium should be given to women of childbearing age only with unequivocal indications, that any such women should practise effective contraception and be told of the risk of malformation, that planned pregnancies should be preceded by withdrawal of lithium, and that women on lithium who become pregnant should discontinue therapy as soon as possible.

Lithium may be resumed after the third months of pregnancy if the psychiatric condition merits it. Initially the dosage may need to be lower than that given habitually to that individual because lithium clearances may be reduced in the first half of pregnancy. However, during the second trimester the converse develops, renal clearance is increased so that larger than usual doses may be required (Schou, Amdisen and Steenstrup, 1973).

Ideally, lithium should be discontinued at 38 weeks. Fetal and maternal bloodstream are in equilibrium as far as lithium is concerned (MacKay, Loose and Glen, 1976), and this avoids any possibility of neonatal lithium toxicity. The fetal thyroid gland is also at risk, so the maternal thyroid function should be monitored to make sure there is no lowering of thyroid hormone as a result of lithium.

Immediately after birth the mother can be restarted on lithium remembering that renal clearance of lithium then returns to 'normal'.

Breast feeding while taking lithium is not absolutely contraindicated as a matter of dogma, but on the whole is not advisable, since breast milk contains 10–50 per cent of the level found in the mother's serum (Schou and Amdisen, 1973). In a mother on low levels of lithium it might be permissible, but it is a case of weighing up the pros and cons, even in such circumstances. If breast feeding is undertaken the parents must be carefully instructed to watch for and discontinue breast feeding at any sign of toxicity in the child—restlessness, fever, vomiting, diarrhoea, sluggishness, until the lithium level has been assayed. In general breast feeding should be discouraged.

Drug interactions

Diuretics

With the thiazides, as discussed above, the lessening of proximal tubular absorption of sodium enhances lithium re-uptake so that toxicity can develop rapidly. It follows that the concurrent use of thiazides with lithium should be avoided when possible. When it cannot, the aim should be to reduce the lithium dosage in preparation for a thiazide-induced rise in lithium, and assays of plasma lithium should be frequent.

Other diuretics, e.g. triamterene and amiloride, may prevent reabsorption of lithium (Singer and Franko, 1973), so that again lithium levels need to be monitored frequently.

Nephrotoxins

Lithium intoxication may follow the parallel administration of drugs which are potentially toxic to the kidney, such as tetracycline and spectinomycin (Conroy, 1978; McGennes, 1978).

Anti-inflammatory drugs

There is a complex relationship between lithium and anti-inflammatory drugs. Indomethacin, and possibly phenylbutazone, inhibit the synthesis of prostaglandins $(PG)E_1$ production, and this potentiates the effects of ADH. Water clearance will be reduced, and both plasma osmolarity and lithium levels will rise (Leftwich *et al.*, 1978). Use of either drug is yet another indication for frequent lithium assays.

Drugs used in cardiovascular diseases

QUINIDINE

In theory quinidine should be avoided during lithium treatment. Although the effect on a-v block is probably small, quinidine can produce partial a-v block which, pending further knowledge, lithium might potentiate slightly.

DIGITALIS

Lithium reduces intracellular potassium, an action whose effects on the myocardium may result in the flattened T-waves as seen in the ECG. If thiazide diuretics are also given, this can lead to further losses of intracellular potassium and sodium. The myocardial hypokalaemia could lead to an increase in the toxicity of digoxin.

In a person in cardiac failure, the combination of digoxin, lithium and Na^+/K^+ depleting diuretics is a therapeutic tangle. Sodium losses are going to enhance lithium toxicity and lithium may be complicating the effect of the cardiac glycoside.

ANTIHYPERTENSIVE COMPOUNDS

Lithium has no effect on blood pressure in patients with hypertension and there are few contraindications to antihypertensive drugs.

The questionable exception may be α-methyldopa which has been reported as possibly increasing side effects during lithium therapy (O'Regan, 1976; Byrd, 1975), but this needs further study.

Drugs acting on the central nervous system

Lithium has no significantly dangerous interactions with moderate amounts of alcohol or analgesics, but may potentiate the anticonvulsant effect of phenytoin (Umberkoman and Joseph, 1974).

Benzodiazepines, other minor tranquillizers, MAOIs, tricyclics and other anti-depressants can be given without problems, although tremor may be more trouble-some when lithium is combined with tricyclics.

Neuroleptics are a special case. Large numbers of patients have received lithium and chlorpromazine, and lithium and haloperidol without serious irreversible side effects but some authors report greater incidence of neurological symptoms on the combined drugs, particularly of extrapyramidal side effects (Krishna, Taylor and Abrams, 1978; Juhl, Tsuang and Perry, 1977; Strayhorn and Nash, 1977; Loudon and Waring, 1976; Rifkin, Quitkin and Klein, 1973; Tyrer et al., 1980). Toxic doses of lithium may produce extrapyramidal symptoms, fits, organic brain syndrome, ataxia, abnormal EEG and finally deepening coma (Tyrer and Shopsin, 1980). Returning to haloperidol and lithium, irreversible brain damage was found where patients were maintained on very high doses of the two drugs (Cohen and Cohen, 1974). Loudon (1980) recommends keeping lithium levels to below 1 mmol if haloperidol is to be given as well, and haloperidol to 20 mg or below if the patient is on lithium. Severe toxicity involving the nervous system can also occur in especially vulnerable individuals at 'normal' serum lithium levels (Speirs and Hirsh, 1978).

Anaesthesia

Lithium can prolong the actions of suxamethonium, pancuronium and *d*-tubo-curarine (Hill, Wong and Hodges, 1976; Borden, Clarke and Katz, 1974; Basuray and Harris, 1977), so whenever possible lithium should be withdrawn 3 d before surgery.

Patients given electroconvulsive therapy while on lithium may have delayed return of respiration.

Unwanted and toxic effects of lithium

Unwanted effects of lithium fall naturally into three phases. There is an initial group present while the body burden of lithium is increasing from zero to the initial chosen end-point, and these differ in some respects from those seen at the intermediate and later stages.

Early unwanted effects

Early side effects (those occurring from the start of treatment to 5–6 d) can be reduced to a minimum by slow induction of therapy with lithium. In prophylactic therapy there is usually no urgent need to establish therapeutic levels in a hurry, so the patient can be allowed to establish equilibrium with the smallest dose, and then raised gradually to their optimum level (lithium clearance or the lithium loading test (Cooper, Bergner and Simpson, 1973) can also be used before treatment) (*see* pp. 284–285).

Age and individual susceptibility are two of the factors which determine the dosage at which side effects appear at all phases of treatment. In general, tolerance diminishes with age both as regards plasma levels and as regards dosage (reduced renal clearance with ageing and loss of body mass mean that a given plasma concentration is achieved at a smaller total input of drug).

The percentage of individuals having side effects depends very much on the characteristics of the sample and how the induction of therapy is achieved. Some side effects may be related to rates of change in plasma levels (Gershon and Shopsin, 1973). Persson (1977) has suggested that this may be important in one early side effect—fine tremor of the hands—where the high concentrations in plasma are also a factor.

Other symptoms encountered at this initial phase include abdominal discomfort, loss of appetite, nausea, loose stools, thirst and polyuria.

Later unwanted effects

Following the initial period of introduction to the drug, patients may have a variety of side effects in the time between 5–6 d of therapy extending to 5–6 weeks. A fairly common complaint is lethargy, muscle weakness, tiredness and sometimes an awareness of emotional blunting—all of which can be quite distressing even if the patient is prepared in advance. Polyuria and thirst may have persisted from the early days of treatment, or may make their debut at this time, and this applies also to the symptoms of fine tremor of the hands. The ECG alters to give a flattened or inverted T-wave and perhaps a broadened QRS complex.

Long-term maintenance therapy

From one and a half months onwards other symptoms appear. There are two forms of weight gain. One, the less common, is due to the presence of slight, mostly peripheral oedema which, while it may be annoying to the patient is not otherwise usually too troublesome. The more commonplace complaint, and one which can lead to refusal to take lithium, is gain in 'solid tissue' in the form of fat. This increase in body mass may be potentiated by other psychotropic drugs—neuroleptics, and antidepressants which conceivably may act in this way by altering central appetite/satiety centres. Craving for carbohydrates is one problem, another is the drinking of quantities of high calorific drinks because of thirst induced by lithium.

A proportion of patients in long-term therapy with lithium develop hypothyroidism or borderline hypothyroidism with or without the presence of goitre (Schou *et al.*, 1968). This is usually managed by thyroid replacement or withdrawal of the drug.

Rare side effects include skin conditions—rashes, exacerbations of psoriasis, acne, and increased white cell counts (neutrophils).

It is of interest that in a survey of 237 patients (Vestergaard, Amdisen, and Schou, 1980) on long-term treatment one-tenth had no complaints, two-thirds had one or two and one-quarter three or more. Thirty per cent complained of tremor of the hands, two-thirds had thirst, one-fifth had diarrhoea, one-fifth weight gain exceeding 10 kg and one-tenth oedema of legs or face. However, even with long continued lithium treatment the risk of renal failure and terminal uraemia was small, even after lithium had been given for many years (Vestergaard *et al.*, 1979) (*see below*).

In a further investigation (Vestergaard, Amdisen and Hansen, 1980), lithium produced little change in creatinine clearance but improvement in renal function after discontinuing lithium was not complete.

Lithium toxicity

As frequently pointed out, the therapeutic index of lithium is low. Toxicity usually develops slowly as a result of the delay in entry of lithium into the brain across the blood–brain barrier. Conversely, a person who has been in lithium toxicity may still be so even though plasma levels are within the therapeutic range. This is because of the delay in exit of the drug from the brain. The slowness of onset of toxicity applies even in patients who have taken an overdose of lithium as a suicide attempt.

These observations imply that in man, the central nervous system is the most vulnerable organ to lithium toxicity. Even in a person in steady state conditions, plasma levels may not be a useful indicant of toxicity in *some* individuals.

Susceptibility to toxicity is very variable between individuals and what is toxic for one person may not be so for another. In general, toxicity usually appears at plasma levels of 1.3–1.4 and above, but elderly people and others with usual susceptibility to the drug may manifest signs at much lower concentrations—0.5–1 mmol·ℓ^{-1}.

Impending toxicity is heralded by diminishing appetite, nausea, vomiting and diarrhoea. There is usually slight impairment of consciousness, incoordination, ataxia, dysarthria and coarse tremor of the hands (to be distinguished from the fine tremor seen as an annoying but non-dangerous side effect).

As toxicity increases the presence of acute brain syndrome becomes more apparent, leading ultimately to coma. There is increased neuronal and neuromuscular excitability as shown by fasciculation of the muscles, myoclonus, hyperreflexia, nystagmus and fits. Urinary output drops as a direct toxic effect on the kidney (leading to a dangerous situation) and in some patients there are cardiac arrhythmias.

Lithium and the kidney

Hestbech *et al.* (1977) described the renal consequences on the kidneys in patients on long-term treatment with lithium, who had had acute lithium intoxication and lithium-induced diabetes insipidus. In renal biopsies there was no evidence of acute lesions but there was focal atrophy of nephrons and/or interstitial fibrosis which was not the product of arteriosclerosis. Taking a non-psychiatric control group matched for age and sex, those who had had lithium had twice as much interstitial fibrosis, and three times as much tubular atrophy. There was also an excess of sclerotic glomeruli. Two individuals who died and came to autopsy had granular scarring and multiple small cysts.

These findings initiated further studies of the renal effects of lithium with somewhat disparate results.

Interstitial nephropathy is often accompanied by lessened ability to concentrate urine and this is a common symptom in patients on lithium who complain of polyuria. It was important to know if patients who had not experienced lithium intoxication but had had the drug long term were at risk for renal damage.

Vestergaard *et al.* (1979) found that over one-third of lithium treated patients had polyuria, 10 per cent had reduced creatinine clearance and nearly 80 per cent of the patients with polyuria had impaired concentrating capacity.

In a further investigation Vestergaard and Amdisen (1981) confirmed the earlier findings, i.e. that stopping lithium led to an improvement in renal function, but not complete 'recovery'. Lithium produced little change in creatinine clearance.

A report on this topic by Bucht and Wahlin (1978) (1980) supported these data. However, they found that patients also on neuroleptics had more severe renal effects, but their ability to draw conclusions was clouded by the fact that these patients had had high doses of lithium. During lithium therapy renal concentrating ability was correlated with dosage, withdrawal was followed by improvement in renal function which, as demonstrated before, stopped short of completion. Thus the deficiency remaining showed that the lesions were not totally reversible.

Rafaelsen *et al.* (1978) described a series of 37 patients containing one group on lithium for over five years, and five for over ten years. A urinary output of 4 ℓ or more was a good predictor of renal damage and was to be anticipated in 8–15 per cent of people treated long term. Such long periods on lithium were not necessary for the appearance of effects on the kidney according to Donker *et al.* (1979) in whose sample treatment for a mean of 3.3 years resulted in 27 per cent with polyuria and 37 per cent with low urine osmolarity. In the series of Wahlin and Alling (1979) polyuria was an indifferent indicator of renal capacity to concentrate, there was a slight relationship between this latter feature and duration of treatment but treatment for 10–15 years induced no serious renal complications. There was some suggestion that matched patients on sustained release formulations of lithium (compared with those on 'normal' release preparations) had fewer deleterious renal effects. Other workers have not replicated these findings.

Grof *et al.* (1980) in an investigation of patients maintained on long-term lithium found no deterioration in filtration rate but a deficiency in renal concentration capacity correlated with the time on lithium treatment. Coppen *et al.* (1980), in a similar investigation, also showed that creatinine clearance was only impaired in a minority (13 per cent) of lithium treated patients. Many had abnormalities in urinary osmolality but there was no significant difference compared with control depressed patients who had never been exposed to treatment with lithium, apart from increased 24-h urinary volumes in 'lithium'-treated males only.

In a recent paper, however, Tyrer *et al.* (1980) found a lower concentrating capacity in patients receiving long-term lithium compared to affectively ill patients maintained on other drugs. However, most of these patients had normal glomerular and tubular function and a later prospective study showed no effect of lithium on inulin and para-amino hippurate clearance when the drug was administered for a mean period of five months (Tyrer *et al.*, 1982).

Hullin *et al.* (1979) studied 30 patients for 8.3 (3–12.4) years and matched them with 30 psychiatric patients taking psychotropic drugs but no lithium. Excretion of arginine vasopressin in the lithium group was enhanced suggesting reduced tubular responsiveness to the peptide, but renal function as assessed by urinary volume, plasma creatinine, creatinine clearance and urine osmolality following 20 h of water deprivation did not support the view that long-term lithium altered renal function significantly. The series had been treated however at relatively low serum levels.

Given the variability in some of the findings, one of the questions remaining is whether lower stable levels of lithium without toxicity might reduce the renal problems to a negligible or non-existent level. In those demonstrating renal lesions the use of non-psychiatric controls may be inappropriate and the effect of other psychotropic drugs requires further study.

In summary there is clear evidence that patients who develop lithium toxicity are likely to have structural renal damage. However, in many cases renal function may not be severely impaired, largely because there is considerable reserve renal capacity. This should not make us complacent. Lithium toxicity is an ominous illness, both because of its immediate effects and long-term sequelae and constant care should be taken to avoid this condition.

The question of renal damage occurring in patients maintained on lithium without toxicity is less plainly answered. Most patients receiving lithium at dosages sufficient to maintain serum lithium levels within the therapeutic range show little renal functional impairment. A sizable minority demonstrate some loss of renal concentrating capacity, to be expected because of the known inhibiting effect of lithium on antidiuretic hormone, but most of these patients have normal glomerular and tubular function. However, the few studies that have involved histological examination in such patients suggest that most have more interstitial nephropathy and tubular atrophy than expected. To what extent these changes are consequent upon prolonged lithium treatment and are likely to progress with continued exposure to the drug remain unanswered questions. We do know, however, that renal failure is a very rare event in patients receiving long-term lithium and we can reassure our patients that maintenance lithium treatment has not been shown to seriously affect kidney function as long as toxicity is avoided.

Acknowledgements

Our thanks are due to Amdi Amdisen, who supplied new information about the early use of lithium. Mrs Gerrie Ballard and Miss Kay Bulmer typed and assembled the joint manuscript and we thank them for their efforts.

References

ABE, K. Lithium prophylaxis of periodic hypersomnia, *British Journal of Psychiatry* **130**, 312–313 (1977)

ALMY, G. L. and TAYLOR, M. A. Lithium retention in mania, *Archives of General Psychiatry* **29**, 232–234 (1973)

AMDISEN, A. Sustained release preparations of lithium. In *Lithium Research and Therapy* (Ed. F. N. JOHNSON), pp. 197–210, Academic Press, London (1975)

AMDISEN, A. Serum level monitoring and clinical pharmacokinetics of lithium, *Clinical Pharmacokinetics* **2**, 73–92 (1977)

AMDISEN, A. Clinical and serum level monitoring in lithium therapy and lithium intoxication. In *Lithium—Controversies and Unresolved Issues* (Eds. T. B. COOPER, S. GERSHON, N. S. KLEIN and M. SCHOU), pp. 304–332, Excerpta Medica, Amsterdam (1979)

AMDISEN, A. and SJÖGREN, J. Lithium absorption from sustained-release tablets (Duretter), *Acta Pharmaceutica Suecica* **5**, 465–472 (1968)

AMDISEN, A., GOTTFRIES, C. G., JACOBSSON, L. and WINBLAD, B. Grave lithium intoxication with fatal outcome, *Acta Psychiatrica Scandinavica* (Suppl.) **255**, 25–33 (1974)

ANGST, J., GROF, P. and SCHOU, M. Lithium, *Lancet* **1**, 1097 (1969)

ANGST, J., WEIS, P., GROF, P., BAASTRUP, P. C. and SCHOU, M. Lithium prophylaxis in recurrent affective disorder, *British Journal of Psychiatry* **116**, 604–614 (1970)

AZAR, I. and TURNDORF, H. Paroxysmal left bundle branch block during nitrous oxide anaesthesia in a patient on lithium: a case report, *Anaesthesia and Analgesia* **56**, 868–870 (1977)

BAASTRUP, P. C. The use of lithium in manic-depressive psychosis, *Comprehensive Psychiatry* **5**, 396–408 (1964)

BAASTRUP, P. C. and SCHOU, M. Lithium as a prophylactic agent. Its effects against recurrent depressions and manic-depressive psychosis, *Archives of General Psychiatry* **16**, 162–172 (1967)

BAASTRUP, P. C., POULSON, J. C., SCHOU, M., THOMSEN, K. and AMDISEN, A. Prophylactic lithium: double-blind discontinuation in manic-depressive and recurrent-depressive disorders, *Lancet* **2**, 326–330 (1970)

BAASTRUP, P. C. Practical problems concerning lithium maintenance therapy. In *Advances in Neuropsychopharmacology* (Eds. O. VINAR, Z. VOTAVA and P. B. BRADLEY), pp. 39–44, North Holland, Excerpta Medica, Amsterdam (1971)

BAASTRUP, P. C., HOLLNAGEL, P., SØRENSEN, R. and SCHOU, M. Adverse reactions in treatment with lithium carbonate and haloperidol, *Journal of the American Medical Association* **236**, 2645–2646 (1976)

BARON, M., GERSHON, E. S., RUDY, V., JONAS, W. Z. and BUCHSBAUM, M. Lithium carbonate response in depression: prediction by unipolar/bipolar illness, average-evoked response, catechol-O-methyl transferase, and family history, *Archives of General Psychiatry* **32**, 1107–1111 (1975)

BASURAY, B. N. and HARRIS, C. A. Potentiation of d-tubocurarine neuromuscular blockade in cats by lithium chloride, *European Journal of Pharmacology* **45**, 79–82 (1977)

BENNIE, E. H., MANZOOR, A. K., SCOTT, A. M. and FELL, G. S. Serum concentrations of lithium after three proprietary preparations of lithium carbonate (Priadel, Phasal and Camcolit), *British Journal of Clinical Pharmacology* **4**, 479–483 (1977)

BERGNER, P-E. E., BERNIKER, K., COOPER, T. B., GRADIJAN, J. R. and SIMPSON, G. M. Lithium kinetics in man: effect of variation in dosage pattern, *British Journal of Pharmacology* **49**, 328–339 (1973)

BORDEN, H., CLARKE, M. T. and KATZ, H. The use of pancuronium-bromide in patients receiving lithium carbonate, *Canadian Anaesthetic Society Journal* **21**, 79–82 (1974)

BROCKINGTON, I. F., KENDELL, R. E., KELLETT, J. M., CURRY, S. H. and WAINWRIGHT, S. Trials of lithium, chlorpromazine and amitriptyline in schizoaffective patients, *British Journal of Psychiatry* **133**, 162–168 (1978)

BUCHT, G. and WAHLIN, A. Impairment of renal concentrating capacity by lithium, *Lancet* **1**, 778–779 (1978)

BUCHT, G. and WAHLIN, A. Renal concentrating capacity in long-term lithium treatment and after withdrawal of lithium, *Acta Medica Scandinavica* **207**, 309–314 (1980)

BYRD, G. J. Methyl dopa and lithium carbonate: suspected interaction, *Journal of the American Medical Association* **233**, 320 (1975)

CADE, J. F. J. Lithium salts in the treatment of psychotic excitement, *Medical Journal of Australia* **2**, 349–352 (1949)

CARTER, T. N. The relationship of lithium carbonate to psoriasis, *Psychosomatica* **13**, 325–327 (1972)

CARROLL, B. J. and FEINBERG, M. P. Intracellular lithium, *Neuropharmacology* **16**, 527 (1977)

CATTELL, W. R., COPPEN, A., BAILEY, J. and RAMA RAO, V. A. Impairment of renal concentrating ability by lithium, *Lancet* **2**, 44–45 (1978)

COHEN, W. J. and COHEN, N. H. Lithium carbonate, haloperidol and irreversible brain damage, *Journal of the American Medical Association* **230**, 1283–1287 (1974)

COLBURN, R. W., GOODWIN, F. K., BUNNEY, W. E. and DAVIS, J. M. Effect of lithium on the uptake of noradrenaline by synaptosomes, *Nature* **215**, 1395–1397 (1967)

CONROY, R. W. Lithium intoxication in a streptomycin-treated patient, *International Drug and Therapeutics Newsletter* **13**, 15 (1978)

COOPER, T. B. and SIMPSON, G. M. The 24-hour lithium level as a prognosticator of dosage requirements: A 2-year follow-up study, *Americal Journal of Psychiatry* **133**, 440–443 (1976)

COOPER, T. B., BERGNER, P.-E. E. and SIMPSON, G. M. The 24-hour serum lithium level as a prognosticator of dosage requirements, *American Journal of Psychiatry* **130**, 601–603 (1973)

COOPER, T. B., SIMPSON, G. M., LEE, J. H. and BERGNER, P.-E. E. Evaluation of a slow-release lithium carbonate formulation, *American Journal of Psychiatry* **135**, 917–922 (1978)

COPPEN, A., BAILEY, J. E. and WHITE, S. G. Slow-release lithium carbonate, *Journal of Clinical Pharmacology* **9**, 160–162 (1969)

COPPEN, A., NOGUERA, R., BAILEY, J., BURNS, B. H., SWANI, M. S., HARE, E. H., GARDNER, R. and MAGGS, R. Prophylactic lithium in affective disorders: Controlled trial, *Lancet* **2**, 275–279 (1971)

COPPEN, A., BISHOP, M. E., BAILEY, J. E., CATTELL, W. R. and PRICE, R. G. Renal function in lithium and non-lithium treated patients with affective disorders, *Acta psychiatrica scandinavica* **62**, 343–355 (1980)

CORCORAN, A. C., TAYLOR, R. D. and PAGE, I. H. Lithium poisoning from the use of salt substitutes, *Journal of the American Medical Association* **139**, 685–688 (1949)

CORRODI, H., FUXE, K., HÖKFELT, T. and SCHOU, M. The effect of lithium on cerebral monoamine neurons, *Psychopharmacologia* **11**, 345–353 (1967)

CORYELL, W. H. and WINOKUR, G. Predicting lithium responders and non-responders: Familial indicators. In *Handbook of lithium therapy* (Ed. F. N. JOHNSON), pp. 137–142, MTP Press Ltd, Lancaster (1980)

CRAMMER, J. L., ROSSER, R. M. and CRANE, G. Blood levels and management of lithium treatment, *British Medical Journal* **3**, 650–654 (1974)

CUNDALL, R. L., BROOKS, P. W. and MURRAY, L. G. A controlled evaluation of lithium prophylaxis in affective disorders, *Psychological Medicine* **2**, 308–311 (1972)

DALE, P. G. Lithium therapy in aggressive mentally subnormal patients, *British Journal of Psychiatry* **137**, 469–474 (1980)

DAWES, P. M. and VIZI, E. S. Acetylcholine release from the rabbit isolated superior cervical ganglion preparation, *British Journal of Pharmacology* **48**, 225–232 (1973)

DEMERS, R. G. and HENINGER, G. Electrocardiographic changes during lithium therapy, *Diseases of the Nervous System* **31**, 674–679 (1970)

DONKER, A. J., PRINS, E., MEIJER, S., SLUITER, W. J., VAN BERKESTIJN, J. W. and DOLS, L. C. M. A renal function study on 30 patients on long-term lithium therapy, *Clinical Nephrology* **12**, 254–262 (1979)

DRUG AND THERAPEUTICS BULLETIN. Lithium updated **19**, 21–24 (1981)

DUNNER, D. L., MELTZER, H. L. and FIEVE, R. R. Clinical correlates of the lithium pump, *American Journal of Psychiatry* **135**, 1062–1064 (1978)

EBSTEIN, R. P. and BELMAKER, R. H. Lithium and brain adenylate cyclase. In *Lithium—Controversies and Unresolved Issues* (Eds. T. B. COOPER, S. GERSHON, N. S. KLEIN and M. SCHOU), pp. 703–729. Excerpta Medica, Amsterdam (1979)

EGLI, H. Erfahrungen mit der Lithiumprophylaxe phasicher affectiver Erkrankungen in einer Psychiatrischen Poliklinik. Erfolge und Nebenwirkungen, *Schweiz. Med. Wschr.* **101**, 157–164 (1971)

ELIASEN, P. and ANDERSEN, M. Sinoatrial block during lithium treatment, *European Journal of Cardiology* **3**, 97–98 (1975)

ERWIN, C. W., GERBER, C. J., MORRISON, S. D. and JAMES, J. F. Lithium carbonate and convulsive disorders, *Archives of General Psychiatry* **28**, 646–648 (1973)

EVRARD, J-L., BAUMANN, P., PERA-BALLY, R. and PETERS-HAEFELI, L. Lithium concentrations in saliva, plasma and red blood cells of patients given lithium acetate, *Acta psychiatrica scandinavica* **58**, 67–79 (1978)

FANN, W. E., DAVIS, J. M., JANOWSKY, D. S., CAVANAUGH, J. H., KAUFMANN, J. S., GRIFFITH, J. D. and OATES, J. A. Effects of lithium on adrenergic function in man, *Clinical Pharmacology and Therapeutics* **13**, 71–77 (1972)

FIEVE, R. R., PLATMAN, S. R. and PLUTCHIK, R. R. The use of lithium in affective disorders II. Prophylaxis of depression in chronic recurrent affective disorders, *American Journal of Psychiatry* **125**, 492–498 (1968)

FRAZER, A., MENDELS, J., BRUNSWICK, D., LONDON, J., PRING, M., RAMSEY, T. A. and RYBAKOWSKI, J. Erythrocyte concentrations of the lithium ion: clinical correlates and mechanism of action, *American Journal of Psychiatry* **135**, 1065–1069 (1978)

FRIEDMAN, E., DALLOB, A. and LEVINE, G. The effect of long-term lithium treatment on reserpine-induced supersensitivity in dopaminergic and serotonergic transmission, *Life Sciences* **25**, 1263–1266 (1979)

FRIEDMAN, E. and GERSHON, S. Effect of lithium on brain dopamine, *Nature* **243**, 520–521 (1973)

GARROD, A. B. *Gout and Rheumatic Gout.* Walton and Maberly, London (1859)

GERBER, C. J., ERWIN, C. W., JAMES, J. F. and MORRISON, D. The use of lithium carbonate in epileptic patients. In *Abstracts 5th World Congress of Psychiatry*, p. 311, Mexico City (1971)

GERSHON, S. and TRAUTNER, E. M. Treatment of shock-dependency by pharmacological agents, *Medical Journal of Australia* **43**, 783–787 (1956)

GERSHON, S. and YUWILER, A. Lithium ion: a specific psychopharmacological approach to the treatment of mania, *Journal of Neuropsychiatry* **1**, 229–241 (1960)

GERSHON, S. Use of lithium salts in psychiatric disorders, *Diseases of the Nervous System* **29**, 51–55 (1968)

GERSHON, S. and SHOPSIN, B. Pharmacology, Toxicology of the lithium ion. In *Lithium: its role in psychiatric research and treatment* (Eds. S. GERSHON and B. SHOPSIN), pp. 107–140, Plenum, New York (1973)

GLESINGER, B. Evaluation of lithium in treatment of psychotic excitement, *Medical Journal of Australia* **41**, 277–283 (1954)

GOODWIN, F. K., MURPHY, D. L. and BUNNEY, W. E. Jr. Lithium, *Lancet* **2**, 212–213 (1969a)

GOODWIN, F. K., MURPHY, D. L. and BUNNEY, W. E. Jr. Lithium carbonate in depression and mania, *Archives of General Psychiatry* **21**, 486–496 (1969b)

GOODWIN, F. K., MURPHY, D. L., DUNNER, D. L. and BUNNEY, W. E. Jr. Lithium response in unipolar versus bipolar depression, *American Journal of Psychiatry* **129**, 44–47 (1972)

GOTTESFELD, Z., EBSTEIN, B. S. and SAMUEL, D. Effects of lithium on concentrations of glutamate and GABA levels in amygdala and hypothalamus of rat, *Nature* **234**, 124–125 (1971)

GREENSPAN, K., GOODWIN, F. K., BUNNEY, W. E. and DURELL, J. Lithium ion retention and distribution: Patterns during acute mania and normothymia, *Archives of General Psychiatry* **19**, 664–673 (1968)

GROF, P., CAKULS, P. and DOSTAL, T. Lithium drop-outs. A follow-up study of patients who discontinued prophylactic treatment, *International Pharmacopsychiatry* **5**, 162–169 (1970)

GROF, P., MacCRIMMON, D. SAXENA, B., PRIOR, M. and DAIGLE, L. Bioavailability and side effects of different lithium carbonate products, *Neuropsychobiology* **2**, 313–323 (1976)

GROF, P., MacCRIMMON, D. J. SMITH, E. K. M., DAIGLE, L., SAXENA, B., VARMA, R., GROF, E., KEITNER, G. and KENNY, J. Long term lithium treatment and the kidney, *Canadian Journal of Psychiatry* **25**, 535–543 (1980)

HAIG, A. *Uric acid as a factor in the causation of disease.* Churchill, London (1892)

HARTIGAN, G. P. The use of lithium salts in affective disorders, *British Journal of Psychiatry* **109**, 810–814 (1963)

HARTITZSCH VON, B., HOENICK, N. A., LEIGH, R. J., WILKINSON, R., FROST, T. H., WEDDEL, A. and POSEN, G. A. Permanent neurological sequelae despite haemodialysis for lithium intoxication, *British Medical Journal* **4**, 757–759 (1972)

HESTBECH, J., HANSEN, H. E., AMDISEN, A. and OLSEN, S. Chronic renal lesions following long-term treatment with lithium, *Kidney International* **12**, 205–213 (1977)

HEWICK, D. S., NEWBURY, P., HOPWOOD, S., NAYLOR, G. and MOODY, J. Age as a factor affecting lithium therapy, *British Journal of Clinical Pharmacology* **4**, 201–205 (1977)

HILL, G. E., WONG, K. C. and HODGES, M. R. Potentiation of succinylcholine neuromuscular blockade by lithium carbonate, *Anaesthesiology* **44**, 439–442 (1976)

HULLIN, R. P. McDONALD, R. and ALLSOPP, M. N. E. Prophylactic lithium in recurrent affective disorders, *Lancet* **1**, 1044–1046 (1972)

HULLIN, R. P., COLEY, V. P., BIRCH, N. J., THOMAS, T. H. and MORGAN, D. B. Renal function after long-term treatment with lithium, *British Medical Journal* **1**, 1457–1459 (1979)

HULLIN, R. P. Minimum serum lithium levels for effective prophylaxis. In *Handbook of Lithium Therapy* (Ed. F. N. JOHNSON), pp. 243–247, MTP Ltd, Lancaster (1980)

ISAKSSON, A., OTTOSON, J-O. and PERRIS, C. In *Das Depressive 'Syndrom'* (Eds. H. HIPPINS and H. SELBAC), pp. 561–574, Schwarzenberg, München, Berlin and Wien (1969)

JAFFE, C. M. First-degree atrioventricular block during lithium carbonate treatment, *American Journal of Psychiatry* **134**, 88–89 (1977)

JAMES, J. F. and REILLY, E. The electrocephalographic recording of short- and long-term lithium effect, *Southern Medical Journal* **64**, 1322–1327 (1971)

JEFFRIES, J. J. and LEFEVRE, A. Depression and mania associated with Kleine-Levin-Critchley syndrome, *Canadian Psychiatry Association Journal* **18**, 439–444 (1973)

JOHNSON, G. S., GERSHON, S. and HEKIMIAN, L. J. Controlled evaluation of lithium and chlorpromazine in the treatment of manic states. An interim report, *Comprehensive Psychiatry* **9**, 563–573 (1968)

JOHNSON, G., GERSHON, S., BURDOCK, E. I., FLOYD, A. and HEKIMIAN, L. Comparative effects of lithium and chlorpromazine in the treatment of acute manic states, *British Journal of Psychiatry* **119**, 267–276 (1971)

JOHNSON, G., HUNT, G., JACKSON, D., RICHARDS, T. and KWAN, E. Pharmacokinetics of standard and sustained-release (Priadel) lithium carbonate preparations, *Medical Journal of Australia* **2**, 382 (1979)

JOHNSON, G. Antidepressant effect of lithium, *Comprehensive Psychiatry* **15**, 43–47 (1974)

JOHNSTON, B. B., NAYLOR, G. J., DICK, E. G., HOPWOOD, S. E. and DICK, D. A. T. Prediction of clinical course of bipolar manic depressive illness treated with lithium, *Psychological Medicine* **10**, 329–334 (1980)

JUHL, R. P., TSUANG, M. T. and PERRY, P. J. Concomitant administration of haloperidol and lithium carbonate in acute mania, *Diseases of the Nervous System* **38**, 675–676 (1977)

JUS, A., VILLENEUVE, A., GAUTIER, J., PIRES, A., CÔTÉ, J. M., JUS, K., VILLENEUVE, R. and PERRON, D. Influence of lithium carbonate on patients with temporal epilepsy, *Canadian Psychiatry Association Journal* **18**, 77–78 (1973)

JUUL-JENSEN, P. and SCHOU, M. Permanent brain damage after lithium intoxication, *British Medical Journal* **4**, 673 (1973)

KEMPEN VAN, G. M. J. and FABIUS, A. J. M. Lithium blood levels on use of various preparations, *Bulletin van de coordinatiecommissie biochemisch* **3**, 74–76 (1978)

KENT, N. L. and McCANCE, R. A. Absorption and excretion of the 'minor' elements in man, *Biochemical Journal* **35**, 837–844 (1941)

KLAWANS, H. L., WEINER, W. S. and NAUSIEDA, P. A. The effect of lithium on an animal model of tardive dyskinesia, *Progress in Neuropsychopharmacology* **1**, 53–60 (1977)

KNAPP, S. and MANDELL, A. J. Short- and long-term lithium administration. Effects on the brains serotonergic biosynthetic systems, *Science* **180**, 645–647 (1973)

KRISHNA, N. R., TAYLOR, M. A. and ABRAMS, R. Combined haloperidol and lithium carbonate in treating manic patients, *Comprehensive Psychiatry* **19**, 119–120 (1978)

KUKOPULOS, A., REGINALDI, D., GIRARDI, P. and TONDO, L. Course of manic-depressive recurrences under lithium, *Comprehensive Psychiatry* **16**, 517–524 (1975)

LANGE, C. *Periodische Depressionzustande und ihre Pathogenesis auf dem Boden der Harnsauren Diathese.* Voss, Hamburg (1896)

LAURELL, B. and OTTOSON, J.-O. Prophylactic lithium? *Lancet* **2**, 1245–1246 (1968)

LEFTWICH, R. B., WALKER, L. A., RAGHEB, M., OATES, J. A. and FROLICH, J. C. Inhibition of prostaglandin synthesis increases plasma lithium levels, *Clinical Research* **26**, 291 (1978)

LENA, B. and BASTABLE, M. D. The reliability of salivary lithium estimations in children, *IRCSJ Medical Science* **6**, 284 (1978)

LINGJAERDE, O., EDLUND, A. H., GORMSEN, C. A., GOTTFRIES, C. G., HAUGSTAD, A., HERMANN, I. L., HOLLNAGEL, P., MÄKIMATTILA, A., RASMUSSEN, K. E., REMVIG, J. and ROBAK, O. H. The effect of lithium carbonate in combination with tricyclic antidepressants in endogenous depression, *Acta psychiatrica scandinavica* **50**, 233–242 (1974)

LOUDON, J. B. and WARING, H. Toxic reactions to lithium and haloperidol, *Lancet* **2**, 1088 (1976)

LOUDON, J. B. Personal communications (1980)

McGENNIS, A. J. Lithium carbonate and tetracycline interaction, *British Medical Journal* **1**, 1183 (1978)

MacKAY, A. V. P., LOOSE, R. and GLEN, A. I. M. Labour on lithium, *British Medical Journal* **1**, 878 (1976)

MAGGS, R. Treatment of manic illness with lithium carbonate, *British Journal of Psychiatry* **109**, 56–65 (1963)

MANDELL, A. J. and KNAPP, S. Asymmetry and mood, emergent properties of serotonin regulation, *Archives of General Psychiatry* **36**, 909–916 (1979)

MARINI, J. L. and SHEARD, N. H. Anti-aggressive effect of lithium ion in man, *Acta psychiatrica scandinavica* **55**, 267–286 (1977)

MATHEW, N. T. Lithium therapy in cluster headache, *Headache* **17**, 92–93 (1977)

MEDICAL RESEARCH COUNCIL DRUG TRIALS SUBCOMMITTEE. Continuation therapy with lithium and amitriptyline in unipolar depressive illness: a controlled clinical trial, *Psychological Medicine* **11**, 409–416 (1981)

MELIA, P. I. Prophylactic lithium, a double blind trial in recurrent affective disorders, *British Journal of Psychiatry* **116**, 621–624 (1970)

MENDELS, J., SECUNDA, S. K. and DYSON, W. L. A controlled study of the antidepressant effects of lithium carbonate, *Archives of General Psychiatry* **26**, 154–157 (1972)

MENDELS, J. Lithium in the treatment of depression, *American Journal of Psychiatry* **133**, 373–378 (1976)

MENDELS, J. and FRAZER, A. Intracellular lithium concentration and clinical response, *Journal of Psychiatric Research* **10**, 9–18 (1973)

MENDELSOHN, M. *Zur Therapie der harnsauren Diathese. Verhandlungen des congresses für innere Medizin.* Zwolfter Congress, Wiesbaden (1893)

MERRY, J., REYNOLDS, C. M., BAILEY, J. and COPPEN, A. Prophylactic treatment of alcoholism by lithium carbonate. A controlled study, *Lancet* **2**, 481–482 (1976)

NEU, C., DiMASCIO, A. and WILLIAMS, D. Saliva lithium levels; Clinical applications, *American Journal of Psychiatry* **132**, 66–68 (1975)

NOACK, C. H. and TRAUTNER, E. M. Lithium treatment of maniacal psychosis, *Medical Journal of Australia* **38**, 219–222 (1951)

NOYES, R. Jr., DEMPSEY, G. M., BLUM, A. and CAVANAUGH, G. L. Lithium treatment of depression, *Comprehensive Psychiatry* **15**, 187–193 (1974)

OGURA, C., OKUMA, T., NADAZAWA, O. and KISHIMOTO, A. Treatment of periodic somnolence with lithium carbonate, *Archives of Neurology* **33**, 143 (1976)

O'REGAN, J. B. Adverse interaction of lithium carbonate and methyldopa, *Canadian Medical Association Journal* **115**, 385–386 (1976)

PEREZ-CRUET, J., TAGLIAMONTE, A., TAGLIAMONTE, P. and GESSA, G. L. Stimulation of brain serotonin turnover by lithium, *Pharmacologist* **12**, 257 (1970)

PERSSON, G. Lithium side effects in relation to dose and to levels and gradients of lithium in plasma, *Acta psychiatrica scandinavica* **55**, 208–213 (1977)

PERT, A., ROSENBLATT, J. E., SIVIT, C., PERT, C. B. and BUNNEY, W. E. Long-term treatment with lithium prevents the development of dopamine receptor supersensitivity, *Science* **201**, 171–173 (1978)

PLATMAN, S. R., ROHRLICH, J. and FIEVE, R. R. Absorption and excretion of lithium in manic-depressive disease, *Diseases of the Nervous System* **29**, 733–738 (1968)

PLATMAN, S. R. A comparison of lithium carbonate and chlorpromazine in mania, *American Journal of Psychiatry* **127**, 351–353 (1970)

PLENGE, P. Lithium effects on rat brain glucose metabolism in long-term lithium-treated rats. In *Lithium in Medical Practice* (Eds. F. N. JOHNSON and S. JOHNSON), pp. 145–152, MTP Ltd, Lancaster (1978)

PRACTITIONER. Quoted in *Squires Companion to British Pharmacopoeia* **1**, 116 (1907)

PRIEN, R. F., CAFFEY, E. M. and KLETT, C. J. Relationship between serum lithium level and clinical response in acute mania treated with lithium, *British Journal of Psychiatry* **120**, 409–414 (1972a)

PRIEN, R. F., CAFFEY, E. M. and KLETT, C. J. Comparison of lithium carbonate and chlorpromazine in the treatment of mania, *Archives of General Psychiatry* **26**, 146–153 (1972b)

PRIEN, P. F., CAFFEY, E. M. and KLETT, C. J. A comparison of lithium carbonate and chlorpromazine in the treatment of excited schizo-affectives, *Archives of General Psychiatry* **27**, 182–189 (1972c)

PRIEN, R. F., CAFFEY, E. M. Jr. and KLETT, C. J. Prophylactic efficacy of lithium carbonate in manic-depressive illness, *Archives of General Psychiatry* **28**, 337–341 (1973)

PRIEN, R. F., KLETT, C. J. and CAFFEY, E. M. Jr. Lithium carbonate and imipramine in prevention of affective episodes, *Archives of General Psychiatry* **29**, 420–425 (1973)

RAFAELSEN, O. J., BOLWIG, T. G., LADEFOGED, J. and BRUN, C. Kidney function and morphology in long-term lithium treatment. Paper read at International Lithium Congress, New York, 1978, pp. 528–583, Excerpta Medica, Amsterdam (1978)

RAMSEY, T. A. and MENDELS, J. Lithium in the acute treatment of depression. In *Handbook of Lithium Therapy* (Ed. F. N. JOHNSON), pp. 17–25, MTP Ltd, Lancaster (1980)

RIFKIN, A., QUITKIN, F. and KLEIN, D. F. Organic brain syndrome during lithium carbonate treatment, *Comprehensive Psychiatry* **14**, 251–254 (1973)

ROOSE, S. P., NURNBERGER, J. I., DUNNER, D. L., BLOOD, D. K. and FIEVE, R. R. Cardiac sinus node dysfunction during lithium treatment, *American Journal of Psychiatry* **136**, 804–806 (1979)

SCHOU, M., JUEL-NIELSEN, N., STRÖMGREN, E. and VOLDBY, H. The treatment of manic psychoses by the administration of lithium salts, *Journal of Neurology, Neurosurgery and Psychiatry* **17**, 250–260 (1954)

SCHOU, M. Lithium studies. 1. Toxicity, *Acta Pharmacologica Toxica* **15**, 70–84 (1958)

SCHOU, M. Lithium in psychiatric therapy and prophylaxis, *Journal of Psychiatric Research* **6**, 67–95 (1968)

SCHOU, M., AMDISEN, A. and TRAP-JENSEN, J. Lithium poisoning, *American Journal of Psychiatry* **125**, 520–527 (1968)

SCHOU, M., AMDISEN, A., JENSEN, S. E. and OLSEN, T. Occurrence of goitre during lithium treatment, *British Medical Journal* **3**, 710–713 (1968)

SCHOU, M., THOMSEN, K. and BAASTRUP, P. C. Studies on the course of recurrent endogenous affective disorders, *International Pharmacopsychiatry* **5**, 100–106 (1970)

SCHOU, M., AMDISEN, A. and STEENSTRUP, O. R. Lithium and Pregnancy. II. Hazards to women given lithium during pregnancy and delivery, *British Medical Journal* **2**, 137–138 (1973)

SCHOU, M. and AMDISEN, A. Lithium and Pregnancy. III Lithium ingestion by children breast-fed by women on lithium treatment, *British Medical Journal* **2**, 138 (1973)

SHAW, D. M., HEWLAND, R., JOHNSON, A. L., HILARY-JONES, P. and HOWLETT, M. R. Comparison of serum levels of two sustained-release preparations of lithium carbonate, *Current Medical Research Opinions* **2**, 90–94 (1974)

SHEARD, M. H. Effect of lithium on foot shock aggression in rats, *Nature (London)* **228**, 284–285 (1970)

SHEARD, M. H. Effect of lithium on human aggression, *Nature (London)* **230**, 113–114 (1971)

SHEARD, M. H. Lithium in the treatment of aggression, *Journal of Nervous and Mental Disorders* **160**, 108–118 (1975)

SHEARD, M. H., MARINI, J. L., BRIDGES, C. I. and WAGNER, E. The effect of lithium on impulsive aggressive behaviour in man, *American Journal of Psychiatry* **133**, 1409–1413 (1976)

SHIMIZU, M. and SMITH, D. F. Salivary and urinary lithium clearance while recumbent and upright, *Clinical Pharmacology and Therapeutics* **21**, 212–215 (1977)

SHOPSIN, B. and GERSHON, S. Cogwheel rigidity related to lithium maintenance, *American Journal of Psychiatry* **132**, 536–538 (1975)

SHOPSIN, B., KIM, S. S. and GERSHON, S. A. A controlled study of lithium versus chlorpromazine in acute schizophrenics, *British Journal of Psychiatry* **119**, 435–440 (1971)

SHOPSIN, B., JOHNSON, G. and GERSHON, S. Neurotoxicity with lithium: differential drug responsiveness, *International Pharmacopsychiatry* **5**, 170–182 (1971)

SIMS, A. Monitoring lithium dose levels: Estimation of lithium in saliva. In *Handbook of Lithium Therapy* (Ed. F. N. JOHNSON), pp. 200–204 (1980)

SINGER, I. and FRANKO, E. A. Lithium-induced ADH resistance in toad urinary bladders, *Kidney International* **3**, 151–159 (1973)

SKOVEN, I. and THORMAN, J. Lithium compound treatment and psoriasis, *Archives of Dermatology* **115**, 1185–1187 (1979)

SPEIRS, J. and HIRSCH, S. R. Severe lithium toxicity with 'normal' serum concentration, *British Medical Journal* **1**, 815–816 (1978)

SRINIVASAN, D. P. and HULLIN, R. P. Current concepts of lithium therapy, *British Journal of Hospital Medicine*, 466–475 (1980)

STALLONE, F., SHELLEY, E., MENDLEWICZ, J. and FIEVE, R. R. The use of lithium in affective disorders. III A double-blind study of prophylaxis in bipolar illness, *American Journal of Psychiatry* **130**, 1006–1010 (1973)

STEFANINI, E., LONGONI, R., FADDA, F., SPANO, P. F. and GESSA, G. L. Inhibition by lithium of dopamine-sensitive adenylate-cyclase in the rat brain, *Journal of Neurochemistry* **30**, 257–258 (1978)

STOKES, P. E., SHAMOIAN, C. A., STOLL, P. M. and PATTON, M. J. Efficacy of lithium as acute treatment of manic-depressive illness, *Lancet* **1**, 1319–1325 (1971)

STRAYHORN, J. M. and NASH, J. L. Severe neurotoxicity despite therapeutic serum lithium levels, *Diseases of the Nervous System* **38**, 107–111 (1977)

SWEDBERG, K. and WINBLAD, B. Heart failure as complication of lithium treatment, *Acta medica scandinavica* **196**, 279–280 (1974)

TANGEDAHL, T. N. and GAU, G. T. Myocardial irritability associated with lithium carbonate therapy, *New England Journal of Medicine* **287**, 867–869 (1972)

THOMSEN, K. and SCHOU, M. Renal lithium excretion in man, *American Journal of Physiology* **215**, 823–827 (1968)

TILKIAN, A. G., SCHROEDER, J. S., KAO, J. and HULTGREN, H. Effect of lithium on cardiovascular performance, *American Journal of Cardiology* **38**, 701–708 (1976)

TIME. Editorial **53**, 27 (1949)

TUPIN, J. P. and SMITH, D. B. Communication to NIMH Early Clinical Drug Evaluation Units meeting, Catonsville, Maryland (1972)

TUPIN, J. P., SMITH, D. B., CLANON, T. L., KIM, L. I., NUGENT, A. and GROUPE, A. The long-term use of lithium in aggressive prisoners, *Comprehensive Psychiatry* **14**, 311–317 (1973)

TURNER, J. G., BROWNLIE, B. E. W. and ROGERS, T. G. H. Lithium as an adjunct to radioiodine therapy for thyrotoxicosis, *Lancet* **1**, 614–615 (1976)

TYRER, P., ALEXANDER, M. S., REGAN, A. and LEE, I. An extrapyramidal syndrome after lithium therapy, *British Journal of Psychiatry* **136**, 191–194 (1980)

TYRER, P., LEE, I. and TROTTER, C. Physiological characteristics of tremor after chronic lithium therapy, *British Journal of Psychiatry* **139**, 59–61 (1981)

TYRER, S. Personal communication (1981)

TYRER, S., HULLIN, R. P., BIRCH, N. J. and GOODWIN, J. C. Absorption of lithium following administration of slow-release and conventional preparations, *Psychological Medicine* **6**, 51–58 (1976)

TYRER, S. and SHOPSIN, B. Neural and neuromuscular side effects of lithium. In *Handbook of Lithium Therapy* (Ed. F. N. JOHNSON), pp. 289–309, MTP Ltd, Lancaster (1980)

TYRER, S. P. Lithium and the kidney. In *Lithium—Controversies and Unresolved Issues* (Eds. T. B. COOPER, S. GERSHON, N. S. KLINE and M. SCHOU), p. 665. Excerpta Medica, Amsterdam (1979)

TYRER, S. P. The choice of lithium preparation and how to give it. In *Lithium in Medical Practice* (Eds. F. N. JOHNSON and S. JOHNSON), p. 395–405, MTP Ltd, Lancaster (1978)

TYRER, S. P., GROF, P., KALVAR, M. and SHOPSIN, B. Estimation of lithium dose requirement by lithium clearance, serum lithium and saliva lithium following a loading dose of lithium carbonate, *Neuropsychobiology* **7**, 152–158 (1981)

TYRER, S. P., KALVAR, M., SHOPSIN, B. and GROF, P. Prediction of lithium dose requirement: comparison of renal lithium clearance and serum lithium estimation. In *Recent Advances in Canadian Neuropsychopharmacology* (Eds. GROF, P. and SAXENA, B.), p. 172–181. Basle, S. Karger (1980)

TYRER, S. P., McCARTHY, M. J., SHOPSIN, B. and SCHACHT, R. G. Lithium and the kidney, *Lancet* **1**, 94–95 (1980a)

TYRER, S. P., McCARTHY, M. J., SHOPSIN, B. and SCHACHT, R. G. The effect of lithium on renal haemodynamic function, *Psychological Medicine* (In press) (1982)

TYRER, S. P., PEAT, M. A., MINTY, P. S. B., LUCHINI, A., GLUD, V. and AMDISEN, A. Bioavailability of lithium carbonate and lithium citrate: a comparison of two controlled-release preparations, *Pharmatherapeutica* **3**, 243–246 (1982)

UMBERKOMAN, B. and JOSEPH, T. Effect of diphenylhydantoin and lithium separately and in combination on electroshock-induced seizures in mice, *Indian Journal of Physiology and Pharmacology* **18**, 29–34 (1974)

URE, A. Observations and researches upon a new solvent for stone in the bladder, *Pharmaceutical Journal* **5**, 71–74 (1843)

VESTERGAARD, P., AMDISEN, A., HANSEN, H. E. and SCHOU, M. Lithium treatment and kidney function. A survey of 237 patients in long-term treatment, *Acta psychiatrica scandinavica* **60**, 504–520 (1979)

VESTERGAARD, P., AMDISEN, A. and SCHOU, M. Clinically significant side effects of lithium treatment. A survey of 237 patients in long-term treatment, *Acta psychiatrica scandinavica* **62**, 193–200 (1980)

VESTERGAARD, P. and AMDISEN, A. Lithium treatment and kidney function, *Acta psychiatrica scandinavica* **63**, 333–345 (1981)

WAHLIN, L. and ALLING, C. Effect of sustained-release lithium tablets on renal function. *British Medical Journal* **2**. 1332 (1979)

WATANABE, S., ISHINO, H. and OTSUKI, S. Double-blind comparison of lithium carbonate and imipramine in treatment of depression, *Archives of General Psychiatry* **32**, 659–668 (1975)

WEINSTEIN, M. R. Lithium treatment of women during pregnancy and in the post delivery period. In *Handbook of Lithium Therapy* (Ed. F. N. JOHNSON), pp. 421–429, MTP Ltd, Lancaster (1980)

WELLENS, H. J., CATS, V. M. and DUREN, D. R. Symptomatic sinus node abnormalities following lithium carbonate therapy, *American Journal of Medicine* **59**, 285–287 (1975)

WILSON, J. R., KRAUS, E. S., BAILAS, M. M. and RAKITA, L. Reversible sinus node abnormalities due to lithium carbonate therapy, *New England Journal of Medicine* **294**, 1223–1224 (1976)

WORRALL, E. P., MOODY, J. P. and NAYLOR, G. J. Lithium in non-manic depressives. Antiaggressive effect and red blood cell lithium values, *British Journal of Psychiatry* **126**, 464–468 (1975)

WORRALL, E. P., MOODY, J. P., PEET, M., DICK, P., SMITH, A., CHAMBERS, C., ADAMS, M. and NAYLOR, G. J. Controlled studies of the acute antidepressant effects of lithium, *British Journal of Psychiatry* **135**, 255–262 (1979)

Chapter 11

Psychostimulants

S. Checkley

Introduction

The history of the use and abuse of each of the psychostimulants has followed a familiar cycle. The discovery of each euphoriant drug has been followed by reports of its widespread use, by reports of dependence, of drug-induced psychoses and finally by legal restrictions on prescribing the drug. Thus cocaine has for centuries been obtained by chewing coca leaves but it was not until the late nineteenth century that cocaine could efficiently be extracted and manufactured. Its stimulant properties were appreciated (Aschenbrandt, 1883) and it was widely abused. Reports of dependence (Erlenmeyer, 1885) and psychosis (Obersteiner, 1886) soon followed and now its use is restricted by the Misuse of Drugs Act.

Ephedrine is another naturally occurring stimulant but although dependence and psychosis have been reported (Herridge and a'Brook, 1968; Kane and Florenzano, 1971) such reports are rare as ephedrine has never been widely abused. However, amphetamine, which was synthesized from ephedrine in 1937, was almost immediately abused and reports of amphetamine psychoses appeared rapidly (Young and Scoville, 1938) and extensively (Connell, 1958; Angrist and Gershon, 1970) until the prescription of amphetamines was restricted.

More recently phenmetrazine, methylphenidate and diethylpropion have been synthesized. All are psychostimulants, all cause dependence and all have been reported to cause psychosis (Bethel, 1957; Bartholomew and Marley, 1959; Clein and Benady, 1962; McCormick and McNeel, 1962).

Thus the most important aspects of the psychostimulants are their propensity to produce dependence and psychosis and it for these reasons that they have been included within this volume. For the same reasons their therapeutic usefulness is limited.

Pharmacology

In normal volunteers amphetamine and methylamphetamine have central stimulant properties in that they increase alertness, decrease fatigue and inhibit sleep (*Figure 11.1a* and *b*) (Weiss and Laties, 1962). They are euphoriant, although in some subjects and particularly at high doses, the drugs can cause anxiety and sadness (von Felsinger, Lasagna and Beecher, 1955). They also cause disinhibition and increase the pressure of talk, and for these reasons can elicit the abreaction of emotionally significant memories (Jonas, 1954). The amphetamines are potent anorectic drugs. They are also sympatho-mimetic, raising blood pressure and causing a reflex bradycardia.

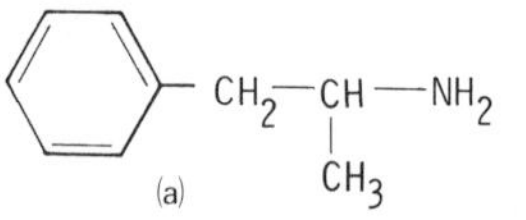

Figure 11.1a Amphetamine

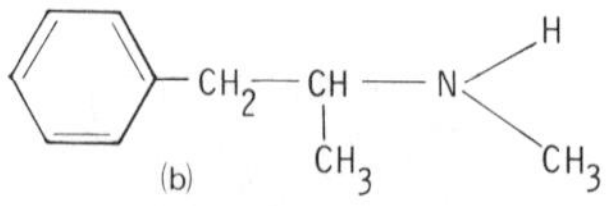

Figure 11.1b Methylamphetamine

When amphetamine is given to experimental animals in clinically relevant doses, then its main pharmacological effects are to inhibit the re-uptake and to stimulate the release of noradrenaline and of dopamine (Moore, 1978). It is likely that these effects explain many of the clinical effects of amphetamines. Thus in animals the motor effects of the amphetamines depend upon the integrity of dopaminergic systems and the availability of newly synthesized dopamine (Moore, 1978). In man dopamine is probably involved in the euphoric effects of methylamphetamine which is inhibited by the dopamine antagonist pimozide (Jönsson, Änggård and Gunne, 1971). In animals the anorectic effect of amphetamine is also dependent upon the normal synthesis of dopamine and the integrity of dopamine pathways (Garattini *et al.*, 1978). Noradrenaline mediates the peripheral sympathomimetic effects of amphetamines and may also be involved in the mediation of the stimulant effect of amphetamines.

When given in larger doses the amphetamines have a number of other biochemical effects in experimental animals. Monoamine oxidase is inhibited: catecholamine receptors are stimulated: catecholamine, indoleamine and acetylcholine stores are depleted (Estler, 1975). However there is no evidence that these effects of amphetamine mediate its clinical effects which appear to depend upon an increased availability of noradrenaline and dopamine at post-synaptic receptors. The effects of the fluorinated amphetamines upon 5-hydroxytryptamine will be discussed in a later section.

Pharmacokinetics

Peak plasma concentrations are reached at 2–3 h after the oral administration of *d*-amphetamine (30 mg), at which time the psychological effects are greatest (Ebert, van Kammen and Murphy, 1974). Under these conditions and with a urinary pH of between 6 and 7.5 the plasma half-life of amphetamine is approximately 10 h (Ebert, van Kammen and Murphy, 1974).

Methylamphetamine is given intravenously: in animals it crosses the blood–brain barrier rapidly (Latini *et al.*, 1977) and in man it produces its psychological effects within minutes. Methylamphetamine is metabolized slowly to amphetamine (Beckett and Rowland, 1965) and the two are excreted in the urine. When amphetamine is administered orally roughly half is excreted in the urine unchanged, the remainder being metabolized in the liver. The urinary excretion of amphetamine is enhanced by acidification of the urine (Beckett and Rowland, 1964).

Clinical efficacy

The hyperkinetic syndrome (Barkley, 1977)

Psychostimulants are the drugs of first choice in the treatment of children with the hyperkinetic syndrome. In the short term the drugs improve attention, reduce restlessness and help to control impulsive behaviour although academic performance and interpersonal functioning are not helped. The drugs have their usual stimulant effects in children and these account for their most important side effects which are insomnia, irritability and anorexia. Tolerance towards these side effects may develop with time or else they may be controlled by reducing the dose. Retarded growth is a persistent problem although this may be prevented by the use of drug holidays. Psychostimulants have no effects upon the long-term natural history of the hyperkinetic syndrome. Methylphenidate and d-amphetamine are given in a daily dose of 10–30 mg.

Narcolepsy

Narcolepsy is a condition which is characterized by brief recurrent episodes of unwanted and inescapable sleep. Traditionally the condition has been treated with amphetamine (5–120 mg daily) although the response is variable (Parkes, 1977).

Other indications

There are no other established indications for the prescription of amphetamines. A 2-d course of both d- and l-amphetamine has been shown to have some antidepressant effect in a carefully conducted placebo controlled study of 11 depressed patients (van Kammen and Murphy, 1975). However a larger study in which amphetamine was given for several weeks failed to detect a useful antidepressant response (General Practitioner Clinical Trials, 1964). There is no study which compares the antidepressant response to amphetamines with that to tricyclic antidepressants and there is no study of the therapeutic usefulness of amphetamines in patients who are resistant to conventional antidepressant treatments.

Methylamphetamine infusions have been used to provoke the abreaction of important memories (Jonas, 1954). Although abreactions are little used nowadays they are occasionally used in patients in whom an acute neurosis with dissociative symptoms results from an extremely stressful event. Similarly methylamphetamine infusions have been used to elicit previously undisclosed psychotic symptomatology in patients in whom such symptoms were suspected (Myerson, 1936; Pennes, 1954). This reviewer does not recommend the use of methylamphetamine for either of these purposes as the same information can be obtained in time without the use of drugs.

Adverse effects

For most patients most of the effects of amphetamines are unwanted. These include insomnia, restlessness, agitation, palpitations, tremulousness, headache, impotence and anorexia.

Tolerance develops to some but not all of these effects. Tolerance to the anorectic and cardiovascular effects of amphetamines develops rapidly but the euphoriant and psychosis-producing effects of amphetamines may increase with repeated drug administration (Angrist and Sudilovsky, 1978).

Withdrawal symptoms

Mild fatigue and depression may follow a marked euphoric response to a single injection of methylamphetamine. After repeated drug administration and after the development of tolerance, the withdrawal phenomena become marked and severe. The main complaints are of hyperphagia, hypersomnia and depression (Angrist and Sudilovsky, 1978).

Dependence

The phenomenon of dependence upon amphetamine can presumably be attributed to the pleasant nature of the drug's initial effects, the unpleasant nature of the withdrawal symptoms and the phenomenon of tolerance.

The amphetamine psychosis

That the amphetamines can cause psychosis has been established by the experimental production of psychoses in normal subjects (Griffith, Oates and Cavanagh, 1968) and in amphetamine addicts (Angrist and Gershon, 1970). Amphetamine was given hourly ($5-10\,\mathrm{mg\cdot h^{-1}}$ to the normal subjects and up to $50\,\mathrm{mg\cdot h^{-1}}$ to the addicts) and psychoses were invariably present within 48 h. The normal subjects developed paranoid delusions, while the amphetamine addicts, who received larger doses of amphetamines, also reported olfactory, auditory and visual hallucinations and thought disorder (Angrist and Sudilovsky, 1978).

Amphetamine psychoses have mostly been studied in amphetamine addicts (Connell, 1958). Occasionally they occur after a single massive dose of amphetamine but normally there has been a progressive escalation of dose. The phenomenology of the psychosis is generally thought to be indistinguishable from that of paranoid schizophrenia. The onset is normally sudden and the patients have evidence of autonomic arousal. It has been suggested (Slater, 1959) that a clinical diagnosis of amphetamine psychosis should be considered when a paranoid psychosis of sudden onset occurs in a patient with psychopathic traits, no family history of schizophrenia with some clouding of consciousness and in whom emotional responsiveness is preserved. However, although as a group patients with amphetamine psychosis lack a family history of schizophrenia, individually they are indistinguishable from patients with acute paranoid schizophrenia. They can only be identified by the detection of amphetamines in their urine and by the resolution of the psychosis as the amphetamines are excreted from the body. When drug treatment has been needed chlorpromazine and haloperidol have been found useful (Angrist and Sudilovsky, 1978).

Methylphenidate

Methylphenidate is a slightly weaker psychostimulant than is amphetamine and for this reason is preferred in the treatment of hyperactive children (*Figure 11.2*). However the differences between methylphenidate and amphetamine are only quantitative and in large doses methylphenidate has been widely abused in Sweden where drug-induced

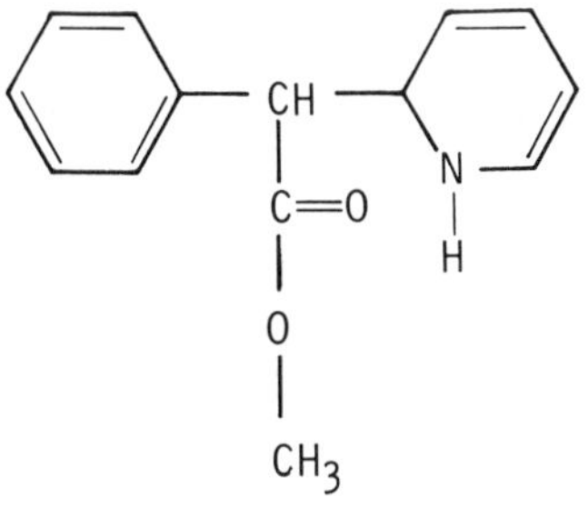

Figure 11.2 Methylphenidate

psychoses have been reported (Angrist and Sudilovsky, 1978). Like amphetamine, methylphenidate has been reported to exacerbate psychotic illnesses (Janowsky and Davis, 1976). Methylphenidate inhibits the metabolism of anticonvulsants such as phenytoin and phenobarbitone.

Other psychostimulants

The drugs shown in *Figure 11.3* have similar biochemical effects. They are all used as anorectic drugs and are all psychostimulants. They are also all prone to abuse and have been reported to cause psychosis. Their general use cannot be recommended.

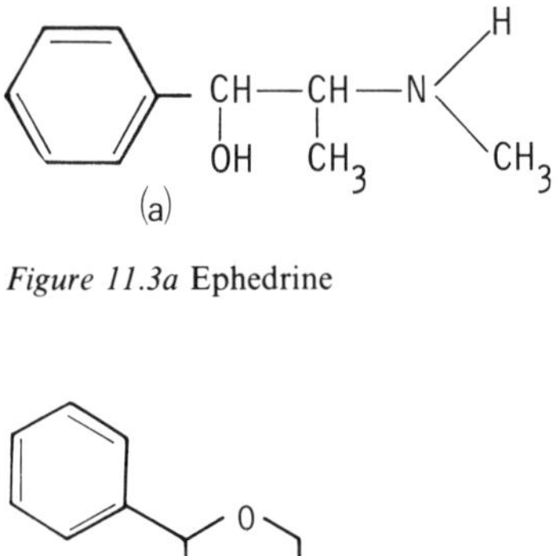

Figure 11.3a Ephedrine

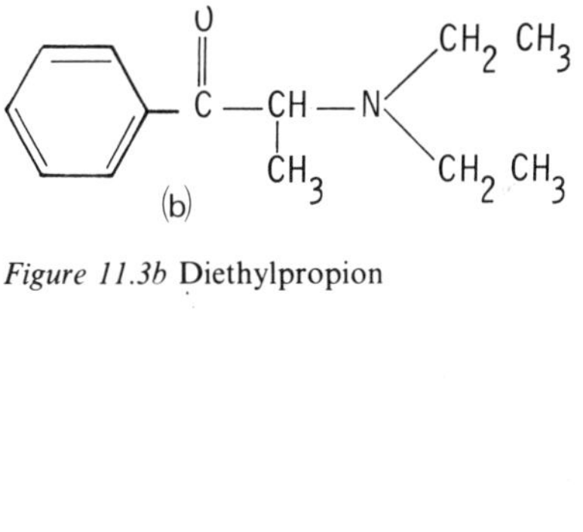

Figure 11.3b Diethylpropion

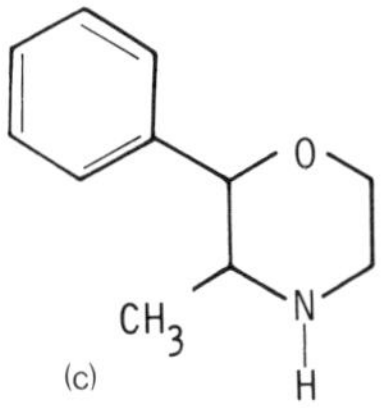

Figure 11.3c Phenmetrazine

Fenfluramine

Fenfluramine is a fluorinated amphetamine (*Figure 11.4*) but it is not a psycho-stimulant. It is included within this chapter to illustrate one of the most striking structure–function relationships that are to be found in clinical psychopharmacology. Apart from being an anorectic drug fenfluramine has little else in common with amphetamine. Fenfluramine is a sedative rather than a stimulant drug and it is not

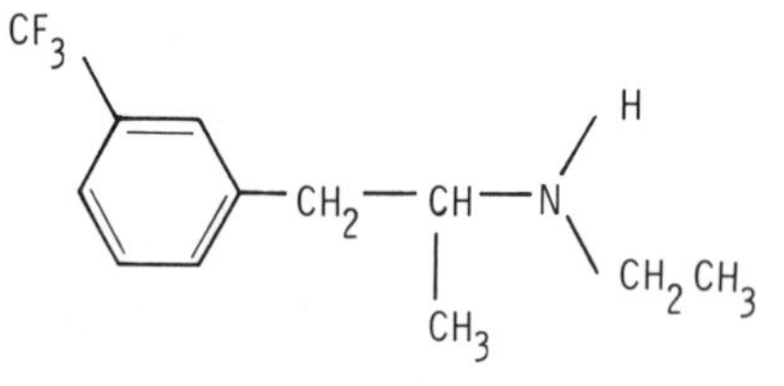

Figure 11.4 Fenfluramine

sympathomimetic. Fenfluramine is not abused and the three single cases of psychosis in association with the prescription of fenfluramine may reflect a chance association (Connell, 1975).

The pharmacology of fenfluramine contrasts with that of amphetamine. At clinically relevant doses fenfluramine predominantly affects 5-hydroxytryptamine (5-HT) (Fuxe *et al.*, 1975) whereas amphetamine predominantly affects noradrenaline and dopamine. The anorectic and behavioural effect of fenfluramine can be antagonized by blocking 5-HT receptors and by inhibiting 5-HT but not catecholamine synthesis (Jespersen and Scheel-Krüger, 1973; Clineschmidt, McGuffin and Werner, 1974) (*Table 11.1*).

TABLE 11.1 Contrasting effects of amphetamine and fenfluramine

Amphetamine	*Fenfluramine*
Anorectic	Anorectic
Stimulant	Sedative
Dependence ⎫	No abuse and probably
Abuse ⎬ common	no psychosis
Psychosis ⎭	
Sympathomimetic	Not sympathomimetic
Increases availability	Increases availability
of DA and NA	of 5-HT

See text for details and *Figure 11.1* for structural differences

Due to the lack of stimulant properties fenfluramine is the anorectic drug of first choice. The daily dose is 40–120 mg. In the short term a modest weight loss of 5–10 lb is expected (Stunkard, Rickeis and Hesbacher, 1973), although controlled studies of the long-term effects of fenfluramine have not been reported. The main side effects are drowsiness, lethargy, nausea, diarrhoea and vomiting, headache and insomnia (Stunkard, Rickels and Hesbacher, 1973).

Caffeine

Caffeine is a mild psychostimulant which shares the general sympathomimetic properties of the other members of this group. However its central effects are restricted to an inhibition of fatigue with a consequent improvement in motor performance (Weiss and Laties, 1962). Few effects upon mood or alertness are noted except when it is taken in excessive quantities. Under these circumstances symptoms of anxiety are frequent and when these symptoms are combined with those resulting from the peripheral effects of caffeine upon the sympathetic nervous system, then the net effects closely mimic those of an anxiety neurosis (Greden, 1974).

Drug interactions

Amphetamines are sympathomimetic drugs which stimulate the release of catecholamines and block their re-uptake. Consequently amphetamine enhances the action of other sympathomimetic drugs. Of these the monoamine oxidase inhibitors are the most dangerous: the combination of amphetamine with a monoamine oxidase inhibitor has probably caused fatalities and should be avoided (Connell, 1975).

Neuroleptic drugs antagonize the effects of amphetamine by blocking post-synaptic catecholamine receptor sites. Ammonium chloride hastens the urinary excretion of amphetamine and sodium bicarbonate has the opposite effect. The combination of an amphetamine with a barbiturate may enhance some of the desired effects of amphetamine (Dickins, Lader and Steinberg, 1965).

References

ANGRIST, B. M. and GERSHON, S. The phenomenology of experimentally induced amphetamine psychosis. Preliminary observations, *Biological Psychiatry* **2**, 95–107 (1970)

ANGRIST, B. and SUDILOVSKY, A. Central nervous system stimulants: historical aspects and clinical effects. In *Handbook of Psychopharmacology* (Eds. L. L. IVERSEN, S. D. IVERSEN and S. H. SNYDER) **11**, 99–165, Plenum Press, New York (1978)

ASCHENBRANDT, T. Die physiologische Wirkung und Bedeutung des Cocain insbesondere auf den menschlichen organismus, klinische Beabachtungen wahrend der Herbstwaftenubung. Quoted by Angrist and Sudilovsky, 1978 (1883)

BARKLEY, R. A. A review of stimulant drug research with hyperactive children, *Journal of Child Psychology and Psychiatry* **18**, 137–165 (1977)

BARTHOLOMEW, A. A. and MARLEY, E. Toxic response to 2-phenyl-3-methyltetrahydro-1,4-oxidazine hydrochloride 'Preludin' in humans, *Psychopharmacologia* **1**, 124–139 (1959)

BECKETT, A. H. and ROWLAND, M. Rhythmic urinary excretion of amphetamine in man, *Nature* **204**, 1203–1204 (1964)

BECKETT, A. H. and ROWLAND, M. Urinary excretion kinetics of methylamphetamine in man, *Journal of Pharmacy and Pharmacology* **17**, 109s–114s (1965)

BETHELL, M. F. Toxic psychosis caused by Preludin, *British Medical Journal* **1**, 30–31 (1957)

CLEIN, L. J. and BENADY, D. R. Case of diethylpropion addiction, *British Medical Journal* **2**, 456 (1962)

CLINESCHMIDT, B. V., McGUFFIN, J. C. and WERNER, A. B. Role of monoamines in the anorexigenic actions of fenfluramine, amphetamine and *p*-chloromethamphetamine, *European Journal of Pharmacology* **27**, 313–323 (1974)

CONNELL, P. H. *Amphetamine psychosis* (Maudsley Monographs), Oxford University Press, London (1958)

CONNELL, P. H. Central nervous system stimulants. In *Meyler's Side Effects of Drugs* (Ed. M. N. G. DUKES), Excerpta Medica, Amsterdam–Oxford (1975)

DICKINS, D. W., LADER, M. H. and STEINBERG, H. Differential effects of two amphetamine-barbiturate mixtures in man, *British Journal of Pharmacology and Chemotherapy* **24**, 14–23 (1965)

EBERT, M. H., VAN KAMMEN, D. P. and MURPHY, D. L. Plasma levels of amphetamine and behavioural response. In *Pharmacokinetics of psychoactive drugs* (Eds. L. A. GOTTSCHALK and S. MERLIS), 157–169, Spectrum Publications, New York (1974)

ERLENMEYER, A. Uber die Wirkung des Cocain bei der Morphium-entziehung. Quoted by Angrist and Sudilovsky, 1978 (1885)

ESTLER, C-J. Effect of amphetamine-type psychostimulants on brain metabolism, *Advances in Pharmacology and Chemotherapy* **13**, 305–357 (1975)

FUXE, K., FARNEDO, L. O., HAMBERGER, B. *et al.* On the *in vivo* and *in vitro* actions of fenfluramine and its derivatives on central monoamine neurons, *Postgraduate Medical Journal* **51**, Supplement 1, 35–44 (1975)

GARATTINI, S., BORRONI, E., MENNINI, T. and SAMARIN, R. Differences and similarities among anorectic drugs. In *Central Mechanisms of Anorectic Drugs* (Eds. S. GARATTINI and R. SAMARIN), pp. 127–143, Raven Press, New York (1978)

GENERAL PRACTITIONER CLINICAL TRIALS. Dexamphetamine compared with an inactive placebo in depression, *Practitioner* **192**, 151–154 (1964)

GREDEN, J. F. Anxiety or caffeinism, *American Journal of Psychiatry* **131**, 1089–1092 (1974)

GRIFFITH, J. D., OATES, J. and CAVANAGH, J. Paranoid episodes induced by drug, *Journal of the American Medical Association* **205**, (11) 39 (1968)

HERRIDGE, C. F. and A'BROOK, M. F. Ephedrine psychosis, *British Medical Journal* **2**, 160 (1968)

JANOWSKY, D. S. and DAVIS, J. M. Methylphenidate, dextroamphetamine and levamphetamine. Effects of schizophrenic symptoms, *Archives of General Psychiatry* **33**, 304–308 (1976)

JESPERSEN, S. and SCHEEL-KRÜGER, J. Evidence for a difference in mechanism of action between fenfluramine and amphetamine-induced anorexia, *Journal of Pharmacy and Pharmacology* **25**, 49–54 (1973)

JONAS, A. D. The adjunctive use of intravenous amphetamine derivative in psychotherapy, *Journal of Nervous and Mental Disease* **119**, 135–147 (1954)

JÖNSSON, L-E., ÄNGGÅRD, E. and GUNNE, L-M. Blockade of intravenous amphetamine euphoria in man, *Clinical Pharmacology and Therapeutics* **12**, 889–896 (1971)

KANE, F. J. and FLORENZANO, R. Psychosis accompanying use of bronchodilator compound, *Journal of the American Medical Association* **215**, 2116 (1971)

LATINI, R., PLACIDI, G. F., RIVA, E., FORNARO, P., GUARNERI, M. and MORSELLI, P. L. Kinetics of distribution of amphetamine in cats, *Psychopharmacology* **54**, 209–215 (1977)

McCORMICK, T. C. JR. and McNEEL, T. W. Acute psychosis and Ritalin abuse, *Texas State Journal of Medicine* **59**, 99–100 (1962)

MOORE, K. E. Amphetamines: biochemical and behavioural actions in animals. In *Handbook of Psychopharmacology* (Eds. L. L. IVERSEN, S. D. IVERSEN and S. H. SNYDER) **II**, 41–98, Plenum Press, New York (1978)

MYERSON, A. Effect of benzedrine sulfate on mood and fatigue in normal and in neurotic persons, *Archives of Neurology and Psychiatry* **36**, 816–822 (1936)

OBSTEINER, H. Uber Intoxication Psychosen. Quoted by Angrist and Sudilovsky, 1978 (1886)

PARKES, J. D. The sleepy patient, *Lancet* **i**, 990–993 (1977)

PENNES, H. H. Clinical reactions of schizophrenics to sodium amytal, pervitin hydrochloride, mescaline sulfate and D-lysergic acid diethylamide (LSD$_{25}$), *Journal of Nervous and Mental Disease* **119**, 95–112 (1954)

SLATER, E. Book review of *Amphetamine Psychosis* by P. H. Connell, *British Medical Journal* **1**, 488 (1959)

STUNKARD, A., RICKELS, K. and HESBACHER, P. Fenfluramine in the treatment of obesity, *Lancet* **1**, 503–505 (1973)

VAN KAMMEN, D. P. and MURPHY, D. L. Attenuation of the euphoriant and activating effects of *d*- and *l*-amphetamine by lithium carbonate treatment, *Psychopharmacologia (Berlin)* **44**, 215–224 (1975)

VON FELSINGER, J. M., LASAGNA, L. and BEECHER, H. K. Drug-induced mood states in man. 2. Personality and reactions to drugs, *Journal of the American Medical Association* **157**, 1113–1119 (1955)

WEISS, B. and LATIES, V. G. Enhancement of human performance by caffeine and the amphetamines, *Pharmacological Reviews* **14**, 1–36 (1962)

YOUNG, D. and SCOVILLE, W. B. Paranoid psychosis in narcolepsy and the possible danger of benzedrine treatment, *Medical Clinics of North America, Boston* **22**, 637–646 (1938)

Chapter 12

Drugs of dependence

P. C. McLean and Patricia Casey

In this chapter we will consider a heterogeneous group of substances which share the common properties of being active in immediately altering aspects of psychic functioning and of inducing dependence. They alter mood, activity, perception, sensation or some or all of these. Many of them are not drugs in that they are not used therapeutically, either because they are of little use or because the dangers of dependence have led to their being totally or partially proscribed (e.g. amphetamines, barbiturates). Others are widely but sparingly used in medicine (e.g. opiates in analgesia) because knowledge of their usefulness is tempered by awareness of the problem of dependence.

The use of pharmacologically active substances for non-medical purposes is more correctly termed abuse. Any non-medical use of therapeutic substances is abuse (opiates, barbiturates, stimulants, hallucinogens) and use of any substance for other than its designed purpose is abuse, (e.g. the use of glue to change the mental state rather than to stick model aeroplanes together). Some substances, e.g. tobacco and alcohol, are used in an acceptable fashion by most people but abused by a minority of others and in these socially acceptable substances abuse is usually a matter of excess in inappropriate settings. Tobacco is perhaps an exception as it is now becoming common to view any tobacco use as unacceptable, particularly since it became known that it was implicated in many chronic disease processes (Royal College of Physicians, 1962) and especially since it also affects those in the vicinity of the smoker and may be viewed by the non-smoker as antisocial.

Substances vary in their ability to induce dependence. Many people, for example, drink large quantities of alcohol without becoming dependent but few escape dependence after even a short spree of heroin abuse. Nicotine in tobacco is probably the most addictive of all (Russell, 1976). There is an obvious relationship between the drug, the drug-taker and his environment, but the drug is the essential and it is the drug that determines the nature of the dependence and to some extent the consequent behaviour, although much of this is shaped by society's attitude to the addicted individual and to the drugs he chooses to take. Dependence is drug-specific and it is nowadays customary to refer to dependence of the morphine type, barbiturate–alcohol type, cocaine type, cannabis type, amphetamine type and hallucinogen (LSD) type, (Eddy *et al.*, 1965) and a volatile solvent inhalent type (WHO, 1973). More recently a syndrome of dependence on benzodiazepines has been described (*see* Chapter 6).

The characteristics of dependence-inducing substances are that they have a perceived, pleasant and desirable effect rapidly after being taken, and they tend to induce tolerance (the need to take increasingly large doses to achieve the desired effect). They induce craving—a pronounced desire (often perceived by the dependent individual as a need) to continue taking that substance. There is often an abstinence syndrome. This is a drug-specific set of physical and psychological symptoms which occur when the drug is withdrawn from the dependent individual. It is always relieved by the administration of the specific substance and sometimes by others for which cross-tolerance has developed. The relative preponderance of physical or psychological symptoms in the abstinence syndrome varies from substance to substance—in amphetamine dependence psychic discomfort is present without physical withdrawal symptoms, whereas in opiates the physical symptoms predominate at least during the early stages of the withdrawal syndrome. It is reasonable to assume that psychological dependence always exists where there is marked physical dependence, but this is not to assume that all dependent individuals will exhibit physical symptoms on withdrawal of their drug of dependence. An interesting example of physical dependence without any psychological component is said to occur with the diuretic drug, frusemide (MacGregor, Tasker and de Wardener, 1975). A reasonable definition of drug dependence is that of the World Health Organization (1969):

'A state, psychic and sometimes physical, resulting from the interaction between a living organism and a drug, characterized by behavioural and other responses that always include a compulsion to take the drug on a continuous or periodic basis in order to experience its psychic effects and sometimes to avoid the discomfort of its absence. Tolerance may or may not be present. A person may be dependent on more than one drug.'

This definition was introduced to overcome the confusion engendered by the previous terms 'addiction' and 'habituation'.

The necessary prerequisite for the development of dependence on any substance is that the individual must have taken too much, too often and for too long. It is unusual for anyone to become dependent, for example, after one or two injections of morphine given for a painful injury, but common for those suffering from terminal illness to be clearly dependent upon the high doses of opiates frequently administered over a prolonged period for the relief of pain.

The essential feature of these drugs, from a neurophysiological point of view, is that they not only affect neuronal functioning but also affect changes in that functioning, leading to adaptive responses from the neurons, which is what underlies tolerance and the withdrawal syndromes. It must also underlie the powerful drive to continue taking the drug that we know as craving. The response to these drugs will therefore differ according to the degree of change which has been induced in the drug-taker, which is, to some extent, a function of the degree of previous exposure to the drug. Thus, the effects of say, heroin on a hardened addict will differ from those on a novice. It is essential to be aware both clinically and in the evaluation of published reports, of the dependence status of the patients or subjects.

Since the nineteenth century when dependence upon opiates came to be recognized as a problem there have been many attempts to control by legal means the use of dependence inducing substances. Various measures have been formulated to deal with the drug problems of various countries. In Great Britain the current legislation is the Misuse of Drugs Act of 1971, which lays down regulations concerning the possession, supply and prescription of certain 'controlled' drugs with appropriate penalties for transgressions of these regulations and allows for the law to change rapidly to take account of changes in fashion in illicit drug taking. The Act introduced restrictions on doctors as to what they could prescribe to addicts and from 1971 doctors required a Home Office Licence to prescribe heroin or cocaine to addicts. It is not generally realized that any registered medical practitioner can prescribe to addicts any drug, including opiates, but with the exception of heroin or cocaine. There is, however, a system by which such prescriptions are monitored. This restriction was in response to the unscrupulous often financially motivated over-prescription of heroin and cocaine by certain doctors to addicts in the London area in the late 1960s. It is necessary under the provisions of current legislation to notify the Home Office* of any person whom a doctor knows or suspects to be addicted to one or more substances on a list of 14 opiates and cocaine, even if he does not treat that individual. For a full discussion of the development of legal controls of drug taking the reader is referred to Bean (1974), Edwards and Busch (1981) and Berridge and Edwards (1982).

Controlled drugs

It is essential for any clinician working in the field of drug dependence to have at least a working knowledge of the current legislation. The following is a list of the commonly occurring drugs whose use is subject to control under the regulations of the Misuse of Drugs Act (1971).

CLASS A CONTROLLED DRUGS

Opium, heroin, methadone, morphine, pethidine, dipipanone (commonly as the proprietary drug Diconal) and other opiates, cannabinol and its derivatives (except as in cannabis and cannabis resin).
Cocaine and all injectable amphetamines.
LSD, mescalin, psilocybin, phencylidine.
Any injectable preparation of a Class B drug.

CLASS B CONTROLLED DRUGS

Cannabis and cannabis resin, codeine, pholcodine, dihydrocodeine (DF 118), methyl-amphetamine, dexamphetamine, methylphenidate.

CLASS C CONTROLLED DRUGS

Methaqualone and some uncommon and less potent amphetamines.

This list is not exhaustive but includes those controlled drugs commonly encountered. Barbiturates are conspicuously missing from this list. In view of the frequency of their abuse and in view of the dangerousness of dependence and abuse of barbiturates there is currently (1982) a recommendation that all barbiturates except phenobarbitone should become Class B drugs. It is also considered that cannabis should become a Class C drug. Since the prescribed penalties for illegal possession, supply or manufacture are greatest for Class A drugs, less severe for Class B drugs and

---

* Notifications can be made within the accepted framework of medical confidentiality to The Chief Medical Officer, Home Office Drugs Branch, Queen Anne's Gate, London, SW1H 9AT. Information is available by phone (01-213 5411). Notification forms including specific information about physical characteristics, scars, tatooes, etc. are also available.

comparatively light for Class C drugs, this indicates a move towards decriminalizing the use of cannabis, a process which is already under way in some parts of the USA and in some countries in Europe.

Dependence cannot be considered solely in terms of the drugs which cause that dependence, especially in clinical practice. Dealing with drug dependents makes it clear that factors in the personality and in the individual's social circumstances contribute towards the drift into the repeated drug abuse which is necessary if dependence is to be established. Other factors, including the withdrawal syndrome conspire to maintain the dependence. Paramount here is the involvement of the person in a drug taking subculture which reinforces the drug taking habit. Vicious circles (van Dijk, 1977) which prevent the easy exit from drug taking are easily established. Van Dijk has described four such vicious circles—the pharmacological, the cerebral, the psychological and the social. It must be emphasized that drug problems occur other than those of dependence, and that it is the social and emotional problems which present to families, to social agencies, the police and the medical profession which constitute the cause for alarm over drug-taking, not the dependence *per se*. It is because of this fact that most cigarette smokers, social drinkers and habitual users of caffeine in tea, coffee, etc. do not regard themselves as 'drug addicts' since they do not create problems in the course of or because of their behaviour in pursuit of their drug of dependence. This is the notion of benign dependence which is endemic, whereas drug abuse which occurs in deviant groups or subcultures is more likely to be epidemic. Hughes and Crawford (1972) have proposed that the spread of heroin dependence is analagous to that of infectious diseases. Like infectious diseases, drug problems undergo change in type, prevalence and apparent intensity, usually in response to changes in the law. The laudanum drinking problems of the nineteenth century had disappeared by the second quarter of the twentieth century and bromism is never now encountered in clinical practice. More recently it has become apparent that stimulant, barbiturate and hallucinogen abuse are becoming less prevalent. Such changes in fashion occurring over a short period in San Francisco have been documented by Gay and Gay (1971). Bean (1974) and Plant (1975) have contributed important overviews of social aspects of drug abuse.

Since drug dependence usually presents clinically as behavioural and emotional problems, its treatment properly falls within the province of the psychiatrist. All psychiatrists should be aware of drug abuse as a possible aetiology of many abnormal mental phenomena, often simulating functional mental illness. The commonest example is delirium tremens as a manifestation of an alcohol or barbiturate withdrawal syndrome but other conditions such as amphetamine psychosis or the effects of hallucinogenic drugs may present as psychotic states and awareness of the possibility of drug abuse in the aetiology of psychoses is essential. Such drug induced states will tend to be atypical psychoses often accompanied by behavioural concomitants out of keeping with the psychoses they mimic. They also tend to be more transient. Nevertheless such conditions can be dangerous to the individual and others and require to be treated seriously.

We will now consider the various groups of substances which constitute the drugs of dependence.

Opiate drugs

Opiate drugs are powerful analgesics whose properties are in general similar to those of opium, the dried juice of the seed heads of the Oriental poppy, *Papaver somniferum*.

Opium has been used for analgesia and for the induction of euphoria and relaxation since the days of the Sumerians (about 3000 BC) and has been present throughout the Far and Middle East since then, eventually spreading throughout the world. Its dependence producing potential has been recognized since the eighteenth century. Opium was readily available on prescription or over the counter in the nineteenth century as tincture (an alcoholic solution) of opium, known as laudanum, leading to a severe problem of addiction which had, however, diminished markedly by the 1920s, only to be resurrected in a different form in the 1960s. In the USA opiate addiction continued to be a severe problem from the mid-nineteenth century to the present time, in spite of total prohibition of non-medical use.

The main constituent (10 per cent by weight) of opium is morphine, first extracted in 1803. Other alkaloids are present in smaller quantities, particularly codeine. Many other compounds have been synthesized which show morphine-like properties (strictly speaking these are opioid compounds) and others have been synthesized which reverse the effects of morphine and the other opiates (the opiate antagonists). Yet another group of drugs have been synthesized which have both agonist and antagonist properties. The more common opiate drugs are listed in *Table 12.1*.

Many effects of these drugs are the same as morphine. They differ mainly in their pharmacokinetics and in their mode of excretion, due to their differing structures. These drugs mediate their analgesic function centrally and in this respect differ from

TABLE 12.1 Common opiate drugs encountered in dependence

Name	Common proprietary preparations	Therapeutic dose (mg)	Legal status (Misuse of Drugs Act)
Codeine	Codeine Linctus	60	Class B
Dextropropoxyphene	Distalgesic (compound with paracetamol)	60	Uncontrolled
Dihydrocodeine	DF.118	30	Class B
Dipipanone	Diconal (compound with cyclizine)	10	Class A
Phenazocine	Narphen	5	Class A
Pethidine	Pethidine hydrochloride BP	100	Class A
Dextromoramide	Palfium	10	Class A
Diamorphine	Diamorphine hydrochloride BP	10	Class A
Morphine	Morphine hydrochloride BP	15	Class A
Methadone	Physeptone	10	Class A
Mixed agonist/antagonists			
Pentazocine	Fortral	30	Not controlled
Buprenorphine	Temgesic	0.3	Not controlled
Levorphanol	Dromoran	1.5	Class A

the peripherally acting aspirin-like analgesics, which accounts in part for their tendency to induce dependence. The production of dependence is also made more likely because their consumption is accompanied by a feeling of intense euphoria. This is a desirable state and leads to a tendency to repeat the experience which then leads to tolerance and dependence.

Morphine will be considered as the prototype of opiate drugs with reference made to specific differences shown by others.

Morphine has both stimulant and depressant actions on the CNS. It depresses respiration, the cough reflex and many spinal reflexes. It depresses the vomiting centre, but concomitant stimulation of the trigger zone accounts for the vomiting often experienced by novice opiate abusers. Due to excitation of the parasympathetic component of the nucleus of the third cranial nerve, morphine produces the characteristic pin-point pupil of the opiate taker. Action on the hypothalamic pituitary axis causes release of the antidiuretic hormone and may induce hypoglycaemia. The heart is slowed and there may be variable body temperature changes. Endocrine changes have been observed in heroin addicts. Ali-Afrasiabi et al. (1979) demonstrated increased thyroid functioning, decreased levels of sex hormones but no alteration in adrenal cortical functioning and Mirin et al. (1980) showed decreased sexual performance in addicts with low levels of luteinizing hormones and consequent lowered levels of plasma testosterone.

Morphine also has effects on the gut giving rise to diminished motility and constipation (codeine or kaolin and morphine mixture are frequently used as antidiarrhoeals), diminished secretions and spasm of the sphincter of Oddi. The bronchi are slightly constricted, the uterus stimulated and the capillaries dilated. Apart from dependence the unwanted effects of morphine are vomiting, constipation and itching, which is partly mediated by histamine release.

The most important effects of the opiates for our purposes are psychic. The euphoria produced by the opiates is accompanied by a sense of tranquillity and detachment. The drug-taker recognizes his problems but is unconcerned by them and feels no anxiety, tending to delay appropriate action which causes much of the self-neglect and social decline of addicts. The addict under the influence of opiates is freed from the sense of urgency to satisfy biological drives—hunger, sexual desire and aggression lose their potency as motivating forces. Bejerot (1977) has described this as 'short-circuiting of the pain–pleasure principle'. By administering a large bolus of drug rapidly by intravenous injection the drug abuser experiences a sensation of an intensity which is said to rival that of the sexual orgasm—and which is far easier to obtain. It is to obtain this 'buzz' or 'rush' that the addict increases the dose of drug. He is continually attempting to re-experience the 'rush' he used to have before tolerance to the drug set in and diminished its intensity.

Tolerance occurs to most of the effects of the opiates. Addicts frequently take doses of opiates sufficient to kill the non-dependent individual several times over. Thomas de Quincy, whose book, Confessions of an English Opium Eater vividly describes the pleasure and pain to be found in drug dependence, took more than 20 g of opium (as laudanum) daily. As tolerance occurs the pleasurable sensations diminish in duration and intensity and the drug becomes necessary mainly to stay 'straight', i.e. in a normal frame of mind and to avoid the onset of withdrawal symptoms.

The opiate withdrawal syndrome is typical of this group of drugs and is the same qualitatively for all opiate drugs (see Table 12.2). It differs in intensity from one drug to another but probably less so than addicts in a clinical situation will claim. Most addicts affect a stance of being highly discriminating connoisseurs of such phenomena but on

TABLE 12.2 Signs of withdrawal syndrome in established opiate addicts in sequential appearance (After Blachly, 1966)

Grade of abstinence syndrome	Signs (seen in cool room with patient uncovered)	Hours after last dose of main drug of addiction				
		Pethidine	Heroin	Morphine	Codeine	Methadone
0	Craving for drug, anxiety	2–3	4	6	8	12
1	Yawning, perspiration, rhinorrhoea, 'Yen' sleep	4–6	8	14	24	34–48
2	Increase in intensity of above plus: mydriasis, piloerection, tremors and muscle twitches, hot and cold flushes, aching bones and muscles, anorexia	8–12	12	16	48	48–72
3	Increased intensity of above plus: insomnia raised blood pressure, increased temperature, increased respiration rate and depth, increased pulse rate, restlessness, nausea	16	18–24	24–36	—	—
4	Increase of above plus: febrile facies. Raised blood sugar, position-curled up on hand surface, vomiting, diarrhoea, eosinopenia, weight loss (5 lb day^{-1}). Spontaneous orgasm or ejaculation. Haemoconcentration–leucocytosis.	—	24–36	36–48	—	—

Note: There is great variability in the syndrome. All the features of any one grade may not be present. Grades 3 and 4 are rarely seen outside prisons.

close examination much of their sophistication is seen to be spurious and based on myth, rumour and an attempt to manipulate the clinical situation. In many respects mild withdrawal symptoms resemble influenza. The duration and severity of the withdrawal syndrome varies according to the addict's habitual dose of drugs and according to how long he has been dependent. His motivation to change and the circumstances with special reference to the ease with which drugs may be obtained to relieve the symptoms also affect the severity of the syndrome and his tolerance of it. Cessation of drug administration is followed by the onset of symptoms—after some 4–8 h in the case of heroin or from 12–24 h in the case of methadone dependence. The patient becomes increasingly agitated, anxious and restless and experiences increasing craving for the drug of choice, or, if that is not available for any similar drug. He then suffers from rhinorrhoea, with the consequent sniffing so characteristic of addicts, and lacrimation. Abdominal cramp-like pain then develops together with profuse sweating at the same time as the patient complains of feeling cold. Diarrhoea and sometimes vomiting accompany these symptoms and throughout there is a restlessness and a difficulty in achieving a comfortable position made worse by muscle twitching and limb pains. Yawning is frequent and prolonged and insomnia is common. The patient is irritable, excitable and easily startled but may withdraw into his own misery. He will emphasize his plight and in turn be aggressively demanding for drugs or grovel and beg for them, being totally preoccupied with his discomfort and need for relief by drugs.

Examination reveals dilated pupils and piloerection, tachycardia and sometimes hypertension, as well as the more obvious behavioural abnormalities. Although the state is physiologically one of CNS hyperexcitability epileptic seizures do not occur. If they do, the questions of concomitant barbiturate or other drug dependence should be considered. Cardiovascular collapse may occur but serious complications are rare. Although uncomfortable and unpleasant the opiate withdrawal syndrome is not the life-threatening emergency it appears to the sufferer. The symptoms reach their most intense at about two days after withdrawal and then ebb away over 10–14 days, but there may be a prolonged abstinence syndrome of low grade lasting for up to three months. Craving for the opiate drug may persist for longer still, often as a feeling of not being normal without drugs.

Metabolism

Variations in the structures of the various opiates give rise to the differing metabolic profiles of the drugs. They vary in their durations of actions, rates of absorption, distribution within the tissues and excretion rates. Basicity and lipophilicity are properties which fundamentally affect these metabolic parameters (Bullingham, 1981).

Opiates are absorbed through the gut, mucosal membranes and the alveolus so they can be taken orally, sublingually or smoked. Addicts prefer the injected route because of the more rapid onset of action and for the increased intensity of the 'rush'. Intravenous injection ('mainlining') is preferred but subcutaneous injection ('skin popping') is often used especially by the more stable, therapeutic or professional, non-deviant addict.

Methadone however is almost as active when taken orally as it is when taken parenterally (van Praag, 1978) which is one of the reasons for its being a drug of choice in the treatment of addicts. The 'buzz' from methadone injection is also rather less intense and euphoric than that from other opiates especially morphine or heroin.

Opiates differ in their ability to pass the blood–brain barrier. Heroin (diacetyl morphine) passes into the brain most rapidly which may account for its being the most addictive of the opiates, and for its popularity.

Excretion of morphine occurs by intrahepatic conjugation with glucuronic acid, 90 per cent being then excreted in the urine where it may be detected for two to three days after the last dose (Jaffé and Martin, 1980). The rest passes into the faeces via the bile. Heroin is detectable in the urine only as morphine. It is deacetylated to monoacetyl morphine and then to morphine which is the active metabolite. Claims for qualitative differences between heroin and morphine must therefore be questioned. Methadone is eliminated by demethylation and cyclization of one of its side chains. Sixty per cent of methadone is detectable unchanged or as its mono N-demethylated derivative (Beckett et al., 1968). After absorption much of the methadone is bound to plasma proteins, which accounts for its longer duration of action.

Pethidine (meperidine) differs from morphine in that it has more excitatory effects and a shorter duration of action. Pethidine itself gives rise to CNS depression with coma, respiratory failure. The excitatory effects which consist of hallucinations, muscle twitches, agitation and even convulsions are attributed to its demethylated metabolite norpethidine. The effects seen in practice will therefore depend on the relative proportions of unchanged pethidine and metabolized norpethidine in the blood. The excitatory effect of pethidine administration are distasteful to many connoisseurs of opiate experience, the 'rush' being described variously as 'edgy', 'jangly' or 'rough'. Pethidine is however the drug of dependence of many 'therapeutic' addicts whose addiction was started iatrogenically by the medical administration of pethidine for the relief of pain, and of many 'professional' addicts. Most of these are doctors and midwives who had easy access to pethidine in the course of their work.

The pharmacology of dextromoramide and dipipanone is similar to that of methadone, and they are structurally similar. There is an increasing problem of dependence on Diconal, a proprietary preparation containing 10 mg of dipipanone together with 30 mg of the antiemetic cyclizine. Diconal is increasingly becoming the drug of first choice of many addicts due to the peculiarly enhanced intense euphoria rapidly following injection followed by a prolonged warm relaxation. This apparent enhancement of opiate effects by cyclizine has received little attention in the literature but we have observed addicts who take large quantities of cyclizine (as the proprietary sea sickness remedy Marzine, purchased over the counter) often by injection in addition to their prescribed methadone in order to achieve results comparable to Diconal. This practice often leads to toxic confusional states with auditory and visual hallucinations and disorientation in an affective setting of relaxed euphoria.

Pentazocine (Fortral, Talwin) and phenazocine (Narphen) are derivatives of benzmorphan, which is roughly half of a morphine molecule. They are powerful analgesics (phenazocine more so than pentazocine). Phenazocine is sometimes used by addicts. Phenazocine is a Class A controlled drug whereas pentazocine is uncontrolled; this reflects accurately their dependence inducing potential. Pentazocine has some opiate antagonist effects and, like other partial agonists, may have some psychotomimetic effects, paranoid delusions, visual hallucinations and affective change being fairly frequent accompaniments of its administration.

Opiate drugs rarely show adverse interactions with other drugs. The main exceptions are the interaction of pethidine with monoamine oxidase inhibitors and the diminution in the effectiveness of methadone in the presence of the antituberculous drug rifampicin (Stockley, 1981).

Opiate antagonists

Some compounds (pentazocine, levorphanol) are partially antagonistic to morphine-like analgesics. Apparently minor changes in the morphine molecule lead to dramatic changes in properties. Naloxone and naltrexone are examples of this in that each is a total morphine antagonist having no agonist properties. These compounds oppose the actions of morphine-like analgesics, including pentazocine and dextropropoxyphene, and have obvious uses in the treatment of opiate overdosage, where the effects are often dramatic, and in the reversal of respiratory depression in the newborn occasioned by over-enthusiastic use of opiates as analgesia in labour. Opiate antagonists will precipitate the withdrawal syndrome in the opiate dependent individual and are of great importance in the assessment of opiate activity in new compounds and in research concerning the mode of action of opiates, which is vital to any understanding of dependence.

The mode of action of opium-like drugs

A great deal of activity has surrounded this topic recently. The elucidation of the action of opiate drugs has had wide ranging implications and has given rise to a multiplicity of hypotheses concerning opiate action, opiate addiction, addictions to most other substances and pleasure seeking behaviours. The mechanism underlying opiate drug actions have been proposed as possibly being involved in the aetiology of major mental illness such as schizophrenia.

Consideration of the molecular structure and stereochemistry of various opiate drugs led to the hypothesis of specific opiate receptor sites on central neurons (Beckett and Casy, 1954). In the 1970s several workers did identify such sites irregularly distributed through the CNS. The binding of opiates to these sites is stereospecific. The sites do not bind to other inactive compounds and the affinity of a site for a specific opiate closely parallels the clinical and experimental effectiveness of the drug. The amount of opiate required to saturate these sites is very small. These manifestations demonstrate that the reactions of neurons with opiates show all the characteristics of agonist–receptor combinations.

The clinical effects of opiates, in particular the analgesia, the euphoria, the induction of sleep and vomiting are related to the distribution of the opiate receptor sites. These are particularly numerous in certain parts of the 'pain pathways' (periaqueductal grey matter, thalamic nuclei and substantia gelatinosa), the limbic system (temporal and frontal lobes, the amygdala and some septal nuclei), the locus caeruleus and parts of the fourth ventricle; areas which are concerned with pain, mood, sleep and vomiting respectively.

The presence in mammals (but not in non-mammals) of a neuronal receptor site specific for substances derived from a fairly obscure oriental plant might be considered surprising. This apparent oddity led to the postulation of endogenous opiate-like substances which acted as central neurotransmitters. Such substances were revealed in 1975 (Hughes, 1975). Initially two such substances, named enkephalins, were isolated and found to be the pentapeptides leucine-enkephalin and methionine-enkephalin (named according to and differing only in the terminal amino acid). These peptides were found to have potent opiate agonist activity (Hughes *et al.*, 1975) and to be antagonized by the specific opiate antagonist naloxone.

The enkephalins are degraded very rapidly *in vitro* by specific enkephalinases. More stable, naturally occurring opioid peptides are present in brain particularly in the pituitary, which is lacking in enkephalins. These are the endorphins and are polypeptide chains of various lengths which are fragments of β-lipotrophin commencing at amino acid position 61 in the amino acid chain. Adrenocorticotrophic hormone and β-lipotrophin are the products of a common precursor, pro-opiocortin. Although the enkephalin chains appear within the endorphin chains the endorphins are not merely precursors of active enkephalins, but have neurotransmitter activity in their own right. Three endorphins, α, β and γ have been described but most published work relates to β-endorphin. Up to six different receptor sites have been described for the various endogenous peptides and these may be receptors of differing affinities. Many opioid-peptides have been synthesized by producing compounds with differing amino acid sequences. Some of these compounds are resistant to the rapid breakdown of enkephalins by enkephalinases and some are up to 1000 times more potent than morphine as an analgesic. However, all show cross-tolerance for opiate drugs and induce tolerance and withdrawal phenomena. Unfortunately addictive and analgesic potency seem to go hand in hand so the hope of synthesizing useful non-addictive yet powerful analgesic agents has yet to be realized.

It is abundantly clear that endogenous opioid peptides play a part in the modulation of naturally occurring pain, possibly by inhibiting the excitatory transmitter, substance P, a polypeptide of 11 amino acids, which may be involved in the transmission of pain impulses in the CNS. Many endogenous opiates have been implicated in many functions of the CNS including temperature homeostasis, food intake and satiety, drinking and control of hydration, hibernation, learning and memory, reward and pleasure, endocrine function and control of motor functions. They are also involved in certain pathological processes such as schizophrenia, Huntington's chorea, Parkinson's disease and other psychoses, ethanol coma, bronchospasm, spinal shock and insulin dependent diabetes mellitus (Schachter, 1981).

The exact mode of interaction between exogenous and endogenous opioid substances is still unclear. The view that exogenous opiates totally block the opiate receptors leading to a diminution in endogenous opiate production and a subsequent lack of these substances at receptor sites on withdrawal of the exogenous opiate is probably naive. Raised levels of endorphins in blood and CSF of heroin addicts in the withdrawal phase have been observed. This is probably a homeostatic attempt at compensation. This paradox seems to point to a change in receptor sensitivity occurring in response to prolonged exposure to large doses of opiates (Clement-Jones et al., 1978). Endogenous and exogenous opiates all have depressant effects on neurons, the possible exception being Renshaw cells and hippocampal pyramidal cells (Beaumont and Hughes, 1979). The inhibitory effect is mediated by an inhibition of adenyl cyclase activity with consequent reduction in cyclic AMP which is responsible for the production of many neurotransmitters. Continuous exposure to opiates rapidly results in tolerance with a restoration of normal cyclic AMP adenyl cyclase and neurotransmitter levels (Jaffé and Martin, 1980). The withdrawal syndrome is a manifestation of neuronal excitation caused by the rebound increase in neurotransmitters following abrupt withdrawal of the exogenous opiate. The transmitters whose release is inhibited by opiates and opioid peptides in the CNS are substance P, dopamine, acetylcholine, and noradrenaline (Beaumont and Hughes, 1979).

From the point of view of treating opiate addiction, the most important neurons are those with opiate receptors which are highly concentrated in the locus coeruleus. At this site there are only about 1400 neurons, the axons of which, however, project ubiquitously and provide the major adrenergic innervation of the CNS (Snyder, 1979). These neurons are inhibited by opiates and also possess α-adrenergic receptors whose stimulation by noradrenaline or clonidine causes a slowing of their firing rate. In morphine tolerant rats showing physical dependence the adrenergic neurons of the locus coereuleus becomes tolerant to the inhibitory effect of morphine but not to that of noradrenaline or clonidine. Withdrawal of morphine in these animals provokes extremely rapid firing of the locus coeruleus neurons (Aghajanian, 1978). Rapid firing of these cells and the accompanying increase of noradrenergenic activity when provoked by α-adrenergic blocking drugs such as piperoxane or yohimbine produces many symptoms in humans which mimic the opiate abstinence syndrome, especially anxiety, agitation and hypertension. These observations provide a reasonable model for explaining the opiate withdrawal syndrome (Gold and Kleber, 1979) and provide a rationale for the use of clonidine in treatment.

Other evidence, however, points to acetylcholine as the neurotransmitter most implicated in the opiate withdrawal syndrome by a mechanism of tolerance to the inhibitory effects of opiates followed by a rebound excessive production of acetylcholine when the opiate is withdrawn (Crossland and Slater, 1968; Crossland, J. 1982, personal communication). These same workers were unable to detect changes in other neurotransmitter systems in any magnitude remotely approaching that of acetylcholine.

It is probable that the endogenous opioid peptides play some part in the regulation of neurotransmitter systems. The massive and supramaximal effects provided by exogenous opiates is likely to be manifested mainly by their effects upon various neurotransmitters. Thus it seems likely that some symptoms may be caused by effects upon one transmitter system and others in the syndrome may be the result of effects on other, different transmitters. Some effects will be mediated directly by endogenous opioids. This differential effect seems the most likely explanation of some of the apparently incompatible results obtained in studies of neurotransmitter levels in opiate addicts, in withdrawing addicts, in addicts and others receiving acupuncture and in other states.

When more clearly elucidated the relationships between exogenous and endogenous opiates and various neurotransmitters will enable treatment of dependence to become more rational with the possibility that certain agents will be found to be specific for certain symptoms or groups of symptoms of the withdrawal or dependence syndromes.

Drug treatment of opiate dependence

Treatment of opiate dependence is a complex process and due attention must be paid to the social, emotional and personality factors operating in any given case. Recent advances in our understanding of the mode of action of the opiates has begun to make it feasible to contemplate the use of pharmacological agents in the treatment of the condition of dependence *per se*.

Treatment falls into two distinct, sometimes incompatible, sometimes complementary parts. The first is the management of the withdrawal syndrome and the second is the management of the addiction with emphasis upon the mastery of the craving for the opiate drug.

A full assessment of each patient is necessary before treatment. Care must be taken to confirm the diagnosis by objective means such as urine or blood analysis to screen for the claimed drugs of dependence (reviewed by Marks and Fry, 1977) and physical examination, being careful to avoid contamination because of the danger of contracting serum hepatitis. Legal requirements regarding notification must be followed. Due to the addicts' life-style and use of often poor intravenous technique when injecting unsuitable material physical disease, especially superficial thrombophlebitis, serum hepatitis, septicaemia, multiple small emboli and gangrene of extremities is common and must be treated appropriately. The morbidity and mortality relating to opiate dependence is well reviewed by Ghodse (1981). The drugs commonly taken and the usual dosage and frequency need to be established, together with the frequency and severity of withdrawal symptoms. Since most drug-takers take many kinds of drugs a check-list approach is useful so that concomitant dependence on substances other than opiates is not missed. This might have serious consequences especially in cases of undetected barbiturate, alcohol or stimulant dependence.

A decision is necessary as to whether the patient is to be withdrawn from opiates (detoxified) and then supported to enable him to live an opiate free life or whether he is to be prescribed opiates to enable him to stabilize his life-style, to keep free from withdrawal symptoms and to avoid the necessity of obtaining illicit drugs and indulging in criminal activities. The basic treatment agreement with the patient should always be that he will be weaned away from opiate drugs, either immediately or in the not too distant future. Indefinite 'maintenance' treatment on opiate drugs may occur but should never be the basis of a contract with the patient.

The use of prescriptions of opiate drugs to attempt to stabilize and decriminalize the addiction is mistakenly referred to as the 'British System' of treatment of addiction. Methadone is the drug of choice for this procedure. It was initially used because it reduced the effectiveness of heroin (methadone blockade) and was thus expected to curtail the 'epidemic' of heroin abuse (Dole and Nyswander, 1965). It is now used because of its pharmacological properties. It is long acting, requiring less frequent dosage. It provides less of a euphoriant effect and is rather a disappointment in comparison with heroin when injected intravenously. Methadone is also as effective when taken orally as it is intravenously. Oral administration is obviously the preferred route in any drug treatment.

The assessment of any patient's dosage requirement is difficult and requires first hand observation to avoid over-prescription and thus potential supply to the illegal market. Patients' statements of their daily intake cannot be accepted as reliable. Our policy is to insist upon admission to a closely observed ward for seven days. Urine specimens are taken regularly and possible injection sites are observed f. equently. A 24 h drug-free period is usually sufficient to allow development of mild withdrawal symptoms and thus more confidently confirm the diagnosis of addiction. Methadone is prescribed in an oral form, usually as a linctus (either 1 mg in 1 ml or 2 mg in 5 ml) on a twice daily basis, adjusting the dose as necessary to obtain a state where the patient is neither intoxicated nor in a state of withdrawal.

Table 12.3 shows approximate dose equivalents of the commonly abused opiates. It

TABLE 12.3

1 mg methadone is equivalent to	3 mg morphine sulphate
	1 mg heroin
	20 mg pethidine
	30 mg codeine
	0.5 mg levorphanol
	0.5 mg dipipanone (approx.)

must be remembered that allowance has to be made for the fact that illicit drugs are often diluted with inert powders such as lactose, talc or brick-dust to increase their profitability so the patient's perception of his dosage may be quite inaccurate in terms of active drug consumption.

The usual requirement is of the order of 30–40 mg of methadone daily and very rarely more than 70 mg daily. The use of methadone linctus is to avoid the possibility of injection. Methadone tablets may be prescribed but can be crushed and dissolved and then injected often with some damage to superficial veins. Sometimes the linctus causes nausea and vomiting and tablets should then be prescribed. In our opinion there is no reason to prescribe injectable drugs—the use of injections and the enjoyment of the ritual surrounding this practice is a habit which can only be extinguished by the instant cessation of its performance. In any case it is the injections, not the long-term use of the drugs, which is responsible for the morbidity and mortality occurring in opiate addicts.

Detoxification of the opiate addicts may be undertaken by stabilization on methadone and then gradual reduction by about 5 mg every two days, with the use of benzodiazepines or other drugs as necessary for symptomatic relief.

Longer-term prescriptions of methadone whilst always aiming at eventual withdrawal from the drug, should involve close supervision of the patient. Quantities prescribed at any one time should be as small as possible and may even be collected on a daily basis. Patients should not be exposed to temptation by being allowed to handle prescriptions which should be posted to chemists or dispensed at a hospital. Prescribing opiate drugs to opiate addicts is a process open to abuse. It is a matter of individual clinical judgement how many transgressions or slip-ups are allowed or of how liberal the treatment policy is to become, in replacing prescribed drugs which have been lost, stolen or may otherwise have strayed.

Other opiate drugs, usually those with a lower addictive potential have been used for detoxification and/or maintainence, e.g. propoxyphene napsylate (Darvon-N) but methadone is currently the common drug of choice.

More recently drugs other than opiate agonists have begun to be used for treatment of addictive states. Opiate antagonists may be prescribed as maintenance therapy after detoxification to block the action of opiates and thereby diminish the reward contingent upon the taking of the illicit drug. Opiate antagonists have few effects when taken by non-dependent individuals, so unwanted effects are not common. The commonest drug used in this way is naltrexone, which has a conveniently long duration of action. Side effects are few and uncommon and consist of mild nausea with occasional abdominal pain. There is no abstinence syndrome when naltrexone is stopped. The main problem in such a regimen is patient compliance (Renault, 1979) which illustrates the importance of motivation, which can only be secured by the skilful manipulation of the doctor/patient relationship. Craving for the feelings engendered by opiate drugs is partly pharmacological and partly psychological in origin and presents problems in the management of the dependent individual. Naltrexone appears to diminish craving but it takes some four to five weeks for this to occur (Siderolf, Charavastra and Jarvik, 1978). Naltrexone, 50 mg daily by mouth, is effective in blocking the effects of up to 25 mg diamorphine for 24 h and depot preparations are being developed to prolong the time of blockade.

Cyclazocine and naloxone have also been used as antagonists in the treatment of opiate dependents.

Non-opiate drugs are being increasingly explored as therapeutic agents. Most attention has been given to clonidine (Dixarit, Catapres), which is a powerful antihypertensive agent with a central action. As we have previously noted many of the symptoms of the withdrawal syndrome are mediated by rebound adrenergic activity in the neurons of the locus coereuleus. This over-activity is reduced by clonidine which is therefore useful in aborting the opiate withdrawal syndrome. The administration of clonidine in a dose of 5 $\mu g \cdot kg^{-1}$ rapidly diminished most of the withdrawal symptoms in a double-blind cross over trial (Gold, Redmond and Kleber, 1978) and has subsequently been shown to be effective over the longer term (Gold *et al.*, 1980). Clonidine detoxification produces less withdrawal symptoms than detoxification with reducing doses of methadone, without itself producing any withdrawal symptoms (Uhde, Redmond and Kleber, 1980). Clonidine produces no opiate-like euphoria and most effectively relieves the chills, lacrimation, rhinorrhoea, yawning, cramps, sweating and muscle/joint pains with a significant but lesser reduction in anxiety and restlessness. Craving is reduced significantly. Side effects of clonidine are sedation, weakness and anergia, dry mouth and a lowering of the blood pressure sometimes enough to cause syncope. Tolerance develops to the sedative effects and the others may be mollified by changes in dosage. Hallucinations, as an effect of clonidine, have been reported (Brown, Salmon and Rendell, 1980). Dosages up to 17 $\mu g \cdot kg^{-1}$ have been used.

Clonidine appears to be a promising treatment in the detoxification of opiate addicts and may be best used as a preliminary to the institution of opiate antagonist maintenance.

Other treatments

The discovery of endogenous opioid peptides led to a resurgence of interest in acupuncture, electro-acupuncture (where the stimulus comes from a pulsed electric current passed through the needle rather than from the rapid manual rotation of the acupuncture needle) and counter irritation. The serendipitous discovery of acupuncture as a means of relieving opiate withdrawal symptoms (Wen and Cheung, 1973) led to the incorporation of acupuncture into some treatment programmes. Wen proceeded to develop a system of pulsed direct current electrical stimulation using surface electrodes, as a means of combating the opiate withdrawal syndrome. Others have claimed that electro-acupuncture is effective in all addictions in removing the withdrawal symptoms and diminishing craving but the evidence is anecdotal. The analgesia induced by acupuncture is reversed by naloxone (Mayer, Price and Rafii, 1977) and electro-acupuncture in withdrawing heroin addicts resulted in a marked increase in CSF met-enkephalin (Clement-Jones *et al.*, 1978). The conclusion that electro-acupuncture is effective in relief of pain and in relief of opiate withdrawal symptoms is inescapable and the effect is probably mediated by central stimulation of production of endogenous opioid peptides—probably met-enkephalin. In spite of relief from symptoms the addicts studied by Wen, Ho and Ling (1980) showed no change in plasma or CSF β-endorphin after electro-acupuncture, nor did the normal subjects. The usefulness of electro-acupuncture in the treatment of opiate addiction is not fully established. It may be that it is most effective when combined with other forms of treatment.

Overall, the treatment of opiate addiction is not very successful and there is a need for continual exploration and evaluation of new treatments, which must be based upon a rational appreciation of the rapidly advancing knowledge in the effects of opiates upon brain mechanisms.

Tobacco smoking and nicotine dependence

Tobacco has been smoked since antiquity and since its introduction has been continuously popular, in spite of alternating between being fashionable and being a dirty and unsociable habit. Following convincing evidence of a causal link between cigarette smoking and cancer of the lung, chronic bronchitis and heart disease, and the increased mortality of smokers, this habit has become less acceptable but hardly less popular in spite of numerous health education campaigns, warning signs on cigarette packets and limitations on advertising. There has recently been a resurgence of interest in the pharmacology and psychology of smoking and in ways of assisting smokers to give up the habit.

Tars (polycyclic hydrocarbons) from tobacco are the carcinogenic agents and the carbon monoxide present is also toxic. The main pharmacological agent is nicotine, the chronic ingestion of which gives rise to disorders of the cardiovascular and nervous system (tobacco amblyopia) which especially afflict smokers.

Nicotine has a biphasic effect dependent upon dose. Its actions are mediated at low dosage by stimulation and, at high dosage, by blockade of acetylcholine receptors at the synapse. Its actions are thus widespread and are manifestations, at the dosage normally encountered in the average cigarette (1 mg) or cigar (about 50 mg) of both sympathetic and parasympathetic stimulation peripherally. The effects on the cardiovascular system are to raise blood pressure and heart rate and to dilate the skeletal muscle vessels but to constrict those of the skin. Nicotine stimulates the smooth muscle of the gut, bladder and uterus, increases salivation, sweating and the secretion of bronchial mucus. The drug also stimulates the adrenal medulla with consequent increase in circulating noradrenaline. Skeletal muscle is stimulated. In the central nervous system the vomiting centre, the respiratory centre, cardiovascular regulating centre, and several centres in the hypothalamus are stimulated. The hypothalamic centre includes that responsible for producing the antidiuretic hormone and the satiety centre, which accounts for the tendency of ex-smokers to increase in weight.

At higher dose levels all the above effects are blocked.

Marked tolerance to the effects of nicotine occur. This is readily apparent when the casual indifference of the chain-smoking veteran is contrasted with the autonomic hyperactivity which produces the unpleasant effects on the novice, taking his first furtive puffs.

Nicotine is rapidly absorbed from skin, buccal and nasal mucosae and from the lungs, but not from the gut where it is rapidly and totally degraded to inert cotinine. Due to its alkalinity (pH 8.5) cigar smoke allows nicotine to be more readily absorbed from the buccal mucosa than the acid (pH 5.3) cigarette smoke. The cigarette smoker therefore needs to inhale to obtain maximal alveolar absorption of nicotine and thus to increase the chances of carcinogenesis.

Because the effects of nicotine are dose related the smoker, by titrating the dose, may produce a mixed state of arousal and relaxation. The cigarette is an ideal device for the fine control of the intake of nicotine (Armitage, Hall and Morison, 1968). Smokers tend to adjust their level of nicotine according to circumstances by altering the rate of puffing and the depth of inhalation and the length of time before expiration (Russell, 1980). This control of nicotine level is automatic, in the sense that smokers are not subjectively aware of their own increased arousal and vigilance (Waller and Levander, 1980).

There is some controversy as to whether smoking constitutes pharmacological or psychological dependence (Stepney, 1980) and this has been reviewed by Schachter *et al.* (1977). Russell (1976) argues cogently that those who smoke and inhale from more than 20 cigarettes daily show physical dependence. The phenomenon of tolerance is clear, the desire or compulsion to continue the habit (craving) is also clear and a tobacco withdrawal syndrome, with both physical and psychological components, is identifiable (Shiffman, 1979). This consists of craving, depression, irritability, restlessness and poor concentration together with sleep disturbance, low blood pressure (which may give rise to dizziness), constipation and bradycardia. This syndrome is variable in duration from days to weeks or even months and in part causes the frequent relapse into smoking. Ex-smokers often gain in weight, due to the absence of chronic stimulation of the satiety centre, with consequent overeating. The rapid arrival at the brain of a bolus of nicotine after the inhalation (about 7.5 seconds) and the consequent arousal are potent reinforcements of smoking behaviour so that there are both psychological and physical components to dependence upon tobacco— 'Cigarette smoking is probably the most addictive and dependence producing form of object specific gratification known to man' (Russell, 1976). 'Many in this kingdom have had such a continued use of taking this unsavoury smoke, they are not now able to resist the same, no more than an old drunkard can abide to be long sober' (King James I, 1604).

The high morbidity and mortality of cigarette smoking coupled with the addictive nature of the habit has led to an increased interest in helping people to overcome it. In 1980 there were 35 smoking clinics in Britain run by the National Health Service.

Many programmes emphasize psychological techniques, either individual or in groups, often using cognitive or behavioural methods. These are well reviewed by Lichtenstein and Brown (1980) and by Ashton and Stepney (1982).

The role of drugs in giving up smoking is not fully evaluated and it is probable that a combined approach using pharmacology within the correct psychological framework will prove to be most effective. Substitution of tobacco by lobeline, a nicotine-like drug, taken orally has been traditional but ineffective (Bernstein and MacAlister, 1976).

A link has been made between smoking and enkephalins, leading to the assessment of the effects of opiate antagonists on cigarette smoking. Naloxone caused a loss of craving and loss of interest in smoking and a reduction in consumption, when continuously infused into subjects (Karras and Kane, 1980) and long-acting opiate antagonists may prove to be useful in this area.

The ingestion of nicotine from chewing gum is proving useful as an aid to stopping smoking. Nicotine impregnated chewing gum, available as Nicorette (Lundbeck), containing either 2 mg or 4 mg per piece, is slowly chewed. The nicotine is absorbed and satisfies the craving for nicotine leading to a reduction in the use of cigarettes. There are obvious analogies here with the process of weaning an addict off opiates by means of methadone. The pharmacological and psychological aspects of smoking are divorced so that any pharmacological need is satisfied but there is no preceding behaviour to reward as no cigarette has been located, lit or sucked. By abandoning the cigarette as the source of nicotine, the smoker causes the decay and extinction of the habitual behaviour of smoking. Since he is not subjectively aware of the arousal state stemming from nicotine, it is relatively easy to abandon the chewing gum after a period which may be more than four months for heavily inhaling smokers. This is a promising technique. In a controlled trial Malcolm *et al.* (1980) found that nicotine gum produced the same abstinence rates after one month as placebo gum but much superior abstinence rates after six months. The nicotine gum was also superior to non gum-chewing controls at both one and six months. After six months however Malcolm *et al.* achieved only a 23 per cent abstinence rate using nicotine gum.

There are problems in this technique. The gum is unpleasant and burns the mouth. Too rapid chewing may cause mild nicotine poisoning, manifest often by hiccoughing. Nonetheless it is a promising development. It is unfortunate that the chewing gum cannot be prescribed under the National Health Service at present.

Amphetamines

Even though amphetamines were synthesized in 1927 and introduced into clinical practice in 1935, amphetamine dependence was not recognized until the 1940s when stocks, accumulated during the Second World War, were released on to the open market. In the early years most of the abusers were women who were prescribed these drugs for depression or slimming. Today, with effective antidepressants and a reluctance to prescribe them as dieting aids, the profile of amphetamine addicts has changed. They are now young people who either abuse them on their own or as an antidote to the depressive symptoms associated with other drug abuse.

Pharmacokinetics

This has been discussed in Chapter 11.

Tolerance

Tolerance develops to some of the effects of amphetamines—notably to the cardio-vascular and appetite suppressant actions, also to the central nervous stimulating effects. With chronic use, some abusers may be taking up to 50 times the initial dose.

In rats chronic administration of amphetamines leads to a reduction of noradrenaline and dopamine in the central nervous system. This reduction parallels the development of tolerance to the excitatory and anorectic effects.

Physical withdrawal symptoms have not been documented although this has been questioned by some (Ellinwood and Petrie, 1977). Oswald and Thacore (1963) also challenge this on their findings of an increase in REM sleep and total sleep time on discontinuing amphetamines. These changes reverted to normal on re-starting them.

Unwanted effects

ACUTE

These depend on the tolerance and dose of amphetamines. Initially euphoria is induced and awareness is heightened. Hunger and tiredness are reduced and the subject becomes more talkative. There is hyperreflexia, tachycardia, mydriasis and dry mouth, tremor, nausea and ataxia can also occur. Intravenous injection produces an intense feeling of well-being referred to as 'whole body orgasm'. In addition there is a tendency to accidents because of the excitement produced by these drugs. The EEG is activated.

LONG TERM

With chronic abuse psychotic illness indistinguishable from acute schizophrenia may develop in a setting of clear consciousness (Connell, 1958). This develops in those using more than 100 mg daily but occasionally may be precipitated by 'therapeutic doses'. This usually fades in a week but occasionally may persist and require long-term treatment. There have been some reports of brain damage following the use of amphetamines in high doses with focal neurological signs and coma (Connell, 1966; Yatsu, Wesson and Smith, 1975). The role of amphetamines in causing congenital malformation has been questioned and it now seems that the association is coincidental rather than causal (Connell, 1972). Psychological symptoms develop during withdrawal or periods of abstinence. Depression is frequent and may be severe enough to lead to a suicide attempt. Barbiturates are sometimes abused at this time as the combination is euphoriant and also induces sleep. Restlessness, hunger and fatigue are also prominent during withdrawal.

MANAGEMENT

Amphetamines may be withdrawn abruptly without physical risk to the patient. If severe restlessness or sleeplessness supervenes phenothiazines may be required. Close supervision is required if the patient becomes depressed and suicidal.

Exploration of the factors which led to the abuse of amphetamines is necessary with psychotherapeutic intervention where applicable. In the long term regular follow-up and the use of social agencies to provide support to the patient and his family are necessary. There have been no comparative studies of the various locations or forms of treatment.

Other amphetamine-like drugs of dependence

Tranylcypromine has a chemical structure similar to amphetamines. There have been individual case reports of tolerance and physical withdrawal symptoms in recent years (Legassicke, 1963; Ben-Arie and George, 1979). These are discussed in Chapter 7, p. 265).

Hallucinogens

The most widely used of these is lysergic acid diethylamide (LSD-25), whose psychoactive properties were first noted by Hoffman in 1955. Mescaline, from the Mexican cactus, has long been known to have hallucinogenic properties—hence its ritual use in pagan rites. It was not until the writings of Huxley that this group of substances became familiar to the western world. In more recent years the illicit use of this group of drugs is associated with Dr Timothy Leary.

Pharmacokinetics

LSD, mescaline and psilocybin are the most commonly found drugs of this group. LSD has a half-life in man of about 3 h. It is concentrated mainly in the hypothalamus and visual and auditory centres of the mid-brain. It is believed to act by increasing the responsiveness of sensory collaterals into the reticular formation of the brain stem. It is thought to alter 5-hydroxytryptamine metabolism by decreasing its synthesis and turnover in the brain. It also interacts with dopamine but this is complex and ill understood. Peripherally it has a sympathomimetic effect causing tachycardia, elevated blood pressure and pupillary dilation. Tolerance develops rapidly, as does psychological dependence. There is no evidence of physical dependence on this group of drugs.

Experimental uses

This has centred around the 'model psychosis' which resulted from ingestion of LSD. This paved the way for much of the psychopharmacological research into schizophrenia. It was prescribed in the 1950s for the treatment of psychotic illnesses. In addition it was used as an adjunct in psychotherapy but was later discredited.

Characteristic effects

ACUTE

LSD is a Class A controlled drug (Misuse of Drugs Act 1971) and invariably obtained on the 'black market'. It is usually taken by mouth. Its somatic effects precede its psychological effects. These consist of rapid pulse, altered salivation, nausea, headache and dizziness. After the prodromal phase, usually 30–60 min, the psychological symptoms develop. These consist of perceptual disturbance—visual hallucinations in which scenic orygeometric forms are prominent. Moving objects may seem still and surface irregularities may seem altered. Colour contrasts are either glaring or delicately blended. The subject is however able to maintain a sense of distance and insight and these perceptual disturbances are best termed pseudohallucinations. Depersonalization and derealization may occur and be prolonged. Auditory illusions with sounds either muted or amplified are common. Distortions of body images and tactile hallucinations occur. There is blending of sensory inputs so that colours may be heard and sounds felt (synaesthesiae). Vivid recollection of the past may lead the subject to believe he is reliving the past and result in delirium. Distractability, indecision and poor concentration are marked. These symptoms fade in about 6 h but residual symptoms, e.g. poor concentration, disinhibition, etc. persist for up to 24 h.

Adverse reactions

The most commonly occurring of these, colloquially known as 'bad trips', occur with unknown frequency and probably relate as much to the setting of abuse and expectation about it as to the drug itself (Mallenson, 1971). This consists of a feeling of panic with fear of imminent insanity. A toxic psychosis may also develop followed by profound depression when suicide is a risk. Sudden and profound mood changes contribute further to this risk. Accidents of a bizarre nature can occur due to delusions, e.g. walking on air.

'Flashbacks' to previous perceptual experiences may occur when the person is abstinent and are not dependent on the duration of abuse (Forrest and Tarala, 1973). They may occur for up to one year after the last dose. These are believed by some to be the most common and serious complications of LSD abuse (Dewhurst and Hatrick, 1972).

Occasionally a psychotic illness similar to schizophrenia supervenes. The duration is variable and it may last from days to years. A 'psychedelic syndrome' with passive and inert behaviour has been described in chronic users (Blacker et al., 1968). The role of LSD in causing epileptiform seizures is uncertain (Forrest and Tarala, 1973). The teratogenic effects are unproven (Robinson *et al.*, 1974) and are based on work which found that LSD produced chromosomal damage in human leucocytes *in vitro* and congenital malformation in rats and mice when injected in early pregnancy (Cohen, Hirschloren and Frosch, 1968).

Management

LSD may be stopped without fear of physical withdrawal. Close observation is necessary at this time, because of the risk of suicide. Tranquillizers may be required if agitation supervenes. Toxic psychotic states and 'bad trips' require sedation with major tranquillizers. When a schizophreniform illness develops management is along conventional lines with phenothiazines, either short or long term. In addition exploration of possible personality factors in the causation of drug abuse is necessary with psychotherapeutic intervention where appropriate. Long-term support as with amphetamine abusers is indicated although its benefit has not been scientifically proven.

Other hallucinogenic drugs

Mescaline is one of the best studied of the central stimulating drugs. Its effects are similar to those of LSD, although it is not produced in sufficient quantities now to be a widespread drug of abuse. Psilocybine is the active ingredient in teonanacatl ('the magic mushroom'), which has been used for many centuries in South American religious ceremonies. Its effects are similar to those of LSD but, unlike it, mescaline is not a widespread drug of abuse. Its effects on the ancient culture of South America have been explored by Heim and Wasson (1959).

Solvent abuse

Solvent sniffing as we know it today has become a widespread problem since the late 1950s when the first cases were reported in the USA. These substances are mainly abused by children and adolescents and are not legally controlled. The, include glues, plastic cements, gasoline, nail polish remover, etc.

Pharmacokinetics

Toluene and acetone are the commonly found organic bases in these substances. Others in addition have benzene, hexane and trichlorethylene. Toluene and acetone have a central nervous system depressant effect, benzene a bone marrow depressant action. Gasoline is a mixture of saturated and unsaturated hydrocarbons with tricresylphosphate added, which is believed to have a toxic effect on peripheral nerves.

Unwanted effects

ACUTE

The initial effects in some respects resemble those of alcohol intoxication with euphoria followed by depression. This can last from a few minutes to a few hours followed by a hangover, described as being milder than that after alcohol intoxication. Visual hallucinations and distorted spatial perception have also been reported. If inhalation continues loss of consciousness occurs. An acute psychosis similar to that caused by hallucinogens has been reported following gasoline sniffing (Tolan and Lingl, 1964). With heavier abuse cardiac arrythmias may occur and death can follow, especially after moderate to strenuous physical exercise.

LONG TERM

With long-term abuse aplastic anaemia may develop due to bone marrow depression. Hepatic and renal damage has been reported, as has peripheral neuritis and a chronic brain syndrome. The latter is thought to be due to alterations in the lipid components of central nervous system cells. EEG studies show transient abnormalities in isolated cases (Knox and Nelson, 1966). Burns have been described as a result of sniffing highly flammable substances such as gasoline. With long-term abuse there is some suggestion that solvent sniffing may be replaced by alcohol abuse (Watson, 1974). The development of physical dependence with withdrawal symptoms has not yet been definitely established (Allen, 1966). There have been single case reports of a withdrawal state similar to delirium tremens with fear, visual hallucinations, paraesthesia and abdominal pain (Merry and Zachariadis, 1962). Tolerance does develop gradually, as does psychological dependence.

Management

Solvents can be discontinued without fear of withdrawal symptoms. Acute psychotic episodes require management in the usual way with major tranquillizers. Long-term management is as for the management of conduct disorders in adolescence generally.

Minor analgesic abuse

Of the population, 2.8 per cent take analgesics daily. However, it is only recently that the extent of the problem of analgesic abuse has been recognized (Murray, 1980). The minor analgesics most frequently abused are aniline derivatives (phenacetin and paracetamol—the substance into which phenacetin is metabolized), and there have been reports of addiction to the proprietary preparation Distalgesic (Wall, Linford and Akhter, 1980). Those abusing analgesics favour ones with caffeine or codeine added (Stewart, 1978). In general simple preparations such as aspirin are taken for appropriate reasons, compound preparations for inappropriate reasons. Minor analgesics are often taken initially for recognizable symptoms, e.g. pain (Abrahams, Armstrong and Whitlock, 1970). The criterion for abuse is set at consumption of 1 g daily for three years or a total consumption of 1 kg in this period (McMillan *et al.*, 1968; Murray, Lawson and Linton, 1971). As with other drugs of abuse there is a tendency to increase the dose, because of tolerance and withdrawal headaches, so commonly experienced, reinforce this tendency further. There is denial of abuse and efforts to conceal it. Some patients will admit to taking mild analgesics because of feelings of pleasure and well being. In this respect it resembles other drugs of abuse and is not due to uninformed self-medication. Common effects of analgesic abuse are peptic ulceration, bleeding and anaemia.

Analgesic nephropathy is a well documented side effect and 500 new cases are reported annually in Great Britain and 47 new cases in the West of Scotland where minor analgesic abuse is common. The microscopic picture of nephropathy consists of papillary necrosis, interstitial fibrosis and intracytoplasmic brown granules (Lee, Davidson and Burston, 1974). Ureteric structures and retroperitoneal fibrosis have also been documented. Rarely malignancy of the urinary tract may occur. Infertility and congenital effects (Murray, 1972), brain damage (Murray, Green and Adams, 1971) and organic psychosis may occur.

Management

The management of this problem lies in its prevention. The withdrawal of phenacetin from preparations in Sweden resulted in a dramatic drop in the incidence of analgesic nephropathy. Unfortunately paracetamol which is metabolized from phenacetin is still readily available. It is likely that stricter control of this will result in a further reduction in analgesic associated renal disease. Public education about the unwanted effects of analgesics and also about their true spectrum of activity (these compounds are often taken for assumed effects, e.g. relief of tension) can only prove beneficial in combating this growing problem.

Non-barbiturate sedatives

Since its introduction in 1957 chlormethiazole has found widespread use especially in the treatment of delirium tremens. Although it is related chemically to thiamine (vitamin B1) its central nervous system effects are very similar to those of the barbiturates. It has become apparent in recent years that this drug also has some of the drawbacks of barbiturates—notably that of causing dependence. At present chlormethiazole is not a widespread drug of abuse and most reports of withdrawal symptoms have been individual case reports (Reilly, 1976). While the earlier studies suggested that it produced only a psychological dependence (Lundquist, 1966) there is now more conclusive evidence of a physiological dependence also (Von Kryspin-Exner and Mader, 1971; Reilly, 1976). In overdose it can cause severe and some-times fatal poisoning (Illingworth, Stewart and Jarvie, 1979). Chlormethiazole induces liver enzymes and, although evidence is inconclusive, there is a likelihood that tolerance to its effects develops.

The drug-seeking behaviour of chlormethiazole abusers is different from that with other drugs of abuse. It consists essentially of patients requesting further prescriptions from their general practitioners. There is little evidence of any criminal activity to procure the drug and there is no black market, in Britain at any rate.

Chlormethiazole is used therapeutically in the treatment of status epilepticus, as a hypnotic, especially in the elderly, and in the treatment of alcohol withdrawal where it is claimed it has some benefit over chlordiazepoxide (McGrath, 1975). However, this must be balanced against its addictive properties (*see* p. 159).

Methaqualone (Mandrax) has been available since the 1960s and is a drug of widespread abuse and dependence. Its main clinical use is as a sedative hypnotic. It is abused mainly by young people and is often preferred to barbiturates as a hypnotic in opiate abusers. It is taken orally and intravenously. Being a social drug it is abused in a similar way to cannabis. Doses of 600–800 mg are generally used to induce a feeling of relaxation and euphoria (a hypnotic dose is 150–300 mg). Tolerance develops and a psychological dependence has been described. The question of methaqualone inducing a physical dependence is still not certain but is likely. As well as the pleasurable feelings mentioned above, unpleasant symptoms can often occur during abuse, e.g. weakness, dizziness, nausea, diarrhoea and headache (Gerald and Schwirian, 1973). Symptoms on withdrawal include anxiety, depression, irritability, tremors and an organic psychosis (Lockhart and Priest, 1967). Methaqualone is commonly used as an agent of self-poisoning—it does not cause respiratory depression like the barbiturates but increases muscle tone and has been noted to cause convulsions and bleeding tendencies.

Glutethimide, like methaqualone, can cause a psychological and possibly a physiological dependence with a withdrawal syndrome resembling delirium tremens. More commonly withdrawal results in tremulousness, anxiety and insomnia. In overdose glutethimide is highly dangerous and can cause respiratory depression, hypotension, pulmonary and cerebral oedema as well as convulsions and apnoea. Coma is fluctuating and is thought to be due to its toxic metabolite 4-hydroxy-2-ethyl-2-phenyl glutarimide (*British Medical Journal*, 1976). In view of the risk of dependence and the dangers associated with overdose this drug should not be prescribed.

Barbiturates

These drugs were introduced into clinical practice in 1903. By 1913 it was recorded that they could cause a 'veronal habit' (Willcox, 1913). It was not until Isbell *et al.* (1950) produced experimental dependence that this danger was appreciated. Barbiturate prescribing increased throughout the 1960s and in 1968 there were 24.7 million prescriptions for this group of drugs. It was estimated at this time that about 0.2 per cent of the population were regularly using these drugs with some degree of dependence. Because of altered prescribing habits and alternative drugs, by 1973 the numbers of barbiturates prescriptions had fallen to 8.8. million (*Practitioner*, 1975).

The stereotype of the barbiturate addict—a middle-aged housewife prescribed barbiturates by her general practitioner—has been altered to some extent by the recognition of a second group of barbiturate abusers. These are young poly drug abusers (Aylett, 1978) who are similar demographically to opiate abusers.

Pharmacokinetics

This has been discussed in Chapter 6. The pharmacokinetic basis of withdrawal is not fully understood but it is believed to be due to a rebound increase in neurotransmitter release when the neurons escape from the inhibitory effects of barbiturates. There is recent evidence of increased cerebral folic acid with chronic barbiturate administration to rats which potentiates withdrawal effects. Tolerance to barbiturates develops with the effect on REM sleep being the first to appear. There is cross-tolerance to alcohol and benzodiazepines.

Unwanted effects

The short-acting barbiturates are the most frequently abused. With low doses, barbiturates have a stimulant effect which may account for their abuse potential. Although it is held that withdrawal symptoms do not occur at low doses there have been individual case reports of this occurring (Epstein, 1980). As tolerance develops and doses increase, physical dependence supervenes. Chronic intoxication produces a state of impaired functioning, often unnoticed, with ataxia, dysarthria and nystagmus.

As tolerance to the respiratory depressant effects does not occur risk of death increases with increasing dosage. On withdrawal a state similar to delirium tremens occurs. Initially the patient will complain of tremor, nausea and weakness followed by fits, hallucinations and delirium. This develops within 24 h of withdrawing the drugs and increases in intensity over the following two to three days. Occasionally, with chronic abuse a state of over-activity and violence develops. The underlying mechanisms for this are not understood (Hofmann and Hofmann, 1975). The mortality from barbiturate dependence is high and barbiturates are frequently used as drugs of self-harm, especially in drug-abusing people (Ghodse, 1976). A barbiturate abstinence syndrome in neonates has been described (Desmond *et al.*, 1972) which begins within the first few days after birth but may sometimes be delayed for up to two weeks. The infants are restless, febrile and tremulous but unlike those born to opiate addicts are not small for dates nor is respiration depressed.

Intravenous use in 'hard drug addicts' is associated with thrombophlebitis, abscesses and gangrene due to intra-arterial injections (Pollard, 1973).

Management

Barbiturate withdrawal requires close supervision. The patient is prescribed a long-acting barbiturate, e.g. phenobarbitone up to 60 mg three times daily regularly until stabilized. Anticonvulsant cover may or may not be included. The barbiturate is then slowly reduced over the next week. If fits supervene sodium amylobarbitone, intravenously up to 1 g, will control these. Alternatively diazepam may be given intravenously.

Cannabis

Cannabis indica (sativa) or Indian Hemp, was introduced into Europe in the nineteenth century by the Napoleonic armies on their return from the East. It became fashionable in Bohemian circles in Paris and was used by the poets Gautier and Baudelaire.

It is a Class B controlled drug (Misuse of Drugs Act 1971). Despite the controversy surrounding this drug and attempts to legalize it, in the USA it is still regarded with circumspection and included among the drugs of abuse (Position Statement on Substance Abuse, 1981). In Britain hashish (resin from the male and female flowers) is more commonly abused than marihuana, (the dried leaves and stems of the plant).

Pharmacokinetics

Cannabis is most commonly smoked but may be ingested in cakes, sweets or drinks. Effects occur within minutes of inhalation and last for several hours. There are at least 20 active cannabinoids but the most active is the 9-transisomer of tetrahydro-cannabinol.

Hashish has a THC content of 5–12 per cent, marihuana of 4–8 per cent. THC is metabolized very rapidly and completely. The principal metabolite is 11-hydroxy-THC which is itself more active than THC. This persists in the urine for up to a week after the last ingestion. The half-life decreases with increasing use. It is 56 h initially decreasing to 27 h. This suggests that it induces its own metabolism. There is still discussion over the possible development of tolerance and dependence. The reduction in half-life observed with increasing use lends weight to the likelihood of tolerance. This is complicated by the fact that with increasing use symptoms of intoxication become more severe—the opposite of what is expected when tolerance develops. Snyder (1971) suggests that this 'reversed tolerance' is due to THC being metabolized to a more active compound. Psychological dependence is present but usually mild. However, in some susceptible individuals serious psychological dependence may develop. Physical withdrawal symptoms have been described under experimental conditions (Jones, Benowitz and Bachman, 1976) but not under normal conditions. The question of escalation has not yet been settled (Graham, 1976; Kraus, 1981), but it seems likely that only a minority of cannabis abusers will progress to 'hard drugs'.

Cannabis has no therapeutic use in psychiatry but may have use as an antiemetic agent in conjunction with antimitotic drugs (*British Medical Journal*, 1982).

Characteristic effects

Within minutes of smoking the subject seems relaxed and contented. Distortions of perception, though not psychotic as with LSD, are very common. Sexual arousal and energy are increased. Hunger and sleep disturbance have also been described. Alterations in mood, e.g. fear, depression, may develop in those prone to such mood changes. Many of these effects are associated with the subjects' expectations and may not arise in naive users. Physiological changes such as increased heart rate, increased respiratory rate and reduced intra-ocular pressure have been recorded. Plasma testosterone levels are reduced.

Unwanted effects

The question of an acute psychotic illness developing has been frequently discussed (*British Medical Journal*, 1976). This seems to be less common in the West than the East and is thought to occur following consumption of large amounts. This may be a confusional state or a schizophreniform illness in which restlessness and violence are prominent features together with delusions and hallucinations. It is probably dose related and fades within a few hours to a few days. Cannabis has been ascribed an aetiological role in chronic psychotic illnesses also (Granville-Grossman, 1979), but as with amphetamines this is still in dispute (Edwards, 1976). Pathological intoxication ('bad trips') and flashback experiences have also been described. The former are characterized by fear, panic, delusions and depersonalization. Occasionally the depersonalization may persist (Szymanski, 1981).

Reports from Canada and the East have described an 'amotivational syndrome' (Campbell, 1976) characterized by apathy, self-neglect and laziness. This issue is still in dispute (Mellinger et al., 1976), and it has been suggested that these features reflect the premorbid personality of the group rather than being the result of cannabis abuse. The question of cerebral atrophy as a result of long-standing cannabis misuse is equally debatable. Campbell and his colleagues (1971) reported memory impairment and personality change suggestive of organic brain damage. CAT scan studies (Kuepnie et al., 1977) failed to confirm this. Impairment of testicular functions with reduced plasma testosterone have been documented, as have oligospermia, impotence and gynaecomastia (Kolodny et al., 1974), and the latter has been produced experimentally. There have been conflicting reports of possible teratogenic effects of this substance, but all reports have been based on animal studies.

Management

Cannabis detoxification is unlikely to occupy much of the clinical psychiatrist's time. His main role is in the management of pathological intoxication. One recommendation is that major tranquillizers be prescribed. However, other sources suggest reassurance and sedation with benzodiazepines rather than phenothiazines (Tinklenberg, 1977). Acute psychotic episodes are managed by sedation with major tranquillizers which may need to be continued if a schizophreniform illness develops.

Cocaine

Cocaine is the active ingredient of the South American plant *Erythroxylon coca*, isolated by Albert Niemann towards the end of the nineteenth century. It was introduced into medicine for its anaesthetic properties in preference to morphine, but was found to have its own problems of dependence. Its name has been closely linked with Sigmund Freud.

Its plasma half-life, when given intravenously, is about 20 min. It acts mainly on all catecholaminergic systems by inhibiting the uptake of these neurotransmitters. It is also a monoamine oxidase inhibitor. Its pronounced effect on dopamine may be responsible for the increased motor activity associated with it. It does not have any therapeutic use now and it is met with in medicine today as a drug of abuse.

Because of its long-standing association with opiate abuse it is governed by the same legislation as opiates. At present it is rarely used on its own but in association with opiates. Cocaine may be injected, swallowed, chewed or inhaled as 'snow', the latter resulting in ulceration of nasal mucosa and perforation of the nasal septum. Neither physical dependence nor tolerance develop but psychological dependence is pronounced. Its effects are very transient and consist of feelings of happiness, confidence and exhilaration. Many of its effects resemble those of amphetamines but are said to be more subtle. In addition to relieving fatigue it reduces hunger, causes pupillary dilatation and an increase in pulse rate. If CNS stimulation is too great, restlessness becomes extreme and may require an antidote. For this reason cocaine is often combined with opiates in drug abusers. With high doses a psychotic state with delusions and hallucinations (visual and haptic—'cocaine bug') can occur. This is potentially a dangerous state particularly if the person has a sociopathic personality, as violence can result. With long-term use, the social effects of cocaine are marked, resulting in personality deterioration with increasing unreliability and loss of self control.

Due to effective legislation and the exorbitant black market price cocaine is much less commonly used now. Management is non-specific and the drug can be discontinued without fear of physical withdrawal symptoms. If psychotic symptoms develop management is with major tranquillizers.

References

ABRAHAMS, M. J., ARMSTRONG, J. and WHITLOCK, F. A. Drug dependence in Brisbane, *Medical Journal of Australia* 2, 397–404 (1970)

AGHAJANIAN, G. Tolerance of locus coereulus neurons to morphine and suppression of withdrawal response by clonidine, *Nature* 276, 186–188 (1978)

ALI-AFRASIABI, M., FLOMM, M., FRIEDLANDER, H. and VALENTA, L. J. Endocrine status in heroin addicts, *Psychoneuroendocrinology*, 145–153 (1979)

ALLEN, A. M. Glue sniffing, *International Journal of Addictions* **1**, 147–149 (1966)

AMERICAN JOURNAL OF PSYCHIATRY. Position statement on substance abuse **138**, 874–875 (1981)

ARMITAGE, A. K., HALL, G. M. and MORISON, C. F. Pharmacological basis for the tobacco smoking habit, *Nature* **217**, 331–334 (1968)

ASHTON, H. and STEPNEY, R. *Smoking: psychology and pharmacology*, Tavistock, London (1982)

AYLETT, P. A. Barbiturate misuse in 'hard' drug addicts, *British Journal of Addiction* **73**, 385–390 (1978)

BEAN, P. T. *The social control of drugs*, Martin Robertson, London (1974)

BEAUMONT, A. and HUGHES, J. Biology of opioid peptides, *Annual Review of Pharmacology and Toxicology* **19**, 245–267 (1979)

BEN-ARIE, O. and GEORGE, G. C. W. A case of tranylcypromine (Parnate) addiction, *British Journal of Psychiatry* **35**, 273–274 (1979)

BECKETT, A. M. and CASY, A. F. Synthetic analgesics: stereo-chemical considerations, *Journal of Pharmacy and Pharmacology* **6**, 986–1001 (1954)

BECKETT, A. M., TAYLOR, J. F., CASY, A. F. and MASSAN, M. M. A. The biotransformation of methadone in man—synthesis and identification of a major metabolite, *Journal of Pharmacy and Pharmacology* **20**, 754 (1968)

BEJEROT, N. The nature of addiction. In *Drug Dependence. Current Problems and Issues* (Ed. M. M. GLATT), MTP Press, Lancaster (1977)

BERNSTEIN, D. A. and MACALISTER, A. The modification of smoking behaviour. Progress and problems, *Addictive Behaviour* **1**, 89–102 (1976)

BERRIDGE, V. and EDWARDS, G. *Opium and the people*, Penguin, Allen Lane, London (1982)

BLACHLY, P. M. Management of the opiate withdrawal syndrome, *American Journal of Psychiatry* **122**, No. 7, 742–743 (1966)

BLACKER, K. H., JONES, R. T., STONE, G. C. and PFEFFERBAUM, D. Chronic users of LSD: the 'acid heads', *American Journal of Psychiatry* **125**, 341–348 (1968)

BRITISH MEDICAL JOURNAL. Cannabis psychosis (2), 1092–1093 (1976)

BRITISH MEDICAL JOURNAL. Glutethimide—an unsafe alternative to barbiturate hypnotics (1), 1424–1425 (1976)

BRITISH MEDICAL JOURNAL. Therapeutic potential of cannabinoids (1), 1211–1212 (1982)

BROWN, M. J., SALMON, D. and RENDELL, M. Clonidine hallucinations, *Annals of Internal Medicine*, 456–457 (1980)

BULLINGHAM, R. E. S. Synthetic opiate analgesics, *British Journal of Hospital Medicine* **25**, 59–64 (1981)

CAMPBELL, A. M. G., EVANS, M., THOMSON, J. L. G. and WILLIAMS, M. J. Cerebral atrophy in young cannabis smokers, *Lancet* **2**, 1219–1224 (1971)

CAMPBELL, I. The amotivational syndrome and cannabis use with emphasis on the Canadian scene, *Annals of the New York Academy of Sciences* **282**, 33–36 (1976)

CLEMENT-JONES, V., McLOUGHLIN, L., LOWRY, P. J., BESSER, G. H., REES, L. M. and WEN, H. L. Acupuncture in heroin addicts: changes in met-enkephalin and β-endorphin in blood and cerebrospinal fluid, *Lancet* **2**, 380–382 (1978)

COHEN, M. H., HIRSCHLORN, K. and FROSCH, W. A. LSD and chromosomes, *New England Journal of Medicine* **278** , 223 (1968)

CONNELL, P. H. *Amphetamine psychosis*. Maudsley Monograph, No. 5, Oxford University Press, Oxford (1958)

CONNELL, P. H. Clinical manifestations and treatment of amphetamine type of dependence, *Journal of American Medical Association* **196**, No. 8, 718 (1966)

CONNELL, P. H. Central nervous system stimulants. In *Side Effects of Drugs. A Survey of Unwanted Effects of Drugs reported in 1968–71* (Eds. P. L. MEYLER and A. HORXHEIMER) **7**, 1–6, Excerpta Medica, Amsterdam (1972)

CROSSLAND, J. and SLATER, P. The effect of some drugs on 'free' and 'bound' acetylcholine content of rat brain, *British Journal of Pharmacology and Chemotherapy* **33**, 42–47 (1968)

DEWHURST, K. and HATRICK, J. A. Differential diagnosis and treatment of lysergic acid diethylamide induced psychosis, *Practitioner* **209**, 327–332 (1972)

DESMOND, M. M., SCHWANECKE, R. P., WILSON, G. S., YASUNAGA, S. and BURGDORFF, I. Maternal barbiturate utilisation and neonatal withdrawal symptomatology, *Journal of Paediatrics* **80**, 190–197 (1972)

DOLE, V. and NYSWANDER, M. A medical treatment for diacetyl morphine (heroin) addiction, *Journal of the American Medical Association* **193**, No. 8, 80 (1965)

EDDY, N. B., HALBACK, H., ISBELL, H. and SEEVERS, M. H. Drug dependence: its significance and characteristics, *Bulletin of the World Health Organisation* **32**, 721–733 (1965)

EDWARDS, G. Cannabis and the psychiatric position. In *Cannabis and Health* (Ed. J. D. P. GRAHAM), Academic Press, London and New York (1976)

EDWARDS, G. and BUSCH, C. (Eds.) *Drug Problems in Britain. A Review of Ten Years*, Academic Press, London (1981)

ELLINWOOD, E. K. and PETRIE, W. M. Dependence on amphetamines, cocaine and other stimulants. In *Drug Abuse, Clinical and Basic Aspects* (Eds. S. N. PRADHAN and S. N. DUTTON), Mosby, St. Louis (1977)

EPSTEIN, R. S. Withdrawal symptoms from chronic use of low dose barbiturates, *American Journal of Psychiatry* **137**, (1), 107–108 (1980)

FORREST, J. A. H. and TARALA, R. Sixty hospital admissions due to reactions to Lysergide, *Lancet* **2**, 1310–1313 (1973)

GAY, A. C. and GAY, C. R. Haight-Ashbury: evolution of a drug culture in a decade of mendacity, *Journal of Psychadelic Drugs* **4**, 81 (1971)

GERALD, M. C. and SCHWIRIAN, P. M. Non-medical use of methaqualone, *Archives of General Psychiatry* **28**, 627–631 (1973)

GHODSE, A. H. Drug problems dealt with by 62 London casualty departments, *British Journal of Preventive Medicine* **30**, 251–256 (1976)

GHODSE, A. H. Morbidity and mortality. In *Drug Problems in Britain. A Review of Ten Years* (Eds. G. EDWARDS and C. BUSCH), Academic Press, London (1981)

GOLD, M. S., REDMOND, D. E. and KLEBER, H. D. Clonidine blocks acute opiate withdrawal symptoms, *Lancet* **2**, 599–602 (1978)

GOLD, M. S. and KLEBER, H. S. A rationale for opiate withdrawal symptomatology, *Drugs and Alcohol Dependency* 419–424 (1979)

GOLD, M. S., POTTASH, A. C., SWEENEY, D. R. and KLEBER, H. D. Opiate withdrawal using clonidine. A safe, effective and rapid non-opiate treatment, *Journal of the American Medical Association* **234**, No. 4, 343–346 (1980)

GRAHAM, J. P. D. (Ed.). *Cannabis and Health*, Academic Press, London and New York (1976)

GRANVILLE-GROSSMAN, K. (Ed.). *Recent Advances in Clinical Psychiatry*, 3rd edn, Churchill Livingstone, Edinburgh, London and New York (1979)

HEIM, R. and WASSON, R. G. Les champignons hallucinogenes du Mexique: etudes ethnologiques, toxonomiques, biologiques physiologiques et cliniques, *Le Museum National d'histoire Naturelle de Paris*, 438 (1959)

HOFMANN, F. G. and HOFMANN, A. D. *A handbook of drug and alcohol abuse. The bio-medical aspects*, Oxford University Press, Oxford (1975)

HUGHES, J. Isolation of an endogenous compound from the bra.n with pharmacological properties similar to those of morphine, *Brain Research* **88**, 295–308 (1975)

HUGHES, J., SMITH, T. W., KOSTERLITZ, H. W., FOTHERGILL, I. A., MORGAN, B. A. and MORRIS, H. R. Identification of two related pentapeptides from the brain with potent opiate agonist activity, *Nature* **258**, 577–579 (1975)

HUGHES, P. M. and CRAWFORD, G. A. A contagious Disease Model for researching and intervening in heroin epidemics, *Archives of General Psychiatry* **27** (2), 149–155 (1972)

ILLINGWORTH, R. N., STEWART, M. J. and JARVIE, D. R. Severe Poisoning with Chlormethiazole, *British Medical Journal* **2**, 902–903 (1979)

ISBELL, H., ALTSCHUL, S., KORNETSKY, C. M., EISENMAN, A. J., FLANARY, H. G. and FRASER, H. F. Chronic barbiturate intoxication, *Archives of Neurological Psychiatry* **64** (i), 416–418 (1950)

JAFFÉ, J. H. and MARTIN, W. R. Opioid analgesics and antagonists. In *The Pharmacological Basis of Therapeutics* (Eds. A. G. GILMAN, I. S. GOODMAN and A. GILMAN), 6th edn, Macmillan, New York (1980)

JONES, R. T., BENOWITZ, N. and BACHMAN, J. Clinical studies of cannabis tolerance and dependence, *Annals of the New York Academy of Sciences* **282**, 221–239 (1976)

KARRAS, A. and KANE, J. M. Naloxone reduces cigarette consumpton, *Life Sciences* **27**, 1541–1545 (1980)

KNOX, J. W. and NELSON, J. R. Permanent encephalopathy from toluene inhalation, *New England Journal of Medicine* **275**, 1494–1496 (1966)

KOLODNY, R. C., MASTERS, W. H., KALODNER, R. M. and TORO, G. Depression of plasma testosterone levels in chronic intensive marijuanha use, *New England Journal of Medicine* **290**, 872–874 (1974)

KRAUS, J. Juvenile drug abuse and delinquency; some differential associations, *British Journal of Psychiatry* **139**, 422–430 (1981)

KUEPNIE, J., MENDESON, J. M., DAVIS, K. R. and NEW, P. F. J. Computed tomographic examination of heavy marijuanha smokers, *Journal of the American Medical Association* **237**, 1231–1232 (1977)

LEE, H. A., DAVIDSON, A. R. and BURSTON, J. Analgesic nephropathy in Wessex. A clinico-pathological survey, *Clinical Nephrology*, 197–207 (1974)

LEGASSICKE, J. Tranylcypromine, *Lancet* 1, 270 (1963)

LICHTENSTEIN, E. and BROWN, R. A. Smoking cessation methods: review and recommendations. In *Addictive Behaviours* (Ed. W. R. MILLER), Pergamon, New York (1980)

LOCKHART, E. R. B. and PRIEST, R. G. Methaqualone addiction and delirium tremens, *British Medical Journal* 3, 92–93 (1967)

LUNDQUIST, G. The risk of dependence on chlormethiazole, *Acta Psychiatrica Scandanavica*, Suppl. 42, 203–207 (1966)

McGRATH, S. D. A controlled trial of chlormethiazole and chlordiazepoxide in the treatment of the acute withdrawal phase of alcoholism, *British Journal of Addiction* 70, Suppl. 1, 81–90 (1975)

MACGREGOR, C. A., TASKER, P. R. W. and DE WARDENER, H. E. Diuretic induced oedema, *Lancet* 1, 489–492 (1975)

McMILLAN, J. M., LAWSON, D. H., PATON, A. M. and LINTON, A. L. The occurrence and clinical features of analgesic abuse in Western Scotland, *Scottish Medical Journal* 13, 382–387 (1968)

MALCOLM, R. E., SILLETT, R. W., TURNER, J. A. M. and BALL, K. P. Use of nicotine gum as an aid to stopping smoking, *Psychopharmacology*, 295–296 (1980)

MALLENSON, N. Acute adversive reactions to LSD in clinical and experimental use in the United Kingdom, *British Journal of Psychiatry* 118, 229–230 (1971)

MARKS, V. and FRY, D. E. Detection and measurement of drugs in biological fluids: Their relevance to the problem of drug abuse. In *Drug dependence. Current Problems and Issues* (Ed. M. M. GLATT), MTP Press, Lancaster (1977)

MAYER, D. J., PRICE, D. D. and RAFII, A. Antagonism of acupuncture analgesia in man by the narcotic antagonist Naloxone, *Brain Research* 121, 368–372 (1977)

MELLINGER, G. D., SOMERS, R. H., DAVIDSON, S. T. and MANHEIMER, D. I. The amotivational syndrome and the college student, *Annals of the New York Academy of Sciences* 282, 37–55 (1976)

MERRY, J. and ZACHARIADIS, M. Addiction to glue sniffing, *British Medical Journal* 2, 1448 (1962)

MIRIN, S. M., MEYER, R. E., MENDELSON, J. H. and ELLINGBOE, J. Opiate use and sexual function, *American Journal of Psychiatry* 137, 909–915 (1980)

MISUSE OF DRUGS ACT 1971. HMSO, London

MURRAY, R. M., GREEN, J. G. and ADAMS, J. H. Analgesic abuse and dementia, *Lancet* 2, 242–245 (1971)

MURRAY, R. M., LAWSON, D. H. and LINTON, A. L. Analgesic nephropathy; clinical syndrome and prognosis, *British Medical Journal* 1, 479–482

MURRAY, R. M. The use and abuse of analgesics, *Scottish Medical Journal* 17, 393–397 (1972)

MURRAY, R. M. Minor analgesic abuse. The slow recognition of a public health problem, *British Journal of Addiction* 75, 9–17 (1980)

OSWALD, I. and THACORE, V. R. Amphetamine and phenmetrazine addiction. Physiological abnormalities in the abstinence syndrome, *British Medical Journal* 2, 427 (1963)

PITT, B. Withdrawal symptoms after stopping phenelzine, *British Medical Journal* 2, 332–333 (1974)

PLANT, M. A. *Drug takers in an English town*, Tavistock, London (1975)

POLLARD, R. Surgical implications of some types of drug dependence, *British Medical Journal* 1, 784–787 (1973)

PRACTITIONER. The freedom to prescribe 215, 567–568 (1975)

REILLY, T. M. Physiological dependence on and symptoms of withdrawal from chlormethiazole, *British Journal of Psychiatry* 128, 375–378 (1976)

RENAULT, P. F. Treatment of heroin dependent persons with antagonist—current status, *Contemporary Drug Problems*, 15–29 (1979)

ROBINSON, J. T., CHITHAM, R. G., GREENWOOD, R. M. and TAYLOR, J. W. Chromosome aberrations and LSD: a controlled study of 90 patients, *British Journal of Psychiatry* 125, 238–244 (1974)

ROYAL COLLEGE OF PHYSICIANS. *Smoking and Health*. Summary of a report of the Royal College of Physicians of London in relation to cancer of the lung and other diseases. Pitman, London (1962)

RUSSELL, M. A. H. Tobacco smoking and nicotine dependence. In *Recent Advances in Drug and Alcohol Dependence* (Ed. R. J. GIBBENS), Wiley and Sons, New York (1976)

RUSSELL, M. A. H. Nicotine intake and its regulation, *Journal of Psychosomatic Research*, 253–264 (1980)

SCHACHTER, M. Enkephalins and endorphins, *British Journal of Hospital Medicine* 25, No. 3, 128–136 (1981)

SCHACHTER, S., SILVERSTEIN, B., KOZLOWSKI, L. T., PERLICK, D., HERMAN, C. P. and LIEBLING, B. Studies of interaction of psychological and pharmacological determinants of smoking, *Journal of Experimental Psychology: General* 106 (i), 3–40 (1977)

SHIFFMAN, S. M. The tobacco withdrawal syndrome. In *Progress in smoking cessation: Proceedings of an international conference on smoking cessation, 1978* (Ed. N. A. KRASNAGOR), American Cancer Society, New York (1979)

SIDEROLF, S. I., CHARAVASTRA, V. C. and JARVIK, M. E. Craving in heroin addicts maintained on the opiate antagonist naltrexone, *American Journal of Alcohol and Drug Abuse*, 415–423 (1978)

SNYDER, S. H. *Uses of marijuanha*, Oxford University Press, New York (1971)

SNYDER, S. H. Clinical relevance of opiate receptor and opioid peptide research, *Nature* **273**, 13–14 (1979)

STEPNEY, R. Smoking behaviour. A psychology of the cigarette habit, *British Journal of Diseases of the Chest*, 325–344 (1980)

STEWART, J. K. Analgesic Abuse and Renal Failure in Australia, *Kidney International* **13**, 72–78 (1978)

STOCKLEY, I. *Drug Interactions*, Blackwell Scientific Publications, London (1981)

SZYMANSKI, M. S. Prolonged depersonalisation after marijuanha use, *American Journal of Psychiatry* **138**, 231–233 (1981)

TINKLENBERG, J. R. Abuse of marijuanha. In *Drug abuse—clinical and basic aspects* (Eds. S. N. PRADMAN and S. N. DUTTA), Mosby, St. Louis (1977)

TOLAN, E. J. and LINGL, F. A. 'Model psychosis', produced by inhalation of gasoline fumes, *American Journal of Psychiatry* **120**, 757–761 (1964)

UHDE, T. W., REDMOND, D. R. and KLEBER, M. D. Clonidine suppresses the opiod abstinence syndrome without Clonidine withdrawal symptoms. A blind inpatient study, *Psychiatric Research*, 37–47 (1980)

VAN DIJK, W. K. Vicious circles in alcoholism and drug dependence. In *Drug Dependence, Current Problems and Issues* (Ed. M. M. GLATT), MTP Press, Lancaster (1977)

VAN PRAAG, H. M. *Psychotropic Drugs*, Macmillan, London (1978)

VON KRYSPIN-EXNER and MADER, R. Withdrawal delirium in Chlormethiazole Addiction, *Wiener Medizinische Wochenschrift* **121**, 811–812 (1971)

WALL, R., LINFORD, S. M. J. and AKHTER, M. I. Addiction to Distalgesic (dextropropoxyphene), *British Medical Journal* **280**, 1213–1214 (1980)

WALLER, D. and LEVANDER, S. Smoking and Vigilance. The effect of tobacco smoking on CCF (critical flicker fusion) as related to personality traits and smoking habits, *Psychopharmacology*, 131–136 (1980)

WATSON, J. M. *A study of solvent sniffing in Lanarkshire 1973/74*, Diploma in Public Health Dissertation, Glasgow University (1974)

WEN, H. L. and CHEUNG, S. Y. C. Treatment of drug addiction by acupuncture and electrical stimulation, *Asian Journal of Medicine* **9**, 138–141 (1973)

WEN, H. L., HO, W. K. K. and LING, N. Immunoassayable B endorphin levels in the plasma and CSF of heroin addicted and normal subjects before and after acupuncture, *American Journal of Chinese Medicine*, 154–159 (1980)

WILLCOX, W. Veronal Habit, *Lancet* **2**, 1178 (1913)

WORLD HEALTH ORGANIZATION. Expert Committee on Dependence. Sixteenth Report, *WHO Technical Reports Series* **407**, 6 (1969)

WORLD HEALTH ORGANIZATION. Expert Committee on Drug Dependence. Nineteenth Report, *WHO Technical Reports Series* **516**, 8 (1973)

YATSU, F. M., WESSON, P. R. and SMITH, D. E. Amphetamine abuse. In *Medical aspects of drug abuse* (Ed. R. W. RICHTER), Harper and Row, New York (1975)

Chapter 13

Alcohol

Anthony P. Thorley

Historical background

Ethanol is the only one of a family of aliphatic alcohols which man can reasonably tolerate in his body. Almost all the other alcohols, for instance methanol, as in wood oil, and heavier alcohols, collectively known as fuel oil, are highly toxic to man and are usually avoided (Ritchie, 1980; Thorley, 1982c).

Natural fermentation generates ethanol concentrations of 13–15 per cent, and for many thousands of years man could not produce a stronger beverage. However, in the ninth century AD, the process of distillation was developed in Persia and the Arab word for the unpalatable and toxic essence or distillate was 'al kohl'; the word has been integrated into most western languages. To render it drinkable, 'al kohl' was diluted to generate a variety of beverages. Thus before 900 AD beverages were based on natural fermentation: ales from barley, beer with hops added, meads from honey, wines from the grape, and so on. The distillation of whisky commenced in Ireland in the twelfth century, and the production of brandy, gins and other spirits developed and organized into a formal industry in the seventeenth and eighteenth centuries (Thorley, 1982c).

Today, next to tobacco, alcoholic beverages are the most widely utilized recreational chemical substances in the western world. The medical damage and social problems they produce are legion so that it is often remarked that alcohol has now replaced syphilis as the great mimic of all diseases. Detailed reviews of the widespread effects and harm from alcohol have been excellently compiled by Sherlock (1982), and Thorley (1982c) has surveyed the consequences and medical, legal and social problems specifically related to regular excessive consumption, intoxication and dependence.

Ethanol metabolism

An understanding of the basic features of ethanol metabolism gives the clinician a framework of the nature of pathology caused by the drug (Sandler, 1980; Peters, 1982; Davis, Cashaw and McMurtrey, 1980). There is a great deal of clinical and lay mythology about the relative damage and strengths of different beverages. For instance it is widely held that spirits are more likely to cause liver disease than beers, whereas it is merely the dose frequency of ethanol which is important. Similarly the role of congeners in intoxication and damage is considered much less important than ethanol itself. Education of clinicians and clients alike, about the various beverage strengths, and the utilization of a unit system of counting beverages, becomes an essential part of good clinical practice (Thorley, 1980; 1982c).

Most healthy adults of average weight require 10 ml of ethanol, or one unit, to produce a blood alcohol concentration of 15 mg per 100 ml blood within 1 h. Such a unit will have 60 calories of energy, and considerably more when sugar and other carbohydrate congeners are present. Although there can be marked individual variation, each hour the average body weight eliminates approximately one unit of ethanol, a very convenient fact for clinical teaching of alcohol self management (Thorley, 1980; 1982c). Unlike many other substances the rate of oxidation of ethanol is constant with time, is only very slightly increased by raising the blood alcohol concentrations (BACs) and is therefore an example of zero order kinetics. Eighty per cent of ingested alcohol is metabolized by the liver, 5 per cent is excreted in the breath and urine, and the remainder is metabolized elsewhere. All these basic metabolic dynamics are subject to variation due to tolerance effects and genetic factors (Murray and Gurling, 1980).

Ethanol oxidation

This fundamental process has been reviewed in detail by Sandler (1980) and Peters (1982). Ethanol is oxidized to acetaldehyde in the liver cells by three principal pathways (*see Figure 13.1*). Almost all this oxidation is by the cytosol enzyme alcohol dehydrogenase, although microsomal ethanol oxidizing systems in the smooth endoplasmic reticulum contribute, and catalase and hydrogen peroxide also play a part. For some time it has been known that in heavy dependent drinkers who show

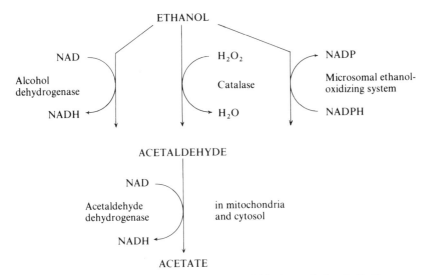

Figure 13.1 The main pathways of ethanol and acetaldehyde metabolism in the liver

enhanced metabolism of ethanol, there is a relatively slow clearance of acetaldehyde (Korsten *et al.*, 1975). In recent years, therefore, considerable interest has focused upon the role of acetaldehyde in causing tissue damage and contributing to dependence (Thomas and Peters, 1981), and some authors have coyly suggested that the clinical condition should in truth not be called alcoholism but 'acetaldehydism'!

The role of acetaldehyde

Acetaldehyde is a very active substance which *in vitro* interferes with mitochondrial ATP production and protein synthesis. Recent evidence suggests that there may be slight impairment of mitochondrial function in early alcoholic liver disease, but in later stages of liver damage, for instance alcoholic hepatitis, mitochondrial damage is definitely present (Peters, 1982). Acetaldehyde may also act as a hapten, binding to tissue protein, and so generating abnormal immunological reactions, which are commonly found in patients with alcoholic liver disease (Bailey *et al.*, 1976). However, clear evidence that acetaldehyde is the major cause of widespread tissue damage at levels of heavy drinking is not, at present, convincing (Thomas and Peters, 1981).

Acetaldehyde also appears to act in the central nervous system, condensing with various biogenic amines to form morphine-like alkaloid compounds: the tetrahydroisoquinolines (Davis, Cashaw and McMurtrey, 1980; Thomas and Peters, 1981). Although this would seem to provide a link between alcohol metabolism, dependence and the endorphin system, particularly as the direct infusion of tetrahydroisoquinolines into rat brains produces a marked and sustained ethanol preference for many months (Meyers, 1978) the evidence is far from clear in man and elucidation must await the huge research effort which is in progress at the moment.

Acetaldehyde is then oxidized to acetate by the single pathway due to acetaldehyde dehydrogenase which probably acts more in the cytosol than in mitochondria. The action of disulfiram, discussed below, is, in part, to inhibit cytosol acetaldehyde dehydrogenase, thus causing a build-up of blood levels of acetaldehyde leading to a variety of uncomfortable symptoms. Finally acetaldehyde is converted to acetyl coenzyme A, which is then oxidized through the citric acid cycle to become carbon dioxide and water.

Both alcohol and acetaldehyde oxidation activities lead to a marked increase in reduced pyridine nucleotides, and the NADH:NAD ratio in liver cells produces profound metabolic sequelae (Peters, 1982). For example, the redox ratio of lactate to pyruvate, involving lactate dehydrogenase, is markedly increased, leading to lactic acidosis. As high blood lactates are associated with feelings of panic and anxiety, some authorities have speculated that the lactic acidosis in heavy drinkers may contribute to their anxiety and altered mood states (Thorley, 1982c). This acidosis, coupled with ketosis, also interferes with urate excretion and leads to gout (Peters, 1982). The altered redox potential has also been implicated in the generation of fatty liver, collagen formation, altered steroid metabolism and impaired gluconeogenesis (Lieber, 1973).

Regular excessive consumption of alcohol leads commonly to hepatomegaly (fatty liver) and this appears to be made up by triglyceride accumulation and increased protein production in liver cells (Lieber, 1980). Peters (1982) has speculated that, in man, as all these unfavourable redox changes of alcohol and acetaldehyde oxidation appear to occur in the cytosol rather than in mitochondria, this may be one reason that man is more susceptible to alcoholic liver disease than many animals in experimental situations.

Problem drinking

In spite of paradoxical acceptance and commercial encouragement of social drinking, throughout history there have always been vast numbers of people in all societies afflicted with alcohol related problems. However, it has only been in the last 20 years with increased public health interest and recognition that an alarming increase in problem drinking in the UK has been widely reported (Thorley, 1982a). Although geographical differences are considerable (Kilich and Plant, 1981), in most parts of the UK between 2 and 5 per cent of the adult population have a serious drinking problem (Cartwright, Shaw and Spratley, 1975; Saunders and Kershaw, 1977) and up to 10 per cent of the population have some form of alcohol problem (e.g. social or legal incidents related to intoxication). A recent survey of drinking in England and Wales amongst a random sample of 2000 adults over 18 (Wilson, 1980), found 6 per cent of men and 1 per cent of women drinking more than the recommended (Royal College of Psychiatrists, 1979) safe upper limit of a weekly consumption of 50 units and 35 units respectively (1 unit = $\frac{1}{2}$ pint of beer = 1 single measure of spirits = 10 ml or 8 g of ethanol).

Elsewhere, Thorley (1982a) has argued for and developed a more pragmatic and problem orientated definition of problem drinker (DHSS, 1978), which recognizes the distinct contributions made to problems from three elements of alcohol use: intoxication, regular excessive consumption and dependence. The definition closely follows the thinking behind the DHSS Advisory Committee on Alcoholism's Pattern and Range of Services report (1978), and is as follows:

> A problem drinker is any person who experiences psychological, physical, social or legal problems related to intoxication and/or regular excessive consumption and/or dependence as a consequence of his or her drinking of alcohol.
>
> (Thorley, 1982a, b)

This problem-orientated model of alcohol use seeks to go beyond mere dependence and is more appropriate to rehabilitation and other forms of treatment (Thorley, 1982a). Problem drinking falls into three parts which may be distinct, but, more commonly, overlap:

(1) intoxication: usually from a single dose taking episode with specifically defined criteria where possible;
(2) regular excessive consumption: more than four days a week of daily alcohol drinking at a level which statistically may lead to excessive morbidity or mortality or other significant harm;
(3) dependence: the basic characteristic is the development of negative effect upon cessation of alcohol use or associated behaviour.

Each of these three elements of alcohol use produces its own characteristic consequences and often these constitute identifiable problems. Thorley (1982c) has detailed these for alcohol elsewhere.

Tolerance and pharmacological dependence

Tolerance and physical dependence with withdrawal symptoms are widely thought to be inextricably related to the problem of alcohol dependence. As is clear elsewhere in this book tolerance is a very general pharmacological phenomenon, seen in a wide range of substances and involves many independent mechanisms. Jaffé (1980) notes that as well as *innate* tolerance to various drugs there are at least three types of *acquired* pharmacological tolerance: dispositional, pharmacodynamic and behavioural. *Drug dispositional tolerance* relates to pharmacokinetic changes of the drug in the organism so that reduced drug concentrations are present at the sites of action, often resulting in an increased rate of metabolism. *Pharmacodynamic tolerance* results from adaptive changes within affected systems such as enzyme induction, so that the response is reduced for the same concentration of the drug.

Behavioural tolerance involves change in the response of a drug due to psychological mechanisms. This is very evident in the high cognitive component related to intoxication in heavy drinking, and must involve features of state dependent learning. Thus it is naïve to consider tolerance phenomena to be centred on one site or mechanism. Rates of absorption, metabolism, excretion and elimination, as well as behavioural responses are all implicated.

Cross tolerance is evidenced when the animal tolerant to one set of drugs (e.g. barbiturates) shows significantly less sedation and ataxia than do non-tolerant animals when challenged with another related drug (e.g. alcohol). Thus whilst alcohol and barbiturates have relatively high cross tolerance, neither has high levels of cross tolerance with opiates, and this can have considerable clinical significance. Further elucidation of cross tolerance and the possibility of common enzymic pathways remains a complex matter discussed more fully by Jaffé (1980).

It is worth mentioning that tolerance in relation to regular excessive consumption over many years of alcohol or barbiturate use tends to diminish. Thus the drinker in his 50s may find that after 30 years of drinking he gets easily drunk after only two to three pints of beer. The reason for this long-term loss of tolerance effect is not known. Clinical impression of both alcohol and opiate pharmacologically dependent users suggests that even after a considerable period of abstinence, tolerance never completely returns to its original baseline level, indicating that some fundamental long-term adjustment has taken place. Where such adjustment is to be found in Jaffé's classification of types of tolerance can only be a matter of speculation.

Pharmacological or *physical dependence* remains elusive to explain at a specific pharmacological level. The key feature of physical dependence is withdrawal symptoms associated with rebound phenomena. The precise symptomatic nature of this rebound differs profoundly from drug to drug, and thus a common neuropharmacological basis is rather dubious. Thus barbiturates elevate the seizure threshold, but spontaneous seizures are seen as withdrawal; opiates depress gut peristalsis, but increased gut motility is a feature of withdrawal; amphetamines elevate mood and activity and suppress appetite, but amphetamine withdrawal is characterized by depression, hyperphagia and general inertia. Similar rebound effects can be specifically described for pharmacological dependence upon alcohol and nicotine. All these rebound hyperexcitability states constitute only a technical pharmacological withdrawal, in that many are not recognized by clinicians or by drug users as constituting withdrawal states or syndromes. There is usually no doubt about alcohol or opiate withdrawal, but many afflicted individuals are less aware of benzodiazepine, nicotine or amphetamine withdrawal.

Finally it is important to recognize that the status of pharmacological dependence does not invariably lead to a major drug or alcohol problem. Patients given opiate analgesics for post-operative pain can develop pharmacological dependence, but as Jaffé (1980) has pointed out 'the overwhelming majority do not develop a psychological dependence, do not become compulsive users, and discontinue when the medical condition is relieved'. Similarly, many individuals who drift into physical dependence on alcohol do not come to the notice of treatment agencies, but spontaneously, or using a little volition, moderate their consumption and lose their dependent status (Thorley, 1982c). It would seem that problems from dependence rely on a great deal more than pharmacological dependence, and that social, cultural, and above all, psychological factors, require to be studied by both research worker and clinician.

Alcohol and women

In the last ten years alcoholic liver disease in the UK has increased markedly among women and there is some evidence that the incidence of serum autoantibodies is markedly high in women, particularly those with alcoholic hepatitis superimposed on cirrhosis (Krasner et al., 1978). There is also evidence that women in general appear to absorb alcohol faster than men, reach higher peak BACs and excrete alcohol more speedily, particularly in the premenstrual and ovulatory phases of the monthly cycle (Ghodse and Tregenza, 1980). Conversely there is some evidence that women using oral contraceptives absorb and metabolize alcohol more slowly and evenly (Ghodse and Tregenza, 1980).

Ethanol and the neuronal membrane

Littleton (1980) has developed an important hypothesis supported by much animal work to explain the generation of tolerance and physical dependence which is based on changes in the integrity of cell membranes due to ethanol. Ethanol causes the fluidization of the neuronal cell membrane allowing the chemical to pass into the cell and disrupt functioning. Tolerance appears related to adaptive changes in this fluidization effect which result in resistance to ethanol transport across the membrane. Continuous ethanol administration leads to increased saturation of membrane phospholipids and an increased cholesterol : phospholipid mole ratio. If it is assumed that the tolerance to ethanol is due to an alteration of the lipid composition of neuronal membranes, then the dissipation of tolerance is presumably due to some reversal of this process. Littleton (1980) has speculated that physical dependence is due to slow dissipation of tolerance and that this may be caused by some inability to adjust brain lipid composition in a normal way.

The fetal alcohol syndrome

There is now wide acceptance that ethanol consumption by pregnant women is related to embryo and fetal damage characterized by, at one extreme, the fetal alcohol syndrome (Sclare, 1980; Pratt, 1982), and at the other extreme, minor retardation of intra-uterine growth, including neural development, resulting in psychological handicaps and enduring behaviour difficulties in later childhood. The relation between ethanol and this range of damage is complex and open to speculation and research endeavour. However, animal studies suggest that both ethanol and acetaldehyde are teratogenic or directly toxic upon dividing cells, and that ethanol may disturb the balance of amino acids in the maternal, and consequently, in the fetal circulation, seriously enough to interfere with the development of the fetal brain. In addition, Pratt (1980) has suggested that ethanol-induced hypoglycaemia generated by even a single episode of marked maternal intoxication, may not be responded to by gluconeogenesis in the naïve fetal liver, and so the sustained fetal hypoglycaemia causes enduring central nervous system dysfunction. The clinical implications are clear. Women planning to become pregnant should avoid drinking alcohol. Pregnant women should avoid drinking alcohol. Pregnant women should avoid intoxication and limit their drinking to no more than one drink (one unit) a day. Wider publicity about this matter is required (Pratt, 1982).

Hangover and the role of congeners

Hangovers merit little attention in a clinical setting, perhaps unfairly, and yet this common consequence of intoxication may have an important aversive effect on most people, such that they moderate their drinking. Hangovers are responded to more by the humourist (Freud, 1981) or the concerned amateur gourmet intent on finding the elusive hangover cure (Outerbridge, 1982). As a consequence of ethanol toxicity interacting with a cocktail of beverage congeners, hangover is an interesting example of an acute toxic syndrome. It is very variable, but commonly characterized by depressed mood, headache, dehydration, nausea and hypersensitivity to outside stimuli, such as noise. It is not possible to give a full pharmacological explanation of hangover, but many of its features are produced by the wide variety of toxic congeners which are added to drinks for their tastes and aroma. In combination with the dehydration directly caused by the diuretic effect of ethanol, the congeners may be particularly responsible for the headache and mood change. There is some evidence that some drinks, or mixtures, contain more congeners than others, and therefore produce a more unpleasant hangover effect. Vodka has very few congeners, whereas brandy, port and rich red wines have many: evidence is strong that mixing drinks is more likely to produce hangover than remaining on a single beverage. Thorley (1982c) has described a simple 'hangover scale' which advises the wary drinker what to avoid. Cures for hangovers are more open to mythology than alcohol beverages themselves (Outerbridge, 1982), but double-blind trials in the USA with pyritinol, a neurotropic derivative of pyridoxine unavailable in the UK, but used in Ireland and Europe, show a significant reduction of hangover symptoms as compared with placebo.

Clinical use of ethanol

In the past alcohol was widely used as a medicine and medical prescriptions of ethanol became a feature of the abstinent temperance campaigns of the past. Today alcoholic beverages are used occasionally in the elderly (*see* Chapter 6, p. 127) as anxiolytics or hypnotics, and as base solvents for externally or topically applied preparations and rubifacients. Dehydrated ethanol may be injected in the proximity of nerves or sympathetic ganglia for the relief of chronic pain as in trigeminal neuralgia or in inoperable carcinoma. Finally, alcohol does occasionally have a place in detoxification and withdrawal management (*see below*). In short, the clinical use of alcohol is limited.

Drug interactions

Ethanol reacts adversely with a number of commonly prescribed drugs, and only a brief outline will be presented here. Alcohol which produces psychomotor effects at a BAC of 40 mg per 100 ml (40 mg%) may be markedly enhanced by a person who has also taken sedatives, hypnotics, anticonvulsants, antidepressants, opiates and tranquillizers. Monamine oxidase inhibitors are contraindicated with alcoholic drinks containing tyramine (*see* Chapter 9, p. 263) due to hypertensive side effects. Oral hypoglycaemic agents in conjunction with ethanol can produce side effects similar to the disulfiram ethanol reaction (*see below*). Ethanol also enhances the activity of the coumarin type of anticoagulant, and may increase gastric mucosal bleeding exacerbated by concomitant use of salicylates. There are so many interactions between ethanol and drugs that it is essential for the physician to clearly advise his patients. An excellent critical survey of evidence of ethanol drug interactions and clinical advice is provided by Pirola (1977).

Drug treatment for problem drinking

Acute intoxication

Intoxication and its effects usually do not require the use of drugs unless the BAC is above 350 mg per 100 ml or 350 mg% and the patient is in coma. The relation between ingested ethanol and BACs for a subject of average weight has been detailed elsewhere (Thorley, 1980). Death due to acute alcohol poisoning is possible at levels above 500 mg% but levels may be higher in problem drinkers with high tolerance. Acute alcohol poisoning in children, up to 8 per cent of all child poisoning in the USA, constitutes a medical emergency as there is often a concomitant acute hypoglycaemia (Rada and Kellner, 1979).

Patients in alcoholic coma require hospital admission and need treatment according to specific needs. General principles involve maintenance of airway and respiration, correction of electrolytic or acid–base imbalance and treatment of shock as required. Intravenous glucose may be required for concomitant hypoglycaemia. High doses of B vitamins, particularly thiamine, may be required to avoid acute onset of Wernicke's encephalopathy (Shaw, 1980). Renal dialysis is occasionally necessary if the BAC is above 500 mg% or if there is a severe metabolic acidosis or coma produced by the additional presence of a dialysable drug (Sellers and Kalant, 1976). In spite of a number of reports of drugs to hasten the metabolism of ethanol, so called 'sobering up' drugs, none has emerged with any safe consistent proven clinical value (Shaw, 1980; Rada and Kellner, 1979).

The alcohol withdrawal syndrome

The alcohol withdrawal syndrome occurs in those patients who stop drinking abruptly or rapidly reduce their BAC, and its manifestation includes complex psychological and pharmacological responses to dependence as discussed above. At a mildest level, and most commonly, it is represented by all or some of the following: mild tremor of hands and feet, nausea and dry retching, perspiration, anxiety and/or mood change (Edwards and Gross, 1976; *British Medical Journal*, 1981). Serious alcohol withdrawal syndromes including stupor, psychomotor restlessness, hallucinosis, convulsions or delirium tremens are only found in a minority, between 3 and 15 per cent, of abruptly abstaining physically dependent drinkers. Feuerlein (1980) in a penetrating review, has pointed out how some of these 'withdrawal' conditions including hallucinosis and delirium tremens, can commence in situations of sustained drinking with high BACs. Feuerlein (1980) concludes that there are many other factors involved in the precipitation of delirium tremens, including concomitant infection, liver damage, personality and cultural factors.

The management of detoxification

Many drugs with tranquillizing and anticonvulsant activity suitably cross tolerant with ethanol have been used for the management of patients in alcohol withdrawal, or elective drying out or detoxification. However it is worth bearing in mind that a large number of cases of physical dependence 'spontaneously' remit as the drinker appreciates his dependent status and related problems and so modifies his daily consumption until the withdrawal symptoms disappear. The relatively low use of tranquillizing medication used by experimental detoxification centres provides similar evidence (Thorley, 1982a). Thus detoxification may not require hospitalization or medical supervision (Thorley, 1980; 1982c).

Where daily medical contact is possible (hospital outpatients, day patients, accident and emergency departments, domiciliary visits or general practitioners' surgeries) and there is no previous history of epilepsy, delirium tremens or other contra-indications, detoxification out of hospital is appropriate. With daily contact the patient can gradually reduce consumption on a contracted basis over a 14-day period, with or without tranquillizers (Thorley, 1980). The use of ethanol itself in a reducing dose is inadequately assessed at present, but in hospital or supervised settings, ethanol is of value for mild withdrawal symptoms. The equivalent of one unit or 8 g of ethanol (*see* p. 353) as beer or spirits can be dispensed every 4–6 h and gradually tailed off in a supervised setting, thus facilitating the use of smaller doses of tranquillizing drugs (*British Medical Journal*, 1981).

Sellers and Kalant (1976) have reported over 100 drugs used in the treatment of withdrawal symptoms and detoxification regimens. Several important double-blind trials have compared the relative efficacy of chlordiazepoxide, chlorpromazine, hydroxyzine, thiamine and placebo on 537 patients (Kaim, Klett and Rothfeld, 1969; Kaim, 1980). Surprisingly, certain symptoms appeared to respond more readily to one or another of the treatments, including the placebo, but there was no consistent superiority of any one treatment. Convulsions developed in 1 per cent of those receiving chlordiazepoxide, 12 per cent receiving chlorpromazine, 8 per cent receiving hydroxyzine, 7 per cent receiving thiamine and 7 per cent receiving placebo. Similarly, delirium tremens developed in 1 per cent of those on chlordiazepoxide, 7 per cent on chlorpromazine, 4 per cent on hydroxyzine, 4 per cent on thiamine and 6 per cent on placebo. Not surprisingly, chlordiazepoxide has emerged as the tranquillizer drug of choice in the USA.

Other drugs are very adequate in controlling withdrawal symptoms but have other disadvantages. Barbiturates, once the drugs of first choice, now run too much risk of generating dependence to be acceptable; chloral hydrate/paraldehyde mixtures have a very high anticonvulsant action, are not a high dependence risk, but are not convenient to store and dispense; phenothiazine tranquillizers such as chlorpromazine are contra-indicated as they may precipitate convulsions and are associated with liver damage; diazepam, with a higher anticonvulsant activity than chlordiazepoxide, is widely used in the UK but appears less acceptable in the USA, possibly because of adverse publicity about dependence. Similarly, chlormethiazole is very popular in the UK, in spite of very real risks of dependence, but has never been licensed for use in the USA; propranolol, as a representative beta blocker, in doses of 40 mg six-hourly, has been used to alleviate autonomic hyperactivity, but beta blockers do not have any anticonvulsant action.

Abrupt abstinence usually requires tranquillizers dispensed daily to avoid risk of overdose or misuse. My own clinical experience favours on balance diazepam as the drug of first choice, and a practical but modifiable regimen is as follows. Diazepam, 10 mg four times daily (three days), 10 mg thrice daily (three days); 5 mg thrice daily (two days); 5 mg twice daily (two days). Many patients can be ambulant, but resting through this period. Ideally, after ten days, no further tranquillizers or hypnotic medication should be prescribed.

Many physicians and psychiatrists favour chlormethiazole, in spite of mounting evidence of problems from dependence (Reilly, 1976). In my experience many patients prone to addiction problems report a euphoric effect from chlormethiazole in therapeutic doses which is rarely reported by patients on appropriate doses of diazepam or chlordiazepoxide, and therefore chlormethiazole has a compelling 'palate effect'. Chlormethiazole also causes physical dependence at regular doses above 3 g daily and withdrawal convulsions in cases entirely uncomplicated by alcohol or other drugs have been my clinical experience on several occasions in spite of very gradual phased withdrawal regimens. My opinion is that chlormethiazole is rapidly developing into a drug with risks of dependence, misuse and problems. Another contraindication is that as this drug increases the secretions in the respiratory tract it should not be used in patients who have respiratory disease (Madden, Jones and Frisch, 1969). For those who continue to favour its use among problem drinkers, a suitable and modifiable regimen is as follows: Chlormethiazole 1.5 g thrice daily (two days); 1 g thrice daily, (two days); 500 mg thrice daily (one day) (Shaw, 1980; *British Medical Journal*, 1981). It should not be given to problem drinkers who are not hospitalized, or prescribed on a maintenance, prophylactic anxiolytic basis as the dependence risks are too high in this group of patients.

Both the diazepam and chlormethiazole regimens should be sufficient to prevent withdrawal convulsions, but where patients are found to be prone to seizures or exhibit myoclonic twitchings, the tranquillizing regimen may be complemented with an antiepileptic such as phenytoin (100 mg thrice daily) or sodium valproate (200 mg thrice daily) for at least four days (Shaw, 1982). Where myoclonic twitchings are associated with low serum magnesium levels, 1–2 mg of magnesium sulphate by intramuscular injection should be given (Shaw, 1980). Where seizures occur in spite of precautions, diazepam 10 mg intramuscularly or intravenously, repeated if necessary, should be adequate in providing control.

Delirium tremens

Delirium tremens is a relatively uncommon syndrome, most usually occurring 48–72 h after cessation of drinking and characterized by disorientation and confusion, vivid hallucinations, severe tremor and agitation, fever and sweating, tachycardia, hypertension, increased respiration rate, possible epileptic seizures and other signs and symptoms of a serious debilitating illness. Hospital admission is essential and large doses of a safe and reliable tranquillizing anticonvulsant by mouth or possibly intravenously (such as diazepam or chlordiazepoxide 100–400 mg, or chlormethiazole 3–7 g in the first 24 h) may be required in a reducing dose over seven to ten days. The patient's general condition must be carefully observed. Concomitant infections may require antibiotics; parenteral B vitamins are essential; electrolytic and fluid deficiencies must be monitored and corrected (Sellers and Kalant, 1976; Rada and Kellner, 1979; Shaw, 1980).

Alcoholic hallucinosis

Alcoholic hallucinoses are a complex group of syndromes which require a more discerning clinical approach and classification (Cutting, 1978). Hallucinations, usually visual and tactile may accompany withdrawal symptoms, but occasionally auditory hallucinations with marked paranoid ideation present both during a spell of sustained drinking, and, more rarely during periods of sustained abstinence and with a clear sensorium. Some of these conditions are very similar to paranoid schizophrenic states but there is no substantial evidence that the acute hallucinosis is itself related to schizophrenia (Shaw, 1982). For persistent or predominant hallucinosis which does not respond to withdrawal regimens, phenothiazines are indicated in antipsychotic dosage (*see* Chapter 4, p. 61) (Rada and Kellner, 1979).

Vitamin supplements

In mild cases of physical dependence, provided the patient has a good dietary history and appears healthy, vitamin supplements are not usually required. However, anaemia from iron or folic acid deficiency may require oral iron or folic acid (15–20 mg daily) once a vitamin B12 deficiency has been excluded. Patients with organic neurological sequelae, or cognitive dysfunction (Acker, 1982) are best prescribed B vitamins especially vitamin B1 (thiamine). It is essential to prescribe parenteral B vitamins for Wernicke's encephalopathy and Korsakoff's psychosis. Reilly (1979), after reviewing the variety of thiamine deficiency conditions related to chronic alcoholism, concludes that all chronic alcoholics should receive thiamine supplementation as standard procedure.

Disulfiram and citrated calcium carbimide

Two drugs have been developed from a variety of reports about drugs and plant substances causing a hypersensitivity to ethanol (Ritchie, 1980); disulfiram and citrated calcium carbimide. Both drugs interfere with acetaldehyde dehydrogenase, possibly competing with NAD for the active centres of the enzyme, and so causing

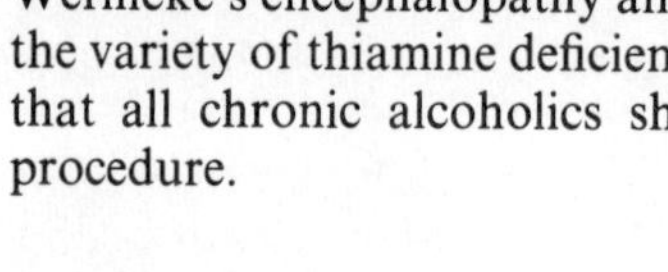

Figure 13.2 Disulfiram

raised blood and tissue levels of acetaldehyde. Most of the effects of the disulfiram ethanol reaction (DER) appear to be the same as produced by experimental injection of acetaldehyde, but there are exceptions and full understanding of the mechanism remains obscure. For instance, DER causes *hypotension*, whereas injection of acetaldehyde in animals produces *hypertension* (Kitson, 1977). Disulfiram also inhibits the enzyme dopamine β-hydroxylase causing an accumulation of dopamine and a depletion of noradrenaline, which may adversely affect mood and myocardial function (Morgan and Cagan, 1974). The characteristic symptoms of the disulfiram ethanol reaction are flushing, dyspnoea, nausea, tachycardia and hypotension. A severe DER may require emergency medical treatment: intravenous fluids, noradrenaline, sodium ascorbate and antihistamines (Kwentus and Major, 1979).

Use of disulfiram is contra-indicated for patients over 60, patients with a history of overdose or impulsive behaviour, ischaemic heart disease, cerebrovascular disease, severe liver or brain damage, asthma, diabetes mellitus and pregnancy. Disulfiram itself is associated occasionally with a number of side effects which are dose related: drowsiness, seizures, depressive and paranoid psychoses, hepatitis, peripheral neuropathy, optic neuritis, myocardial infarction and allergic skin rashes (Kwentus and Major, 1979).

These drugs have earned a significant place as an adjunct to the management of abstinence, but should not be presented as a panacea for drinking problems or prescribed without careful consideration. However, where abstinence is indicated and the patient is stable and well motivated, disulfiram 200 mg taken each morning, or citrated calcium carbimide 50 mg taken once or twice a day, can aid the patient's resolve not to drink. It is no longer the usual practice to elicit a disulfiram ethanol reaction from a test dose, but the patient should be clearly informed that a reaction with ethanol will occur up to 80 h after 200 mg of disulfiram, and up to 36 h after citrated calcium carbimide, and may be serious or even lethal. The patient must also learn to avoid disguised forms of alcohol: culinary sauces, fermented vinegars, cough syrups and cosmetics such as after-shave lotions. Attempts to develop an effective slow release disulfiram capsule have not been very successful. Disulfiram implants are relatively expensive to insert, do not provide effective blood levels after two to three weeks, and thus any benefit in supporting abstinence has to be regarded as a placebo effect (Malcolm, Madden and Williams, 1974; Kwentus and Major, 1979). An oral, once a week slow release drug, related to metronidazole, a drug which is known to reduce craving for ethanol and to cause a disulfiram-like response (Goodwin and Reinhard, 1972), is being developed in Germany but is not at present available in the UK.

Lithium carbonate

Winokur, Rimmer and Reich (1971) are particularly associated with the view that dependent problem drinking is the alternative expression of a depressive affective illness type and many severely handicapped problem drinkers certainly have a significant affective component. Where this is a marked depressive illness, it has been suggested that lithium could be a prophylactic drug and recent reviews suggest a useful role in selected cases (McMillan, 1981; Coppen, 1980). Early prospective double-blind trials (Kline, Wren and Cooper, 1974; Merry et al., 1976) found that abstaining depressed drinkers on normal therapeutic doses of lithium (0.6–1.2 mmol · ℓ^{-1}) were less likely to relapse and less likely to become depressed than those of placebo. McMillan (1981) has reviewed less firm evidence which suggests that lithium may act directly on intoxication effects by reducing general drug euphoria. Further studies are clearly required, but it appears that lithium does confer significant benefit on drinking behaviour and mood in problem drinkers with concurrent and significant affective disturbances.

Other psychotropic medication

Most authorities agree that long-term 'replacement' medication such as a benzo-diazepine tranquillizer, or hypnotic, or other similar medication, should be avoided after the period of withdrawal. Most problem drinkers rapidly develop some degree of dependence on the new drug or hypnotic, and the resumption of a natural sleep pattern and diurnal rhythm will only be postponed further by such medication. Similarly there is only a limited place for conventional tricyclic antidepressant medication. The high suicide rate amongst problem drinkers, up to 80 times the normal rate, makes prescription of any medication a matter of careful consideration. Much severe affective illness is caused by or intensified by regular excessive ethanol consumption. Where a clear cut depressive illness predates excessive drinking and continues after de-toxification, conventional antidepressants may be prescribed in the normal way (*see* Chapter 7).

References

ACKER, W. Objective psychological changes in alcoholics after the withdrawal of alcohol. In *Alcohol and Disease* (Ed. S. SHERLOCK), Churchill-Livingstone, London (1982)

BAILEY, R. J., KRASNER, N., EDDLESTON, A. L. W. F., WILLIAMS, R., TEE, D. E. H., DONIACH, D., KENNEDY, L. A. and BATCHELOR, J. R. Histocompatability, antigens, antibodies and immunoglobulins in alcoholic liver disease, *British Medical Journal* 2, 727–729 (1976)

BRITISH MEDICAL JOURNAL. Management of alcohol withdrawal symptoms (Leader) 1, 282, 502 (1981)

CARTWRIGHT, A. K. J., SHAW, S. J. and SPRATLEY, T. A. Designing a comprehensive community response to problems of alcohol abuse, Maudsley Alcohol Pilot Project, London (1975)

COPPEN, A. Lithium in the treatment of alcoholism. In *Psychopharmacology of Alcohol* (Ed. M. SANDLER), Raven Press, New York (1980)

CUTTING, J. A reappraisal of alcoholic hallucinosis, *Psychological Medicine* 8, 285–295 (1978)

DAVIS, V. E., CASHAW, J. L. and McMURTREY, K. M. Catecholamine derived alkaloids in dependence. In *Addiction and Brain Damage* (Ed. D. RICHTER), Croom Helm/University Park Press, London and New York (1980)

DHSS. Advisory Committee on Alcoholism: The pattern and range of services for problem drinkers, DHSS, London (1978)

EDWARDS, G. and GROSS, M. Alcohol dependence: provisional description of a clinical syndrome, *British Medical Journal* 1, 1058–1061 (1976)

FEUERLEIN, W. Alcohol withdrawal syndrome. In *Psychopharmacology of Alcohol* (Ed. M. SANDLER), Raven Press, New York (1980)

FREUD, C. *Clement Freud's book of Hangovers*, Sheldon Press, New York (1981)

GHODSE, A. H. and TREGENZA, A. The physical effects and metabolism of alcohol. In *Women and Alcohol*, Camberwell Council on Alcoholism, Tavistock, London (1980)

GOODWIN, D. W. and REINHARD, J. Disulfiram-like effects of trichomonacidal drugs: A review and double blind study, *Quart. J. Stud. Alcohol* 33, 734–740 (1972)

JAFFÉ, J. H. Drug addiction and drug abuse. In *The Pharmacological Basis of Therapeutics*, 6th edn (Eds. A. G. GILMAN, L. S. GOODMAN and A. GILMAN), Macmillan, New York (1980)

KAIM, S. C., KLETT, C. J. and ROTHFELD, B. Treatment of the acute alcohol withdrawal state: a comparison of four drugs, *American Journal of Psychiatry* 125, 1640–1646 (1969)

KAIM, S. C. Treatment of alcoholism: experience with benzodiazepines. In *Benzodiazepines today and tomorrow* (Eds. R. G. PRIEST, U. VIANNA FILHO, R. AMREIN and M. SKRETA), pp. 175–185, MTP Press, Lancaster (1980)

KILICH, S. and PLANT, M. A. Regional variations in the levels of alcohol related problems in Britain, *British Journal of Addiction* 76, 47–62 (1981)

KITSON, T. M. The disulfiram-ethanol reaction, *Journal of Studies on Alcohol* 38, 96–113 (1977)

KLINE, N. S., WREN, J. C. and COOPER, T. B. Evaluation of lithium therapy in chronic and periodic alcoholism, *American Journal of Medical Sciences* 268, 15–22 (1974)

KORSTEN, M. A., MATSUZAKI, S., FEINMAN, L. and LIEBER, C. S. High blood acetaldehyde levels after ethanol administration, *New England Journal of Medicine* 292, 386–389 (1975)

KRASNER, N., DAVIS, M., PORTMANN, B. and WILLIAMS, R. The changing pattern of alcoholic liver disease in Great Britain—relationship to sex and immunological factors, *British Medical Journal* **1**, 1497–1499 (1978)

KWENTUS, J. and MAJOR, L. F. Disulfiram in the treatment of alcoholism: A review, *Journal of Studies in Alcohol* **40**, 428–446 (1979)

LIEBER, C. S. Hepatic and metabolic effects of alcohol (1966–1973), *Gastroenterology* **65**, 821–846 (1973)

LIEBER, C. S. Alcohol, protein metabolism, and liver injury, *Gastroenterology* **79**, 373–390 (1980)

LITTLETON, J. Development of membrane tolerance to ethanol may limit intoxication and influence dependence liability. In *Psychopharmacology of Alcohol* (Ed. M. SANDLER), Raven Press, New York (1980)

McMILLAN, T. M. Lithium and the treatment of alcoholism: a critical review, *British Journal of Addiction* **76**, 245–258 (1981)

MADDEN, J. S., JONES, D. and FRISCH, E. P. Chlormethiazole and trifluoperazine in alcohol withdrawal, *British Journal of Psychiatry* **115**, 1191–1192 (1969)

MALCOLM, M. T., MADDEN, J. S. and WILLIAMS, A. E. Disulfiram implantation critically evaluated, *British Journal of Psychiatry* **125**, 485–489 (1974)

MERRY, J., REYNOLDS, C. M., BAILEY, J. and COPPEN, A. Prophylactic treatment of alcoholism by lithium carbonate: a controlled study, *Lancet* **1**, 481–482 (1976)

MEYERS, R. D. Tetrahydroisoquinolines in the brain: the basis of an animal model of alcoholism, *Alcoholism: clinical and experimental research* **2**, 145–154 (1978)

MORGAN, R. and CAGAN, E. J. Acute alcohol intoxication, the disulfiram reaction, and methyl alcohol intoxication. In *The Biology of Alcoholism*, Vol. III, *Clinical Pathology* (Eds. B. KISSIN and H. BEGLEITER), Plenum Press, New York (1974)

MURRAY, R. M. and GURLING, H. M. D. Genetic contribution to normal and abnormal drinking. In *Psychopharmacology of Alcohol* (Ed. M. SANDLER), Raven Press, New York (1980)

OUTERBRIDGE, D. *The Hangover Handbook. The definitive guide to the causes and cures of mankind's oldest affliction*, Pan Books, London (1981)

PETERS, T. J. Ethanol and metabolism. In *Alcohol and Disease* (Ed. S. SHERLOCK), Churchill-Longman, London (1982)

PIROLA, R. C. *Drug Metabolism and Alcohol. A survey of Alcohol—Drug Reactions—Mechanisms, Clinical Aspects, Experimental Studies*, Adis Press, New York (1977)

PRATT, O. E. The fetal alcohol syndrome: Transport of nutrients and transfer of alcohol and acetaldehyde from mother to fetus. In *Psychopharmacology of Alcohol* (Ed. M. SANDLER), Raven Press, New York (1980)

PRATT, O. E. Alcohol and the developing fetus. In *Alcohol and Disease* (Ed. S. SHERLOCK), Churchill Livingstone, London (1982)

RADA, R. T. and KELLNER, R. Drug treatment in alcoholism. In *Psychopharmacology Update: New and neglected areas* (Eds. J. M. DAVIS and D. GREENBLATT), Grune and Stratton, New York (1979)

REILLY, T. M. Physiological dependence on, and symptoms of withdrawal from, chlormethiazole, *British Journal of Psychiatry* **128**, 375–378 (1976)

REILLY, T. M. The value of thiamine replacement in chronic alcoholism: a reminder, *British Journal of Addiction* **74**, 205–207 (1979)

RITCHIE, J. M. The aliphatic alcohols. In *The Pharmacological Basis of Therapeutics*, 6th edn (Eds. A. G. GILMAN, L. S. GOODMAN and A. GILMAN), Macmillan, New York (1980)

ROYAL COLLEGE OF PSYCHIATRISTS. *Alcohol and Alcoholism*, Tavistock, London (1979)

SANDLER, M. *Psychopharmacology of Alcohol* (Ed. M. SANDLER), Raven Press, New York (1980)

SAUNDERS, W. M. and KERSHAW, P. W. The prevalence of problem drinking and alcoholism in the west of Scotland, *British Journal of Psychiatry* **133**, 493–499 (1978)

SCLARE, A. B. The foetal alcohol syndrome. In *Women and Alcohol*, by Camberwell Council on Alcoholism, Tavistock, London (1980)

SELLERS, E. M. and KALANT, H. Alcohol intoxication and withdrawal, *New England Journal of Medicine* **14**, 757–762 (1976)

SHERLOCK, S. (Ed.). Alcohol and Disease, *British Medical Bulletin*, Churchill-Livingstone, London (1982) Livingstone, London (1982)

SHAW, G. K. A guide to drug treatment of alcoholism. In *Psychopharmacology of Alcohol* (Ed. M. SANDLER), Raven Press, New York (1980)

SHAW, G. K. Alcohol dependence and withdrawal. In *Alcohol and Disease* (Ed. S. SHERLOCK), Churchill-Livingstone, London (1982)

THOMAS, M. and PETERS, T. J. Acetaldehyde: Its role in alcohol toxicity and dependence, *British Journal of Addiction* **74**, 375–378 (1981)

THORLEY, A. Medical responses to problem drinking, *Medicine* (3rd series) **35**, 1816–1822 (1980)

THORLEY, A. Rehabilitation of problem drinkers and drugtakers. In *Principles of Psychiatric Rehabilitation* (Eds. F. WATTS and D. BENNETT) (In press), John Wiley, London (1982a)

THORLEY, A. Drug problems. In *Essentials of Postgraduate Psychiatry*, 2nd edn (Eds. P. HILL, R. MURRAY and A. THORLEY) (In preparation), Academic Press, London (1982b)

THORLEY, A. The effects of alcohol. In *Drinking and Problem Drinking* (Ed. M. A. PLANT), Junction Books, London (1982c)

WILSON, P. Drinking in England and Wales, *O.P.C.S.*, HMSO, London (1980)

WINOKUR, G., RIMMER, J. and REICH, T. Alcoholism. iv. Is there more than one type of alcoholism? *British Journal of Psychiatry* **118**, 523–531 (1971)

Chapter 14

Drugs in child psychiatry

P. J. Tyrer

Drugs are used to some extent in the treatment of childhood psychiatric disorders but are usually thought of as secondary measures to treatment based on social and psychotherapeutic lines. There is some reluctance to resort to drug therapy because it is perceived as crossing the Rubicon into the territory of neuropathology and long-term disability. This is understandable, because one of the delights of child psychiatry is its continual change. Many of the children who come to psychiatric care have only temporary emotional and behavioural disturbance that can be thought of as developmental in nature, and it would be quite wrong to use the drug sledgehammer to crack a nut that will naturally crack itself in time.

There are other concerns that also inhibit the use of drugs. One is the ethical perennial of informed consent. A young child is incapable of giving informed consent and this has to be provided by the parents or guardians. If, as so often happens, the parents are at least partly responsible for the child's problems, it is difficult for the psychiatrist to regard the parents' consent as always in the best interests of the child. The prescription of a drug, more than any amount of psychotherapy, also confers the label of 'illness' on the child in the parents' eyes, leading to attitudinal changes that may be pathological and reinforce the problem.

It is also relevant that doctors attracted towards child psychiatry are in the main not interested in drug therapy and the biological aspects of psychiatry. They will therefore turn to drug treatment out of necessity rather than preference and tend to regard it as a second order of treatment that is inferior to their main psychotherapeutic skills. Whilst the statement that in child psychiatry 'psychotropic drugs are degraded to a rather irritating interference with the therapist's desire for psychotherapeutic omnipotence' (Van Praag, 1978, p. 407) might be considered a little too strong, it is not surprising that child psychiatrists are less at ease with drugs than with their other modes of treatment. The disorders in which drug treatment is common are ones which are considered to have a putative organic basis, including the hyperkinetic disorders of childhood, particularly when there is a history of brain damage, childhood schizophrenia and infantile autism. These are not necessarily the most appropriate for drug treatment but the therapist need not feel uncomfortable about prescribing drugs for them. The literature on drug therapy in some other childhood disorders is embarrassingly small and thus it is often necessary to fall back on individual experience in deciding how, when and what to treat.

Pharmacokinetics

The pharmacokinetics of drugs in children is not a scaled-down version of that in adults and it is unwise to extrapolate too much from adult data. Unfortunately there have been virtually no pharmacokinetic studies of psychotropic drugs in children and one is compelled to rely on data derived from older patients. The pharmacokinetics of drugs in the first two years of life is quite different from that in older children but as most psychotropic drugs are seldom prescribed in very young children this does not usually influence therapy. Older children tend to require larger dosages of drugs than younger children but even this obvious prediction does not always hold. Fortunately most psychotropic drugs prescribed in childhood have a rapid onset of action so it is reasonable to titrate dosage by clinical response. In deciding on dosage it is conventional to recommend a formula based on $mg \cdot kg^{-1}$ of body weight but this should be taken as a rough guide only. If time permits it is best to start with a low dose, about one-quarter of that used in adults, and increase this as necesary. Because metabolism and excretion of drugs can be very rapid in children the timing and frequency of dosage is critical. By recording the time interval between drug administration and clinical effects the drugs can be given more economically and effectively.

Pharmacodynamics

Antipsychotic drugs

Schizophrenia and manic-depressive illness can begin in adolescence and drug therapy with antipsychotic drugs may be needed. In such instances the drugs used and dosage required are similar to that described in Chapter 4 with only some revision of dosage depending on the patient's weight and age. A more common use of antipsychotic drugs is in the treatment of the 'hyperkinetic syndrome'. This term is not entirely satisfactory as it is variously interpreted as a simple description of overactive children, a syndrome of increased motor activity and reduced attention presenting between the ages of 5–10 years, or a specific neuropsychiatric diagnosis often associated with brain damage. In this chapter the term is used to describe a combination of overactivity and restlessness occurring in a wide range of situations, inability to concentrate on a task for long enough to complete it, and haphazard impulsive behaviour leading to social handicap. The disorder usually presents between the ages of four and eight.

Phenothiazines have been compared with placebo in the treatment of hyperactive children and in the studies which involved adequate sample sizes chlorpromazine ($30–150\,mg \cdot d^{-1}$) and thioridazine ($100–200\,mg \cdot d^{-1}$) were significantly superior (Werry et al., 1966; Kenny, Badie and Baldwin, 1968; Greenberg, Deem and McMahon, 1972; Gittelman-Klein et al., 1976). Similar superiority has been shown for haloperidol in comparison with placebo (Werry and Aman, 1975). Haloperidol in a dose of $0.05\,mg \cdot kg^{-1}$ body weight was more effective than a dose of $0.025\,mg \cdot kg^{-1}$ body weight in reducing hyperactivity. Taking the studies as a whole, when higher dosage is used (at levels equivalent to antipsychotic dosage in adults) greater efficacy is found. Although the evidence shows that short-term treatment with antipsychotic drugs is effective in controlling hyperkinesis there is no indication of the right duration of treatment. The iatrogenic syndrome of tardive dyskinesia does not seem to occur in children but there are doubts about the effects of antipsychotic drugs on intellectual function in children. In this respect the psychostimulants are superior, as they either have no effect on intellectual performance or improve speed and efficiency of cognitive function.

Antipsychotic drugs have also been used in the treatment of infantile autism and psychotic disorders of early childhood (presenting between the ages of three and ten). Results in childhood autism have generally been disappointing. Although in one study by Campbell and her colleagues haloperidol in a daily dose of 2–4 mg was superior to placebo in aiding word learning using a behavioural approach (Campbell *et al.*, 1978) there was little improvement in the core features of autism. In other psychotic disorders of childhood the same disappointing results are shown. Although some improvement in behaviour follows treatment the changes are not of great clinical significance and much less marked than in adult schizophrenia (Campbell *et al.*, 1970; Engelhardt *et al.*, 1973; Saletu *et al.*, 1975). There is no evidence that any single drug or antipsychotic drug group is superior to others in clinical efficacy, with the possible exception of Gilles de la Tourette syndrome, the relatively rare combination of motor and vocal tics associated with echolalia and coprolalia, in which haloperidol is specifically effective (Connell *et al.*, 1977).

Antipsychotic drugs have also been used in the treatment of childhood behaviour disorders. Antiaggressive effects have been demonstrated with haloperidol in a dose of 3 mg daily (Cunningham, Pillai and Blachford Rogers, 1968) and when other methods of coping with aggression have failed it is worth considering haloperidol and other antipsychotic drugs.

Antianxiety drugs

Anxiety is a common symptom in child psychiatry and only when it becomes severe and persistent is drug therapy considered. If persistent free-floating anxiety is to be treated with drugs, barbiturates, as in adults, should be avoided, and the usual choice is between benzodiazepines, chloral hydrate and antihistamine drugs such as diphenhydramine and promethazine.

Benzodiazepines are effective antianxiety drugs in children but there are no published controlled studies evaluating their use in anxiety. The indications from open studies suggest that similar response to that in adult anxiety is shown with benzodiazepines (Kraft *et al.*, 1965) and these authors also noted the paradoxical release of aggressive behaviour in some children. Benzodiazepines also have some effect in reducing hyperkinesis but are less effective than psychostimulants (Zrull *et al.*, 1963).

One of the antihistamines, diphenhydramine, has been widely used as a sedative for children for reasons that are not fully clear from its pharmacological profile. It appears to be an effective night time hypnotic drug (Fish, 1960) and may be of particular use in anxious children because of its antinauseant and antiallergic properties. Other antihistamines such as promethazine, cyclizine, chlorpheniramine and mepyramine are probably equally effective. Antihistamines are also used to treat the dystonic reactions produced by antipsychotic drugs although no formal comparisons have been made with the more conventional antiparkinsonian drugs used in adult psychiatry.

Chloral hydrate, usually given as an elixir (500 mg$\cdot$5 ml^{-1}) in a dose of 50 mg$\cdot$kg^{-1} of body weight is a commonly used hypnotic in children. A lower dosage strength (200 mg$\cdot$5 ml^{-1}) is available for children under one year. Benzodiazepines are not often prescribed as hypnotics in children although there is no reason why they should not be used. Tolerance and dependence to antianxiety drugs is fortunately rare in children and seldom constitutes a clinical problem.

Tricyclic antidepressants

Severe depression in children below the age of 12 is uncommon and it is unwise to place too much reliance on the single feature of depressed mood (Graham, 1974). Studies of the efficacy of antidepressants in depressed children are often handicapped by diagnostic confusion and no satisfactory controlled trials have been carried out. Frommer (1968) separates depressive illness in childhood into pure depression, phobic depression and enuretic depression. She claims the MAOIs are specific therapy for the first two groups and the tricyclic antidepressants are indicated for the enuretic depressions. However, Gittelman-Klein and her colleagues in New York have produced good evidence that phobic disorders in childhood are also responsive to imipramine (Rabiner and Klein, 1969; Gittelman-Klein and Klein, 1971). In a well-designed double-blind study, 35 children aged between 7 and 15 with school refusal were treated with imipramine in substantial dosage (up to $200\,mg\cdot d^{-1}$). Eighty-one per cent of those on imipramine returned to school whereas only 47 per cent of those on placebo did so. Gittelman-Klein does not regard the improvement as indicative of the antidepressant actions of imipramine, because separation anxiety was the symptom that was predominantely improved. She therefore regards the beneficial effect of imipramine as anxiety-reducing in a similar way to the reduction of phobic anxiety and panic in adult anxious patients (Klein, 1964; Gittelman-Klein and Klein, 1973).

The use of tricyclic antidepressants in treating nocturnal enuresis in children has been discussed earlier by Professor Mindham (Chapter 7). Other psychotropic drugs, including dexamphetamine, MAOIs, antihistamines and anticholinergic drugs, are ineffective in preventing enuresis. The reasons for the therapeutic specificity of tricyclic antidepressants is not known and is likely to be due to a combination of anticholinergic and antidepressant actions and drug effects on sleep. Comparisons of conditioning procedures (e.g. pad and bell) with imipramine suggests that drug treatment is more effective in the short term and conditioning in the long term (McConaghy, 1969). This is in keeping with the effects of most drug treatments. In treating nocturnal enuresis it is best to start with a relatively low dose of imipramine or amitriptyline (12.5 mg or 25 mg nightly), increasing to 50 mg or 75 mg nightly if necessary in resistant cases. It takes at least a week for the full clinical effects to be shown so dosage should not be raised too rapidly. Treatment should be continued for up to six months and then tailed off gradually.

Tricyclic antidepressants have also been used in the treatment of hyperkinesis. In general the results show that both amitriptyline and imipramine are superior to placebo in reducing hyperactivity and aggression (Yepes et al., 1977) but less effective than psychostimulants such as methylphenidate (Rapoport et al., 1974). The mechanism of therapeutic action in reducing hyperactivity is far from clear and has no parallel in adult psychiatry. Relatively high doses (e.g. $100-150\,mg\cdot d^{-1}$ of imipramine or amitriptyline) are needed to have significant clinical effects.

The newer antidepressants have not been used to any appreciable extent in child psychiatry but it is reasonable to suppose that they have some place in the treatment of depressive disorders, enuresis and hyperkinesis. In particular, the sedative, anticholinergic and potential cardiotoxic effects of tricyclic antidepressants may be troublesome if high dosage is needed, and replacement with mianserin, nomifensine or trazodone might alleviate these adverse effects without loss of clinical efficacy.

Monoamine oxidase inhibitors

Monoamine oxidase inhibitors (MAOIs) are only used to a very limited extent in child psychiatry. Most evidence for their efficacy comes from the work of Eva Frommer at St Thomas's Hospital in London. She was impressed by the beneficial effects of MAOIs in adult 'atypical depression' reported by her hospital colleague Dr Sargant (1961) and therefore used MAOIs (mainly phenelzine) in similar disorders presenting in childhood. In a double-blind study using a cross-over design with 32 depressed children she found that the combination of phenelzine and chlordiazepoxide for two weeks was significantly superior to the combination of phenobarbitone and placebo for the same period. Both primarily phobic and primarily depressed patients improved on the MAOI—benzodiazepine combination, and Frommer concluded that phenelzine had valuable antidepressant effects in such children (Frommer, 1967). Unfortunately it is not really possible to make such a conclusion from the data, as two combinations of treatments were used. Specific effects of each combination as well as interaction between the drugs after the cross-over period could therefore affect the results. Nevertheless, extrapolation from use of MAOIs in adult patients supports the beneficial properties that Frommer ascribed to phenelzine, particularly in children over the age of ten. Whether it is generally wise to use MAOIs in these disorders is another question, and most child psychiatrists are too concerned about the dangers of food and drug interactions to risk using this class of drugs.

No comparison has been made between MAOIs and tricyclic antidepressants in the affective disorders of childhood and it is not possible to say which is superior. There is also no indication for how long treatment should be continued after clinical response is achieved but six months' duration of treatment seems an appropriate maximum.

Amine precursors

Levodopa has been used in the treatment of autistic children, mainly in order to test the theory that there were abnormalities of 5-hydroxytryptamine in this disorder. No appreciable benefit has been noted (Ritvo et al., 1971; Campbell et al., 1976) although levodopa produced some increase in energy and initiative. L-5-Hydroxytryptophan has also been used together with carbidopa in the treatment of childhood autism without any benefit being noted (Sverd et al., 1978). On present evidence there is no place for amine precursors in child psychiatry.

Lithium carbonate

Lithium carbonate is only occasionally used in children. Early reports suggesting that it is effective in the treatment of manic and depressive disorders in children (Frommer, 1968; Annell, 1969) are difficult to evaluate because of their anecdotal nature and diagnostic uncertainty. Because of the rarity of manic-depressive illness in childhood it is unlikely that a controlled trial could be carried out without multicentre cooperation. Manic-depressive illness may begin in adolescence and in this group it is reasonable to consider prophylaxis with lithium if the episodes are frequent.

The antiaggressive effects of lithium have already been described in Chapter 10. Some support for a similar action in explosively aggressive children has come from two studies (Campbell et al., 1972; Gram and Rafaelsen, 1972). Some of the children described in these studies were autistic, but it is unlikely that the beneficial effects of lithium extend to the central features of the autistic syndrome.

A possible variant of manic-depressive psychosis in childhood, emotionally unstable character disorder (EUCD), has been described by Rifkin and his colleagues (1972). It consists of mood swings associated with behaviour disturbance in adolescents and responds significantly better to lithium than to placebo. Serum lithium levels are maintained within the adult prophylactic range of $0.6-1.5\,mmol \cdot \ell^{-1}$ and the drug appears to act as in adults by preventing the mood and behaviour disturbance. However, the patients studied were all in in-patients and with this type of disorder it is unlikely that good compliance could be achieved with out-patients.

Psychostimulants

The use of psychostimulants in the hyperkinetic syndrome of childhood has already been mentioned in Chapter 11. This is the main clinical use of psychostimulants in psychiatry. At first sight it seems paradoxical that drugs that stimulate mental and physical activity should be used to treat a disorder in which mental and physical overactivity are the main clinical features. When it is appreciated that the central effects of drugs such as amphetamine are often opposite to their peripheral effects the rationale becomes clearer. The hypothesis that hyperkinesis results from cerebral underactivity rather than overactivity is also a plausible one. Nonetheless it has to be admitted that the use of psychostimulants in this group of disorders is entirely empirical and is difficult to sustain on purely pharmacological grounds.

In evaluating the efficacy of different psychostimulants in hyperkinetic syndromes it is important to be aware of the differences between hyperkinesis, minimal brain dysfunction (MBD) and overactivity occurring in conduct disorders. Minimal brain dysfunction is not a satisfactory term because although it implies central nervous pathology it does not require any neurological signs to be present. Any child with disturbed behaviour could therefore be classified as having minimal brain dysfunction without fear of contradiction. The term hyperkinetic syndrome is now often described as attention deficit disorder with hyperactivity. Fuller accounts of the classification of hyperkinesis in childhood are found in other texts (Cantwell, 1975; Klein et al., 1980).

Both dextro and laevo-isomers of amphetamine, methylamphetamine, methylphenidate, caffeine, deanol and magnesium pemoline are all stimulants that have been used in the treatment of hyperkinesis. Antipsychotic and antidepressant drugs have also been used and were mentioned earlier. Despite the diagnostic difficulties the results from a large number of studies are fairly consistent, leading to the unusual luxury in child psychiatry of clear guidelines based on experimental data. Caffeine and deanol have only weak therapeutic activity and do not have a significant place in treating hyperkinesis. The other psychostimulants are all effective in reducing hyperactivity and improving attention and are generally superior to antipsychotic and antidepressant drugs (Greenberg, Deen and McMahon, 1972; Rapoport et al., 1974; Gittelman-Klein et al., 1976). Magnesium pemoline (marketed as pemoline in the UK) is an effective treatment in a dosage of 50–125 mg daily but its effects take between three and eight weeks to be fully shown (Conners et al., 1972; Page et al., 1974). The initial dosage is 20 mg daily increasing to a maximum of 120 mg daily. It is not as reliably effective as methylphenidate and amphetamine and is best considered as a second-line treatment. Dexamphetamine and laevo-amphetamine have been known to reduce hyperactivity in children for many years. Indeed, the demonstration of the effectiveness of dexamphetamine was one of the first controlled drug studies in child psychiatry (Zrull *et al.*, 1963). Laevo-amphetamine is of the same order of efficacy as dexamphetamine but offers no particular advantages (Arnold *et al.*, 1972). The effects of amphetamine are normally shown within a few hours of starting treatment and are therefore substantially more rapid than magnesium pemoline. Methylamphetamine is not as potent as the isomers of amphetamine and may be considered when children respond well to amphetamine but are greatly troubled by its side effects, particularly anorexia and insomnia.

Methylphenidate has been demonstrated to be an effective drug in treating hyperkinesis in many studies. Response is partly dependent on dosage, with higher dosage ($0.5–1.0$ mg·kg^{-1} of body weight) more effective than lower dosage ($0.1–0.3$ mg·kg^{-1} body weight) (Werry and Sprague, 1974). Using still higher dosage of up to 2 mg·kg^{-1} of body weight the effectiveness of methylphenidate is even more apparent (Lewis and Young, 1975; Schain and Reynard, 1975). Better response to methylphenidate was found in patients with psychophysiological measurements suggesting low arousal, supporting the hypothesis that hyperkinesis responds to psychostimulants because it is a state of central under-arousal (Satterfield *et al.*, 1972). Methylphenidate apparently improves the children's span of attention and this allows better learning and concentration as well as less disorganized behaviour. Most children with hyperkinesis treated with psychostimulants are in the 7–12 age group. Younger children with hyperkinesis are not so responsive to treatment although one study suggests methylphenidate is also beneficial in treating hyperkinesis in children aged between three and five (Schleifer *et al.*, 1975).

Methylphenidate and dexamphetamine are the drugs of choice in the treatment of hyperkinesis. Once the decision has been made to give drug therapy either methylphenidate (2.5–7.5 mg) or dexamphetamine (1.25–2.5 mg) is given in a single dose in the morning (to avoid the risk of insomnia at night). Some response is normally shown within 1 h and the effects of a single dose last up to 6 h. Dexamphetamine can be given in the form of a spansule to extend the duration of effect. Dosage is gradually increased to produce the optimum therapeutic effects; this is much easier to achieve than with other psychotropic drugs because the psychostimulants act so rapidly. It is unwise to increase the dosage of methylphenidate beyond 100 mg daily and dexamphetamine beyond 50 mg daily. The ideal duration of treatment is not known but it averages many months. It is advisable to stop treatment at least once a year to determine if continuation is still needed. The effects of medication wear off quickly so that it is easy to determine whether the hyperkinetic behaviour has returned but it is important to distinguish this from withdrawal effects (*see below*).

Megavitamins have also been used in child psychiatry to treat autistic and schizophrenic children. The results are no different from similar therapy in adult schizophrenia; they are ineffective and have no place in therapy (American Academy of Paediatrics, 1976).

Summary of clinical use

The use of drugs in child psychiatry is only a small fraction of treatment but in some disorders, particularly hyperkinesis, it is a very important part. The choice of drug treatment often has to be based on less than adequate evidence but a summary of first and second-line treatments is given in *Table 14.1*. As there is no fundamental difference in efficacy between individual members of the antipsychotic, benzodiazepine and tricyclic antidepressant drug groups the generic name is listed, although it should be

TABLE 14.1 Summary of use of psychotropic drugs in child psychiatry

Childhood disorder	Drug treatment of first choice	Other effective drug treatments	Average duration of treatment
Childhood autism	None	Antipsychotic drugs	Intermittent for several months at a time
Hyperkinetic syndrome (for other synonyms see text)	Dexamphetamine Methylphenidate	Laevo-amphetamine Magnesium pemoline Antipsychotic drugs Tricyclic antidepressants Methylamphetamine	Intermittent for several months at a time
Anxiety states	Benzodiazepines	Antihistamines	Intermittent for 7–14 d
Insomnia	Benzodiazepines Chloral hydrate	Antihistamines	Intermittent for 7–21 d
Depressive illness	Tricyclic antidepressants	Monoamine oxidase inhibitors Lithium carbonate (for manic-depressive illness)	Several weeks
Phobic anxiety (including school refusal)	Tricyclic antidepressants	Monoamine oxidase inhibitors	Several weeks
Conduct disorders	Antipsychotic drugs	Lithium carbonate	Intermittent up to several months
Nocturnal enuresis	Tricyclic antidepressants	None	Up to 6 months

added that chlorpromazine, thioridazine and haloperidol of the antipsychotic drugs, chlordiazepoxide and diazepam of the benzodiazepines, and imipramine of the tricyclic antidepressants, have been the most widely studied drugs. Many improvements on this list are possible as much of the data on which it is founded were derived from studies completed many years ago. In particular, the newer antidepressants and antianxiety drugs deserve further study.

Unwanted effects of psychotropic drugs in children

There are special problems in evaluating the benefits of psychotropic drugs in children, including the ethical problems of controlled trials, the transient nature of many childhood psychiatric disorders and the hazards of unwanted effects in developing children, who may not show evidence of these effects until some years later. Any doctor who prescribes drugs to children has to be especially sensitive to unwanted effects because of possible criticism by others who would not normally use drug therapy for the same condition. A small gain in clinical status may be more than offset by the loss produced by an untoward effect that might be regarded as acceptable in adult psychiatric practice.

The use of antipsychotic drugs leads to similar unwanted effects in adults and children, with extrapyramidal symptoms, the anticholinergic side effects of dry mouth, constipation and blurred vision, and increased appetite predominating. Drowsiness may also be a problem, and haloperidol may be preferred to chlorpromazine or thioridazine in such instances. In general, children can tolerate higher dosage levels of antipsychotic drugs than adults before developing extrapyramidal symptoms. When extrapyramidal symptoms do develop they often do so suddenly in the form of acute dystonic reactions, particularly involving the head, neck and trunk. These may be successfully treated with intramuscular benztropine (0.5–1 mg) or procyclidine (2.5–5 mg). The use of diphenhydramine and other antihistamine drugs is a less preferable alternative.

As mentioned earlier, tardive dyskinesia as described in adults does not occur in children, confirming the importance of increasing age as an aetiological factor in the condition. Nevertheless, withdrawal of antipsychotic drugs after prolonged treatment is sometimes associated with dystonic movements of the head, neck and trunk (Polizos et al., 1973). These normally disappear within 1–3 weeks and are best avoided by withdrawing antipsychotic drugs slowly. These reactions are more likely to occur after withdrawal from long-term use, emphasizing that treatment with antipsychotic drugs should always be kept under close review and wherever possible long-term continuous therapy should be avoided.

Antianxiety drugs do not cause any serious side effects in children. If dosage is excessive drowsiness and impaired concentration can lead to learning difficulties. By using clinical response as the main criterion for dosage this can usually be prevented. Neither tolerance nor dependence have been reported with benzodiazepines, antihistamines or chloral derivatives in children but this may be due to most treatments being for short periods only. Care should be exercised in prescribing antianxiety drugs during the later years of adolescence because long-term use may be a prelude to abuse of other more addictive drugs.

Tricyclic antidepressants, as in adults, can cause anticholinergic side effects and drowsiness, but these are not normally a serious problem in children. Postural hypotension can be a particular problem in children because of their greater activity and frequent changes of posture. Epileptogenic effects have also been reported in children (Brown et al., 1973) and it is best to avoid tricyclic antidepressants in children with a history of epilepsy. Although appetite stimulation is usually a problem with adults, in children anorexia is more common. This may be associated with nausea and can be severe enough to stop therapy. There has been greatest concern over the possible cardiotoxic effects of tricyclic antidepressants in children, particularly in the USA. Cardiotoxicity with imipramine has been responsible for at least one death (Saraf et al., 1974) and ECG changes, including the characteristic widening of the PR interval and, less commonly, widening of the QRS complexes, has been noted in many children treated with imipramine in dosages above $3.5\,\text{mg}\cdot\text{kg}^{-1}$ (Saraf et al., 1978). Small increases in systolic and diastolic blood pressure have also been noticed in children treated with imipramine (Saraf et al., 1974); there is nothing to suggest that these are precursors of true hypertension but they are understandably disturbing.

Monoamine oxidase inhibitors have not been reported as causing any unusual unwanted effects in children. Nevertheless, the danger of drug and food interactions need to be explained carefully to both parents and children and warning cards issued to all those likely to be concerned with preparing the children's meals. Anticholinergic side effects and postural hypotension occur with approximately the same frequency as the tricyclic antidepressants.

Lithium carbonate has also not been used to any extent in child psychiatry and so there is little literature on its adverse effects. Tremor and minor gastrointestinal disturbance (nausea, anorexia and, less commonly, diarrhoea) may occur and if long-term therapy is considered it is prudent to check thyroid function at regular intervals.

Psychostimulants can produce several side effects of sufficient severity to alter or curtail treatment. Anorexia and insomnia are predictable symptoms that usually affect all patients at some time or another. The anorexia itself does not usually lead to a significant loss of weight because at the times when the psychostimulant is least effective, usually in the evening, appetite often returns and a hearty meal is eaten. Insomnia is also partly dependent on the timing of dosage; it is almost always shown as delay in getting to sleep although with some children there is a reduction of the average sleeping time.

Most psychostimulants are sympathomimetic so there is an increase in heart rate and sometimes a small rise in systolic blood pressure, but these rarely lead to symptoms. Amphetamines and methylphenidate are mildly epileptogenic and if their use is considered essential in children with definite brain damage and a history of epileptic seizures (which is sometimes associated with hyperkinesis) it is best to combine them with anticonvulsant drugs. Tics may also appear during treatment but it

TABLE 14.2 Serious and minor unwanted effects of psychotropic drugs in children

Drug group	Serious unwanted effects	Minor unwanted effects
Antipsychotic drugs	Acute dystonia	Drowsiness Appetite increase and weight gain Dry mouth and other anticholinergic effects Photosensitivity (with chlorpromazine) Withdrawal dyskinesias
Antianxiety drugs	—	Drowsiness
Tricyclic antidepressants	Cardiotoxicity Hypertension	Anticholinergic side effects Sweating Drowsiness Postural hypotension Anorexia
Monoamine oxidase inhibitors	Nil if correct drug and food restrictions observed	Anticholinergic side effects Postural hypotension
Lithium carbonate	Hypothyroidism	Tremor Gastrointestinal disturbances
Psychostimulants	Impaired growth Tics Hallucinations	Withdrawal effects Insomnia Anorexia

is difficult to know whether these are specific unwanted effects of psychostimulants or whether the drugs predispose to their manifestations in susceptible children.

It is surprising that frank addiction to psychostimulants almost never occurs in children, despite prolonged therapy and frequent high dosage. This, and a lack of addictive potential in children with other psychotropic drugs, suggests that psychological factors and physiological immaturity of the central nervous system protect against dependence. Rarely, hallucinations may occur but these are not accompanied by other psychotic phenomena (Lucas and Weiss, 1971). Withdrawal effects are shown in a small percentage of children if psychostimulants are withdrawn suddenly; they usually last only a few days and often appear as an exaggerated form of the hyperkinesis. Such children could be regarded as mildly addicted to their drugs in a similar way to benzodiazepine dependence. A possibly serious unwanted effect is the inhibition of growth with psychostimulants, which is most likely to occur with dexamphetamine and least with pemoline (Roche *et al.*, 1979). For this reason height should be regularly measured in all children on psychostimulants and long-term therapy avoided. It is not yet known whether children who remain on psychostimulants regain their decrement in height after the drugs are stopped or are permanently shorter than their peers.

The unwanted effects produced by psychotropic drugs in children are summarized in *Table 14.2*. The milder untoward effects can usually be treated by altering the timing or dosage of the drug, but when the serious ones are shown it is preferable to stop the offending drug.

References

AMERICAN ACADEMY OF PEDIATRICS—COMMITTEE ON NUTRITION. Megavitamin therapy for childhood psychoses and learning disabilities, *Pediatrics* **58**, 910–912 (1976)

ANNELL, A. L. Lithium in the treatment of children and adolescents, *Acta Psychiatrica Scandinavica*, Suppl., **207**, 19–30 (1969)

ARNOLD, L. E., WENDER, P. H., McCLOSKEY, K. and SNYDER, S. H. Levoamphetamine and dextroamphetamine: comparative efficacy in the hyperkinetic syndrome: assessment by target symptoms, *Archives of General Psychiatry* **27**, 816–822 (1972)

BROWN, D., WINSBERG, B. G., BIALER, I. and PRESS, M. Imipramine therapy and seizures: three children treated for hyperactive behavior disorders, *American Journal of Psychiatry* **130**, 210–212 (1973)

CAMPBELL, M., FISH, B., SHAPIRO, T. and FLOYD, A. Jr. Thiothixene in young disturbed children: a pilot study, *Archives of General Psychiatry* **23**, 70–72 (1970)

CAMPBELL, M., FISH, B., KOREIN, J., SHAPIRO, T., COLLINS, P. and KOH, C. Lithium and chlorpromazine: a controlled crossover study of hyperactive severely disturbed young children, *Journal of Autism and Child Schizophrenia* **2**, 234–263 (1972)

CAMPBELL, M., SMALL, A. M., COLLINS, P. J., FRIEDMAN, E., DAVID, R. and GENEISER, N. B. Levodopa and levoamphetamine: a crossover study in schizophrenic children, *Current Therapeutic Research* **19**, 70–86 (1976)

CAMPBELL, M., ANDERSON, L. T., MEIER, M., COHEN, I. L., SMALL, A. M., SAMIT, C. and SACHAR, E. J. A comparison of haloperidol and behaviour therapy and their interaction in autistic children, *Journal of the American Academy of Child Psychiatry* **17**, 640–655 (1978)

CANTWELL, D. P. (Ed.). *The Hyperactive Child. Diagnosis, Management, Current Research*, Spectrum Publications, New York (1975)

CONNELL, P. H., CORBETT, J. A., HORNE, D. J. and MATHEWS, A. M. Drug treatment of adolescent tiqueurs; a double-blind trial of diazepam and haloperidol, *British Journal of Psychiatry* **113**, 375–381 (1967)

CONNERS, C. K., TAYLOR, E., MEO, G., KURTZ, M. A. and FOURNIER, M. Magnesium pemoline and dextroamphetamine: a controlled study in children with minimal brain dysfunction, *Psychopharmacologia* **26**, 321–336 (1972)

CUNNINGHAM, M. A., PILLAI, V. and BLACHFORD ROGERS, W. J. Haloperidol in the treatment of children with severe behaviour disorders, *British Journal of Psychiatry* **114**, 845–854 (1968)

ENGELHARDT, D. M., POLIZOS, P., WAIZER, J. and HOFFMAN, S. A double-blind comparison of fluphenazine and haloperidol in outpatient schizophrenic children, *Journal of Autism and Childhood Schizophrenia* **3**, 128–137 (1973)

FISH, B. Drug therapy in child psychiatry: pharmacological aspects, *Comprehensive Psychiatry* **1**, 212–227 (1960)

FROMMER, E. A. Depressive illness in childhood. In *Recent Development in Affective Disorders* (Eds. A. COPPEN and A. WALK), pp. 117–136, Headley, Ashford (1968)

FROMMER, E. A. Treatment of childhood depression with antidepressant drugs, *British Medical Journal* **1**, 729–732 (1967)

GITTELMAN-KLEIN, R. and KLEIN, D. F. Controlled imipramine treatment of school phobia, *Archives of General Psychiatry* **25**, 204–207 (1971)

GITTELMAN-KLEIN, R. and KLEIN, D. F. School phobia: diagnostic considerations in the light of imipramine effects, *Journal of Nervous and Mental Diseases* **156**, 199–215 (1973)

GITTELMAN-KLEIN, R., KLEIN, D. F., KATZ, S., SARAF, K. and POLLACK, E. Comparative effects of methylphenidate and thioridazine in hyperkinetic children, *Archives of General Psychiatry* **33**, 1217–1231 (1976)

GRAHAM, P. Depression in pre-pubertal children, *Developmental Medicine and Child Neurology* **16**, 340–349 (1974)

GRAM, L. F. and RAFAELSEN, O. J. Lithium treatment of psychotic children and adolescents, *Acta Psychiatrica Scandinavica* **48**, 253–260 (1972)

GREENBERG, L. M., DEEM, M. A. and McMAHON, S. Effects of dextroamphetamine, chlorpromazine and hydroxyzine on behavior and performance in hyperactive children, *American Journal of Psychiatry* **129**, 532–539 (1972)

KENNY, T. J., BADIE, D. and BALDWIN, R. W. The effectiveness of a new drug, mesoridazine, and chlorpromazine with behavior problems in children, *Journal of Nervous and Mental Diseases* **147**, 316–321 (1968)

KLEIN, D. F. Delineation of two drug-responsive anxiety syndromes, *Psychopharmacologia* **5**, 397–408 (1964)

KLEIN, D. F., GITTELMAN, R., QUITKIN, F. and RIFKIN, A. *Diagnosis and Drug Treatment of Psychiatric Disorders: Adults and Children*, 2nd edn, Williams and Wilkins, Baltimore (1980)

KRAFT, I. A., ARDALI, C., DUFFY, J. H., HART, J. T. and PEARCH, P. A clinical study of chlordiazepoxide used in psychiatric disorders of children, *International Journal of Neuropsychiatry* **1**, 433–437 (1965)

LEWIS, J. A. and YOUNG, R. Deanol and methylphenidate in minimal brain dysfunction, *Clinical Pharmacology and Therapeutics* **17**, 534–540 (1975)

LUCAS, A. E. and WEISS, M. Methylphenidate hallucinosis, *Journal of the American Medical Association* **217**, 1079–1081 (1971)

McCONAGHY, N. A controlled trial of imipramine, amphetamine, pad-and-ball, conditioning and random awakening in the treatment of nocturnal enuresis, *Medical Journal of Australia* **2**, 237–239 (1969)

PAGE, J. G., JANICKI, R. S., BERNSTEIN, J. E., CURRAN, C. F. and MICHELLIS, F. A. Pemoline (Cylert) in the treatment of childhood hyperkinesis, *Journal of Learning Disorders* **7**, 498–503 (1974)

POLIZOS, P., ENGELHARDT, D. M., HOFFMAN, S. P. and WAIZER, J. Neurological consequences of psychotropic drug withdrawal in schizophrenic children, *Journal of Autism and Childhood Schizophrenia* **3**, 247–253 (1973)

RABINER, C. J. and KLEIN, D. F. Imipramine treatment of school phobia, *Comprehensive Psychiatry* **10**, 387–390 (1969)

RAPOPORT, J. L., QUINN, P. O., BRADFORD, G., RIDDLE, D. and BROOKS, E. Imipramine and methylphenidate treatments of hyperactive boys, *Archives of General Psychiatry* **30**, 789–793 (1974)

RIFKIN, A., QUITKIN, F., CORRILLO, C., BLUMBERG, A. G. and KLEIN, D. F. Lithium carbonate in emotionally unstable character disorder, *Archives of General Psychiatry* **27**, 519–523 (1972)

RITVO, E., YUWILER, A., GELLER, E., KALES, A., RASHKIS, S., SCHICOR, A., PLOTKIN, S., AXELROD, H. and HOWARD, C. Effects of L-dopa in autism, *Journal of Autism and Childhood Schizophrenia* **1**, 190–205 (1971)

ROCHE, A. F., LIPMAN, R. S., OVERALL, J. E. and HUNG, W. The effects of stimulant medication on the growth of hyperkinetic children, *Pediatrics* **63**, 847–850 (1979)

SALETU, B., SALETU, M., SIMEON, J., VIAMONTES, G. and ITIL, T. M. Comparative symptomatological and evoked potential studies with *d*-amphetamine, thioridazine, and placebo in hyperkinetic children, *Biological Psychiatry* **10**, 253–275 (1975)

SARAF, K. R., KLEIN, D. F., GITTELMAN-KLEIN, R. and GROFF, S. Imipramine side effects in children, *Psychopharmacologia* **37**, 265–274 (1974)

SARAF, K. R., KLEIN, D. F., GITTELMAN-KLEIN, R., GOOTMAN, N. and GREENHILL, P. EKG effects of imipramine treatment in children, *Journal of the American Academy of Child Psychiatry* **17**, 60–69 (1978)

SARGANT, W. Drugs in the treatment of depression, *British Medical Journal* **1**, 225–227 (1961)

SATTERFIELD, J. H., CANTWELL, D. P., LESSER, L. I. and PODOSIN, R. L. Physiological studies of the hyperkinetic child, *American Journal of Psychiatry* **128**, 1418–1424 (1972)

SCHAIN, R. J. and REYNARD, C. L. Observations on effects of a central stimulant drug (methylphenidate) in children with hyperactive behaviour, *Pediatrics* **55**, 709–716 (1975)

SCHLEIFER, M., WEISS, G., COHEN, N., ELMAN, M., CVEJIC, H. and KRUGER, E. Hyperactivity in preschoolers and the effect of methylphenidate, *American Journal of Orthopsychiatry* **45**, 38–50 (1975)

SVERD, J., KUPIERZ, S. S., WINSBERG, B. G., HURWIC, M. J. and BECKER, L. Effects of L-5-hydroxytryptophan in autistic children, *Journal of Autism and Childhood Schizophrenia* **8**, 171–180 (1978)

VAN PRAAG, H. M. *Psychotropic Drugs: a Guide for the Practitioner*, MacMillan, London (1978)

WERRY, J. S. and SPRAGUE, R. L. Methylphenidate in children: effect of dosage, *Australian and New Zealand Journal of Psychiatry* **8**, 9–19 (1974)

WERRY, J. S. and AMAN, M. G. Methylphenidate and haloperidol in children: effects on attention, memory and activity, *Archives of General Psychiatry* **32**, 790–795 (1975)

WERRY, J. S., WEISS, G., DOUGLAS, V. and MARTIN, J. Studies on the hyperactive child, 111. The effect of chlorpromazine upon behavior and learning ability, *Journal of the American Academy of Child Psychiatry* **5**, 292–312 (1966)

YEPES, L. E., BALKA, E. B., WINSBERG, B. G. and BIALER, I. Amitriptyline and methylphenidate treatment of behaviorally disordered children, *Journal of Child Psychology and Psychiatry* **18**, 39–52 (1977)

ZRULL, J. P., WESTMAN, J. C., ARTHUR, B. and BELL, W. A. A comparison of chlordiazepoxide, d-amphetamine and placebo in the treatment of the hyperkinetic syndrome in children, *American Journal of Psychiatry* **120**, 590–591 (1963)

Chapter 15

Drugs in psychogeriatrics

C. Trotter

Introduction

The elderly are the major consumers of drugs and the major source of unwanted effects of drugs (Hurwitz, 1969). In a recent community survey of psychotropic drug use (Williams, 1980) 14 per cent of men and 22 per cent of women over the age of 65 years admitted to taking at least one psychotropic drug in the previous two weeks. In the age 45–64, 9 per cent of men and 17 per cent of women were taking psychotropic drugs. In another study (Williamson and Chopin, 1980) the use of all drugs in nearly 2000 patients admitted to geriatric hospitals was examined. About 25 per cent of the patients were taking psychotropic drugs on admission. A similar percentage were taking analgesics, and the only group of drugs being taken by more patients (35 per cent) was the diuretics. In some 12 per cent of patients taking psychotropic drugs, adverse reactions to the drugs played a major part in the reason for admission. The authors estimated that nearly 4000 geriatric admissions per annum in England, Wales and Scotland are due solely to adverse drug reactions, and in another 11 000 cases adverse reactions contribute to the admissions.

A similar situation occurs in other countries. Chapman (1976) in Australia showed that pensioners, who make up 9 per cent of the population, were consuming 45 per cent of psychotropic drugs issued under the Australian National Health Service. In another Australian study of mental disorders induced by psychotropic drugs (Learoyd, 1972), two years of admissions to a psychogeriatric unit in a psychogeriatric hospital were reviewed. About 20 per cent of admissions were thought to be directly due to the effects of psychotropic drugs, and rapid improvement occurred on withdrawal of the medication. Three types of adverse reaction to psychotropic drugs were seen. Firstly, simple drug intoxications resulting in lethargy, confusion and disorientation. Secondly, physical side effects such as respiratory depression leading to chest infection, hypotension, urinary retention, constipation and falls. Thirdly, disinhibition reactions of restlessness, agitation and aggression. This study illustrates the common problem of sedative drugs being prescribed to control the behaviour that may be being induced or worsened by the very same drug.

In Canada 1400 over-65-year-old referrals to a Health Council, for assessment of long-term institutional or community care, were reviewed (Achong, 1978). All drugs being prescribed at the time of referral were recorded. Twenty-five per cent of patients were receiving one psychotropic drug and another 6.6 per cent were being prescribed two or three simultaneously. Of the patients receiving psychotropic drugs, 76.2 per cent were taking hypnotics/sedatives/anxiolytics, mainly benzodiazepines, 29.7 per cent major tranquillizers and only 4.2 per cent antidepressants. This last group of patients comprised 14 patients only one of whom was thought to be markedly depressed at the time of referral. However another 81 patients (6 per cent of the total referrals) were noted to be markedly depressed at the time of referral, none of whom were receiving antidepressant medication, but 22 of whom were receiving tranquillizers. This latter problem of the prescribing of inappropriate medication for depression, is commonly seen in clinical practice. The anxiety symptoms and insomnia of a depressed old person are recognized and treated but the depression is missed, perhaps because of the generally pessimistic view of ageing propagated in our culture.

The main principle in the psychotropic drug treatment of the elderly should be to avoid over-treatment and under-treatment. Over-treatment leads to falls, over-sedation, strokes, confusion, dehydration and hypotension. Under-treatment leads to partial improvement only, and a great deal of unnecessary suffering for patients and their relatives.

Pharmacokinetic and pharmacodynamic aspects of ageing

Pharmacokinetics refers to the process of absorption, metabolism, distribution and elimination of drugs and pharmacodynamics includes study of the sensitivity of receptor sites to the actions of drugs. All of these processes may be altered by age, but the end result depends on a variety of other factors including the properties of the drug, the physical and psychological state of the indi.vidual, and the interaction with other drugs that are being prescribed.

Absorption of drugs might be expected to be reduced in the elderly, due to reduced intestinal blood flow. This has not been demonstrated, however, and overall drug absorption is not affected by age (van Praag, 1977; Hollister, 1979). In individual cases the rate of absorption may be reduced or increased. Increased gastric motility and emptying increases the rate of absorption of most drugs. The presence of food in the stomach, and anticholinergic drugs, delay gastric emptying, and slow the rate of absorption of drugs. Thus tricyclics, antiparkinsonian drugs and major tranquillizers delay the rate of absorption of other drugs. Congestive cardiac failure may delay the absorption of some drugs due to mucosal oedema and reduced splanchnic blood flow. Apart from disease states involving severe malabsorption, illness has little effect on the overall absorption of drugs. Changes in the rate of absorption of drugs have important consequences only when immediate therapeutic effect is required (Scott and Hawksworth, 1981).

There may be changes in the metabolism of drugs by the liver in elderly patients. Hepatic enzyme induction is reduced in the aged (Castleden, 1978; van Praag, 1977) which may lead to higher blood levels of ingested drugs. However this effect is variable; for example there is evidence that oxidation is reduced for some drugs (chlormethiazole, phenylbutazone) but not for others (digoxin, warfarin). Hydrolysis, reduction and conjugation are unchanged as far as is known (Ramsay and Tucker, 1981).

The distribution of a drug depends on its lipid solubility, regional blood flow to the target organ and degree of plasma protein binding (Smith and Rawlins, 1973). Body fat increases with age, and lipid soluble drugs have an increased distribution volume and decreased blood levels (Ramsay and Tucker, 1981). Most psychotropic drugs are lipid soluble (Bowden and Giffen, 1978a). Highly water soluble drugs have reduced distribution volume and higher blood levels in the aged. Because plasma albumin falls with increasing age, plasma protein binding is reduced in the elderly. Protein binding of drugs is influenced by disease states and the binding properties of other drugs. Renal disease causes reduced binding due to the accumulation of endogenous metabolities. Liver disease may cause hypoalbuminaemia and reduce binding. Rheumatoid arthritis also leads to reduced plasma albumin. The higher circulating levels of the free drug consequent on reduced binding, leads to enhanced pharmacological effects and increased glomerular filtration of the drug (Lindup and L'E. Orme, 1981).

Elimination of drugs takes place in the kidney and the liver. Glomerular filtration and tubular excretion of drugs decreases with age, although there may be no evidence of renal failure. Individuals aged 80 and above have reduced creatinine clearance of 50–60 ml·min^{-}1 (Castleden, 1978). Creatinine production is reduced in old age, and therefore serum creatinine levels do not tend to reflect creatinine clearance rates and this must be taken into account when assessing renal function in the elderly. Reduced renal clearance is of particular consequence for drugs with a narrow therapeutic range such as lithium, nitrofurantoin and digoxin.

Available evidence indicates that receptor site sensitivity is increased in the elderly (Castleden, 1978; Prescott, 1979). This is particularly true for the benzodiazepines and anticoagulants, although there appears to be reduced receptor sensitivity to beta-blockers in the elderly (Ramsay and Tucker, 1981).

Other aspects of ageing of relevance to psychotropic drug therapy

Physical ill health

There is an association between physical illness and psychiatric disorder (Lloyd, 1977). The impact of physical illness can have adverse psychological consequences and can either precipitate psychiatric disorder, or worsen existing psychiatric illness. Unrecognized somatic disease can present as psychiatric illness and psychiatric illness can worsen existing somatic disease. Finally the drugs used in the treatment of somatic disease can give rise to psychiatric disorders, or interact with the drugs used to treat the psychiatric disorders.

A list of common physical disorders in the elderly which have particular relevance to psychogeriatrics is shown (*Table 15.1*). Heart failure is particularly common in the elderly and diuretics the most commonly prescribed drugs in patients referred to geriatric hospitals (Williamson and Chopin, 1980). It is quite possible that oedema of the ankles is frequently taken to be a symptom of heart failure when a more likely diagnosis might be immobility, varicose veins or a pelvic mass such as constipation (Jarvis, 1981).

TABLE 15.1 Common physical disorders in the elderly

Heart failure	Prostatic hypertrophy
Organic brain disease	Constipation
Parkinson's disease	Glaucoma
Renal failure	Diabetes
Liver disease	Infections
Arthritis	Hypertension

Parkinson's disease may be associated with dementia in some cases, and depression is commoner in patients with Parkinson's disease (Mindham, 1978). Antiparkinsonian drugs are well known to cause confusional states (*see* p. 100).

It is well documented that chronic pain can be caused by depression, and that depression and anxiety can make pain of organic origin worse (Merskey, 1977). It is not uncommon to be able to reduce the dose of analgesic medication in patients with chronic pain when antidepressant therapy is commenced. Over-investigation of complaints of chronic pain can occur when underlying depression is not recognized and treated.

Renal and liver disease interferes with the metabolism and excretion of drugs. Urinary retention can occur when tricyclic antidepressants, major tranquillizers or anticholinergic drugs are given to patients with prostatic hypertrophy. Glaucoma can be precipitated by tricyclic antidepressants although this problem is over-emphasized (*see* Chapter 7).

Constipation is worsened by all drugs with anticholinergic side effects. The hypoglycaemic effects of oral diabetic agents may be potentiated by major tranquillizers. Infections, which may be chronic and undiagnosed, can present as confusional states. Homeostatic mechanisms for the correction of postural hypotension are impaired in the elderly (Ramsay and Tucker, 1981; Prescott, 1979) and particularly in the elderly with hypertension. These patients are very sensitive to the postural hypotensive effect of tricyclic antidepressants and major tranquillizers (*Drugs and Therapeutics Bulletin*, 1975b).

Interactions with other medications

Some common drug interactions are listed in *Table 15.2*. These interactions may occur in any age group but elderly patients are more likely to be taking other groups of drugs, particularly analgesics, antihypertensives, diuretics and antiparkinsonian drugs. Some of the more important interactions will be mentioned later in the chapter.

Problems with compliance

An old person may have difficulty in grasping instructions relating to their medication. The difficulty may not be due to the presence of organic or functional psychiatric illness but to deafness, or to benign senescence. Deafness is common in the elderly. One community study using audiometric techniques (Herbst and Humphrey, 1980) found a point prevalence of 60 per cent for hearing impairment in their sample of over 70 year olds. They also found an association between deafness and depression although not between deafness and dementia.

Agitated and depressed patients may stop medication too soon as they think that their deterioration is due to the drug, and by the nature of agitation they are impatient to feel better.

Arthritis of the hands may cause difficulty in unscrewing bottle tops, particularly the childproof variety, and in halving small tablets. The writing on the label of the bottle may be impossible to read for an old person with poor eye-sight. Mistrust of tablets of any sort is common in the elderly, particularly when unsteadiness or falls have occurred or been exacerbated by previous medication. These problems can be minimized by enlisting the help of responsible relatives or friends. Hurried instructions given in passing in a busy surgery or brief visit must be avoided. Written instructions in large writing giving the name of the drug, what it is to be used to treat (in lay terms) and

TABLE 15.2
Important psychotropic drug interactions in the elderly

	Drug	Effect
Tricyclic antidepressants	Bethanidine ⎫ Debrisoquine ⎬ Guanethidine ⎭ Clonidine	Uptake of these drugs into noradrenergic neurons is blocked by tricyclics and antihypertensive effect is reduced.
Monoamine oxidase inhibitors	Tyramine ⎫ Barbiturates ⎪ Antidiabetic drugs ⎪ Pethidine ⎬ Amphetamine ⎪ Levodopa ⎪ Ephedrine ⎭	Discussed in Chapter 9 (p. 266).
Barbiturates	Coumarin anticoagulants ⎫ Chloramphenicol ⎪ Corticosteroids ⎬ Phenylbutazone ⎪ Tricyclics ⎭	Enzyme induction reduces effects of these drugs.
Benzodiazepines	Alcohol ⎫ Sedatives ⎭	Addition of cerebral depressant effects.
Chloral hydrate	Coumarin anticoagulants	Increase in anticoagulant effect due to displacement from protein binding sites.
Major tranquillizers	Tricyclics ⎫ Anticholinergic anti-⎬ parkinsonian drugs ⎭	Anticholinergic side effects potentiated.
	Levodopa ⎫ Antiparkinsonian drugs ⎭	Antiparkinsonian effect of these drugs is diminished.
Lithium	Thiazide diuretics ⎫ Potassium sparing diuretics ⎭	Lithium retention with increased serum levels of lithium.

when it is to be taken, should be left with the patient. Small quantities at a time should be prescribed and dosage regimens should be simplified as much as possible to once or twice daily dose. Possible side effects should be discussed and some idea of the time scale of expected response should be given. All out-of-date medication should be removed from the patient's home. Whenever possible the patient should be followed up after a few days of starting medication to observe compliance, monitor side effects, encourage perseverance with the medication where appropriate or discontinue or reduce the dose of a drug that has caused an idiosyncratic adverse reaction. This approach is inevitably time consuming. From the hoards of barely touched out of date medication frequently found in the homes of old persons, it is plain to see that failure to spend that initial time is wasteful of effort and money in the long run.

The 'fitting in' syndrome

A high level of socially disruptive behaviour has been reported in Local Authority Part III homes (Masterton, Holloway and Timbury, 1979). In one study of 100 consecutive referrals to a psychiatric service from 20 old peoples' homes (Margo, Robinson and Corea, 1980) 86 per cent were referred because of behavioural disturbance. In the milieu of old peoples homes where there may be more than 50 residents with very few care staff, even mild behavioural disturbance may be difficult to tolerate. A mildly demented old person, thrust into an environment so different from his own home is likely to take some time to settle into the routine of the institution. It is unfortunate that chemical (*Table 15.2*) rather than interpersonal means of controlling behaviour are frequently used in such an environment.

Unwanted effects of psychotropic drugs—some general principles

Unwanted effects of drugs are of various types. They may be due to the pharmacological effects of the drug itself, either an exaggeration of the wanted effect of the drug as in oversedation in the tranquillizer group, or some other unavoidable pharmacological action of the drug as in the anticholinergic properties of tricyclic antidepressants. Occasionally the patient has an allergic reaction to the drug such as a skin rash. Other unwanted effects may occur when one drug interacts with another, or when the patient has taken too large a dose of a drug, or where the patient's target organ is particularly sensitive to the effects of the drug. Some apparent unwanted effects may not be due to the drug itself but to anxiety or resentment on the part of the patient who is apprehensive about the effects of the drug. A placebo adverse response may occur when a patient is expecting to experience an unwanted effect. Occasionally a drug may appear to produce an unwanted drug effect that is in fact due to the withdrawal effects of another drug recently stopped. Finally, concurrent physical illness may produce symptoms that may appear to be unwanted effects of a drug.

Most adverse reactions occur on the first day of treatment and two-thirds develop within 4 d (Prescott, 1979). Other adverse effects may take months or years to develop; for example, hypothyroidism and renal changes from lithium, and tardive dyskinesia from phenothiazines. With the benzodiazepines, accumulation of active metabolites may give rise to unwanted effects several days after commencement of therapy, and the lack of improvement for several days after the drug is stopped may confuse the clinician (Prescott, 1979).

Polypharmacy, or the concurrent administration of more than one drug at a time, makes side effects more likely to occur. Concurrent administration of more than one psychotropic drug at a time is recognized to be hazardous, often unnecessary and has been shown to be a common problem in general practice (Tyrer, 1978). Psychiatrists are probably equally at fault. In a survey of psychotropic drug prescribing in psychiatric hospitals, half the patients receiving medication were on two or more psychotropic drugs, and major and minor tranquillizers were commonly prescribed together (Michel and Kolakowska, 1981). Over half of the 511 patients in this survey were over the age of 65 years.

The 'repeat prescription' is a notorious cause of patients receiving drugs unnecessarily. These patients may be rarely seen by their general practitioners. As many as half of patients over the age of 70 who are receiving drugs do so on repeat prescriptions (Ramsay and Tucker, 1981). This has particular implication for those unwanted effects that are of late onset.

Antidepressant drugs and the treatment of depression

Depression is more common in the elderly than in those under 65 years. The prevalence of depression in the general population is probably around 8 per cent for women and between 5 and 7 per cent for both sexes (Paykel and Rowan, 1979; Wing, 1976; Weissman and Myers, 1978). The prevalence of moderate to severe depression in two community surveys of elderly people was 14.1 per cent (Kay, Beamish and Roth, 1964; Kay et al., 1970). An active and comprehensive psychogeriatric unit can expect over half of admissions in the 65–75 age group, and at least one-third of the over 75 year olds to have depression (Jolley and Arie, 1976). It has in the past been rare for elderly people to be referred for specialist psychiatric advice (Hopkins and Cooper, 1969) although this is very much determined by the general practice involved and the availability of psychiatric help for the elderly. The elderly respond well to antidepressant drugs, although relapse is common (Post, 1972). Antidepressant drugs should be used with caution but their potential usefulness is often hampered by over-cautious dosage or by failure to even attempt antidepressant therapy.

Many elderly depressed patients perform poorly on tasks of cognitive function, and there may be some reluctance to prescribe antidepressants lest the depression is complicated by an underlying dementia. Certainly patients with failing cerebral function are more likely to become confused as a result of antidepressant therapy, particularly tricyclics. This is probably due to the anticholinergic effects of tricyclics. Central cholinergic deficits have been implicated in normal ageing and in Alzheimer's disease (Perry et al., 1977; Sitaram and Weingartner, 1979) and it is therefore not surprising that additional anticholinergic drug effects give rise to confusional states and poor memory. However the relationship between depression and dementia is probably overemphasized. Some studies indicate a weak relationship between depression and dementia (Cawley, Post and Whitehead, 1973; Davies et al., 1978; Henrickson, Levy and Post, 1979). Post (1962) found a 12 per cent prevalence of cerebrovascular disease in elderly depressives, but the incidence of new cerebrovascular disease over an eight year follow-up was low. A study of computed tomography scans in elderly depressed patients (Jacoby and Levy, 1980) found no significant difference in cerebral atrophy scores in depressed patients and controls. A small group of depressed patients did have enlarged ventricles, however, and in these patients their first depression had begun in late life. Interestingly this study confirmed that tests of cognitive function in depressed patients are notoriously bad at predicting the presence of organic brain disease, as there was no correlation between the atrophy score and the severity of cognitive impairment. It is likely therefore that many depressed patients are labelled demented and are deprived of the opportunity of a trial of adequate doses of antidepressants. In any case dementia is not a contraindication to the use of antidepressant drugs. These drugs may be effective in the control of depression occurring in dementing patients, at the expense of a temporary decrease in cognitive functioning.

Tricyclic antidepressants

Plasma levels after a fixed daily dose of some tricyclic antidepressants have been shown to increase with age. This appears to be true for imipramine and desipramine (Nies *et al.*, 1977) and clomipramine (Moyes, 1980). There is some disagreement as to whether amitriptyline levels are raised in the elderly, but nortriptyline levels are similar in all age groups (Nies *et al.*, 1977; Moyes, 1980). Although there may be some impairment of liver metabolism in the elderly, which leads to generally slightly raised serum levels of tricyclics, the more likely reason for the increase of unwanted effects of these drugs in the elderly is increased target organ sensitivity. The cardiovascular system is more sensitive to the hypotensive and cardiac conduction side effects of the drugs, the brain to the sedative effects, and the bowels to the constipating effects.

The two most commonly prescribed drugs in the tricyclic group are amitriptyline and imipramine. Sedation is a common problem with amitriptyline but less so with imipramine. Sedation may be used to good advantage if most of the dose is prescribed at night to help with the problem of depressive insomnia. As agitated depression with much anxiety is a common form of depression in the elderly (Jacoby, 1981) then some sedation in the daytime may be helpful. However a mixture of sedation and hypotension leads to dizziness and falls in the elderly. The most common cause of falling in one study of elderly psychiatric outpatients was the combination of tricyclics with other hypotensive drugs such as diuretics and major tranquillizers (Blumenthal and Davie, 1980).

The unwanted effects of tricyclic drugs are essentially the same in the elderly as in younger patients, but more likely to occur and with more serious consequences. Hypotension is the most common of the cardiovascular effects; 75 per cent of patients of all ages will experience dizziness from the postural hypotension (*Drug and Therapeutics Bulletin*, 1979). ECG changes of prolonged PR interval, ST segment depression and T wave flattening are usually benign, but the arrhythmias that can occur may give rise to problems in patients with existing cardiac dysfunction. In one study (Coull *et al.*, 1970) there were 13 sudden deaths in 119 patients with pre-existing cardiac dysfunction taking amitriptyline. This compared with only three deaths in a matched drug-free group of patients. Ventricular arrhythmias are particularly common after serious overdosage with tricyclics. Even at therapeutic levels the contractile force of the heart muscle is reduced, conduction is interfered with and tachycardia occurs. The tachycardia is due to the interference of tricyclics with the re-uptake of noradrenaline leading to facilitation of sympathetic transmission. Ectopics may occur due to the anticholinergic (atropine-like) action which increases the speed of diastolic repolarization (*Drug and Therapeutics Bulletin*, 1979). The increased sympathetic activity may give rise to an exaggerated physiological tremor, which may prove troublesome in the elderly with senile tremor or Parkinson's disease.

Hypertension and depression are two commonly occurring disorders in the elderly and may well both be present in the same patient and require treatment. Methyldopa and clonidine can cause depression, or worsen pre-existing mild depression (*Drug and Therapeutics Bulletin*, 1975c). These drugs therefore should be avoided in a depression-prone individual. Guanethidine, bethanidine, debrisoquine and other adrenergic neuron depleting drugs can also cause depression but less commonly. The hypotensive effects of guanethidine, bethanidine and debrisoquine are antagonized by tricyclics which block the uptake of these drugs into noradrenergic neurons. These antihypertensive drugs therefore are less effective in patients taking tricyclics. Where depression and hypertension co-exist, then whenever possible antihypertensive treatment should be by diuretics and beta-blockers, in combination if necessary. Tricyclic antidepressants do not interfere with the antihypertensive action of these agents.

All tricyclic drugs have potent anticholinergic effects and in the elderly can cause confusion and memory impairment as already mentioned. Frequently the elderly are receiving other drugs with anticholinergic effects such as antiparkinsonian drugs and major tranquillizers and in them constipation may present severe problems. Blurred vision may worsen already poor eyesight, and in elderly males with mild prostatic enlargement, urinary retention may occur. Acute glaucoma may be precipitated in certain susceptible individuals but this is thought to be rare (Davidson, 1980). Patients who have had closed angle glaucoma treated by peripheral iridectomy are protected from the effects of pupillary dilatation as are those patients receiving miotic eye drops. In chronic simple glaucoma the small rise in intra-ocular pressure that may be caused by the anticholinergic properties of tricyclics is barely enough to cause problems (*Drug and Therapeutics Bulletin*, 1975a). Glaucoma therefore is not a contraindication to the use of tricyclic antidepressants.

Maintenance tricyclic antidepressants have been shown to be effective in preventing relapse, and as the elderly are more prone to developing recurrent depression, maintenance therapy for prolonged periods may be useful (Jacoby, 1981). Preliminary reports on the newer antidepressants such as mianserin hydrochloride, suggest that anticholinergic and cardiovascular effects are rare with this group (*see* Chapter 8). They do, however, cause drowsiness.

The monoamine oxidase inhibitors

The major and most troublesome unwanted effect of this group in the elderly is postural hypotension. As in younger patients hypertensive crisis can occur with ingestion of tyramine- or dopamine-containing foods. Interaction of MAOIs with other drugs is a particular problem in the elderly. Levodopa, used to treat Parkinson's disease, depends on monoamine oxidase for its metabolism, and may produe a hypertensive crisis in patients taking MAOIs. The MAOIs also inactivate other liver enzymes such as hydroxylases and as these are responsible for the metabolism of barbiturates, tricyclic antidepressants and phenytoin, all these drugs are potentiated in patients taking MAOIs. Glucose tolerance is increased by MAOIs therefore the hypoglycaemic effect of antidiabetic drugs are potentiated (van Praag, 1977).

Both MAOIs and tricyclic drugs can precipitate epilepsy in susceptible individuals, particularly in patients with multi-infarct dementia where the occurrence of convulsions is not uncommon. Despite their problems MAOIs can be useful in the treatment of depression in the elderly (Ashford and Ford, 1979).

Minor tranquillizers and the treatment of anxiety and insomnia

Anxiety states are unlikely to occur for the first time in old age. When an elderly patient complains of anxiety then a diagnosis of depression must be carefully excluded before anxiolytic drugs are prescribed. In a community study of neuroses in the elderly (Bergmann, 1971) depressive neurosis was found to predominate over anxiety neurosis. Eleven per cent of this sample of elderly persons developed neurosis after the age of 60. A small group of these patients did seem to have developed a true anxiety neurosis for the first time in old age, usually following an episode of physical illness.

Minor tranquillizers are the most commonly prescribed psychotropic drugs in the elderly (Achong et al., 1978; Salzman, 1979; Chapman, 1976). The most commonly prescribed drugs of the minor tranquillizers are the benzodiazepines and these are used primarily as hypnotics. There is an increased risk of adverse reactions to benzodiazepines with age (Achong et al., 1978; Tideiksaar, 1978). This may not be due to higher blood levels of these drugs in the elderly. In fact in one study concentrations of diazepam and desmethyldiazepam were lower for equivalent doses of diazepam the older the patient (Rutherford, Okoko and Tyrer, 1978). However this effect may have been due to the liver enzyme induction produced by other prescribed drugs. Chlordiazepoxide would seem to have lowered peak levels in the elderly than in younger patients (Shader et al., 1977). The clearance of nitrazepam and diazepam has been shown to be similar in older and younger patients (Castleden, 1978). Other studies have shown an increased half-life of diazepam (Klotz et al., 1975) and temazepam (Huggett et al., 1981) in the elderly. The most likely explanation for the increased risk of adverse reactions to benzodiazepines in the elderly may be the increased sensitivity of the ageing brain to the depressant action of these drugs, and the slow accumulation of active metabolites (Salzman, 1979). The side effects of these drugs experienced by elderly people are tremor, ataxia, confusion and hypotension. (*Drug and Therapeutics Bulletin*, 1980). It would seem reasonable to prescribe shorter acting benzodiazepines (*see* p. 141) if any in the elderly to minimize the cumulative effect of active metabolites.

Useful alternatives to benzodiazepines as hypnotics in the elderly are the chloral hydrate derivatives and chlormethiazole. For behavioural disturbance, or for anxiety and agitation in the elderly, small doses of major tranquillizers such as thioridazine (which has less parkinsonian side effects than others of this group) may be appropriate.

Barbiturates should be avoided in the elderly as in any age group. They can cause paradoxical excitation and confusion (Bowden and Giffen, 1978b) and have been implicated in causing nocturnal falls and fractured femurs in the elderly (McDonald and McDonald, 1977).

Major tranquillizers and the treatment of paranoid states

Paranoid states in the elderly may accompany early dementia or may occur in the absence of any organic disorder (Lazarus, 1979). Deafness and isolation may be aetiological factors in the latter, and these patients respond well to major tranquillizers. Pure paranoid states in the elderly make relatively little demand on in-patient facilities (Jolley and Arie, 1976). A prevalence of 1.7 per cent of previously unidentified paranoid states in a community sample of elderly people was found by Kay et al. (1970). Post (1966) followed up a series of paranoid patients and found that provided adequate treatment with major tranquillizers could be instigated and maintained, then almost all types of paranoid symptoms could be controlled. It is interesting that the 93 patients in his study were shown to be no more likely to develop cognitive impairment than other persons of their age group.

The elderly are particularly sensitive to the parkinsonian side effects of the major tranquillizers and 50 per cent of 60–80 year olds on major tranquillizers will experience extrapyramidal side effects (Ayd, 1961). Again this is in part due to the increased sensitivity of the ageing brain to the effects of dopamine blockade and the disturbance of the balance between dopamine and acetylcholine. Treatment of the parkinsonian side effects by antiparkinsonian drugs is at the expense of adding to the anticholinergic effects that the major tranquillizers themselves cause. Hence parkinsonian side effects are best avoided by using low doses of major tranquillizers such as thioridazine, which have less propensity to cause parkinsonism. The long-acting intramuscular major tranquillizers such as flupenthixol decanoate and fluphenazine decanoate must be used with care in the elderly, but may provide an invaluable means of treating paranoid states in patients who have no insight into their problems and who are reluctant to comply with medication. Very small doses administered more frequently than in younger patients, provide a better safety margin with these intramuscular drugs. Haloperidol has been reported to cause less sedative effects than many other major tranquillizers (Pitt, 1979; Rosen, 1979).

The occurrence of tardive dyskinesia also increases with age, independently of duration of treatment with major tranquillizers (Jus et al., 1976; Crane, 1968). Work with rats has shown that aged rats are more sensitive to the stereotypic inducing effects of dopamine agonists, which is the animal model of tardive dyskinesia (Smith and Leelavathi, 1980). Antiparkinsonian drugs appear to make tardive dyskinesia worse (Klawans, 1973; Gerlach and Thorsen, 1976; Perris et al., 1979) but it is possible that patients most likely to develop tardive dyskinesia are also more sensitive to the parkinsonian side effects and have received more antiparkinsonian drugs (Fann, 1980). Some studies have suggested that brain damage predisposes patients to developing tardive dyskinesia (Perris et al., 1979); if so, demented patients will be particularly at risk. There is also evidence that the elderly are more susceptible to developing the irreversible form of tardive dyskinesia (Gerlach and Faurbye, 1980). Spontaneous orofacial dyskinesia and senile chorea occur in the elderly and may be confused with tardive dyskinesia (Weiner and Klawans, 1973). Elderly patients are less likely, however, to develop an acute dystonic reaction or oculogyric crisis in response to major tranquillizers (Ayd, 1972).

Major tranquillizers block alpha-adrenergic receptors and may cause troublesome postural hypotension (George, 1978). They also potentiate the effects of antidepressants, minor tranquillizers, analgesics and alcohol. As with antidepressants the antihypertensive effect of some hypotensive drugs may be antagonized.

The drug treatment of organic brain syndrome

The prevalence of organic brain syndrome in a community study of over 65 year olds was 10 per cent (Kay, Beamish and Roth, 1964). Eight per cent of the sample were thought to be suffering from dementia and 2 per cent from confusional states. Extension of this study gave a revised figure of a prevalence of 6.2 per cent for dementia in the over 65 year olds (Kay et al., 1970) and 22 per cent in the over 80 year olds.

Infections, adverse reactions to drugs and cardiovascular disease are important causes of acute confusional states in the elderly, and particularly in the elderly with early dementia. Treatment of acute confusional states depends on the underlying cause, but management of the behavioural disturbance such as restlessness, irritability and insomnia relies on the use of major tranquillizers, as does the behavioural disturbance in dementia. Control of behaviour by major tranquillizers may be at the expense of further impairment of cognitive function, as drugs with anticholinergic effects have been shown to reduce performance in tests of memory even in young healthy individuals (Davies *et al.*, 1978; Drachman, 1977). Pitt (1979) advises the use of thioridazine or haloperidol to control abnormal behaviour, thioridazine as it has less parkinsonian side effects and haloperidol as it causes less drowsiness. All major tranquillizers themselves can cause akathisia or motor restlessness and it is difficult in some cases to ensure that the tranquillizers are not adding to the behavioural problems. For in-patients, well designed wards, reality orientation and a high staff/patient ratio may reduce the need to use tranquillizers. It is unfortunate that lack of resources often dictates that such management is not possible, and frequently patients remain in the community or in inadequately staffed institutions and are prescribed inappropriately high doses of medication.

The use of major tranquillizers in dementia must be carefully monitored but remains the major drug treatment of a disorder that as yet is progressive and irreversible.

It is now well established that a deficit in cholinergic neurons exists in senile dementia of Alzheimer's type (SDAT) (Kendall, 1979). This form of dementia predominates in the very elderly whereas arteriosclerotic dementia predominates in the 65–75 year age group (Kay, Beamish and Roth, 1964). Loss of cholinergic nerve cells has been demonstrated in the temporal lobe of patients with SDAT as has loss of acetylcholinesterase activity in the hippocampus (Bowen and Davison, 1980). Some studies show slight improvement in the behaviour of demented patients given choline chloride (Boyd *et al.*, 1977; Etienne *et al.*, 1978; Smith *et al.*, 1978). Others have shown no improvement (Mohs *et al.*, 1979). Physostigmine, which as an anticholinesterase blocks the breakdown of acetylcholine, is reported to produce improvement in tasks of memory function in younger subjects (Davis *et al.*, 1978). To date, however, sustained and significant effects of treatment with choline agonists have been disappointing.

The place of dopamine in SDAT is uncertain. Some studies (Yates *et al.*,1979; Mann *et al.*, 1980) showed no difference in the enzymes involved in the synthesis of dopamine or of dopamine itself in the dopamine system in SDAT. In a recent study (Cross, 1981) two enzyme markers for dopamine, dopa beta hydroxylase (DBH) and methoxyhydroxyphenyl glycol (MHPG) were found to be reduced in the temporal cortex of patients who died of SDAT compared with control patients with multi-infarct dementia or depression. DBH was also reduced in the frontal lobe and hippocampus. The DBH levels correlated with the severity of the SDAT as measured by senile plaque count. In a study of 13 patients with SDAT degenerative changes have been reported in the noradrenergic system (Mann *et al.*, 1980). The underlying mechanism of the development of senile dementia of Alzheimer's type is therefore uncertain but is the focus of considerable research at the present time, and may provide other avenues for treatment in the future.

Reviews of the use of vasodilators and stimulants of neuronal metabolism in dementia (Yesavage *et al.*, 1979; *Drug and Therapeutics Bulletin*, 1975d) conclude that the value of these drugs is doubtful. Drugs on the market at the present time include the following:

(1) Cyclandelate (Cyclospasmol), a vasodilator which can improve certain intellectual functions, but in the studies which showed it to be of benefit, the improvement had little practical significance (van Praag, 1977).

(2) Dihydroergotoxine mesylate (Hydergine) is a vasodilator and increases energy producing metabolic processes in the brain. Some improvement of intellectual processes and mood has been reported but trials in the main have been uncontrolled (Glen, 1980).
(3) Isoxsuprine (Duvadilan, Defencin, Vasotran) is a beta-receptor stimulator causing vasodilatation, but has potent peripheral effects which may in fact decrease cerebral blood flow (*Drug and Therapeutics Bulletin*, 1975d).
(4) Meclofenoxate (Lucidril), naftidrofuryl (Praxilene) and fencamfamin (Reactivan) have shown a marginal improvement only in the few trials of their use (*Drug and Therapeutics Bulletin*, 1975d).

Lithium and the treatment of mania and recurrent depression

Hypomania is not uncommon in the elderly and from clinical impression is frequently misdiagnosed. The elderly overactive hypomanic individual quickly becomes confused and his garrulous overactivity may be labelled confusional state. A report by Foster, Gershall and Goldfarb (1977) of the use of lithium in 30 elderly bipolar manic-depressive patients found the antimanic therapeutic effect to be just as good as in younger patients. Therapeutic and toxic effects occurred at lower serum levels than in younger patients and serum levels of $0.4–0.7\,\text{mEq}\cdot\ell^{-1}$ were found to be adequate. A few patients in this study were extremely sensitive to lithium and the authors recommend a very cautious and slow introduction of lithium therapy, commencing with a test dose of 50 mg, to be repeated in a few hours by not more than 300 mg. Increases thereafter they advise to be in the region of 75–150 mg every other day until 500–600 mg is being given at day 5. Serum levels are then awaited before increasing dosage.

The use of lithium in elderly patients with recurrent depressive illness is limited.

Because of side effects, compliance problems, fluctuating physical ill health, interaction with other drugs and the nuisance of obtaining regular serum lithium estimations, many clinicians are reluctant to use lithium in the elderly. Toxic effects are reported to occur at much lower serum levels in the elderly (*Drug and Therapeutics Bulletin*, 1981) and intoxication at normal to low therapeutic serum levels has been reported (Speirs and Hirsch, 1978) even in younger patients (Thornton and Pray, 1975). The elderly with dementia and Parkinson's disease, and some relatively fit elderly, are prone to suffer ataxia, tremor, impaired concentration and confusion at normal to low serum levels (*Drug and Therapeutics Bulletin*, 1981). Because of this, divided doses are advised with all lithium preparations to minimize the side effects occurring at peak levels, and an upper limit of $1.0\,\text{mEq}\cdot\ell^{-1}$ is advocated.

Lithium is excreted by the kidney and impaired renal function leads to reduced excretion and higher serum lithium levels. The half-life of lithium increases with age from 24 h in middle age to 36–48 h in old age. This is due to reduced glomerular filtration rate with age (van Praag, 1977). Unstable renal function is a contraindication to lithium therapy, but consistently impaired renal function is not necessarily so, provided that lower doses of lithium are used (Jefferson and Griest, 1979).

Thiazide diuretics and potassium sparing diuretics cause lithium retention and as diuretics are so commonly prescribed in the elderly this may present problems. Frusemide and other loop diuretics do not have this effect (Jefferson and Griest, 1979). A patient receiving lithium may be given a thiazide diuretic if the dose of lithium is reduced a few days earlier. A patient receiving a steady dose of diuretic may be given lithium at a low dose provided serum levels are monitored carefully and the diuretic dose is not changed. Stopping a diuretic in a patient who is also receiving lithium leads to a fall in serum lithium levels.

Structural renal changes have been shown to occur in patients on long-term lithium (Hestbech *et al.*, 1977) but studies of the renal effects of lithium have not included many patients over the age of 65. Renal function appears to return to normal after cessation of lithium therapy and permanent renal damage is very rare if lithium toxicity is avoided (Chapter 10). Lithium-induced polyuria may cause particular problems in an elderly patient who is prone to urgency or stress incontinence.

Lithium interferes with thyroid function and can produce lowering of TSH levels, goitre and in some patients hypothyroidism. Hypothyroidism may be of sudden onset after several months of treatment. Serum T_3 concentration decreases with age and the elderly are therefore more susceptible to developing hypothyroidism (van Praag, 1977). Hypothyroidism is not necessarily a contraindication to lithium therapy provided replacement thyroid therapy is undertaken (*Drug and Therapeutics Bulletin*, 1981).

Lithium can induce extrapyramidal side effects, particularly tremor, in all ages (Loudon and Waring, 1976; Kane *et al.*, 1978; Johnels, Wallin and Wålinder, 1976; Tyrer *et al.*, 1980). These reports have mainly involved patients in middle age. Bech *et al.* (1979) found tremor to be a particular problem in the over 60 year olds in a study of the use of lithium in Ménière's disease. He found that the occurrence of tremor, thirst and polyuria bore no relationship to serum lithium levels, and did not show any tendency to disappear over the six months' follow up. Chronic tremor induced by lithium has a lower frequency than physiological tremor (Tyrer, Lee and Trotter, 1981) close to the parkinsonian frequency of antipsychotic drugs (Collins, Lee and Tyrer, 1979). Acute lithium tremor may respond to beta blocking drugs and Bateman (1979) suggests that it may be an exaggeration of physiological tremor. The extrapyramidal side effects of lithium therapy, mainly tremor and rigidity, have been reported to be worsened by antiparkinsonian drugs (Kane *et al.*, 1978; Tyrer *et al.*, 1980) for reasons that are not clear.

Irreversible brain damage, and dyskinesia have been reported in a few patients taking lithium and haloperidol (Cohen and Cohen, 1974). However a large study of over 400 patients taking lithium and haloperidol, reported no increase in side effects of lithium alone, or haloperidol alone when these drugs were used in combination (Baastrup *et al.*, 1976). Interactions between lithium and diuretics, neuroleptics, nephrotoxic antibiotics, digoxin, antihypertensives, anticonvulsants, levodopa, hypoglycaemic agents and anti-inflammatory drugs have been reported (*Drug and Therapeutics Bulletin*, 1981). Lithium can be safely combined with tricyclic and tetracyclic antidepressants.

Non-psychotropic drugs causing psychiatric problems

Antihypertensive drugs particularly methyldopa and clonidine can cause depression, sedation and confusion in the elderly. This is due to reduced compensatory mechanisms regulating blood flow to the CNS. Forty per cent of patients taking diuretics will complain of fatigue (Hammond and Kirkendall, 1979). Propranolol can cause nightmares, hallucinations and delusions. The action of guanethidine, bethanidine and debrisoquine is antagonized by antidepressants.

Antiparkinsonian drugs of the anticholinergic type such as benzhexol, benztropine, orphenadrine and procyclidine may cause confusion. Benzhexol is particularly prone to cause confusional states (Lishman, 1978). Levodopa causes postural hypotension dyskinesias, mild depression, anxiety, severe depression, paranoid psychosis, confusional states and hypomania. Thirty per cent of patients taking levodopa will experience some disturbance of mood (Mindham, 1978). Digoxin has been reported to cause confusion and paranoid states in the elderly (Doherty *et al.*, 1979). This is due to the prolonged half-life, diminished excretion and decreased volume of distribution of digoxin in the elderly. Steroid drugs can cause depression and paranoid psychosis. Cimetidine may cause reversible confusional states (Blain, 1980).

Conclusions

The effects of drugs in the elderly are influenced by the properties of the drug, the psychological and physical state of the elderly person, and interaction with other drugs the patient may be taking. The situation is complex and varies from patient to patient and within the same patient and responses to drugs may be unpredictable. Clinicians should not be reluctant to prescribe drugs in the elderly as almost all problems can be overcome by commencing with small doses after careful assessment of the physical state and other medication. Attention then must be paid to careful follow-up to ensure that adequate therapeutic drug levels are eventually reached. Psychotropic drugs form only part of the treatment of psychiatric disorder in the elderly. The psychiatry of old age is a challenging and rewarding field. The elderly with functional psychosis respond well to treatment and the organically ill elderly and their relatives require the psychiatrist not only to be an alert physician, social worker, administrator and psychotherapist but also to have a thorough knowledge of the use of drugs in old age.

References

ACHONG, M. R., BAYNE, J. D. R., GERSHON, L. W. and GOLSHANI, S. Prescribing of psychoactive drugs for chronically ill elderly patients,*Canadian Medical Association Journal* **118**, 1503–1508 (1978)

ASHFORD, J. W. and FORD, C. V. Use of MAO inhibitors in elderly patients, *American Journal of Psychiatry* **136**, 1466–1467 (1979)

AYD, F. J. A survey of drug-induced extrapyramidal reactions, *Journal of the American Medical Association* **175**, 1054–1060 (1961)

AYD, F. J. Haloperidol: fifteen years of clinical experience, *Diseases of the Nervous System* **33**, 459–469 (1972)

BAASTRUP, P. C., HOLLNAGEL, P., SØRENSEN, R. and SCHOU, M. Adverse reactions in treatment with lithium carbonate and haloperidol, *Journal of the American Medical Association* **236**, 2645–2646 (1976)

BATEMAN, D. N. Drug induced movement disorders, *Adverse Drug Reaction Bulletin* **79**, 284–287 (1979)

BECH, P., THOMSEN, J., PRYTZ, S., VENDSBORG, P. B., ZILSTORFF, K. and RAFAELSEN, O. J. The profile and severity of lithium-induced side effects in mentally healthy subjects, *Neuropsychobiology* **5**, 160–166 (1979)

BERGMANN, K. The neuroses of old age. In *Recent Developments in Psychogeriatrics, British Journal of Psychiatry Special Publication No. 6* (Eds. KAY and WALK), pp. 39–50, Headley Brothers, Kent (1971)

BERGMANN, K. Neurosis and personality disorder in old age. In *Studies in Geriatric Psychiatry*, (Eds. ISAACS and POST), pp. 41–75, John Wiley, Chichester (1978)

BLAIN, P. G. Unwanted effects of cimetidine, *Adverse Drug Reaction Bulletin* **83**, 300–303 (1980)

BLUMENTHAL, M. D. and DAVIE, J. W. Dizziness and falling in elderly psychiatric outpatients, *American Journal of Psychiatry* **137**, 203–206 (1980)

BOWDEN, C. L. and GIFFEN, M. B. Drug treatment in elderly. In *Psychopharmacology for Primary Care Physicians* (Ed. BOWDEN), pp. 67–68, Williams and Wilkins, USA (1978a)

BOWDEN, C. L. and GIFFEN, M. B. Organic brain syndrome. In *Psychopharmacology for Primary Care Physicians* (Ed. BOWDEN), pp. 65–66, Williams and Wilkins, USA (1978b)

BOWEN, D. M. and DAVISON, A. N. Biochemical changes in the cholinergic system of the ageing brain and in senile dementia, *Psychological Medicine* **10**, 315–319 (1980)

BOYD, W. D., GRAHAM-WHITE, J., BLACKWOOD, G., GLEN, I. and McQUEEN, J. Clinical effects of choline in Alzheimer senile dementia, *Lancet* **2**, 711 (1977)

CASTLEDEN, C. M. Prescribing for the elderly, *Prescribers Journal* **18**, 90–94 (1978)

CAWLEY, R. H., POST, F. and WHITEHEAD, A. Barbiturate tolerance and psychological functioning in elderly depressed patients, *Psychological Medicine* **3**, 39–52 (1973)

CHAPMAN, S. F. Psychotropic drug use in the elderly. Public ignorance or indifference?, *Medical Journal of Australia* **2**, 62–64 (1976)

COHEN, W. J. and COHEN, N. H. Lithium carbonate, haloperidol and irreversible brain damage, *Journal of the American Medical Association* **230**, 1283–1287 (1974)

COLLINS, P., LEE, I. and TYRER, P. Finger tremor and extrapyramidal side effects of neuroleptic drugs, *British Journal of Psychiatry* **134**, 488–493 (1979)

COULL, D. C., CROOKS, J., DINGWALL-FORDYCE, I., SCOTT, A. M. and WEIR, R. D. A method of monitoring drugs for adverse reactions II. Amitriptyline and cardiac disease, *European Journal of Clinical Pharmacology* **3**, 51–55 (1970)

CRANE, G. E. Tardive dyskinesia in patients treated with major neuroleptics: a review of the literature, *American Journal of Psychiatry* **124**, No. 8, Suppl. 40–48 (1968)

CROSS, A. J. Loss of adrenergic neurons in some cases of Alzheimeres disease. Presented at Royal College of Psychiatrists Biological Psychiatry Group Meeting, 11th February, 1981

DAVIDSON, S. I. Drug induced disorders of the eye, *British Journal of Hospital Medicine* **24**, 24–28 (1980)

DAVIES, G., HAMILTON, S., HENDRICKSON, D. E., LEVY, R. and POST, F. Psychological test performance and sedation thresholds of elderly dements, depressives and depressives with incipient brain change, *Psychological Medicine* **8**, 103–109 (1978)

DAVIS, K. L. MOHS, R. C., TINKLENBERG, J. R., PFEFFERBAUM, A., HOLLISTER, L. E. and KOPELL, B. S. Physostigmine: improvement of long-term memory processes in normal humans, *Science* **201**, 272–274 (1978)

DOHERTY, J. E., DE SOYZA, N., KANE, J., MURPHY, M. L., SCOVIL, J. and WATSON, J. Cardiac glycosides. In *Neuropsychiatric Side Effects of Drugs in the Elderly* (Ed. LEVENSON), Raven Press, New York (1979)

DRACHMAN, D. A. Memory and cognitive function in man: does the cholinergic system have a specific role?, *Neurology (Minneapolis)* **27**, 783–790 (1977)

DRUG AND THERAPEUTICS BULLETIN. Tricyclic antidepressants and glaucoma. What's the risk? **13**, 7–8 (1975a)

DRUG AND THERAPEUTICS BULLETIN. Treatment of depression in elderly. **13**, 21–23 (1975b)

DRUG AND THERAPEUTICS BULLETIN. Treating depression in patients with hypertension. **13**, 25–26 (1975c)

DRUG AND THERAPEUTICS BULLETIN. Drugs for dementia. **13**, 85–87 (1975d)

DRUG AND THERAPEUTICS BULLETIN. Cardiac effects of antidepressive drugs. **17**, 13–14 (1979)

DRUG AND THERAPEUTICS BULLETIN. The CRM on benzodiazepines. **18**, 97–98 (1980)

DRUG AND THERAPEUTICS BULLETIN. Lithium updated. **19**, 21–24 (1981)

ETIENNE, P., GAUTHIER, S., JOHNSON, G., COLLIER, B., MENDIS, T., DASTOOR, D., COLE, M. and MULLER, H. F. Clinical effects of choline in Alzheimer's disease, *Lancet* **1**, 508–509 (1978)

FANN, W. E. Tardive dyskinesia and other drug induced movement disorders. In *Tardive Dyskinesia, Research and Treatment* (Eds. FANN, SMITH, DAVIS and DOMINO, Spectrum Publications, New York (1980)

FOSTER, J. R., GERSHALL, W. J. and GOLDFARB, A. I. Lithium treatment in the elderly. 1. Clinical usage, *Journal of Gerontology* **32**, 299–302 (1977)

GEORGE, C. F. Adverse effects of psychotropic drugs, *Prescribers Journal* **18**, 75–83 (1978)

GERLACH, J. and FAURBYE A. Pathophysiological aspects of reversible and irreversible tardive dyskinesia. In *Tardive Dyskinesia, Research and Treatment* (Eds. FANN, SMITH, DAVIS and DOMINO), Spectrum Publications, New York (1980)

GERLACH, J. and THORSEN, K. The movement pattern of oral tardive dyskinesia in relation to anticholinergic drugs and antidopaminergic treatment, *International Pharmacopsychiatry* **11**, 1–7 (1976)

GLEN, A. I. The pharmacology of dementia, *Hospital Update* **6**, 977–988 (1980)

HAMMOND, J. J. and KIRKENDALL, W. M. Antihypertensive agents. In *Neuropsychiatric Side Effects of Drugs in the Elderly* (Ed. LEVENSON), Raven Press, New York (1979)

HENDRICKSON, E., LEVY, R. and POST, F. Averaged evoked responses in relation to cognitive and affective state of elderly psychiatric patients, *British Journal of Psychiatry* **134**, 494–501 (1979)

HERBST, K. G. and HUMPHREY, C. Hearing impairment and mental state in the elderly living at home, *British Medical Journal* **281**, 903–905 (1980)

HESTBECH, J., HANSEN, H. E., AMDISEN, A. and OLSEN, S. Chronic renal lesions following long-term treatment with lithium, *Kidney International* **12**, 205–213 (1977)

HILLESTAD, L., HANSEN, T. and MELSOM, H. Diazepam metabolism in normal man. II Serum concentration and clinical effect after oral administration and cumulation, *Clinical Pharmacology and Therapeutics* **16**, 485–489 (1974)

HOLLISTER, L. E. Psychotherapeutic drugs. In *Neuropsychiatric Side Effects of Drugs in the Elderly* (Ed. LEVENSON), Raven Press, New York (1979)

HOPKINS, P. and COOPER, B. Psychiatric referral from a general practice, *British Journal of Psychiatry* **115**, 1163–1174 (1969)

HUGGETT, A., FLANAGAN, R. J., COOK, P., CROME, P. and CORLESS, D. Chlormethiazole and temazepam, *British Medical Journal* **282**, 475 (1981)

HURWITZ, N. Predisposing factors in adverse reactions to drugs, *British Medical Journal* **1**, 536–539 (1969)

JACOBY, R. J. Depression in the elderly, *British Journal of Hospital Medicine* **25**, 40–47 (1981)

JACOBY, R. J. and LEVY, R. Computed tomography in the elderly. 3. Affective disorder, *British Journal of Psychiatry* **136**, 270–275 (1980)

JARVIS, E. H. Drugs and the elderly patient, *Adverse Drug Reaction Bulletin* **86**, 312–315 (1981)

JEFFERSON, J. W. and GREIST, J. H. The cardiovascular effects and toxicity of lithium. In *Psychopharmacology Update. New and Neglected Areas* (Eds. DAVIS and GREENBLATT), Grune and Stratton, New York (1979)

JOHNELS, B., WALLIN, L. and WÅLINDER, J. Extrapyramidal side effects of lithium treatment, *British Medical Journal* **2**, 642 (1976)

JOLLEY, D. J. and ARIE, T. Psychiatric service for the elderly: how many beds?, *British Journal of Psychiatry* **129**, 418–423 (1976)

JOLLEY, D. J. and ARIE, T. Organisation of psychogeriatric services, *British Journal of Psychiatry* **132**, 1–11 (1978)

JUS, A., PINEAU, R., LACHANCE, R., PELCHET, G., JUS, K., PIRES, P. and VILLENEUVE, R. Epidemiology of tardive dyskinesia. Part 1, *Diseases of the Nervous System* **37**, 210–213 (1976)

KANE, J., RIFKIN, A., QUITKIN, F. and KLEIN, D. F. Extrapyramidal side effects with lithium treatment, *American Journal of Psychiatry* **135**, 851–853 (1978)

KAY, D. W. K., BEAMISH, P. and ROTH, M. Old age mental disorders in Newcastle upon Tyne. Part 1. A study of prevalence, *British Journal of Psychiatry* **110**, 146–158 (1964)

KAY, D. W. K., BERGMANN, K., FOSTER, E. M., McKECHNIE, A. A. and ROTH, M. Mental illness and hospital usage in the elderly: a random sample followed up, *Comprehensive Psychiatry* **11**, 26–35 (1970)

KENDALL, M. J. Will drugs help patients with Alzheimer's disease?, *Age and Ageing* **8**, 86–92 (1979)

KLAWANS, H. L. The pharmacology of tardive dyskinesias, *American Journal of Psychiatry* **130**, 82–86 (1973)

KLOTZ, U., AVANT, G. R., HOYUMPA, A., SCHENKER, S. and WILKINSON, G. R. The effects of age and liver disease on the disposition and elimination of diazepam in adult man, *Journal of Clinical Investigation* **55**, 347–359 (1975)

LAZARUS, L. W. Management of organic psychoses in the elderly. In *Psychopharmacology Update New and Neglected Areas* (Eds. DAVIS and GREENBLATT), Grune and Stratton, New York (1979)

LEAROYD, B. M. Psychotropic drugs and the elderly patient, *Medical Journal of Australia* **1**, 1131–1133 (1972)

LINDUP, W. E. and L'E. ORME, M. C. Clinical pharmacology. Plasma protein binding of drugs, *British Medical Journal* **282**, 212–214 (1981)

LISHMAN, W. A. Other disorders affecting the nervous system. In *Organic Psychiatry*, Blackwell Scientific Publications, Oxford (1978)

LLOYD, G. G. Psychological reactions to physical illness, *British Journal of Hospital Medicine* **18**, 352–358 (1977)

LOUDON, J. B. and WARING, H. Toxic reactions to lithium and haloperidol, *Lancet* **2**, 1088 (1976)

MANN, D. M. A., LINCOLN, J., YATES, P. O., STAMP, J. E. and TOPER, S. Changes in the monoamine containing neurons of the human CNS in senile dementia, *British Journal of Psychiatry* **136**, 533–541 (1980)

MARGO, J. L., ROBINSON, J. R. and COREA, S. Referrals to a psychiatric service from old people's homes, *British Journal of Psychiatry* **136**, 396–401 (1980)

MASTERTON, G., HOLLOWAY, E. M. and TIMBURY, G. C. The prevalence of organic cerebral impairment and behavioural problems within local authority homes for the elderly, *Age and Ageing* **8**, 226–230 (1979)

McDONALD, J. B. and McDONALD, E. T. Nocturnal femoral fractures and continuing widespread use of barbiturate hypnotics, *British Medical Journal* **2**, 483–485 (1977)

MERSKEY, H. Psychiatric management of patients with chronic pain. In *Persistent Pain: Modern Methods of Treatment* (Ed. LIPTON), 113–128, Academic Press, London (1977)

MICHEL, K. and KOLAKOWSKA, T. A survey of prescribing psychotropic drugs in two psychiatric hospitals, *British Journal of Psychiatry* **138**, 217–221 (1981)

MINDHAM, R. H. S. Relevance of research in Parkinson's disease to psychiatry. In *Current Themes in Psychiatry 1* (Eds. GAIND and HUDSON), Macmillan Press, London (1978)

MOHS, R. C., DAVIS, K. L., TINKLENBERG, J. R., HOLLISTER, L. E., YESAVAGE, J. A. and KOPELL, B. S. Choline chloride treatment of memory deficits in the elderly, *American Journal of Psychiatry* **136**, 1275–1277 (1979)

MOYES, I. *The Psychiatry of Old Age* 3, No. 2, p. 7, Smith Kline & French Publication (1980)

NIES, A., ROBINSON, D. S., FREIDMAN, M. J., GREEN, R., COOPER, T. B., RAVARIS, C. L. and IVES, J. O. Relationship between age and tricyclic antidepressant plasma levels, *American Journal of Psychiatry* **134**, 790–793 (1977)

PAYKEL, E. S. and ROWAN, P. R. Affective disorders. In *Recent Advances in Clinical Psychiatry 3* (Ed. K. GRANVILLE-GROSSMAN), pp. 37–90, Churchill Livingstone, Edinburgh (1979)

PERRIS, C., DIMITRIJEVIC, P., JACOBSSON, L., PAULSSON, P., RAPP, W. and FRÖBERG, H. Tardive dyskinesia in psychiatric patients treated with neuroleptics, *British Journal of Psychiatry* **135**, 509–514 (1979)

PERRY, E. K., PERRY, R. H., BLESSED, G. and TOMLINSON, B. E. Necropsy evidence of central cholinergic deficits in senile dementia, *Lancet* **1**, 189 (1977)

PITT, B. The current state of senile dementia. In *Current Trends in Psychiatry 2* (Eds. GAIND and HUDSON), Macmillan Press, London (1979)

PITT, B. Management problems in psychogeriatrics, *British Journal of Hospital Medicine* **24**, 39–46 (1980)

POST, F. *The Significance of Affective Symptoms in Old Age*, Oxford University Press, London (1962)

POST, F. *Persistent Persecutory States in the Elderly*, Pergammon Press, Oxford (1966)

POST, F. The management and nature of depressive illnesses in late life: a follow-through study, *British Journal of Psychiatry* **121**, 393–404 (1972)

PRESCOTT, L. F. Factors predisposing to adverse drug reactions, *Adverse Drug Reaction Bulletin* **78**, 280–283 (1979)

RAMSAY, L. E. and TUCKER, G. T. Drugs and the elderly, *British Medical Journal* **282**, 125–127 (1981)

ROSEN, H. J. Double blind trial of haloperidol and thioridazine in geriatric outpatients, *Journal of Clinical Psychiatry* **40**, 17–20 (1979)

RUTHERFORD, D. M., OKOKO, A. and TYRER, P. J. Plasma concentration of diazepam and desmethyldiazepam during chronic diazepam therapy, *British Journal of Clinical Pharmacology* **6**, 69–73 (1978)

SALZMAN, C. Update on geriatric psychopharmacology, *Geriatrics* **34**, 87–90 (1979)

SCOTT, A. K. and HAWKSWORTH, G. M. Clinical pharmacology: drug absorption, *British Medical Journal* **282**, 462–463 (1981)

SHADER, R. I., GREENBLATT, D. J., HARMATZ, J. S., FRANKE, K. and KOCH-WESER, J. Absorption and disposition of chlordiazepoxide in young and elderly male volunteers, *Journal of Clinical Pharmacology* **17**, 709–718 (1977)

SITARAM, N. and WEINGARTNER, H. Cholinergic mechanisms in human memory. In *Alzheimer's Disease* (Eds. GLEN and WHALLEY), pp. 159–162, Churchill Livingstone, Edinburgh (1979)

SMITH, C. M., SWASH, M., EXTON-SMITH, A. N., PHILIPS, M. J., OVERSTALL, P. W., PIPER, M. E. and BAILEY, M. R. Choline therapy in Alzheimer's disease, *Lancet* **2**, 318 (1978)

SMITH, R. C. and LEELAVATHI, D. E. Behavioural and biochemical effects of chronic neuroleptic drugs: interaction with age. In *Tardive Dyskinesia, Research and Treatment* (Eds. W. E. FANN, R. C. SMITH, J. M. DAVIS, E. F. DOMONO), Spectrum Publications, MTP Press, New York (1980)

SMITH, S. E. and RAWLINS, M. D. Drug metabolism: general principles. In *Variability in Human Drug Response*, Butterworths, London (1973)

SPEIRS, J. and HIRSCH, S. R. Severe lithium toxicity with 'normal' serum concentrations, *British Medical Journal* **1**, 815–816 (1978)

STRADA, S. J. Antiparkinsonian drugs. In *Neuropsychiatric Side Effects of Drugs in the Elderly* (Ed. LEVENSON), Raven Press, New York (1979)

THORNTON, W. E. and PRAY, B. J. Lithium intoxication—a report of two cases, *Canadian Psychiatric Association Journal* **20**, 281–282 (1975)

TIDEIKSAAR, R. Drugs and the elderly, *Canadian Medical Association Journal* **119**, 415–416 (1978)

TYRER, P. Drug treatment of psychiatric patients in general practice, *British Medical Journal* **2**, 1008–1010 (1978)

TYRER, P., ALEXANDER, M. S., REGAN, A. and LEE, I. An extrapyramidal syndrome after lithium therapy, *British Journal of Psychiatry* **136**, 191–194 (1980)

TYRER, P., LEE, I. and TROTTER, C. Physiological characteristics of tremor after chronic lithium therapy, *British Journal of Psychiatry* **139**, 59–61 (1981)

VAN PRAAG, H. M. Psychotropic drugs in the aged, *Comprehensive Psychiatry* **18**, 429–441 (1977)

WEINER, W. J. and KLAWANS, H. L. Lingual-facial-buccal movements in the elderly. II. Pathogenesis and relationship to senile chorea, *Journal of the American Geriatrics Society* **21**, 318–320 (1973)

WEISSMAN, M. M. and MYERS, J. K. Affective disorders in a United States urban community: the use of research diagnostic criteria in an epidemiological survey, *Archives of General Psychiatry* **35**, 1304–1311 (1978)

WILLIAMS, P. Prescribing antidepressants, hypnotics, tranquillizers, *Geriatric Medicine* **10**, 50–55 (1980)

WILLIAMSON, J. and CHOPIN, J. M. Adverse reactions to prescribed drugs in the elderly: a multicentre investigation, *Age and Ageing* **9**, 73–80 (1980)

WING, J. K. A technique for studying psychiatric morbidity in in-patient and out-patient series and in general population samples, *Psychological Medicine* **6**, 665–671 (1976)

YATES, C. M., ALLISON, Y., SIMPSON, J., MALONEY, A. F. and GORDON, A. Dopamine in Alzheimer's disease and senile dementia, *Lancet* **2**, 851–852 (1979)

YESAVAGE, J. A., TINKLENBERG, J. R., HOLLISTER, L. E. and BERGER, P. A. Vasodilators in senile dementia: a review of the literature, *Archives of General Psychiatry* **36**, 220–223 (1979)

Chapter 16

Other uses of psychotropic drugs in psychiatry

P. J. Tyrer

Although the main usage of psychotropic drugs has been described in previous chapters there are some less common psychiatric disorders in which drug treatment may play an important part. In some, a normally unwanted effect of a drug is used as treatment, and in others, drugs that are not normally considered to be primarily psychotropic are given for psychiatric purposes. Because of these considerations the drug treatment is best described under the headings of the relevant psychiatric disorders rather than, as in the rest of this book, in drug groups.

Anorexia nervosa

In anorexia nervosa the central feature is an irrational fear of putting on weight. Deliberate starvation follows and there is also a distorted body image; an emaciated figure is perceived as desirable and a normal figure as grossly obese. In women amenorrhoea occurs as body weight falls and secondary hormonal changes ensue. The psychopathology of anorexia nervosa is complex and much still needs to be discovered. The reasons why it is so much more common in women than men, has its maximum incidence in the immediate post-pubertal years, and predominantly affects social classes 1 and 2 are far from clear. These issues are described in more detail elsewhere (Dally, Gomez and Isaacs, 1979; Crisp, 1980). Drug treatment is but a small part of management, and in recent years has been replaced by other forms of treatment, including conditioning techniques (Bhanji and Thompson, 1974) and psychodynamic approaches (Crisp, 1980).

It is natural that appetite stimulants are the major drugs used in anorexia nervosa. Unfortunately, it is easy to deduce from the symptoms of the illness that as reduction of appetite is a minor or even non-existent part of the syndrome the value of appetite stimulation is limited. However, some of these agents, particularly the antipsychotic drugs, also reduce drive and the will to resist food, and so are often used in the initial stages of treatment. Experimental lesions of the hypothalamus may also simulate the symptoms of anorexia nervosa (Russell, 1965) and as many appetite stimulants act at the hypothalamic level it is also possible that they modify symptoms more fundamentally than by improving appetite alone.

The antipsychotic drugs have the longest period of use in the therapy of anorexia nervosa. Despite their established appetite stimulating properties and popularity they have not been subjected to proper controlled trials of their efficacy. In the 1960s the initial treatment of anorexia nervosa almost invariably included the recommendation that chlorpromazine (virtually no other antipsychotic drug has been investigated systematically) be prescribed in a dosage between 100 and 1000 mg daily (Dally and Sargant, 1966; Crisp, 1966). There is no doubt that in-patients with anorexia nervosa do achieve considerable weight gain when treated with chlorpromazine but similar results can be achieved by bed-rest and skilled nursing care without drug therapy. Even if more rapid weight gain is obtained through drug therapy it is of no advantage if it is perceived by the patient as obscene flesh that has to be removed again as soon as possible. According to Russell (1977) investigators into the treatment of anorexia nervosa often forget two basic facts, 'firstly, the most immediately effective method of treatment is simply to admit the patient to hospital', and secondly, 'the criteria for a fundamental improvement in the course of the illness require a much more radical change in the patient than gain in weight over the course of a few weeks'.

In recent years this more realistic appraisal of treament has led to a falling off of interest in appetite stimulants. Another concern has been the discovery that antipsychotic drugs block dopamine receptors and, secondarily stimulate prolactin secretion, with consequences that are described in more detail by Dr Mackay in Chapter 4. Hyperprolactinaemia interferes with the normal ovarian cycle and may induce amenorrhoea and galactorrhoea (Beaumont et al., 1974b). It is therefore possible that treatment with antipsychotic drugs may delay the return of normal menstrual function even after adequate weight has been regained (Williams, 1977). There is no compensatory adjustment to chronic treatment with phenothiazines and prolactin levels remain high irrespective of the duration of therapy (Beumont et al., 1974a). As the metabolites of antipsychotic drugs persist for many months hyperprolactinaemia may continue to interfere with menstrual function long after the drug has been stopped. However, it should be added that only a small minority of women with normal menstrual function develop amenorrhoea when prescribed antipsychotic drugs although hyperprolactinaemia is an invariable accompaniment of drug treatment. There is some evidence that menstrual problems are more likely to ensue if patients are receiving more than one antipsychotic drug simultaneously (Beumont et al., 1974b) so it is preferable to use only one antipsychotic drug in the treatment of anorexia nervosa. If this is chosen it is best to fix on the duration of therapy before beginning treatment, and in most cases this period will not be longer than a few weeks.

The monoamine oxidase inhibitors and tricyclic depressants are known to stimulate appetite and often lead to weight gain. The tricyclic antidepressants are sometimes used in the treatment of anorexia nervosa. Again results have been claimed from studies that are methodologically unsound (Needleman and Waber, 1976; Mills, 1976) with differing interpretations of the mechanism of action of the antidepressants. Despite the known appetite stimulating properties of tricyclic antidepressants the hypothesis that patients with anorexia nervosa are fundamentally depressed is an enticing one, particularly as tricyclic antidepressants can then be recommended as primary treatment. As nothing approaching a controlled trial has been carried out with tricyclic antidepressants in anorexia nervosa their value cannot be judged. The distinction between depressive illness and anorexia nervosa is seldom difficult but if there are clear-cut depressive symptoms present in a patient with anorexia nervosa (excluding pathological guilt over weight gain) it is reasonable to use tricyclic antidepressants. Mills' cases are mainly students whose anorexia was precipitated by an impending examination and in such patients minor affective symptoms may be common. Nortriptyline and amitriptyline have been most often used in doses between

20–100 mg·d^{-1} (nortriptyline) and 50–200 mg·d^{-1} (amitriptyline). When, as is often the case, such patients suffer from insomnia it is better to give the amitriptyline in a single dose at night.

Levodopa has also been used in the treatment of anorexia nervosa but only one favourable report has been published (Johansen and Knoor, 1974). Treatment is based on the somewhat curious premise that the rigidity of parkinsonism is akin to the rigid personalities of patients with anorexia nervosa. As only six patients were studied (with four improving on levodopa) no assessment of the drug's value can be made.

The drug that has produced the most encouraging results in the treatment of anorexia nervosa is cyproheptadine (*Figure 16.1*). This is an antihistamine that has a

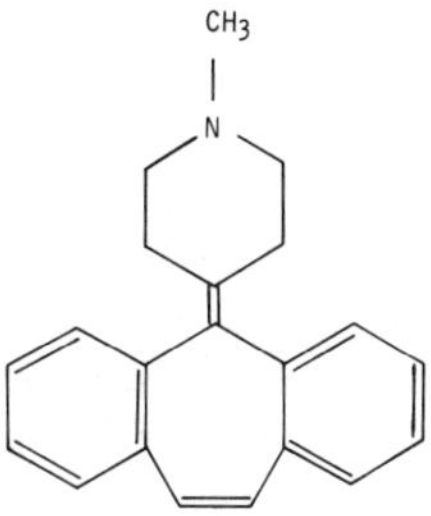

Figure 16.1 Cyproheptadine

place in the treatment of allergies as well as an appetite stimulant but can probably be regarded as more specific than the other drugs used in anorexia nervosa. Although one study showed it to have little value in a double-blind trial against placebo (Vigersky and Loriaux, 1977) only 24 patients were studied and greater responses were shown in patients on cyproheptadine. Subsequently a larger study in which 81 patients were treated with behaviour therapy but also received cyproheptadine or placebo, showed that cyproheptadine was significantly better than placebo in producing weight gain (Goldberg *et al.*, 1979). Patients with birth delivery complications responded preferentially to cyproheptadine and the authors argue that these and other patients who respond to cyproheptadine probably represent the more serious form of anorexia nervosa. Patients were treated with 12 mg daily at first increasing up to 32 mg daily as a maximum. On this dosage there are very few unwanted effects (as one might expect with an antihistamine given in moderate dosage). It is not known whether other antihistamines, such as promethazine, are of similar value in anorexia nervosa. Cyproheptadine differs from other antihistamines in being an antagonist of 5-hydroxytryptamine (5-HT) and this may be the important pharmacological factor associated with appetite stimulation. It is also uncertain whether cyproheptadine can affect other hypothalamic and pituitary functions as do phenothiazines. Promethazine can inhibit lactation and cyproheptadine probably has the same propensity.

The hydantoin group of anticonvulsant drugs has also been used in anorexia nervosa. Green and Rau (1974) reported good results with phenytoin, particularly in patients with bulimia and self-induced vomiting, which is usually considered to be of serious prognostic significance (Russell, 1979). However, their patients could not be regarded as typical of anorexia nervosa as almost all had abnormal electroencephalograms and the rationale for using phenytoin was that the patients' anorexia was secondary to brain dysfunction.

The choice of drug treatment in anorexia nervosa lies between cyproheptadine and one of the antipsychotic drugs. Cyproheptadine appears to be marginally superior on the grounds of fewer side effects but antipsychotic drugs may be a useful adjunct to initial treatment if given for a few weeks only. A phenothiazine with a sedative action such as thioridazine (100–300 mg daily) or chlorpromazine (150–400 mg daily) is likely to be preferred in overactive restless patients.

Insulin has a long history of use in stimulating appetite. It was termed 'modified insulin therapy' to distinguish it from deep insulin coma treatment of schizophrenia. Small amounts (e.g. 10–30 units of soluble insulin) were given subcutaneously to depressed and 'neurasthenic' patients to reawaken their interest in food. This treatment is rarely used nowadays.

Obesity

Obesity is a disorder which no speciality in medicine regards as its own. Its effects straddle medicine, surgery, endocrinology, gastro-enterology, neurology and psychiatry and there are some who believe it is a social rather than a medical disorder. The success of organizations such as Weight-watchers in treating the condition primarily through the help of enthusiastic lay people shows that doctors are often redundant when it comes to management. Nevertheless, psychiatric patients are frequently overweight. This is sometimes a constituent part of their symptoms but all too often is a direct consequence of treatment as antipsychotic drugs, antidepressants and MAOIs all stimulate the appetite. Treatment for obesity is therefore a frequent topic in psychiatric practice.

The decision to treat with drugs should only be made after other methods have been tried and failed; there are no indications for drugs as a first-line treatment (Craddock, 1978). The safest drugs, but unfortunately the least effective, are the bulk-forming drugs. These have no nutritive value but expand in the stomach and small bowel to produce the sensation of fullness. These feelings are alleged to reduce appetite and so less food is eaten. Methylcellulose and sterculia are the most commonly used. They have no serious side effects but a reasonable level of fluid intake must be maintained to allow expansion of the drug to take place in the stomach.

The main appetite suppressants are all centrally acting drugs. They are all psychostimulants with the exception of fenfluramine and have been mentioned earlier by Dr Checkley in Chapter 11. Dexamphetamine, methylamphetamine, diethyl-propion, mazindol, phentermine, phenmetrazine are all effective in suppressing appetite (Silverstone, Cooper and Begg, 1970; McKay, 1973; Smith, Innes and Munro, 1975; Craddock, 1978) but their addictive potential is such that they cannot be recommended. Although they are still used to some extent in the treatment of chronic and severe obesity as an adjunct to other forms of treatment this should not mislead the psychiatrist into using them in a similar way. Unfortunately psychiatric patients as a group show a greater predilection to dependence than other individuals and what may originally begin as a 'short course to get you started' can easily become a chronic iatrogenic problem with addiction spreading to involve other drugs. Each new compound has been introduced with the claim that it is less addictive than its predecessors, but this optimism is dashed as gradually reports of escalation of dosage, inability to stop the drug because 'its the only thing that keeps me going', and withdrawal reactions are reported. The final mark of addictive approval comes when the drug gets a price tag in the illegal drug market.

Fenfluramine does not carry the same dangers as the stimulant appetite suppressants, almost certainly because it reduces appetite without central stimulation. Its
pharmacology is discussed in Chapter 11. It is as effective as amphetamine,
phentermine and diethylpropion in reducing weight (Pinder *et al.*, 1975) and yet its
main unwanted effects are those of sedation and dizziness. It also acts as a mild
anxiolytic drug but may make pre-existing depression worse (Gaind, 1969). For
pharmacological purposes it should still be regarded as an amphetamine-like drug
and interacts with MAOIs to produce a confusional state (Brandon, 1969). Although
frank addiction to fenfluramine does not occur there are withdrawal effects after
stopping treatment, depressed mood being the most prominent. The symptoms begin
4 d after stopping treatment and rapidly resolve afterwards (Oswald *et al.*, 1971; Steel
and Briggs, 1972). Because the initial psychological effects of fenfluramine are sedative
and certainly not euphoriant Oswald regards fenfluramine as 'a drug of dependence
but not of abuse'. Experience since these reports suggests that if fenfluramine is
reduced slowly withdrawal symptoms do not occur. The daily dosage is between 40 and
60 mg, rising to a maximum of 120 mg daily after three weeks. It is usually given
three times daily but sustained release capsules (60 mg) are available. Fenfluramine
potentiates hypotensive drugs and also has mild hypoglycaemic effects. It may
therefore be valuable in reducing weight in diabetic patients.

Obesity is a particular problem in maturity-onset diabetes. The biguanide hypoglycaemic drugs, metformin and phenformin, are also effective in reducing weight as
well as treating the diabetes and these drugs, together with fenfluramine, are the ones of
choice in this type of obesity (Silverstone and Turner, 1974).

Sexual disorders

Antisocial sexual behaviour

Inappropriate sexual behaviour may be considered for drug treatment when increased
sexual drive is felt to be contributory. This is not always easy to assess, but
exhibitionism, rape, indecent assault, buggery, paedophilia and fetishism may all be
associated with abnormal sexual drive. Clearly a simple reduction in sexual activity is
only a small part of management as the main aims are to divert sexual interest into
normal channels and to explore and uncover the motivation behind the abnormal
behaviour. Unfortunately none of the techniques for treating sexual aberration is
particularly successful and reluctantly it is decided that reduction of sexual interest is
the only way to reduce or prevent the behaviour in many cases.

Three groups of drugs have been used for this purpose, sex hormones, antipsychotic
drugs and the anti-androgen, cyproterone acetate. There are particular difficulties in
evaluating the effectiveness of drugs in sexual disorders (Bancroft, 1976) and it is not
surprising that few good studies have been published. Sex hormones are superficially
the most obvious choice in reducing sexual drive. Antisocial sexual behaviour in
women frequently involves increased sexual activity but this is motivated by factors
that are independent of sexual drive, so androgens and other male sex hormones are
not used. Oestrogens have been used for many years in the treatment of sexual
offenders (Golla and Hodge, 1949) and progestogens, such as medroxyprogesterone,
are also claimed to be effective (Money, 1970). Ethinyl oestradiol, a synthetic
oestrogen that is pharmacologically similar to naturally secreted oestrogen, significantly lowers sexual interest and activity in a dose of 0.01–0.03 mg daily (Bancroft *et
al.*, 1974) and is probably the oestrogen of choice if this form of treatment is to be used.

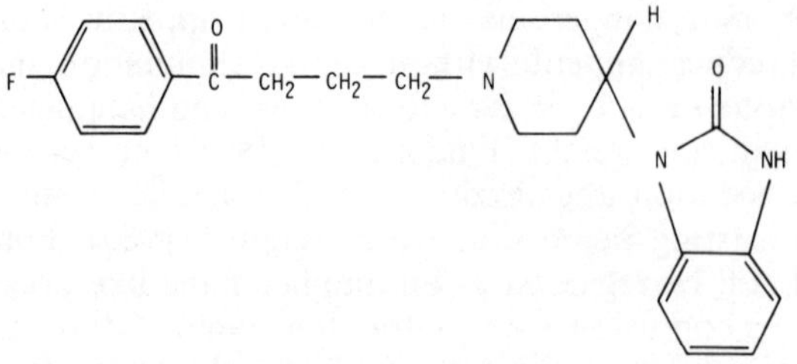

Figure 16.2 Benperidol

The main disadvantages of all female sex hormones and their synthetic analogues is their unwanted feminizing effects, including painful breasts and gynaecomastia, predisposition to carcinoma of the breast and thromboembolism, nausea and vomiting.

Antipsychotic drugs have also been used for many years to reduce sexual interest. The depot preparations such as fluphenazine enanthate have been advocated (Bartholomew, 1968) and thioridazine has also been recommended. It is difficult to find out whether these drugs act as global tranquillizers, reducing sexual interest at the same time as other features of personal initiative, or are specifically acting on sexual behaviour. As reduction in libido is occasionally a serious unwanted effect of antipsychotic drugs in some patients and entirely absent in others their effects in sexual deviation are also likely to be idiosyncratic.

The only antipsychotic drug specifically marketed to reduce sexual interest is the butyrophenone, benperidol. This is structurally similar to haloperidol and droperidol (*Figure 16.2*) and its pharmacological actions in animals are very similar. The claim that it is a specific antilibidinous drug is not adequately authenticated, but in one study, in which benperidol was compared with chlorpromazine and placebo, benperidol was significantly more effective than placebo in reducing sexual thoughts although did not differ significantly from chlorpromazine (Tennent, Bancroft and Cass, 1974).

Cyproterone acetate is an anti-androgen that inhibits the effects of androgens both centrally and peripherally. It is therefore much more specific than oestrogen therapy, which only partly reduces the release of androgens and also has feminizing properties. Cyproterone acetate is a synthetic compound whose pharmacological effects cannot be predicted from its structure (*Figure 16.3*). It inhibits spermatogenesis and leads to the production of abnormal sperm forms. Infertility is consequently common but is reversible. Sexual thoughts and activity are both reduced and penile erection and

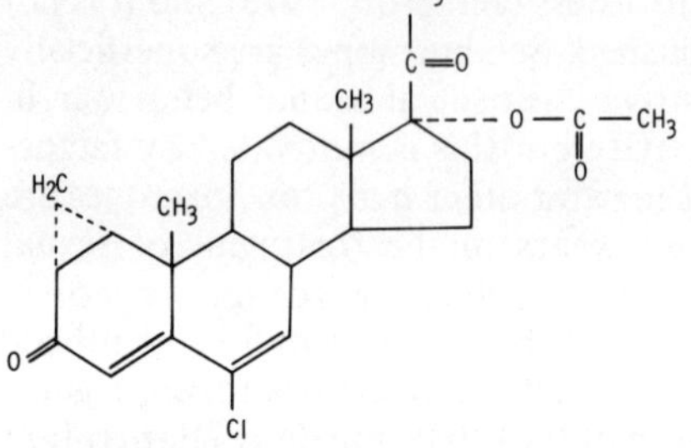

Figure 16.3 Cyproterone acetate

sexual interest are less when the subject is exposed to erotic stimuli (Cooper *et al.*, 1972; Bancroft *et al.*, 1974). Clinical studies suggest that it is probably no more effective than ethinyl oestrodiol (Bancroft *et al.*, 1974) but it has a much lower incidence of unwanted effects. Minor mood disturbances are the most common adverse reactions and growth is inhibited by premature fusion of the epiphyses in adolescents, but as this drug is rarely considered in such young people this is not a serious problem. The drug is normally given in a dose of 50 mg twice daily but may be increased to a maximum of 300 mg daily in some cases.

In making the choice of drug for treating antisocial behaviour it is important to distinguish between sexual thoughts, arousal and performance. If the main problem is perceived to be abnormal sexual thoughts that cause distress to the patient without being acted upon, benperidol in a dosage of 0.25–0.5 mg twice or three times daily is probably the drug of choice. It does not produce the physiologically dramatic changes of cyproterone acetate and normal sexual function may be retained. Patients who have committed a single sexual offence and have recurrent thoughts of committing another despite no action being taken may therefore be considered for treatment. Some patients with obsessional ruminative neurosis whose recurrent thoughts are primarily sexual may also benefit from treatment with benperidol but are more likely to do so if their sexual thoughts are also accompanied by penile erection and other signs of sexual arousal.

Repeated sex offenders who have particular difficulty in controlling their sexual drive are more likely to need treatment with cyproterone acetate. Duration of treatment is very difficult to decide. The full antilibidinous effects are normally delayed for several weeks and there is no evidence that tolerance develops on repeated use. Some patients are treated for several years but it is best to withdraw treatment at least once a year to assess progress. There is also some doubt that the infertility induced by cyproterone acetate is always reversible and so prolonged therapy should be avoided. No depot preparations of benperidol or cyproterone acetate exist and so out-patients who refuse drugs or who take them irregularly are a particular problem, not least because these are often the most likely to re-offend. Depot injections of the progestogen, medroxyprogesterone (50–150 mg intramuscularly every 2–4 weeks), or oestrogen implants (mainly of oestradiol) may be used if compliance to oral medication is suspect. Medroxyprogesterone by depot injection is also an effective contraceptive in women who are sexually promiscuous and either cannot, or will not, tolerate other contraceptive methods.

Drugs to improve sexual performance

The search for a safe and effective aphrodisiac is one of the oldest quests in medicine. Impotence and frigidity are the psychiatric disorders that most commonly present in clinical practice and here the main task is not to gain greater pleasure from the sexual act but to complete it physiologically. Impotence is the inability to maintain an erection for long enough to complete intercourse and has long been thought of in the public mind to be due to an insufficiency of sex hormones. But the key feature of impotence is the disparity between high sexual interest and poor performance, whereas the hypogonadal male who has insufficient circulating androgens has little or no sexual interest so does not complain of poor sexual performance. Hypogonadism can be treated with testosterone given sublingually, by mouth (testosterone undecanoate), intramuscular injection or by a testosterone implant.

Methyltestosterone is less well absorbed by mouth and offers no advantages. There is nothing to be gained by using combinations of testosterone or its analogues with alleged aphrodisiacs such as yohimbine or strychnine (e.g. Potensan Forte). The chief disadvantage of the testosterone group of drugs is their tendency to cause cholestatic jaundice. For this reason they should not be prescribed without adequate evidence that hypogonadism is present, through estimation of plasma and urinary testosterone levels. Testosterone can also lead to growth reduction by premature fusion of the epiphyses in adolescents and dosage should be kept to a minimum in this age group.

The anti-oestrogen drug, clomiphene, is normally used to stimulate gonadotrophin release and thereby induce ovulation in anovulatory women, but it also increases the secretion of testosterone. It can therefore be used in hypogonadism but, predictably, it fails to improve psychogenic impotence despite raising plasma testosterone levels (Cooper et al., 1972).

Although many drugs interfere with sexual performance through their anti-cholinergic and antiadrenergic activity they seldom produce impotence of long duration and the main precipitating factors are psychological or due to physical illness (Ansari, 1975). In general the alpha-noradrenergic blockade produced by most hypotensive drugs that are not beta-blockers (e.g. methyldopa, bethanidine, debrisoquine) leads to delayed ejaculation, whereas the anticholinergic effects of tricyclic antidepressants, monoamine oxidase inhibitors and antiparkinsonian drugs lead to impaired erection. Antipsychotic drugs have both alpha-noradrenergic blocking and anticholinergic activity and might be expected to produce most impairment of sexual function, but comparative data do not exist. The delay in ejaculation produced by antipsychotic drugs may occasionally be used therapeutically in the treatment of premature ejaculation, but the squeeze technique and other behavioural methods of delaying ejaculation are preferable.

Reduced sexual responsiveness in women is now usually treated by behavioural and psychotherapeutic methods, usually in conjunction with their male partners. Relaxation techniques and other anxiolytic therapies are often employed and amongst these are antianxiety drugs such as the benzodiazepines. Because many women with these problems have reduced sexual interest hormone therapy is also used, particularly testosterone in small doses to avoid its virilizing effects. In one impressively designed controlled study diazepam and testosterone were compared in 32 women with reduced sexual responsiveness, who were separated into high and low anxiety groups (Carney, Bancroft and Mathews, 1978). Testosterone was used in a sublingual dose of 10 mg daily and 10 mg of diazepam was given daily in the other drug group. The testosterone group had greater sexual satisfaction and arousal but the diazepam-treated patients in the high anxiety group had a better response than those with low anxiety. The important difference between this work and other studies of drugs in sexual disorders is that all the women received counselling together with their partners so that their problems were not dealt with in isolation. This emphasizes the importance of using drugs as adjuncts to other therapy in sexual disorders, a facet that has often been ignored in earlier studies.

Other uses of hormones in psychiatry

Anabolic steroids (e.g. nandrolone, ethyloestrenol, oxymetholone) lead to greater synthesis of protein and at one time were used to treat patients after debilitating illnesses, including psychiatric ones. Their tendency to produce cholestatic jaundice and their interference in normal physiological functions precludes their use.

Dexamethasone is a powerful synthetic corticosteroid that suppresses corticol secretion for 24 h after a single dose of only 1 mg. It has long been used as a diagnostic test for Cushing's syndrome, as the increased secretion of cortisol in this condition 'escapes' the suppression by dexamethasone. For reasons that are far from clear some patients with depressive illness also continue to secrete cortisol after dexamethasone. The dexamethasone test involves giving 1 mg of dexamethasone at 11 pm and taking blood for plasma cortisol estimation at 8 am, 4 pm and 11 pm the following day. Normal subjects and some depressed patients have cortisol secretion suppressed over all this period so that plasma cortisol levels are less than $5 \mu g \cdot d\ell^{-1}$ in all three blood samples. An abnormal result in depressive illness usually leads to temporary suppression so that the sample taken at 8 am contains no cortisol but by 4 pm (and certainly by 11 pm) plasma cortisol levels have risen again. Carroll (1980) and his colleagues have advocated the dexamethasone suppression test as a diagnostic tool in depressive illness as the separation of suppressors from non-suppressors may be important in treatment and prognosis. To date, however, it is not widely used. Dexamethasone has no use in psychiatric treatment.

The treatment of enuresis has been discussed in Chapters 4 and 13. Although tricyclic antidepressants are the drugs of choice not all patients respond. Recently synthetic hormones similar to those secreted by the posterior lobe of the pituitary gland have been introduced for the treatment of pituitary diabetes insipidus (i.e. polyuria and polydipsia due to insufficient secretion of antidiuretic hormone, vasopressin). One of these, desmopressin, has a duration of action of 24 h when given intramuscularly and one of 12 h when given intranasally. In nocturnal enuresis a single intranasal dose of $10-20 \mu g$ of desmopressin (marketed as DDAVP in a solution of $100 \mu g \cdot m\ell^{-1}$) invariably produces complete antidiuresis overnight and therefore prevents urine entering the bladder, so no enuresis occurs (Lehotská, Lichardus and Némethová, 1979). Further studies are necessary but desmopressin appears to be a valuable therapy for resistant nocturnal enuresis.

References

ANSARI, J. M. A. A study of 65 impotent males. *British Journal of Psychiatry* **127**, 337–341 (1975)

BANCROFT, J. H. J. Evaluation of the effects of drugs on sexual behaviour, *British Journal of Clinical Pharmacology* 3, Suppl. 1, 83–90 (1976)

BANCROFT, J., TENNENT, G., LOUCAS, K. and CASS, J. The control of deviant sexual behaviour by drugs: I. Behavioural changes following oestrogens and anti-androgens, *British Journal of Psychiatry* **125**, 310–315 (1974)

BARTHOLOMEW, A. A. A long-acting phenothiazine as a possible agent to control deviant sexual behaviour, *American Journal of Psychiatry* **124**, 917–923 (1968)

BEUMONT, P. J. V., CORKER, C. S., FRIESEN, H. G., KOLAKOWSKA, T., MANDELBROTE, B. M., MARSHALL, J., MURRAY, M. A. F. and WILES, D. H. The effects of phenothiazines on endocrine function: II. Effects in men and post-menopausal women, *British Journal of Psychiatry* **124**, 420–430 (1974a)

BEUMONT, P. J. V., GELDER, M. G., FRIESEN, H. G., HARRIS, G. W., MACKINNON, P. C. B., MANDELBROTE, B. M. and WILES, D. H. The effects of phenothiazines on endocrine function: I. Patients with inappropriate lactation and amenorrhoea, *British Journal of Psychiatry* **124**, 413–419 (1974b)

BHANJI, S. and THOMPSON, J. Operant conditioning in the treatment of anorexia nervosa: a review and retrospective study of eleven cases, *British Journal of Psychiatry* **124**, 166–172 (1974)

BRANDON, S. Unusual effect of fenfluramine, *British Medical Journal* 4, 557–558 (1969)

CARNEY, A., BANCROFT, J. and MATHEWS, A. Combination of hormonal and psychological treatment for female sexual unresponsiveness: a comparative study, *British Journal of Psychiatry* **133**, 339–346 (1978)

CARROLL, B. J. Neuroendocrine aspects of depression: theoretical and practical significance. In *The Psychobiology of Affective Disorders* (Eds. J. MENDELS and J. D. AMSTERDAM), pp. 99–110, Karger, Basle (1980)

COOPER, A. J., ISMAIL, A. A. A., HARDING, T. and LOVE, D. N. The effects of clomiphene in impotence: a clinical and endocrine study, *British Journal of Psychiatry* **120**, 327–330 (1972)

COOPER, A. J., ISMAIL, A. A. A., PHANJOO, A. L. and LOVE, D. L. Anti-androgen (cyproterone acetate) therapy in deviant hypersexuality, *British Journal of Psychiatry* **120**, 59–64 (1972)

CRADDOCK, D. *Obesity and its Management*, 3rd edn, Churchill-Livingstone, Edinburgh (1978)

CRISP, A. H. A treatment regime for anorexia nervosa, *British Journal of Psychiatry* **112**, 505–512 (1966)

CRISP, A. H. *Anorexia Nervosa: Let Me Be*. Academic Press, London (1980)

DALLY, P. and SARGANT, W. Treatment and outcome of anorexia nervosa, *British Medical Journal* **2**, 793–795 (1966)

DALLY, P., GOMEZ, J. and ISAACS, A. *Anorexia Nervosa*, Heinemann, London (1979)

GAIND, R. Fenfluramine (Ponderax) in the treatment of obese psychiatric out-patients, *British Journal of Psychiatry* **115**, 963–964 (1969)

GOLDBERG, S. C., HALMI, K. A., ECKERT, E. D., CASPER, R. C. and DAVIS, J. M. Cyproheptadine in anorexia nervosa, *British Journal of Psychiatry* **134**, 67–70 (1979)

GOLLA, F. L. and HODGE, S. R. Hormone treatment of the sexual offender, *Lancet* **1**, 1006–1007 (1949)

GREEN, R. S. and RAU, J. H. Treatment of compulsive eating disturbances with anticonvulsant medication, *American Journal of Psychiatry* **131**, 428–432 (1974)

JOHANSEN, A. J. and KNOOR, N. J. Treatment of anorexia nervosa by levodopa, *Lancet* **2**, 591 (1974)

LEHOTSKÁ, V., LICHARDUS, B. and NÉMETHOVÁ, V. Poúzitie *l*-deamino-8-D-arginin vazopresínu (DDAVP) na symptomatickú liečbu enuresis nocturna, *Bratislavské lékařske listy* **72**, 670–676 (1979)

McKAY, R. H. G. Long-term use of diethylpropion in obesity, *Current Medical Research Opinions* **1**, 489–493 (1973)

MILLS, I. H. Amitriptyline therapy in anorexia nervosa, *Lancet* **2**, 687 (1976)

MONEY, J. Use of an androgen-depleting hormone in the treatment of male sex offenders, *Journal of Sex Research* **6**, 165–172 (1970)

NEEDLEMAN, H. L. and WABER, D. Amitriptyline therapy in patients with anorexia nervosa, *Lancet* **2**, 580 (1976)

OSWALD, I., LEWIS, S. A. DUNLEAVY, D. L. F., BREZINOVA, V. and BRIGGS, M. Drugs of dependence though not of abuse: fenfluramine and imipramine, *British Medical Journal* **3**, 70–73 (1971)

PINDER, R. M., BROGDEN, R. N., SAWYER, R. R., SPEIGHT, T. M. and AVERY, G.S. Fenfluramine: a review of its pharmacological properties and therapeutic efficacy in obesity, *Drugs* **10**, 241–323 (1975)

RUSSELL, G. Bulimia nervosa: an ominous variant of anorexia nervosa, *Psychological Medicine* **9**, 429–448 (1979)

RUSSELL, G. F. M. Metabolic aspects of anorexia nervosa, *Proceedings of the Royal Society of Medicine* **58**, 811–814 (1965)

RUSSELL, G. F. M. General management of anorexia nervosa and difficulties in assessing the efficacy of treatment. In *Anorexia Nervosa* (Ed. R. A. VIGERSKY), pp. 277–289, Raven Press, New York (1977)

SILVERSTONE, J. T., COOPER, R. M. and BEGG, R. R. A comparative trial of fenfluramine and diethylpropion in obesity, *British Journal of Clinical Practice* **24**, 423–425 (1970)

SILVERSTONE, T. and TURNER, P. *Drug Treatment in Psychiatry*, Routledge and Kegan Paul, London (1974)

SMITH, R. G., INNES, J. A. and MUNRO, J. F. Double-blind evaluation of mazindol in refractory obesity, *British Medical Journal* **3**, 284 (1975)

STEEL, J. M. and BRIGGS, M. Withdrawal depression in obese patients after fenfluramine treatment, *British Medical Journal* **3**, 26–27 (1972)

TENNENT, G., BANCROFT, J. H. J. and CASS, J. The control of deviant sexual behaviour by drugs: a double-blind controlled study of benperidol, chlorpromazine and placebo, *Archives of Sexual Behaviour* **3**, 261–271 (1974)

VIGERSKY, R. A. and LORIAUX, D. L. The effect of cyproheptadine in anorexia nervosa: a double-blind trial. In *Anorexia Nervosa* (Ed. R. A. VIGERSKY), pp. 349–356, Raven Press, New York (1977)

WILLIAMS, P. Anorexia nervosa and the secretion of prolactin, *British Journal of Psychiatry* **131**, 69–72 (1977)

Index of drug interactions

The page numbers of the most important interactions are given in italic type. Several of the interactions are mentioned more than once in the text but the page numbers given here refer to those pages where interactions are described in more detail.

Index of international trade names

Each of the trade names for the psychotropic drugs is indexed and the approved name is given afterwards. References to the approved name in the text are found in the main index. For simplicity the main approved drug name only is given although it may be marketed in one or more of its salts (e.g. lithium). Trade names of drugs containing two or more compounds are not included here. Those mentioned in the text are included in the main index.

Abilit—Sulpiride
Abstem—Citrated calcium carbimide
Abstinyl—Disulfiram
Acetaminophen—paracetamol
Acetexa—Nortriptyline
Adanon—Methadone
Adapin—Doxepin
Adepril—Amitriptyline
Adiparthol—Dexamephetamine
Adonal—Phenobarbitone
Adumbran—Oxazepam
Agrypnal—Phenobarbitone
Akineton—Biperiden
Akinophyl—Biperiden
Akitan—Benztropine
Aldomet—Methyldopa
Algaphan—Dextropropoxyphene
Alival—Nomifensine
Allegron—Nortriptyline
Althose—Methadone
Altilev—Nortriptyline
Altinal—Amylobarbitone
Amal—Amylobarbitone
Amepromat—Meprobamate
Amfe-din—Dexamphetamine
Amfetasul—Amphetamine
Amipolen—Meclofenoxate
Amiprol—Diazepam
Amizol—Amitriptyline
Amobarbital—Amylobarbitone
Amosene—Meprobamate
Amphamed—Amphetamine
Amphate—Ampetamine
Amphedrine—Amphetamine
Amphedroxyn—Methylamphetamine
Amsal—Amylobarbitone

Amsebarb—Amylobarbitone
Amycal—Amylobarbitone
Amydorm—Amylobarbitone
Amylbarb—Amylobarbitone
Amylobeta—Amylobarbitone
Amylosol—Amylobarbitone
Amytal—Amylobarbitone
Anadep—Chlorpromazine
Anafranil—Clomipramine
Analux—Meclofenoxate
Anametrin—Nomifensine
Anatensol—Fluphenazine
Androcur—Cyproterone
Aneural—Meprobamate
Annolytin—Amitriptyline
Anorex—Phenmetrazine
Anquil—Benperidol
Ansietan—Meprobamate
Ansilan—Medazepam
Ansiolin—Diazepam
Ansiolina—Diazepam
Ansiopax—Dibenzepin
Ansopal—Chloral hydrate
Antabuse—Disulfiram
Antadine—Amantadine
Antalvic—Dextropropoxyphene
Antergan—Phenbenzamine
Antietil—Disulfiram
Anti-spas—Benzhexol
Antitrem—Benzhexol
Anxiolit—Oxazepam
Anxitol—Medazepam
Anxium—Diazepam
Anxon—Ketazolam
Anzepam—Diazepam
Aparkan—Benzhexol

Dormir—Methaqualone
Dormodor—Flurazepam
Dormona—Quinalbarbitone
Dormytal—Amylobarbitone
Dorsital—Pentobarbitone
Dosulepine—Dothiepin
Doxal—Doxepin
Doxedyn—Doxepin
Doxyfed—Methylamphetamine
D-Pam—Diazepam
Dridol—Droperidol
Drinalfa—Methylamphetamine
Drocode—Dihydrocodeine
Droleptan—Droperidol
Dromoran—Levorphanol
D-Tran—Diazepam
Ducene—Diazepam
Dumolid—Nitrazepam
Duromine—Phentermine
Duromorph—Morphine
Durophet—Amphetamine
Duvadilan—Isoxsuprine
Dymoperazine—Trifluoperazine
Dynaprim—Imipramine

Ecatril—Dibenzepin
Edenal—Meprobamate
Effisax—Tybamate
Efroxine—Methylamphetamine
Eglonyl—Sulpiride
Elavil—Amitriptyline
Elatrol—Amitriptyline
Elastonon—Amphetamine
Eldopar—Levodopa
Elenium—Chlordiazepoxide
Eliranol—Promazine
Elmarine—Chlorpromazine
Elrodorm—Glutethimide
Embutal—Pentobarbitone
Emergil—Flupenthixol
Emotival—Lorazepam
Enadine—Clorazepate
Enbol—Pyritinol
Encefort—Pyritinol
Encephabol—Pyritinol
Endep—Amitriptyline
Enerbol—Pyritinol
Enidrel—Oxazepam
Ensidon—Opipramol
Ensobarb—Phenobarbitone
E-Pam—Diazepam
Epanutin—Phenytoin
Epidorm—Phenobarbitone
Epikur—Meprobamate
Epilim—Sodium valproate
Epilol—Phenobarbitone
Epinephrine—Adrenaline
Epsylone—Phenobarbitone
Equadrate—Meprobamate
Equanil—Meprobamate
Equibral—Chlordiazepoxide

Equipertine—Oxypertine
Equipose—Hydroxyzine
Erantin—Dextropropoxyphene
Eridan—Diazepam
Eritab—Diazepam
Errecalma—Dextromoramide
Esbatal—Bethanidine
Eserine—Physostigmine
Eskabarb—Phenobarbitone
Eskalith—Lithium
Eskazine—Trifluoperazine
Eskazinyl—Trifluoperazine
Esmail—Medazepam
Esmind—Chlorpromazine
Esperal—Disulfiram
Etamyl—Amylobarbitone
Ethanol—Alcohol
Ethyl alcohol—Alcohol
Eudatine—Pargyline
Eudorm—Chloral hydrate
Euhypnos—Temazepam
Eunoctal—Amylobarbitone
Eunoctin—Nitrazepam
Euphorin—Diazepam
Eusidon—Opipramol
Eusulpid—Sulpiride
Eutimin—Lithium
Eutimox—Fluphenazine
Eutonyl—Pargyline
Evacalm—Diazepam
Evadyne—Butriptyline
Evronal—Quinalbarbitone

Fastin—Phentermine
Faustan—Diazepam
Feinalmin—Imipramine
Fellowzine—Promethazine
Felsules—Chloral hydrate
Fenactil—Chlorpromazine
Fenatsokin—Phenazocine
Fensed—Phenobarbitone
Fentazin—Perphenazine
Fluanxol—Flupenthixol
Fluazine—Trifluoperazine
Flunox—Flurazepam
Flupentixol—Flupenthixol
F-Mon—Perphenazine
Forit—Oxypertine
Fortral—Pentazocine
Fortuss—Dihydrocodeine
Frenactil—Benperidol
Frenil—Promazine
Frisin—Clobazam
Frisium—Clobazam

Galatur—Iprindole
Ganphen—Promethazine
Gardenal—Phenobarbitone
Gene-bamate—Meprobamate
Gene-poxide—Chlordiazepoxide
Gerobit—Methylamphetamine
Gihitan—Diazepam

Lioresal—Baclofen
Liskonum—Lithium
Litarex—Lithium
Lithane—Lithium
Lithea—Lithium
Lithicarb—Lithium
Lithiofor—Lithium
Lithionit—Lithium
Lithizine—Lithium
Lithocarb—Lithium
Lithomyl—Lithium
Lithonate—Lithium
Lithotabs—Lithium
Liticar—Lithium
Litin—Lithium
Lito—Lithium
Lixin—Chlordiazepoxide
Lodosyn—Citrated calcium carbimide
Lorans—Lorazepam
Lorapam—Lorazepam
Lorax—Lorazepam
Lorinal—Chloral hydrate
LSD—Lysergide
Lucidril—Meclofenoxate
Lucidryl—Meclofenoxate
Ludiomil—Maprotiline
Luminal—Phenobarbitone
Luminaletten—Phenobarbitone
Lunipax—Flurazepam
Lutiaron—Meclofenoxate
Luvatren—Moperone
Lycoral—Chloral hydrate
Lyogen—Fluphenazine
Lyrodin—Fluphenazine
Lysantin—Orphenadrine
Lysivane—Ethopropazine

Mabertin—Temazepam
Madar—Desmethyldiazepam
Madrine—Methylamphetamine
Magrilan—Mazindol
Majeptil—Thioproperazine
Mallorol –Thioridazine
Manegan—Trazodone
Manialith—Lithium
Maniprex—Lithium
Mantadix—Amantadine
Marbate—Meprobamate
Mardon—Dextropropoxyphene
Mareline—Amitriptyline
Marevan—Warfarin
Marezine—Cyclizine
Marplan—Isocarboxazid
Marsilid—Iproniazid
Marsin—Phenmetrazine
Marucotol—Meclofenoxate
Marzine—Cyclizine
Masmoron—Hydroxyzine
Maximed—Protriptyline
Maxolon—Metoclopramide
Mayeptil—Thioproperazine

Mebaral—Methylphenobarbitone
Mebutina—Mebutamate
Medaurin—Medazepam
Medianox—Chloral hydrate
Medilium—Chlordiazepoxide
Mediphen—Phenobarbitone
Meditran—Meprobamate
Mefenal—Methylphenobarbitone
Megadon—Nitrazepam
Megalectil—Butaperazine
Megaphen—Chlorpromazine
Megasedan—Medazepam
Melipramin—Imipramine
Melipramine—Imipramine
Mellaril—Thioridazine
Melleril—Thioridazine
Melleretten—Thioridazine
Menta-bal—Methylphenobarbitone
Mepavlon—Meprobamate
Mep-E—Meprobamate
Meperidine—Pethidine
Mephenamin—Orphenadrine
Mephenon—Methadone
Mephobarbital—Methylphenobarbitone
Mephytal—Methylphenobarbitone
Mepriam—Meprobamate
Meproban—Meprobamate
Meprocompren—Meprobamate
Meprocon CMC—Meprobamate
Meprodil—Meprobamate
Mepronel—Meprobamate
Meprosa—Meprobamate
Meprosan—Meprobamate
Meprospan—Meprobamate
Meprotabs—Meprobamate
Meprotil—Meprobamate
Meprox—Meprobamate
Mequelon—Methaqualone
Meripramine—Imipramine
Meriprobate—Meprobamate
Merital—Nomifensine
Merival—Nomifensine
Metalex-P—Leptazol
Metamide—Metoclopramide
Metamin—Flupenthixol
Metamsustac—Methylamphetamine
Methalone—Methaqualone
Methamphetamine—Methylamphetamine
Methased—Methaqualone
Methedrinal—Methylamphetamine
Methedrine—Methylamphetamine
Methidate—Methylphenidate
Methohexital—Methohexitone
Methyloxan—Methixene
Methyprylon—Methyprylone
Metid—Perphenazine
Metrazol—Leptazol
Metsapal—Chlormezanone
Metynal—Methylphenobarbitone
Mezepan—Medazepam
Microbamate—Meprobamate

Seda-Tablinen—Phenobarbitone
Sedipam—Diazepam
Sediston—Promazine
Sednotic—Amylobarbitone
Sedonal—Quinalbarbitone
Sedrena—Benzhexol
Seduxen—Diazepam
Semap—Penfluridol
Semoxydrine—Methylamphetamine
Sensaval—Nortriptyline
Sensival—Nortriptyline
Sentil—Clobazam
Seotal—Quinalbarbitone
Seral—Quinalbarbitone
Serax—Oxazepam
Serazone—Chlorpromazine
Serenace—Haloperidol
Serenack—Diazepam
Serenamin—Diazepam
Serenase—Haloperidol
Serenid—Oxazepam
Serenium—Medazepam
Serentil—Mesoridazine
Serezin—Diazepam
Serepax—Oxazepam
Seresta—Oxazepam
Serophene—Clomiphene
Serpasil—Reserpine
Serpax—Oxazepam
Sertofren—Desipramine
Setran—Meprobamate
Sevinol—Fluphenazine
Sidenar—Lorazepam
Sigmadyn—Pemoline
Simpamina—Amphetamine
Sindepress—Nitrazepam
Sinequan—Doxepin
Sinquan—Doxepin
Sintodian—Droperidol
Siplarol—Flupenthixol
Siqualone—Fluphenazine
SK-Bamate—Meprobamate
SK-Lygen—Chlordiazepoxide
SK-Pramine—Imipramine
SK-65—Dextropropoxyphene
Sleepinal—Methaqualone
Sodepent—Pentobarbitone
Sodital—Pentobarbitone
Sodium amytal—Amylobarbitone
Sofro—Pemoline
Solacen—Tybamate
Solazine—Trifluoperazine
Solfoton—Phenobarbitone
Solis—Diazepam
Solium—Chlordiazepoxide
Soma—Carisoprodol
Somasedan—Diazepam
Sombutal—Pentobarbitone
Somide—Glutethimide
Sominat—Dichloralphenazone
Somipra—Imipramine

Somitran—Nitrazepam
Somlan—Flurazepam
Somnafac—Methaqualone
Somni-sed—Chloral hydrate
Somnite—Nitrazepam
Somnopentyl—Pentobarbitone
Somnos—Chloral hydrate
Somnotol—Pentobarbitone
Sonacon—Diazepam
Sonazine—Chlorpromazine
Soneryl—Butobarbitone
Sonistan—Pentobarbitone
Sonja—Chlordiazepoxide
Sonollin—Nitrazepam
Sopental—Pentobarbitone
Sopor—Methaqualone
Sordenac—Clopenthixol
Sordinol—Clopenthixol
Sotacor—Sotalol
Sowell—Meprobamate
Sparine—Promazine
Spasepilin—Phenobarbitone
Spiroperidol—Spiperone
Spiropitan—Spiperone
Stadadorm—Amylobarbitone
Stangyl—Trimipramine
Starazine—Promazine
Stelazine—Trifluoperazine
Stemetil—Prochlorperazine
Stental—Phenobarbitone
Sterium—Chlordiazepoxide
Stesolid—Diazepam
Stesolin—Diazepam
Stimul—Pemoline
Stimulol—Pemoline
Stinerval—Phenelzine
Stresso—Meprobamate
Sumial—Propranolol
Supotran—Chlormezanone
Surem—Nitrazepam
Surmontil—Trimipramine
Surplix—Imipramine
Symmetrel—Amantadine
Symoron—Methadone
Syndrox—Methylamphetamine

Tacitin—Benzoctamine
Tagamet—Cimetidine
Talamo—Amylobarbitone
Talofen—Promazine
Talpheno—Phenobarbitone
Talwin—Pentazocine
Tamate—Meprobamate
Taractan—Chlorprothixene
Tarasan—Chlorprothixene
Tasmolin—Biperiden
Tavor—Lorazepam
Tega-flex—Orphenadrine
Tementil—Prochlorperazine
Temesta—Lorazepam

Subject index

423